EMPOWER
your flower

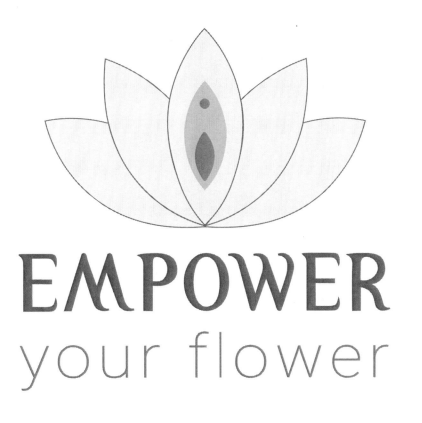

EMPOWER
your flower

Identify the patterns in your body, mind, and life
to empower you to overcome
female pelvic floor dysfunction

Denise Conway

ERYT500, YACEP
Certified Personal Trainer
Creator of TheFlowerEmpowered.com

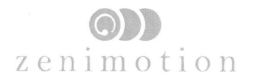

zenimotion

Zenimotion AB
Box 1720, Stockholm
SE-11674, Sweden.

Empower your Flower

First printed 2021.

Zenimotion
https://empoweryourflower.com

Cover and interior design by Arianna Oliviero
Illustrated by Denise Conway
Photography by Aaron Conway and Arianna Oliviero
Edited by Joanna Booth

ISBN 978-91-987097-0-4

Disclaimer

This book is not a medical text and is for informational purposes only. The ideas, opinions and concepts presented are the opinions of the author and are intended to provide information that is both helpful and informative in relation to the subject matter. The resources in this book should not be used to replace specialized training and the professional judgement of a healthcare professional. The content is not a substitute for professional medical advice, nor is it intended to be used to diagnose or treat any medical condition(s). It is imperative that you seek medical advice if you believe you have any conditions mentioned in this book. Always work with your healthcare provider and seek their guidance as to the relevant treatments, exercises and practices for you and your body. A global directory of specialists is available at https://specialists.theflowerempowered.com.

Neither the author nor the publisher assumes any responsibility or liability whatsoever on behalf of the consumer or reader of this material. The author and publisher specifically disclaim, so far as is allowed by law, any responsibility, loss or risk (personal or otherwise) which is incurred, either directly or indirectly, as a consequence of the use and applications of any of the contents of this book.

The author and publisher do not have any control over, or responsibility for, any third-party websites that are referred to in this book. All web addresses provided in this book were correct at the time of going to press. The author and publisher regret any inconvenience caused if these web addresses are offline or no-longer available but can accept no responsibility for any such changes.

Any reference to or mention of specific manufacturers, commercial products or brands should not be interpreted as an endorsement, advertisement or recommendation for any company or product.

Names and identifying information of individuals mentioned in this book have been altered and any similarity to a person living or dead is merely coincidental. Any perceived slight of any individual or organization is purely unintentional.

Some of the material in this book has been previously shared online on The Flower Empowered website.

Dedication

This book is dedicated to my children. Before putting finger to keyboard, I asked if they would be ok with me talking about this taboo subject. Above all else, I wanted to be sure that my passion for breaking the taboo surrounding pelvic floor dysfunction would not negatively affect them. Their support has been complete and unwavering. They are three amazing young individuals who encourage me to be the best person I can. They keep me grounded, they keep me humble, and they show me love each and every day.

To Aaron, Ciarán and Dearbhla,
I love each of you with all of my heart.

In memory of my coach—the legendary
John "Mountain Dog" Meadows

Table of Contents

Part One

The seed of Knowledge - learning to see patterns and connect the dots

Part Two

Empower your flower - Nourish, develop, grow, and blossom

Part Three

Symptom management, tools and strategies for empowerment

My Story

In the spring of 2015, during a visit with my urogynecologist, I received the worst news of my life. I had been living with daily pain since November 2013, following minimally invasive surgery to treat mild stress incontinence. The pain was unbearable and made me feel desperate and broken. Unable to have sex, my relationship was in dire straits, and I needed the suffering to end. Having eliminated every other possibility, I returned to my urogynecologist knowing that there was only one possible remaining cause—the mesh sling he had implanted. I assumed he would just remove it to make the pain stop. Implantation had taken just fifteen minutes; surely, removal would be simple and equally fast.

That's when he dropped the bomb.

"The device is permanent. It cannot be removed." The look on his face implied that I was a dumb blonde. "Don't you understand how many nerves and blood vessels sit close to that device? If I try to remove it, I could kill you."

Oh my God, could this be true? I pushed back with, "You told me it was the *gold standard*, that it was safe, that there are no risks aside from the surgery itself."

He thought for a minute before responding, "You are a very rare case. It is extremely unusual for women to have issues with this device."

I subsequently discovered that I was not a rare case; in fact, one in every ten women implanted with a mesh device has to live with devastating side effects. Life, as I knew it, was over.

He offered to cut the offending device in half. "Maybe that will relieve the pain." He sounded very unsure. This guy was a reputable urogynecologist and I was in Sweden, a country with a world-class healthcare system. How could this be happening? What should I do? The mesh sling felt like it was slicing into my bladder. The thought of two sharp ends, roaming around freely inside my pelvis, filled me with dread. Why hadn't I done proper research? Why did I just blindly trust this medical professional when he told me I needed the surgery? I was dizzy. Shaking. Completely in shock. I left his office and returned home to cry. My life was over. I would never have sex again and would be left to live my life in constant pain. All because of some shitty plastic mesh that took only fifteen minutes to implant but could never be removed.

At that point in time, I was not aware of the level of suffering some women have to endure because of mesh implants. It was not clear to me that I was one of the lucky ones. Mesh creates devastation. If you are one of the women who is now confined to a wheelchair or who has lost your bladder or bowel, and left to live with a stoma, your current reality is far from the life you were expecting to live. My story may seem trivial to you, and, for that, I am sorry. I cannot ease your pain, but I hope to help to raise awareness to save the lives of those who have yet to go under the knife.

At the time that the doctor had agreed that the cause of my pain was the mesh, it had been in place for over one year. Initially, I had believed the pain was due to healing. The surgery had left me with severe bruising on my genitals, legs, and backside. It looked like my nether regions had taken twelve rounds with Mike Tyson. I could only imagine that my bladder and pelvic organs must also have been bruised. When the painful symptoms failed to subside after six weeks, I blamed what I was drinking. I stopped drinking alcohol, coffee, juice (aside from cranberry), and anything carbonated. This made no difference so, I moved my focus to my diet, opting to eat foods that would make me less acidic, believing that my extreme bladder irritation could be stemming from my choice of food. I stopped running, believing that pounding the pavements could be hurting my bladder, but all to no avail.

In the fall of 2014, I started a new relationship and quickly found sex to be difficult and painful. I had returned to my urogynecologist during that fall and was instructed to use vaginal dilators to expand my vagina as he believed my issues to be related to perineal repairs he had done during the same surgery when implanting the mesh. He believed I just needed to "stretch out" my vagina to be able to receive my partner's package. The dilators didn't help.

How Did I End Up Here?

I was a single parent with three kids. I had experienced some injuries during the first birth—an episiotomy (cutting of the perineum), some tearing, and a fractured tailbone. Episiotomy is common practice in many countries as it can reduce the severity of tearing (which is also common). Tailbone pain does affect some women after delivery, however, a fracture is extremely rare. Those injuries had healed, and life went on. My second birth was an elective cesarean section, due to my son being breech, and my third was a natural birth with no tearing or additional injuries. I didn't notice problems with my pelvic floor until I started running.

My daughter was almost one year old when I decided I would run a marathon. Friends laughed when I said I would run twenty-six miles. "You won't make it to the corner!" I was a bit of a couch potato and found myself getting breathless when running around after my kids. I needed to get fit and running seemed to be the logical choice; after all, it was free, I could do it anywhere, and it involved putting one foot in front of the other. What could be easier than that?

For those of you who have run long distances, you may know that the body's fight or flight instinct can kick in while on the road. It's like some sort of primitive response where your body tries to lighten the load, so you can escape that saber tooth tiger that is chasing you. This instinct can result in an urgent need to empty the bladder or bowels. It seems contradictory as digestion and the movement of food through the intestines is halted as part of the fight or flight response, however, absorption is also reduced, and this allows the contents of the large intestine and bowels to get very wet. Combine that with the friction from the movement of running and the result can be very slippery poop looking to make an exit!

Maybe you have seen footage of Paula Radcliffe who did a stop-and-drop poop on her way through the 2005 London Marathon in which she won gold. Shocking and embarrassing as it might seem, this is a perfect example of a natural and instinctual bodily function that is shunned.

Paula was ridiculed, even though she steadfastly pushed to achieve her goal—a result to which most will never come close. I experienced the same urgent need to poop while running; however, my races were never important enough to warrant a stop-and-drop public poop. I wasn't running to compete; I was running to complete. With that said, coming to the end of my races, the encouragement from the crowds would spur me to run as fast as I could, and I would sprint to the finish. This was when I had the first sign of weakness in my pelvic floor as occasionally, I would leak a few drops when sprinting to the finish.

Following my first marathon, I decided to take up triathlons. I signed up to do the Chicago Olympic-distance triathlon as a charity fundraiser for a local children's hospital. I didn't know much about training and had only learned to swim as an adult to allow me to enjoy pool time with my kids. I had a fear of open water and felt really uncomfortable when out of my depth. This is where I learned that fear can lead you or it can present you with a challenge to conquer. Over the course of my life, I had learned that the only way to overcome fear was to stand and face it head-on. To conquer my fear of open water, I committed to swimming 1.5 km in Lake Michigan. To do this, I would need to swim in open water frequently in the months leading up to the race, whether it was cold, raining, or any other unpleasant weather. If I could make it through the swim, the remainder of the race would be a breeze.

When race day came, I entered the water and had to take many deep breaths in an attempt to calm the irrational panic that was the product of my fear. I was on the verge of getting out of the water when I noticed that two of the people beside me were doggy paddling. Neither actually knew how to swim. They had no technique but appeared determined to make it to the end. Fear was my demon but my angel and saving grace was my swim technique. In the pool, I had learned a smooth and efficient stroke. Inspired by those two doggy paddling guys, I reached deep within and found the courage to ignore the demon of fear. The panic subsided, and I began to swim. It was a tough swim, but I pushed through, finishing strong, and exiting the water almost ecstatically.

The 30°C heat in Chicago on that sunny day brought exhaustion at an earlier point than I would have expected. Midway through the final 10 km run, the heat zapped my strength, making those final kilometers the toughest I had ever endured. It was so difficult to continue putting one foot in front of the other. That's when it happened. Not a few drops but a full-on flow. I completely wet myself. I wanted to cry. If it hadn't been for the fact that I was running the race for charity, I would have stopped there and then. Embarrassed, but determined not to let my sponsors down, I accepted my predicament and kept running. After the event, I mentioned this episode of incontinence to a few of the girls in my group and, much to my surprise, I discovered I was not alone. Why had no one had ever mentioned this before?

Following that race, I participated in many other races; short fast races, long slow races, triathlons, duathlons, and endurance races over mountains on bikes. For the most part, I had no issues. In extreme circumstances, when I pushed myself far beyond normal limits, I would struggle with bladder control. I realized that maybe I should do something about it.

My First Attempt to Find a Solution

I asked Mr. Google why I was leaking when running. He told me I had stress incontinence and offered Kegel exercises as a remedy. Basic Kegel exercises involve a squeeze and lift of all pelvic floor muscles while relaxing the rest of the body and breathing normally. They are named Kegels after Dr. Arnold Kegel who first identified the importance of strengthening the pelvic floor. I started working on my Kegels right away. I even purchased vaginal weights and a pelvic-toning device that used electrical currents to stimulate pelvic floor muscle contractions. I carried on with my running and my episodes of mild stress incontinence remained few and far between, happening only under extreme exertion.

In 2011, I moved to Stockholm, Sweden. I didn't manage to find a triathlon club due to the language barrier (I was not familiar with the Swedish "hurdy-gurdy" language). I continued with running to maintain my fitness. My good friend Lisa came to visit. She was a keen yogi and was eager to try hot yoga. We booked a class and endured a full ninety minutes in the sweltering heat that is unique to this style of yoga. During the class, I discovered that I could no longer touch my toes, making me feel I had grown old too soon. I believed myself to be fit and strong, but this was a tough practice and my body felt tight and inflexible. I signed up for a one-month pass and began the journey to touch my toes. This was the beginning of my path into yoga.

Many times, I have seen the quote, "It's not about touching your toes, it's about what you learn on the way down." The journey to touching my toes was just six weeks, and to be honest, I didn't learn anything on my way there. The learnings came much further along. What I did learn was that there was a new love in my life and it was yoga. I practiced hot yoga for several months sometimes going twice per day. I was obsessed; it was addictive! Then, one evening, I turned up for my class only to discover that they were teaching Ashtanga yoga.

I found Ashtanga very challenging, even with my increased flexibility from practicing hot yoga. Ashtanga made me feel stiff and inflexible. You may think that practicing yoga for six months would make you flexible, but change happens slowly over time. To go from where I was then to where I am now, took very many small consistent steps. Determination carried me through the class and I enjoyed trying a headstand at the end of the practice. Trying to stand on my head reminded me of being a child. I could see the potential for some serious fun with this type of practice.

I decided to sign up for an Ashtanga course to see what I could achieve. Maybe you're thinking that I'm going to tell you about the wonderful lessons I learned from yoga, or about the profound experience I had when starting my yoga journey; not quite. I would like to share another experience that is a little less profound.

During those early days of my yoga practice, I began to experience another embarrassing phenomenon. The Ashtanga yoga primary series includes a shoulder stand in the closing sequence. On many occasions, my vagina would draw in a large breath of air on entering the shoulder stand. Coming out of the pose, my vagina would loudly, and proudly expel the air like a trumpet of triumph!

The yoga fart…the vart…the yart…the queef… whatever you want to call it. It was as though my womb was a lung and my vagina determined to breathe into it. At this point in my life, I was intermittently practicing Kegels. My relationship was great, and we had a very active and enjoyable sex life. I couldn't understand how I could be so fit, active, and healthy, and yet suffer these embarrassing yoga farts. To make matters worse, Ashtanga is a class without music. There is no background noise to mask the sound of the trumpet. I considered practicing with a tampon to muffle the sound but would always forget to wear one until I was in the shoulder stand with my little trumpet playing its tune.

From Yoga Farts to Surgery

I was one year into my yoga journey when I visited my urogynecologist to have my intra-uterine device (IUD) checked. During the visit, I mentioned the "yoga farts" that were disturbing my practice. The Swedish doctor smiled and in an almost matter-of-fact manner proclaimed, "Yes, but you are quite open down there."

What! Eh… hello, what? Shock. I felt shocked. I needed an explanation.

He clarified that the muscles around my perineum had not been properly repaired following my episiotomy. On further examination, he confirmed that I also had a stage one rectocele; a type of pelvic organ prolapse (POP). I had no idea what a POP was.

I soon discovered it was a hernia in the pelvic region where the organs are pulled from their correct anatomical position. In my case, an increase in intra-abdominal pressure would pull my rectum slightly into my vaginal passage. It is hard to convey the level of dismay I felt on hearing this. None of my boyfriends had ever mentioned any difference between my vagina and that of their former lovers.

My eldest son was already in his final year in college. It had been almost twenty-one years since his birth, which was the only birth that had required an episiotomy. Had I spent my entire adult life walking around with a broken vagina? The doctor explained that he would have to repair the perineum and during the same operation, he would repair the rectocele. That was when I mentioned my occasional bouts of stress incontinence. I explained that they were very occasional and mild. He recommended having the mesh sling fitted during the same operation.

When I asked about risks, he assured me it was a very common and safe procedure that is routinely performed on thousands of women every day. He called it "the gold standard" for resolving stress incontinence. He described it as a "ribbon" that would sit underneath my urethra. As my incidents of stress incontinence were so rare and mild, he suggested it would be more a "preventative measure" than anything else. Almost as quickly as I had discovered that my vagina was broken, I was going to have it fixed. Surgery would take place just three weeks later and would stop the yoga farts AND prevent any future bouts of stress incontinence—I would never have to do Kegels again. Doesn't this sound too good to be true?

Fear and How It Exposed My Emotional Trauma

Even though I had experienced childbirth, the thought of having surgery on this part of my body brought with it a deep fear. I view this delicate area like a flower. This flower is the source of deep passionate pleasure. It is both fragile and strong. How could I have lived my adult life without realizing that my flower was damaged? So many thoughts raced through my mind. I felt so vulnerable. I believed that this surgery was something I needed to do, and I was very afraid.

In facing this fear, some emotional wounds came to the surface. Believing that I had walked around my entire life with a broken vagina exposed my deepest insecurities. Issues that I had buried and emotions that I had suppressed came bubbling up. By far, my greatest challenge would be to face these deeply buried emotional wounds. Symbolism has always appealed to me. I knew I would feel the physical pain with this surgery and decided to work to heal the emotional wounds while dealing with the physical pain. The result would see me stepping forth into my future with a lightness of foot, having left the weight of my insecurities in the past.

The surgery itself took just thirty minutes and I was soon in the recovery room preparing for my return home. Recovery from surgery is seldom without issue. Cystitis, a condition that irritates the bladder, was something I had experienced once or twice before. From the very day of my surgery, I felt the harsh symptoms of cystitis. Burning pain in my bladder continued every single day. The only relief I could find was to sit on the toilet and release the few dribbles that were burning to come out. It was excruciating, and "pretend peeing" was the only way to relieve the pain. To add insult to injury, I was plagued by constant urinary infections.

Waking Up to Discover the Roots of My Trauma

A few months later, just when it seemed like things couldn't get any worse, my relationship ended. We had been together for over two years and I had lived in Sweden for three years at that point. The ending of this relationship came at a time when I was deep in the process of introspection. It came as a momentous shock, making me feel as though I had been knocked out of my own skin. I was beside myself, feeling as though I had awakened from a lifelong sleep. Suddenly, all those suppressed emotions and insecurities didn't seem so true anymore.

When I had lived in Ireland as an unmarried mother, Catholic Irish society had made me feel like a tainted woman. In this state of deep vulnerability, I could clearly see that I had continued to harshly judge myself long after Catholic Irish society had forgotten my "sins". My deeply buried emotional suffering was my responsibility. In the months following this breakup, I had epiphany after epiphany, with each day bringing more clarity drawing me closer to my center. There was an excitement within. Finding myself awake and seeing clearly, the possibilities seemed endless. So much potential for life to blossom with this newfound view over my emotions.

Yet there hung a dark cloud; the physical pain from surgery that was refusing to subside. I needed to learn more about my body. My desire to learn was so strong that I signed up for yoga teacher training. I needed to understand my anatomy and the wonderful organism that held my energy. The shock of the breakup had led me to see that I had lived in my head and was very much disconnected from my body. I used my yoga practice to help reconnect to my body. Yoga is a very subtle practice, drawing the practitioner away from the restless mind into the grounded body.

Although I had run marathons and triathlons, my yoga practice revealed the feebleness of my mind-to-body connection. The practice of yoga allowed me to tap into a subtler connection. A more precise pathway between the mind and the muscle can be subtly felt when you quiet the mind and bring single-pointed focus to that single point in space where the muscle you are trying to control exists. In the weeks before my fortieth birthday, I completed my first teacher training and began teaching right away.

It is said that life begins at forty. For me, a new version of life definitely began around then. I had studied hard to learn more about my body and mind. I was in a state of deep mindful peace, having healed my emotional wounds. But, physically, I was tortured. The unbearable pain was having an immensely negative impact on my quality of life. It was around this time that I started the relationship, which led to that fateful day when my surgeon dropped the "It's permanent" bombshell. I returned from that appointment believing I would never have sex again. For the rest of my life, I would be left to suffer, endlessly depositing burning dribbles into the toilet bowl.

Unsurprisingly, my budding relationship came to an end. My ex was determined that I shouldn't have to accept this predicament. He did some research and found a UK surgeon who was performing complete removals, and promptly arranged an appointment. I made the trip to Oxford where the surgeon confirmed that I needed complete removal. The "gold standard" mesh was tearing up my insides, causing damage to the neck of my bladder and eroding through my vaginal wall creating a hole (a very common side effect of polypropylene—the mesh material). The mesh acted much like a cheese grater, scraping against delicate tissues abrasively while my body fought hard to expel it.

Mesh Removal—the Cornelian Dilemma

Mesh removal is very high-risk surgery as there is no consideration in the design for removal. Removing mesh from the body is much like trying to remove chewing gum from hair; it is impossible to take away the offending mesh without also removing healthy tissues, leaving structures substantially weakened. My removal surgeon had explained that I could be permanently incontinent following removal, due to the extensive tissue damage.

This was one of the most difficult decisions of my life. Choosing between two evils. Evil one: living a life of celibacy in constant pain. Evil two: living a life in nappies, possibly still with the same pain, and possibly still unable to have sex. I wanted to go back in time, so I could unmake the decision to have the device implanted. To undo the damage that I had so blindly signed up for. Unfortunately, that was not an option.

I choose evil two; hoping that the 51%[1] chance I would be pain-free would pay off. I had learned through my yoga teacher training that the body is a self-healing organism. It is constantly communicating its needs as it surrenders to the irresistible force of healing. It asks for what it needs, and if you provide the right ingredients, it responds positively. Through my athletic training and then yoga, I had learned how to develop strength where before there was weakness. I knew that my determination, coupled with my anatomical knowledge, could potentially empower me to heal my pelvic floor. There was a chance I could recover, and it was a gamble I was willing to take.

In May 2015, I placed my life in the hands of my mesh-removal surgeon, and she successfully performed complete removal of the device without complications. From the very moment it was removed, I felt relief. The cystitis symptoms disappeared instantly. I can't begin to explain the relief I felt when my body was mesh-free. It was the end of the daily trauma and pain. Anyone who has had to live with pain for even a short time can imagine how momentous this was. At last, I had hope; hope that life could begin again; hope that the best of my life was yet to come.

For the first few weeks following surgery, I was quite swollen, and suffered only mild incontinence. As the swelling subsided, my belief that I had escaped a life of incontinence was eradicated as complete incontinence ensued. The feeling of urinating had changed dramatically. I can liken urination pre-removal to water coming out of a pressure hose. Urination post-removal can be likened to that of water being poured from a cup. It felt like my pee was just falling out of my body with no resistance from my pelvic floor. It was soul-destroying. If I walked really slowly, there was a chance I could hold it, but the minute I picked up my pace beyond that of a snail, I would leak. No one should ever have to experience this. It made me want to lock myself in my apartment; never again to go outside and face the world.

The Journey to Empower My Flower

Determined to regain bladder control, I started researching all possible methods. My pelvic floor wasn't responding to my calls and I knew I needed to rebuild strength so, I started on a journey. My search for a solution was relentless. I went through hundreds of hours of additional yoga teacher training and participated in the *Anatomy Trains* courses by Tom Myers, one of the pioneers in the fascial system (connective tissue). These learnings would prove pivotal to my success. I tried to leave no stone unturned on my quest, going so far as to participate in human dissection so as to see with my own eyes how the pelvic floor looks from within.

While others were saying, "Winter is coming" and discussing the thickening plots from *Game of Thrones*, I was wading through my own harsh winter, where the seed of my flower seemed to be buried so deeply that a blossom would never come. In order to heal, I would have to take complete responsibility for my pelvic health, essentially becoming an investigator, and conducting an inquiry into the workings of my body.

Through this endeavor, I discovered the patterns that govern the human organism. Zooming down to the smallest elements within the body reveals a pattern. Zooming out and observing your daily life, also reveals a pattern. Even watching the movement of thoughts in your mind reveals a pattern. Organized patterns contribute to function. If the pattern is chaotic, dysfunction ensues. This is also true when it comes to software. Luckily for me, I had worked many years as a software engineer and decided to use this experience to help decode my own patterns.

Thankfully, the ubiquitous internet exposed a world of scientific research, enabling me to connect the dots as I unearthed the potential root cause of my symptoms. I tapped into the subtlety of yoga to enhance the connection between my brain and my pelvic floor.

Finding My Superpower

I discovered that we all have a superpower hidden in the subtle communication of the body. This language that your body speaks in the form of reflexes and sensations, can be used to develop your superpower—the ability to communicate with the nervous system through thought, movement, and touch. Communication is a two-way street. Over the course of the first year following removal, I learned to communicate with my body, giving it what it was asking for and asking for it to give me what I needed—continence. You can do this too.

This journey of empowerment has subsequently changed the course of my life, bringing me all the way down to earth and teaching me humility, which I feel I had lost somewhere along the way. Pelvic floor dysfunction (PFD) can happen to any of us. One in three women and one in ten men will suffer the condition. It is hidden beneath a cloak of taboo. This taboo serves only to isolate those who endure the embarrassing symptoms, preventing them from seeking help. Failure to deal with mild symptoms can lead to severe symptoms further down the line because these symptoms are your body's way of communicating that your pattern is not optimal.

Lifting the Cloak of the Taboo

I feel compelled to speak openly about my experiences for the benefit of others; to share what I have learned and to work tirelessly to break the taboo. We are still in the darkness of winter. So, here I am, lifting the cloak of darkness, and trying to let the sunlight in. I am exposing my female flower to the world. A flower that has seen the sunshine and is now in full bloom.

I invite you to join me on a journey to find your own superpower. We will step back in history, discovering the roots of this taboo. We will set goals for the future that will help you to optimize your pelvic floor health. We will undertake a journey that encourages you to take responsibility for your own investigation, identifying your unique patterns, and creating a plan to empower your flower. Together we can work to remove the cloak of this taboo and instead we can use it as a cape (shouldn't all superpowers come with a cape?).

About This Book

This book has been written for those suffering from PFD. PFD is an umbrella term covering a multitude of symptoms including stress incontinence, overactive bladder, POP, fecal incontinence, chronic pelvic pain, vaginismus, and dyspareunia among others. The book offers an eight-phase program to empower your flower, with each phase having five modules covering the pelvic floor, breathing, movement, relaxation, and meditation/mind. These five modules ensure you are approaching your PFD from multiple directions to enhance your potential for empowerment. It is not intended to diagnose or treat any medical condition(s) nor to be used as a substitute for professional medical advice.

How to Use This Book

This book has been written in three parts:

Part 1—The seed of Knowledge—learning to see patterns and connect the dots

In Part One, we plant the seed of knowledge by revealing the patterns at play and connecting the dots between body, mind, and life. This part references the scientific research that can lead you toward empowerment. If you are one of those people who likes to understand how things work, this section is for you! This knowledge provides a foundation for understanding *why* the eight-phase program empowers you to regain control.

Part 2—Empower your flower—Nourish, develop, grow, and blossom

Your empowerment begins from where you are now; a place that is unique to you. This part of the book helps you to measure that place by conducting a baseline assessment. The output of this assessment is utilized for goal setting, which helps determine your starting phase in the eight-phase plan, allowing you to address your specific patterns, thus providing the conditions needed for your flower to blossom.

After setting goals, you will be shown *how* to use the assessments in Part Two to choose your starting phase. It is important to understand that big changes take time. If your goal is to eat a hamburger,

Part Two will help you break that down into small bites that you can properly chew before swallowing, instead of trying to swallow the hamburger whole. These small incremental steps are designed not to overwhelm.

Within each phase, you will work on five different modules simultaneously: pelvic floor, breathing movement, relaxation, and mind/meditation. This holistic approach will help to ensure your success.

Part Three—Symptom Management and Life Strategies

Part Three is packed with useful symptom management and life strategies as well as more detailed information on PFD. This part also provides valuable explanations of the conditions that fall under the umbrella of PFD, as well as detailing the treatments offered (both non-surgical and surgical). Information is provided on the tools and devices that can be used as you work toward optimized pelvic floor function. You will also fund a summary of the types of healthcare professionals and therapists that may support you on your journey. This section explains *what* you can do to manage or alleviate your symptoms, and find true empowerment.

Free Support Materials

DOWNLOAD

Register your book on empoweryourflower.com to access free materials relating to this book. Just scan the QR code or go to empoweryourflower.com for more details. Resources include full color figures, a blank assessment booklet for the assessments in Part Two, sequence sheets for the eight-phase training, audio for meditations and more.

What Is Not Covered in This Book?

This book does not cover menstruation, conception, pregnancy or menopause. Although these are important topics in relation to pelvic health; I believe they are very widely and adequately covered in many other books.

For Men

This book has been written with a focus on female PFD; however, the exercises and many of the symptom management strategies detailed are also valid for men. My male clients have benefitted greatly from the information shared in this book. If you would prefer to read a book that is dedicated to male PFD, I would recommend *Pelvic Pain: The Ultimate Cock Block* by Dr. Susie Gronski.

Part
one

The Seed of Knowledge
Learning to see patterns and
connect the dots

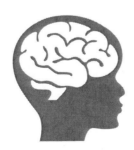

Overview of Part One

The goal with Part One of this book is for you to gain the foundational knowledge needed to empower your flower. I have tried to structure this section of the book in such a way that it brings you on a journey that has the potential to reveal the patterns at play within your own body, life, and mind. I have made every effort to provide good sources for the scientific research that is relevant to this journey. When I started my own journey, every healthcare specialist I consulted focused on the isolated symptom that was related to their specialty. These professionals played an important role in my investigation and subsequent recovery, however, without personally taking responsibility for identifying my patterns and gaining an understanding of the cause and effect of these patterns, I believe I would still be incontinent today.

Root Cause Analysis

When working through this part of the book, you will be learning to identify potential root causes for your PFD. In software engineering, we always look for the root cause of a given problem. Software engineering requires an understanding of conditional logic, structured thinking, pattern recognition, and attention to detail. We zoom in looking for patterns in the log files and zoom out to explore the infrastructure that supports the software. There are many potential points of failure.

To become empowered as an engineer, you need to understand not only the inner workings of your code but also the components that interact with your software. With the relevant data at your fingertips, it is easier to identify the root cause. This part of the book will attempt to provide you with the inner workings of your body, the external factors that can impact how your body functions, and an insight into patterns at play in your body, mind, and life. There are seven chapters:

Chapter One: Looking back and looking down

This first chapter begins your journey by looking back to find the root of the taboo surrounding PFD. You will be encouraged to explore how this relates to your own thoughts and beliefs regarding your genitals and sexuality. This is one of the first steps in identifying patterns at play within your mind. As well as looking back, Chapter One also looks down, exploring the anatomy of the vulva both pre- and post-birth.

Chapter Two: Getting to grips with muscles and your pelvic floor

In Chapter Two, we enhance our anatomy knowledge by exploring muscle function while giving you an understanding of muscle hyper- and hypo- tonicity, which can help you to better understand your specific PFD. You will also learn about the different muscles that make up the pelvic floor and how hyper- and hypo- tonicity of these muscles can impact your pelvic floor function.

Chapter Three: The Business of Your Body's Movement

Chapter Three focuses on the business of your body's movement, beginning with intra-abdominal pressure, and the hydraulics of breathing. This chapter builds on the knowledge from Chapter Two by reaching out into the body to explore relationships between the pelvic floor and other muscle groups. You will also learn about the relationship between muscle and bone before exploring how the nervous system manages movement, which is of particular importance for those suffering from pain conditions. This chapter also introduces the connective tissue system and biotensegrity in relation to POP.

Chapter Four: How Movement Creates Your Shape

When we begin Chapter Four, we explore both build-up and breakdown of muscles, before exploring connective tissue organization, which provides foundational knowledge when trying to identify the movement patterns that contribute to your posture. This chapter provides fuel for thought in relation to your movement, how it is reflected in your shape, and how the pattern of your daily life contributes to function/dysfunction.

Chapter Five: Emptying the Pelvic Bowl and Orgasm

In Chapter Five, we delve a little deeper into the key functions of the pelvic organs; urination, defecation, and sexual function. Simple analogies are used to explain the various functions and you will learn how PFD can impact urination, defecation, and sexual function. These learnings are valuable when reviewing the symptom management and life strategies that are explored in Part Three of this book.

Chapter Six: Connecting Your Mind to Your Muscles

This short thought-provoking chapter attempts to explain how you can use thought and touch to communicate with your nervous system. This can enhance your mind-to-muscle connection helping to change your patterns while manifesting a physical change in your body. This information will be used in both the pelvic floor and mind/meditation modules of the eight-phase program.

Chapter Seven: Empowering Your Mind to Heal

Your thoughts can greatly impact what manifests in your body. Chapter Seven helps you to identify patterns in your thoughts and explains the nervous system's "fight or flight" and "rest and digest" modes of operation. The information within this chapter is key to your empowerment and will be heavily utilized in the mind/meditation modules of the eight-phase program in Part Two.

Once you have read the seven chapters in this part of the book, you should have a foundation for understanding *why* the eight-phase program has five modules that should be worked on concurrently:

Eight-Phase
program modules

Pelvic Floor

This module helps you to optimize pelvic floor resting tone while increasing strength or relaxation (depending on your goals)

Breathing

This module helps you to restore functional breathing while enhancing the relationship between the pelvic floor and diaphragm.

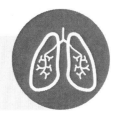

Movement

This module helps to rebalance the distribution of tension through movement, while controlling intra-abdominal pressure and building general strength.

Relaxation

This module helps to rebalance the distribution of tension through relaxation, while encouraging the release of hypertonicity, and relaxing the body.

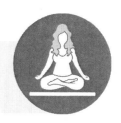

Mind & Meditation

This module uses mind exercises and meditation to address the emotional aspects of PFD while striving to help you achieve equanimity.

By working concurrently on these modules in each phase of training, you will greatly enhance your ability to empower your flower. Good luck!

Chapter One:
Looking back and looking down

The most important learning on my journey of empowerment was that *what you think impacts what manifests in your body*. When the body part that is most impacted is your pelvic floor, chances are, you have thoughts that include guilt or shame. If words such as "impure," "indecent," "shameful," and "dirty" in any way relate to your thoughts about your genitals or sexuality, the history portion of this chapter will be critical for you as we try to uncover the root of the taboo. The purpose of *looking back* is to help you to question your own thoughts and beliefs with regards to your genitals and sexuality before you *look down* at your genitals (which we will also do in this chapter).

When I started my journey, I met the taboo at every turn. Issues surrounding female genitals are somewhat of a *dirty secret*. Taboos prevent clear and relevant information from being freely available, and this is something that needs to change. We look back with a view to beginning the process of changing our minds regarding our genitals and sexuality. We will also begin the exploration of the female anatomy both pre- and post-birth. By the end of this chapter, you should have a renewed appreciation for your feminine flower.

This exploration was a pivotal step in my own journey of empowerment, and I will use my own history as an example to provoke thought in this chapter, helping you to discover the lens of your own conditioning. This process of looking back and looking down is the first step in overcoming any fear, guilt, or shame you may have in relation to your flower, which is an especially important step when trying to overcome PFD.

The History Behind the Taboo

When I first tried to figure out why PFD and female sexuality are shrouded in taboo, I expected to find that guilt and shame relating to female genitals had been around forever. Then I stumbled upon Catherine Blackledge's book *The Story of V: A Natural History of Female Sexuality*, where she uncovers the vulva's historical journey in fine detail. She highlights practices that worshiped the vulva, such as the Hindi worship of the *Yoni* and *ana suromai* (skirt lifting, a practice in Japan and Egypt, which was believed to increase harvests and ward off evil). I was so happy to see that female genitals had once been worshiped. So how did it become taboo?

In her book, Blackledge states that, "Before Western religion introduced the pesky concept of shame, female genitalia were venerated in ancient mythology." I decided to delve a little deeper and found a quote, circa 200AD, by Tertullian, a theologian noted as being "the father of Latin Christianity"[2]. Tertullian wrote, "Woman is the gate to hell and her gaping genitals the yawning mouth of hell." Very harsh words indeed, and not at all how the female flower should be viewed.

Christianity brought with it many morals that have positively changed the world, offering guiding principles that have contributed greatly to life as we know it. Unfortunately, Christianity also propagated corrupt views in relation to women and female sexuality, which is very evident in Tertullian's words.

I cannot say that the taboo is confined to Christianity, nor would I say that the taboo should impact your faith. Instead, I will say that female suppression has taken place over many centuries and is a global problem. The accumulation of female suppression has conditioned us to view our genitals and sexuality through a corrupt lens. My own experience of this suppression has its roots in Catholicism and it is through that lens that I will explain my experience. I would like you to keep an open mind as you read through this section. It is very personal, but I am sharing in the hope that it will help you to identify the lens of your own conditioning, regardless of your faith (or lack thereof).

The Corrupted View Caused by the Taboo

Being raised as an Irish Catholic, I was conditioned to use a corrupt lens. I had first-hand experience of the learned shame surrounding female genital organs and sexuality. As a young girl, I was taught to hide my body and not to talk about my "private" parts. The secrecy and shame associated with sexuality make the transition from child to adult unnecessarily difficult. When a subject is taboo, with words like "impure, "indecent," "shameful," and "dirty" associated, how can you possibly blossom?

As a child, I conformed to my conditioning, agreeing not to talk about my genitals or my sexuality, not even with my closest friends. This secrecy has a knock-on effect regarding access to contraception, which I believe directly contributes to teenage pregnancy and was one of the reasons why, at sixteen years of age, I had to rely on the feather-light condoms my eighteen-year-old boyfriend had stolen from his father. My shameful teenage pregnancy saw me banished to a home in Limerick, run by the Catholic church. All the while, I was rumored to be "working in Dublin." I remained hidden, like a taboo, in that home for five months.

When I gave birth at the age of seventeen, my shameful circumstances impacted the level of care I received at the maternity hospital. I was one of "those girls." Compassion was not to be found in the faces of the hospital staff that were charged with my care. The brutal delivery of my son resulted in a fractured tailbone and botched episiotomy. These injuries were overshadowed by the fight to be allowed to breastfeed my son, a fight that I lost due to my shameful predicament, which the nurse said denied me the right to bond with my son.

Thankfully, I subsequently won the battle to keep my son, avoiding a forced adoption, and managing to bring him back into my arms when he was five weeks old. Unfortunately, the ostracism didn't end there. I was forced to live in a society that constantly reminded me that I was a tainted woman. That dirty, shameful part of my body was to blame, and it caused me tremendous pain.

I had never seen how my genitals looked prior to the birth. I mean, why would I look? Why would anybody look at this hidden and shameful place? I first took a mirror to look "down below" when I was almost twenty-three. I was not impressed by what was reflected in the mirror. My view over my own genitals was corrupt. It was a corruption that had its roots in the religion that taught me it was "dirty." This corruption was further contorted by pictures I had happened upon during my youth from a glossy top-shelf magazine, probably the stash of one of my brothers. My flower was very different from those pictures. I didn't like it. Comparison tends to breed contempt. It implies superiority and inferiority, creating separation, and spawning the illusion that things should be different from how they actually are.

To highlight the impact of this illusion, I could tell you that in the UK, children as young as nine years of age are seeking genital reconstructive surgery[3] to change the appearance of their vulva. Something is fundamentally wrong in a society where children are led to believe that as they are, they are not good enough. It is imperative that we come together to change this negative view.

Access to a world of images and videos, social media, and pornography leads people, of all ages, across the world to believe they need to change their appearance. Of course, this is not just the appearance of the vulva. The beauty industry thrives on our inability to accept ourselves as we are. Modern life is plagued with the obsession to look a particular way. Yoyo-dieting for that "perfect" figure, and obsession with having skin that is without blemishes, appearing airbrushed, making you wish you could apply a Snapchat filter to your everyday face. Change is needed. The time has come for women all around the world to embrace the body they are graced with; lumps, bumps, and all.

Seeing Beyond the Corruption

By looking back in history, for me, the corruption is clear. The idea that we should feel guilt and shame around our genitalia was cultivated in a society that disempowered women. It is clear that we should not accept the guilt and shame that were the product of this suppression. We must empower ourselves, and that begins with you. The most important relationship in your life is the one you have with yourself. Every step you take in life, you have to be there for yourself, like your very own cheerleading squad.

Looking out to the world to see how you should look, serves only to demean either yourself or those to whom you look. As a single parent, I had learned to ignore the perception of society when making decisions relating to myself and my children. This same wisdom must be applied when it comes to appearance. Someone who seems to share this view is the artist, Jamie Mc Cartney.

Jamie undertook the task of quelling the shame associated with the female flower through his "Great wall of vagina."[4] He used plaster casts to create sculptures of vulvas with the very noble goal of freeing women from anxiety relating to the appearance of their vulvas. Figure 1.1 shows just one of many walls of plaster casts created by Jamie.

The Great Wall of Vagina (panel 1 of 10) by Jamie McCartney ©2011

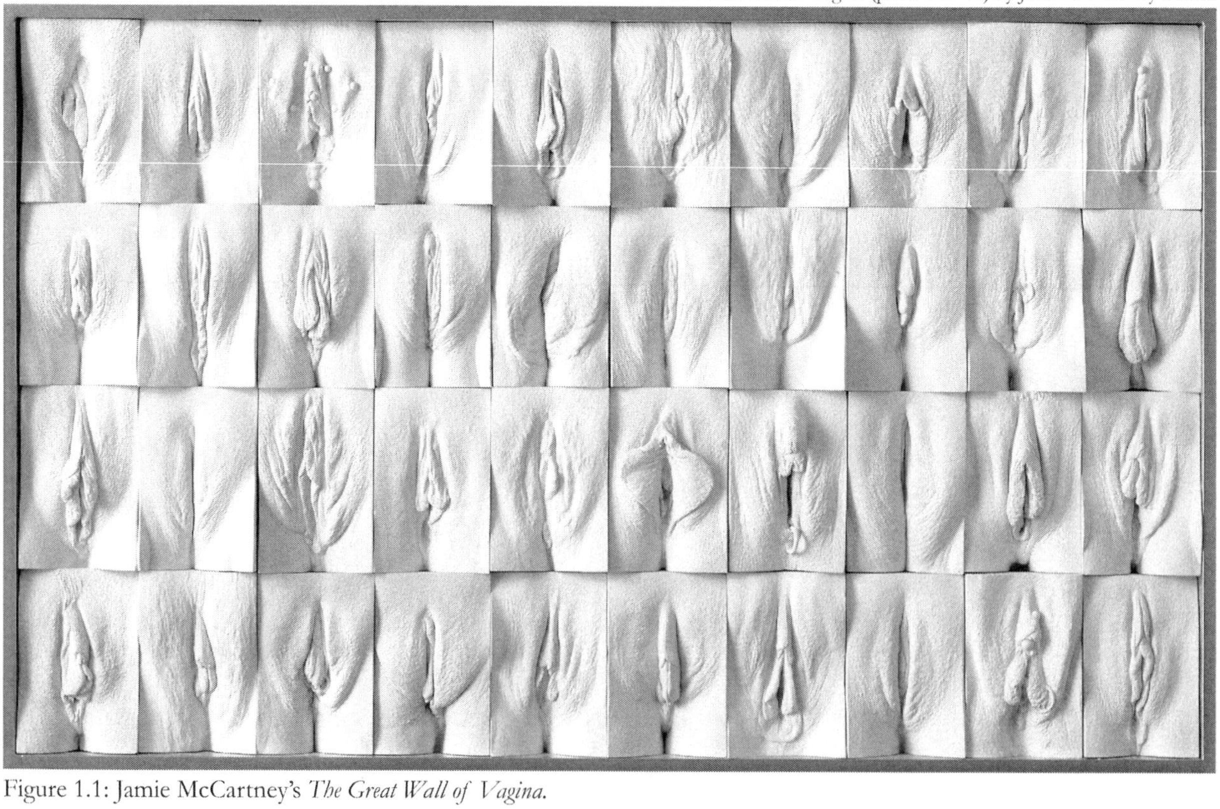

Figure 1.1: Jamie McCartney's *The Great Wall of Vagina.*

Figure 1.1 shows a vast variety of shapes and sizes, all different, and all beautiful in their own ways.

Many people believe the vagina is the proper name for the female genitals, however, the vagina is actually the internal portion that extends from the vaginal opening to the cervix (neck of the womb). The external female genital organ is known as the vulva. The fact that Jamie's wall is called *The Great Wall of Vagina* when it is actually a great wall of vulvas just highlights the lack of common knowledge around the actual name for the external female genitals.

He is not the only artist to attempt to amplify the emancipation of the female genitals. In her play *The Vagina Monologues*[5], Eve Ensler confronts the taboo head-on and gives specific focus to heightening awareness on violence against women. The play gives the vulva a voice, in all its shapes, and forms. It is performed in theaters across the world by three monologists, typically celebrities.

I was lucky to have the opportunity to see the play back in 2002 at London's West End, performed by Melanie B (from the Spice Girls), Rhona Cameron, and Ingeborga Dapkunaite. This was an important step in my own journey of empowerment. When I left the show, I had a little more love and appreciation for my flower than when I took my seat. I was still miles away from having an uncorrupted view, but my journey had started, and my view over my unmentionables was beginning to change.

I stood on the shoulders of Jamie Mc Cartney, Eve Ensler, Catherine Blackledge, and all others who have used words, symbols, and sculptures to bring light to the true beauty of the feminine flower. Now, I encourage you to do the same as we march forth toward empowerment.

Removing the Lens of Your Conditioning

You are now in possession of a brief overview of how history may have shaped the taboo that prevents you from talking openly about PFD. The society in which you were raised has conditioned you to conform to that taboo by shaping your beliefs. This conditioning creates a filter through which you view the world and thus your perception of reality is impacted by these beliefs.

A fundamental change of mind is required to eradicate the negative views you may harbor toward your vulva. Changing your beliefs is not always easy; for me, it was a struggle and took some time, but I did it. I encourage you to approach your beliefs like an engineer, questioning the logic behind them.

There is a strong correlation between beliefs and emotions. Negative emotions, such as guilt and shame around female genitalia and sexuality, are the consequence of corrupt beliefs that have been passed down through the ages. Our current generation is responsible for what we pass to the next generation and so, it is our responsibility to change our beliefs, thus changing the emotional associations and breaking the taboo.

Negativity associated with the taboo can cause stress and fear, which act like barriers, preventing you from seeking much-needed help and support. Stress and fear can impact how your PFD is manifesting in your body. We must eliminate this negativity and build a positive relationship with ourselves on every level.

Relationships take time to blossom, whether that be a relationship with another person, yourself, or even a part of your body. The process of accepting your natural form is accelerated if you apply logic to wipe away the nonsensical concepts of your conditioning. The human body is one of nature's most amazing feats. When you view your lady parts as though you are an engineer, taking great delight in exploring this intricate multifunctional system, it is easier to find love.

Aptitude tests have shown that I have great spatial awareness, something that made it easy for me to work as a software engineer. I absolutely love symmetry and have an eye for patterns. Can you imagine my apprehension when I first saw that my flower was asymmetrical? I could not see beauty. The scarring from my episiotomy was clearly visible. When I first looked, I lacked the knowledge, and understanding to explore my nature through a clear lens. This was in the late nineties before Jamie Mc Cartney's *Wall of Vagina* existed.

I wish someone had told me to look toward this sacred place with love, gratitude, and appreciation. Your genitals are as unique as your face. Anatomically, we have the same parts but visually, they look dramatically different. Following my first exploration, and in the absence of a mature internet, I went to the nearest bookstore and purchased *Everywoman, a genealogical guide for life* a book written by Derek Llewellyn-Jones. It covers female development including puberty, pregnancy, childbirth, and menopause.

This book had an image of female genitals before and after birth, which provided some relief as my post-birth genitals were not dissimilar to those in the book. I did not love how my vulva looked in the mid-nineties, but at least it seemed more normal thanks to those pictures.

Exploring the External Female Anatomy

The pre-birth vaginal opening is typically smaller than post-birth (if you have experienced vaginal delivery). The hymen, a small stretchy band of tissue that sits just inside the vaginal passage, has been the subject of much controversy. Just like we have different shapes of lips, the hymen can be smaller or larger. In some cases, it breaks during the first sexual encounter where intercourse is achieved, in others, it doesn't. After birth, it is typically broken leaving you with small skin tags known as carunculae myrtiformes. Figure 1.2 shows the comparison between a pre-birth and post-birth vulva with the hymen and carunculae myrtiformes marked.

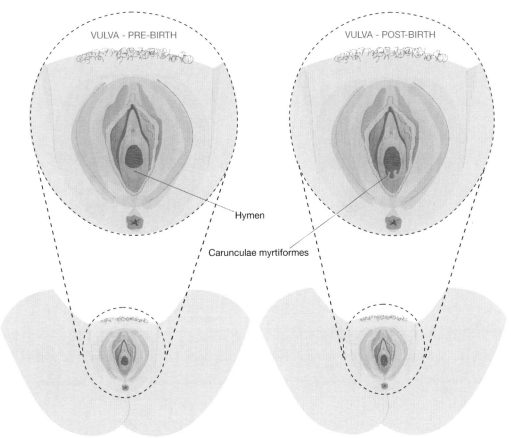

Figure 1.2: Vulva pre- and post-birth.

The vulva to the left, in Figure 1.2, zooms in to show the hymen intact. The vulva on the right in Figure 1.2, zooms in to show the carunculae myrtiformes following birth. We will now take a closer look at the female vulva using Figure 1.3 to identify the parts we can see externally as well as those beneath the skin.

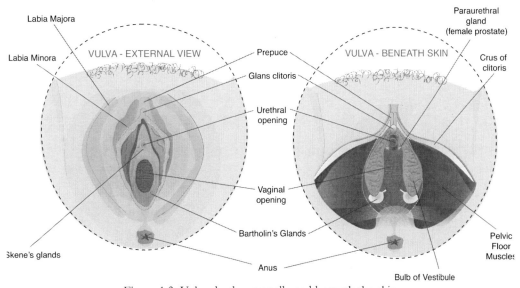

Figure 1.3: Vulva, both externally and beneath the skin.

In Figure 1.3, we see both the external view of the genitals on the left side, as well as the glands beneath the skin on the right side. The various parts of the vulva are labeled in Figure 1.3 and the text that follows gives more detail on these parts. You can refer back to this figure as you review the details.

There are two sets of lips on the vulva: the labia majora, which are the external lips covered in skin, and the labia minora, which are the internal lips. These labia minora are generally pink in color, although sometimes they can appear to look brown, gray, or even a bluish tone.

Derek Llewellyn-Jones comments in his book that "it was once believed that large labia minora were due to masturbation, which at that time was considered evil. It is now understood that this is nonsense."[6] Yet another ludicrous belief that has been quashed. If you take a look back at Jamie McCarthy's *Great Wall of Vagina*, you will see that these lips really do vary greatly in shape and size.

The clitoris is at the top of the vulva where the labia minora are joined in a fold of skin called the clitoral hood. The clitoris feels like a small bean beneath the skin. The clitoris is the female equivalent of the penis, however, don't be fooled by its small size. Whereas the male organ has some 4000 nerve endings, the clitoris boasts double that with some 8000 nerve endings[7].

I like to call the clitoris the *on* switch for sexual arousal. One study explains how "The vaginal tissue responds to sexual arousal by relaxing and lengthening."[8] If you suffer from vaginismus or dyspareunia (two conditions that cause painful sex), you should really learn about how to stimulate your clitoris to orgasm as it switches *on* relaxation, lubrication, and vaginal opening in preparation for sex. We will explore this in more detail in Part Three of this book.

A little below the clitoris, you will find a small hole, which is the opening to the urethra (the pee pipe). It's sometimes hard to identify, particularly after childbirth if there has been stretching or tearing of the vestibule (the space between the urethra and the vagina). Below the opening to the vagina, you will find the perineum, which is an area of skin that stretches from the back of the vagina to the anus (the opening to the rectum). This space can be quite small in some females.

Exploring the Clitoris and Glans

As well as understanding the external physical structures, it is important to understand the glans beneath the skin. To the right in Figure 1.3, you can see that the clitoris is more than just the little bean that you can feel. It has a "crus," which is a large wishbone-shaped structure. The vestibule are large glands that are composed of erectile tissues that swell during sexual arousal.

At the bottom of the bulb of vestibule, you will see a small gland on each side known as Bartholin's Glands. These are responsible for excreting fluid that lubricates the vagina during sex. At the top of the vestibule just above the urethra, there are two small glands known as the skene's glands or paraurethral glands (female prostate). These glands also secrete fluid during sex and, in some women, they are responsible for female ejaculation, which is the expulsion of a few milliliters of thick milky fluid during orgasm.

Maybe you have heard of squirting? Well, female ejaculation is not squirting! Squirting is a different phenomenon that is sometimes combined with female ejaculation. In both cases, secretions are from the skene's glands. However, with squirting, the expelled liquid comes from within the urethral opening.[9] It is not urine but instead, "a larger amount of changed and diluted urine." If you happen to squirt during intercourse, don't be embarrassed. Give yourself and your partner a pat on the back and consider yourself an alpha female.

Having gained an understanding of the root of the taboo, the lens of your conditioning, and the anatomical parts that make up your female anatomy, we will move to the next chapter where our journey into anatomy accelerates.

Chapter Two:
Getting to Grips with Muscles and Your Pelvic Floor

Having seen the external beauty of this life-giving flower and the glands that participate in delightful orgasms, let us go deeper beneath the skin to explore the muscles, bones, and connective tissue structures as well as the organs that they support. I will attempt to explain these anatomy fundamentals in a way that is simple and easy to understand. This should provide you with a foundation that will empower you on your journey toward optimal pelvic health.

In this chapter, you will get to grips with muscles, particularly those within your pelvic floor. We will review the names of muscles, organs, and bones, as well as their relationships and functions. Analogies are used, which should make it easier to understand these sometimes complex relationships. When discussing anatomy, it is typical to use specific language to explain where the body part exists in relation to other parts (e.g., superior and inferior for the upper and lower body, anterior and posterior for the front and back, etc.).

Many of my yoga students and even some teachers get confused with this terminology and, therefore, I will use top, bottom, front, and back to make it easier for you to understand. Try not to feel intimidated or overwhelmed by this chapter. You do not have to commit the details to memory. If your pelvic area was a software program, you could view this chapter as the manual that explains the various components and functions. You can refer back to this chapter at any time should you require troubleshooting!

The Importance of Connection

The pelvic area is made up of muscles, bones, nerves, blood vessels, internal organs (reproductive, digestive, and urological), and connective tissue (fascia). In high school, I was an A+ student in biology, and believed I possessed a great understanding of the different bodily systems and their functions.

To my surprise, when I began to investigate the root cause of my incontinence, I discovered a fundamental flaw in my knowledge. This was due to viewing bodily systems in isolation with no consideration for cross-functional interaction. A view of the body being composed of independent bits and pieces is a corrupt view. Prior to facing my incontinence, I would have viewed a pain in the knee as there being something wrong with my knee. However, this is not necessarily the case.

The body is an intelligent self-healing organism. It may appear that parts work independently but in reality, when you lift your hand, it is just a single note in a harmonious symphony. Your muscles do not act independently. Your brain sends neurological signals. Your heart pumps blood that sustains those muscles. Your digestive system provides the fuel to create energy that powers you. When you make the movement of your hand, other muscles, bones, and connective tissue will also participate in that movement.

There is a sweet harmony to the working of this fantastic organism. When everything works as it should, the bones, muscles, connective tissue, and bodily systems (neurological, cardiovascular, lymphatic, etc.) perform a delightful dance to the symphony of your life. When this dance falls out of rhythm, the ensuing chaos can trigger a chain of symptoms, which result in a tumultuous impact on your quality of life.

By bringing awareness to the subtlety of movement and the biomechanics of your body, you can begin to hear your very own symphony. The more awareness you can create, the louder the volume of your symphony. By understanding this harmonious dance, you can begin to see your patterns.

When you can see your patterns, you can change them, moving you away from dysfunction toward function.

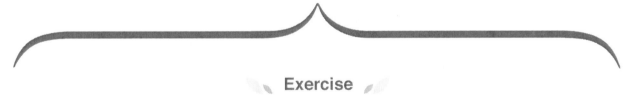

Exercise
to feel the subtle connectivity at play within your body

The purpose of this exercise is for you to feel the connectivity at play within your own body.

➡ To do this ⬅

1. Sit squarely in a chair, relaxing your body for a moment.
2. Raise one hand above your head while bringing your awareness to your feet and legs
3. Feel the subtle activation of muscles in your lower extremities.

4.   Lower your arm again while feeling the sensation in your legs and feet

You should feel that there is subtle movement in your lower limbs even though it is your arm that you are moving. The sensation of these subtle movements marks the very beginning of you tuning in to the language of your body.

Exploring Muscle Basics

To begin our anatomical journey, we will explore some muscle basics. Muscles are considered to be responsible for motion and stability. They utilize the body's energy to create movement. Everything you do with your body involves the use of your muscles. Even automated tasks such as breathing and digesting food involve muscles, albeit those that are involuntarily controlled.

There are three main types of muscle in the body, which are shown in Figure 2.1.

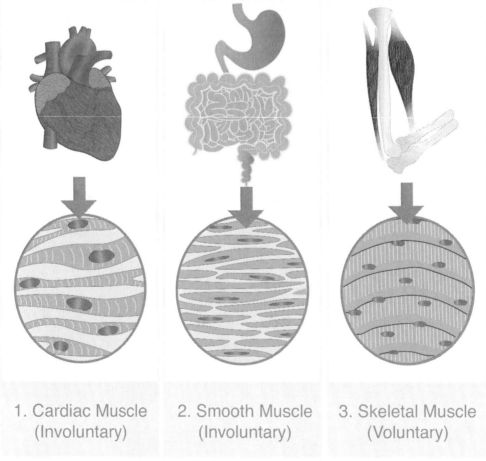

1. Cardiac Muscle   2. Smooth Muscle   3. Skeletal Muscle
   (Involuntary)   (Involuntary)   (Voluntary)

Figure 2.1: Three types of muscle.

Figure 2.1 shows a graphical representation of the pattern of tissues for the three types of muscle. The pattern of a muscle's tissue, optimizes that muscle's function. The three muscle types are:

Muscle Types

1. **Cardiac muscle**: Cardiac muscle has a pattern that is optimized for repeated contraction without fatiguing. Heart muscles are responsible for contracting to pump blood around your body.

2. **Smooth muscle**: Smooth muscle has a pattern that allows both longitudinal and circular contraction, allowing for lengthening, shortening, and squeezing of the colon. This is an involuntary muscle that facilitates bodily functions such as digestion, urination, and defecation. Your hollow organs; including the stomach, the bladder, and the bowel, among others, are constructed of smooth muscle tissues.

3. **Skeletal muscle**: Skeletal muscle has a pattern of long cells that are almost parallel in arrangement. These cells are also known as muscle fibers (a bit like elastic threads). Skeletal muscles cover the skeleton and are responsible for the movement of the body. Simply put, skeletal muscles are utilized to help flex your joints by moving your bones, thus creating the motion of your body. A skeletal muscle's job is to contract (shorten) and it is that contraction that creates the movement. As we progress through this chapter, we will explore how the pattern of tissues in skeletal muscle can impact function.

The contractions of skeletal muscles are controlled by the nervous system, which can be considered the electrical system of the body. The wires of this electrical system (the nerves) reach out to all muscles. A signal to contract can be viewed as switching on the "contract" switch on the muscle's motor. Sometimes, you turn on the contractions by deciding to move (this is known as phasic control). At other times, your nervous system will manage the turning on and off of the "contract" switches to resist gravity and maintain balance (this is known as proprioceptive control).

Muscle Fiber Types

When we talk about PFD, it is important to understand that there are different types of skeletal muscle fibers. We will not delve deeply, but I would like you to know that there are two main skeletal muscle fiber types. They are as follows:

i. **Slow twitch**: built for endurance—the contract switch for this muscle fiber is always on like a car engine when it is ticking over without going anywhere.

ii. **Fast twitch**: built for fast reaction—the contract switch for this muscle fiber is off and switches on only when needed. This fiber type provides lots of power but for shorter periods; it's like the car engine when you press hard on the accelerator.

Most skeletal muscles have some fibers of each type but many muscles will have a dominant fiber type.

During my first yoga teacher training, I learned that each muscle can be viewed as an organ comprising muscle tissue, connective tissue, nerves, and blood vessels. Each complete muscle has a filament of connective tissue surrounding it. This connective tissue allows muscles to slide/glide against each other helping to facilitate fluid movement.

Zooming in on Muscle

In Figure 2.2, we will zoom in on skeletal muscles to get a closer look at how they are comprised:

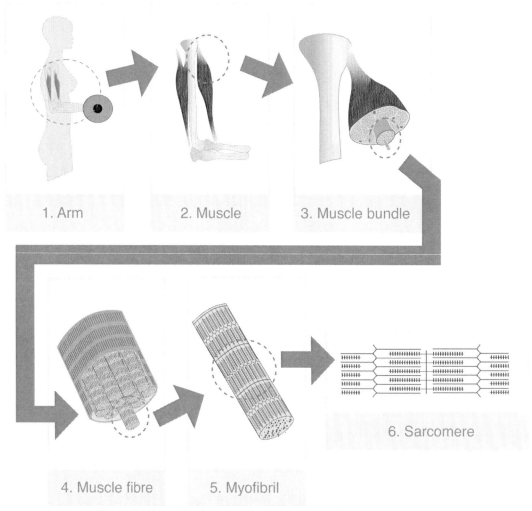

Figure 2.2: Zooming in to see the composition of skeletal muscle.

Figure 2.2 shows a blue dotted circle around the area that is magnified on the subsequent image in this flow. The following numbered list explains the content of each image of Figure 2.2:

1. **Arm**: Shows the muscles and bones of the arm beneath the skin.

2. **Muscle**: Shows the muscles and bones of the arm. The muscles are connected to bones by tendons (part of the connective tissue network). Each muscle is surrounded by a layer of connective tissue.

3. **Muscle Bundles (fascicles)**: This shows a dissected view of the muscle, which allows you to see the muscle bundles; each of these bundles contains multiple muscle fibers (cells). These bundles are surrounded by a thin layer of connective tissue and each fiber is also surrounded by a thin layer of connective tissue. These connective tissue layers help to facilitate fluidity of movement. Within the muscle bundles, you will also find the blood vessels and nerves that serve that muscle.

4. **Muscle Fiber**: This shows a single muscle fiber. We can see that each fiber contains multiple individual myofibrils (each surrounded by a thin layer of connective tissue).

5. **Myofibrils**: Myofibrils are components of muscle fibers, which are composed of protein filaments that form a repeating structural pattern. These structural patterns within myofibrils are known as sarcomeres and are the elastic components of the muscle fiber. Each myofibril is surrounded by a thin layer of connective tissue.

6. **Sarcomere**: A sarcomere is an individual functional unit of elasticity, which contracts and relaxes to create movement.

Understanding Muscle Lenght-Tension Relationships

To gain an understanding of muscle elasticity, we have to understand the function of sarcomeres. Sarcomeres are like tiny stretchy building blocks that are only around 2.2 micrometers in length. Each sarcomere has a number of filaments, which are attracted to each other, much like Velcro. These filaments are called actin and myosin. It is the interactivity between these filaments, which creates elasticity, allowing muscles to contract and stretch.

In Figure 2.3, we can see the interaction of actin (red) and myosin (blue) in a normally functioning sarcomere:

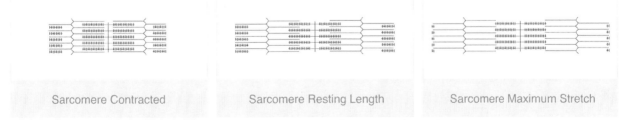

Sarcomere Contracted   Sarcomere Resting Length   Sarcomere Maximum Stretch

Figure 2.3: Sarcomeres contracted, resting, and stretched.

Figure 2.3 shows a contracted sarcomere on the left, a sarcomere at rest in the center, and a sarcomere at maximal stretch on the right. The amount of overlap between the actin and myosin filaments, when a sarcomere is at rest, is known as the length-tension relationship. An optimal length-tension relationship in a normally functioning muscle would have sufficient overlap (at rest) to allow the muscle to contract or stretch quickly when required.

If the resting length is increased, this is indicative of hypotonicity (meaning that the muscle is lax or weak/underactive). In this case, the overlap between actin and myosin would not be sufficient to produce a good contraction.

If the resting length is decreased, this is indicative of hypertonicity (meaning that the muscle is tight or in spasm/overactive). In this case, the overlap between actin and myosin would be too much, leaving no room for further contraction.

Figure 2.4 shows a graphical representation of the length-tension relationship for sarcomeres that are hypotonic, optimal, and hypertonic.

Length-Tension Relationship (Resting Length)

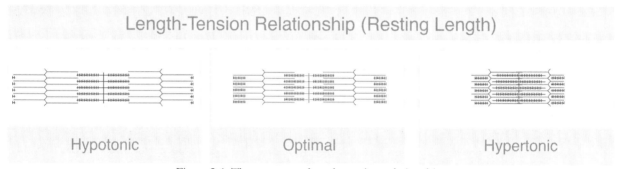

Hypotonic   Optimal   Hypertonic

Figure 2.4: The sarcomere length-tension relationship.

You can see in the sarcomere on the left in Figure 2.4 that there is little overlap between the actin (red) and myosin (blue). It would be hard to contract with this pattern. In the sarcomere to the right of Figure 2.4, there is a lot of overlap, leaving no space for further contraction. It would be difficult to contract with this pattern. The optimal pattern, shown in the center, leaves sufficient overlap to both contract (shorten) and stretch (lengthen).

In the business of your body's movement, the management of the length-tension relationship is governed by your nervous system. When we undertake the training in Part Two of this book, we will utilize movement to communicate with your nervous system to help to strengthen muscles that are hypotonic and to release tension in muscles that are hypertonic

Many people believe that incontinence is a sign of a hypotonic pelvic floor, however, hypertonic muscles can also cause urinary leakage, pelvic pain, and sexual dysfunction. Zooming in to see your pattern of tension provides valuable data for rehabilitation. Of course, it is not possible for you to measure your individual sarcomeres. However, we will use touch to assess the tone of muscles in the assessments in Part Two of this book.

There can be many causes of muscle hypertonicity. In many cases, hypertonic contractions remain in order to compensate for bad posture or a previous injury. With hypertonic muscles, you could imagine that the *contract* switch is constantly on. Muscles that are overly contracted at rest cannot react when there is a sudden force, such as a sneeze or a cough. The following exercise will help to demonstrate this.

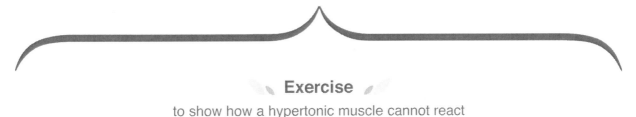

Exercise

to show how a hypertonic muscle cannot react

➡ To do this ⬅

1. Create a fist and squeeze as hard as you can (this is your hypertonic muscle)
2. Now try to contract your fist.

You will notice that you cannot contract your fist further as it is already contracted. This is the same for hypertonic muscles.

Understanding Muscle Contraction

We have learned that muscles are controlled by the nervous system, which turns *on* contraction to shorten the muscle. The length-tension relationship is not the only factor to consider when it comes to contraction. Your muscles require energy to initiate contraction. This energy is provided by a molecule known as adenosine triphosphate (ATP). If your muscles were a car, ATP would be the fuel. ATP is manufactured from the food you eat (fats, carbs, and proteins) along with the air you breathe (oxygen).

First, a muscle receives the signal from its nerve that turns *on* the contraction, and then chemical reactions initiate the action. ATP enables the myosin motors to move along the actin filaments, like car wheels turning to create movement along the road. When the ATP is no longer available (fuel has run out), the contraction releases (contract switch turns *off*) allowing the filaments to slide back to their original resting positions (the sarcomeres resting length), like the car reversing back into its parking spot.

Of course, if the muscle that is trying to contract is hypertonic or hypotonic, this will impact the muscle's ability to contract, which also has an impact on other local muscles. We will explore this later in this chapter. For now, let's assume that muscles have an optimal length-tension relationship and, with that information to hand, we will begin to explore the types of muscle contraction.

Types of Muscle Contraction

The type of contraction is based on the muscle's length when under tension. You can add tension to a muscle by adding resistance (e.g.: weight). In our example, we will add a dumbbell. Figure 2.5 shows the three different types of muscle contraction: isometric, concentric, and eccentric.

In the first image of Figure 2.5, the biceps is at its resting length (neither shortened nor lengthened) while under tension. The weight of the dumbbell is adding resistance and so the biceps needs to contract to counteract the resistance in order to maintain the 90-degree angle at the elbow. This is an isometric contraction.

If you shorten the biceps by flexing your elbow to bring the dumbbell up toward your shoulder, this is known as a concentric contraction as the muscle is shortening while under tension. This is demonstrated in the second image of Figure 2.5.

Finally, if you extend your elbow so your arm is straight while holding the dumbbell, as shown in the third image of Figure 2.5, then your bicep is lengthening while under tension thus producing an eccentric contraction.

It is important to understand these different contraction types when training the pelvic floor as

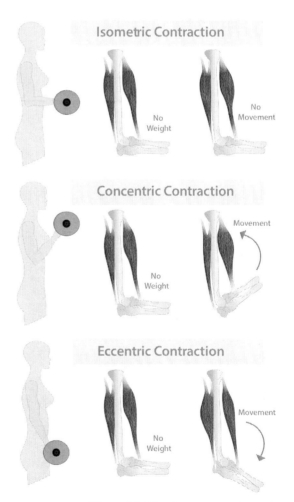

Figure 2.5: The three types of muscle contraction—Isometric, concentric, and eccentric.

utilizing these contractions can enhance the effect of pelvic floor muscle training. We will use these contraction types in the pelvic floor, movement, and relaxation modules of the eight-phase training in Part Two. As well as the types of contractions, it is important to understand the relationships between muscles. The business of your body's movement involves synergy between different muscles where they cooperate to complete the intended movement.

Understanding Muscle Relationships

Your muscles are part of a unified system, therefore, they must have good relationships with one another to ensure fluidity of movement. The two types of muscle relationships that we need to understand are the antagonistic relationship and the synergistic relationship.

With the antagonistic relationship, muscles work, interacting as a pair, in order to control the movement of a specific joint. With antagonistic pairs, one muscle contracts as the other one relaxes/stretches (also known as reciprocal inhibition, which we will discuss later). Typically, these pairs are muscles that control the movement of the same joint but on opposite sides.

We can use the example of the elbow joint, where we have the biceps on one side and the triceps on the other. Both are responsible for moving the elbow and thus participate in an antagonistic relationship. When one contracts (agonist), the other relaxes (antagonist). You do not have to think about relaxing your triceps when contracting your biceps as it happens automatically. The following exercise will help you to feel this antagonistic relationship in your own body.

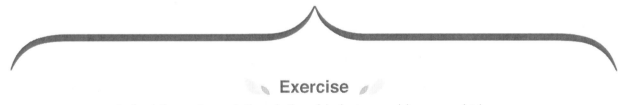

Exercise
to feel the antagonistic relationship between biceps and triceps

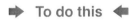

To do this

1. Flex your biceps by bending your elbow
2. Keeping the biceps contracted, feel your triceps on the back of your arm, and notice how it is relaxed/stretched

3.   Now, straighten your elbow by contracting your triceps and notice how the biceps is relaxed/stretched.

This relationship is demonstrated in Figure 2.6.

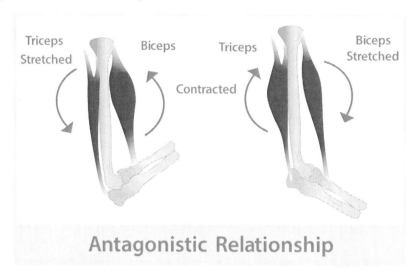

Figure 2.6: The antagonistic relationship between biceps and triceps.

You can see in Figure 2.6 how the contracted muscle is thicker while the relaxed/stretched muscle is thinner. Bodybuilders utilize muscle contractions to show off their physique, flexing to show how much thickness they have in their muscles when they contract.

With a synergistic relationship, muscles work in synergy to perform an action. For example, the muscles on the front of your thigh (the quadriceps and sartorius). There are four quadriceps muscles, and they work together along with the sartorius muscle to perform movements of the hip and knee thus participating in a synergistic relationship.

Your pelvic floor muscles are skeletal muscles that also participate in relationships with other muscles. We will explore some of these relationships later in this chapter but, first, let's explore the bones onto which the pelvic floor muscles are attached.

Bones in the Pelvic Girdle

The bones that exist in the pelvic area, are collectively known as the pelvic girdle. The pelvic floor muscles attach to the pelvic girdle thus influencing pelvic stability, which plays a pivotal role in maintaining a balanced posture. The bones of the pelvic girdle are shown in Figure 2.7 which shows

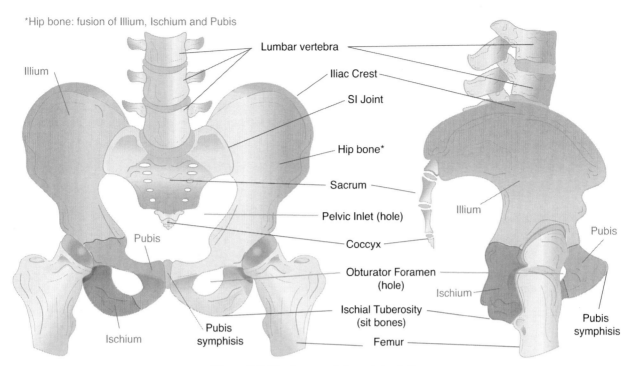

Figure 2.7: The bones of the pelvic girdle.

the pelvis from a front-facing view on the left and a side-facing view on the right. At the base of the spine in Figure 2.7, you will see a triangular bone known as the sacrum, which is a fusion of five vertebrae (S1 to S5). The top side of the sacrum connects to the lowest lumbar vertebra (also known as L5 due to it being the fifth lumbar vertebra). The left and right sides of the sacrum connect to the left and right sides of the pelvis. These joints are known as the sacroiliac joints or SI joints.

The pelvis has two identical sides (hip bones) that are constructed from three bones that fuse during early adulthood, the ilium at the top (highlighted in green), the pubis, at the front (highlighted in pink) and the ischium at the base (highlighted in purple). The hole between the pubis and ischium is known as the obturator foramen. The base of the ischium is known as the ischial tuberosity, which is often referred to as a "sitting bone" or even the "sitz bone" (that one makes me laugh!).

At the front of the pelvis is the pubis symphysis, a thick piece of cartilage that connects the left and right pubis. At the base of the sacrum is the coccyx, which is the small fusion of bones at the base of the spine, often referred to as the tailbone. Due to the way the coccyx curls inwards, it is prone to injury during childbirth.

The space (hole) at the base of the pelvis, known as the pelvic outlet, is the space through which the baby travels during delivery. Your pelvic organs sit just above this space. This space where your organs sit is often referred to as the "pelvic bowl." If nature has done its job correctly, your baby should fit through the pelvic outlet without issue.

I was one of the unfortunate women who suffered the trauma of a fractured coccyx during the birth of my first child. This is an uncommon birth injury, which can happen due to a number of factors, from the size of the pelvic outlet to the position of the sacrum and coccyx during birth. The sacrum is not rigidly held in place and has some degree of movement. If you deliver a child while lying on your back, your pelvic outlet is reduced in size by up to 30%. Many midwives and doulas recommend that you take an upright, squatting, or all-fours position as this helps to extend the sacrum, maximizing the size of the pelvic outlet during delivery.

As well as impacting the size of the pelvic outlet, the hip bones and sacrum have an impact on postural alignment, which we will explore more in the next chapter. Understanding the positioning of the hips and pelvis is important when assessing pelvic floor function. The muscles of the pelvic floor attach to these bones to form an elastic base on the pelvic bowl.

The remaining bones that connect to the pelvic girdle are the femurs (left and right) and the spine. The femurs are the large bones on the top of your legs, connected to the knees at the bottom while inserting into the hip socket at the top (it's a ball joint that inserts into the hip socket).

It is worth noting that our bones, like our faces, vary greatly in shape and size. This has a bearing on the range of motion (ROM) achievable by your joints. For some people, a full split will never be possible due to the shape and position of their hip sockets and femurs. The ROM of the hip bones also has an impact on posture and movement.

The Pelvic Floor and Organs

The muscles of the pelvic floor form three different layers. These layers each perform their own unique function, forming an intricate network of support for the organs that rest in the pelvic bowl. Figure 2.8 shows the bladder, uterus, and rectum resting in the pelvic bowl.

If you look closely at Figure 2.8, you will notice that the pubic bone acts like a little platform onto which the bladder rests. The pelvic floor muscles shown in this image are the outermost muscles that stretch front to back. In order to get a clear visualization of the actual muscles, we will use more detailed images that show the layers from above and below.

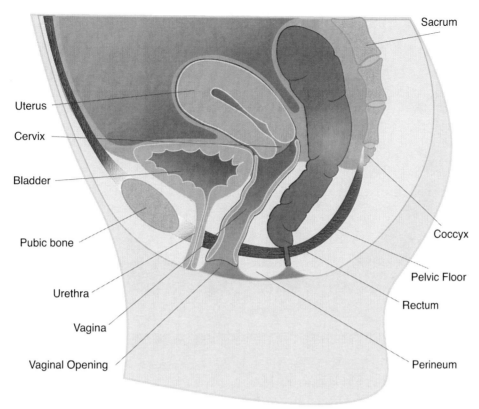

Figure 2.8: Female pelvic organs in their normal position.

As we explore the different layers, try to imagine where they exist in space in relation to your own pelvis. This will be of benefit when we review posture, and will also aid you when completing the baseline assessment of pelvic floor strength in Part Two of this book. To make it easier for you to understand the orientation of these muscles, look at Figure 2.9.

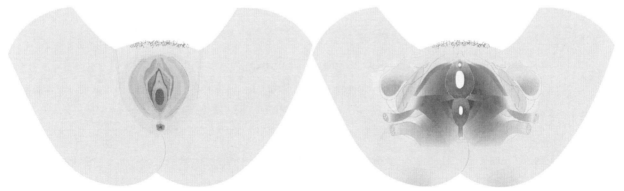

Figure 2.9: Side by side images, showing external genitals and pelvic floor muscles beneath the skin.

The left image in Figure 2.9 shows the external genitals, and the right image shows the pelvic floor muscles beneath the skin. You should be aware that the pelvic floor muscles (like all other muscles) are encased in connective tissue which, in turn, is connected to the connective tissue structures that surround the pelvic organs supporting their correct anatomical position.

I have often heard of the pelvic floor described as a hammock stretching from front to back. This is an extreme over-simplification that, in my opinion, creates the wrong visualization in the mind, lending itself to the typical vagueness of traditional pelvic floor exercises that suggest you just "squeeze and lift" or "pretend to hold your pee."

I believe that a deeper understanding of the different layers of the pelvic floor musculature can help to create a visualization that allows you to connect to the various muscles in a subtler way, enhancing the potential for increased function (either contracting or relaxing).

We will use this knowledge to take a subtle approach to pelvic floor activation so as to increase the mind-to-muscle connection. This also provides the opportunity to identify specific parts of the pelvic floor, which may not be reacting as they should.

There are three layers that form the pelvic floor muscles and these are the:

1. Superficial perineal layer (outermost layer)
2. Urogenital diaphragm (middle layer)
3. Pelvic diaphragm (deepest layer)

We will explore each layer, its muscles, and their functions. By gaining an understanding of these layers and how the muscles function, you will be empowered to enhance your own muscle function when you begin the training detailed in Part Two of this book.

Superficial Perineal Layer—the Pelvic Floor Outer Layer

The first layer, shown in is known as the superficial perineal layer. Figure 2.10 shows each of the muscles that form part of this is the outermost layer of the pelvic floor which provides support beneath the urogenital hiatus, the space in which your urinary and vaginal passages exit.

This layer has a band that stretches from the pubic symphysis bone at the front, to the tailbone at the back, with an additional band of muscle that provides support from left to right, reaching from the sitting bone on each side and meeting in the middle at the perineum. The perineum is the space between the back of the vaginal opening and the front of the anal sphincter.

This layer also covers the clitoris and glans, which we viewed in Figure 2.2. There are four muscles in this layer which are highlighted in green in Figure 2.10.

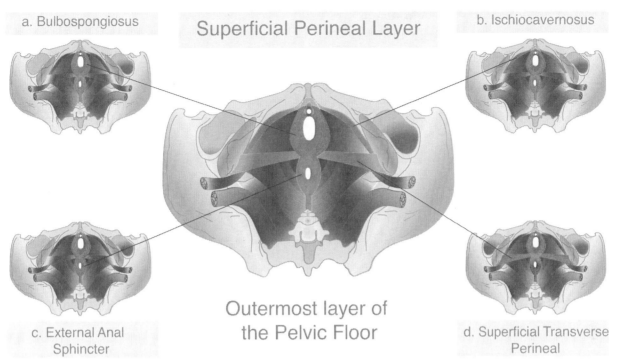

Figure 2.10: Pelvic floor superficial perineal layer muscles.

a. **Muscle: Bulbospongiosus** (also known as bulbocavernosus).

Role: Consists of two symmetrical parts that form the external perineal body, starting above the clitoris and ending at the perineal body. This muscle covers the bulbs of vestibule and is one of the key muscles involved in sexual function, contributing to the strong contractions during orgasm. It is also responsible for closing the vagina and although it is relaxed during urination, it activates at the end of urination to squeeze out the last few drops.

Hypotonicity implication: Hypotonicity can reduce the strength of orgasmic contraction.

Hypertonicity implication: Hypertonicity can cause general urogenital pain and referral pain in the perineum. Hypertonicity can also contribute to painful sex, pain with orgasm, or clitoral pain.

b. **Muscle: Ischiocavernosus.**

Role: You have two of these muscles running along the left and right sides of the front of the pelvis along the ischium bones. The ischiocavernosus covers the crus of the clitoris and maintains clitoral erection during arousal. It participates with the bulbospongiosus during orgasm.

Hypotonicity implications: Same as bulbospongiosus.

Hypertonicity implications: Same as bulbospongiosus.

c.   **Muscle: External anal sphincter.**

> **Role**: Responsible for keeping the anal canal closed. This muscle is typically in a tonic state of contraction and relaxes to allow emptying of the bowel.
>
> **Hypotonicity implication**: Hypotonicity can result in uncontrollable flatulence and anal incontinence.
>
> **Hypertonicity implication**: Hypertonicity in this muscle can cause referral pain in the anus/rectum and back part of the pelvic floor as well as burning and tingling sensations before, during, or after defecation. It can contribute to coccydynia (tailbone pain).

d.   **Muscle: Superficial transverse perineal.**

> **Role**: Stretching on both sides from the internal portion of the sitting bone, connecting to the perineal body, this muscle forms a central junction within the pelvic floor, between the vaginal opening and the anal sphincter. The integrity of the pelvic floor is very much dependent on the stability of this muscle.
>
> **Hypotonicity implication**: Hypotonicity results in less structural support, which can contribute to incontinence and POP.
>
> **Hypertonicity implication**: Hypertonicity can contribute to painful sex.

These muscles have a combination of slow and fast-twitch fibers that typically react well to Kegel exercises. Strengthening these muscles can help produce stronger orgasms. Prior to my repair surgery and subsequent rehabilitation, I was very happy with the strength of my orgasms. Training this external layer made a dramatic difference to the strength of contraction I was able to achieve. My orgasms prior to rehabilitation can be compared to giggling when tickled with a feather. Orgasms today are so powerful that they can be equated to being ferociously tickled and having a huge belly laugh!

Studies show that sexual function can improve dramatically with just a few weeks of consistent pelvic floor muscle training. You will be delighted with the difference you can achieve if you properly train this outermost layer of muscle, the superficial perineal layer.

Urogenital Diaphragm: The Pelvic Floor Middle Layer

The second layer is known by many names including the urogenital diaphragm, urogenital triangle, and triangular ligament. Figure 2.11 shows each of the muscles that form part of this is the middle layer of the pelvic floor. Its triangular formation stretches from the pubis symphysis at the front of the pelvis to an inner portion of the sitting bones (ischial tuberosity's) on the left and right sides. The main function of this layer is to support the pelvic organs and seal the urethra to prevent leakage of urine.

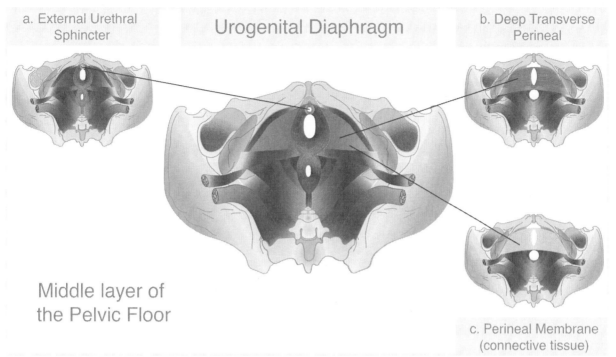

a. External Urethral Sphincter

Urogenital Diaphragm

b. Deep Transverse Perineal

Middle layer of the Pelvic Floor

c. Perineal Membrane (connective tissue)

Figure 2.11: Pelvic floor urogenital diaphragm.

This layer is constructed from two main muscles plus the perineal membrane. (Note: some medical texts mention the compressor urethrae, however, it is my understanding that this is not a separate muscle but a group of directional muscle fibers within the deep transverse perineal muscle). The muscles in this layer, shown from below, and highlighted in green in Figure 2.11 are:

a. **Muscle: External urethral sphincter.**

> **Role**: This is the muscle responsible for sealing the urethra closed to maintain continence. This muscle participates in the reflexes of urination, which we will explore in the next chapter.
>
> **Hypotonicity implication**: Hypotonicity can contribute to incontinence.
>
> **Hypertonicity implication**: If the sphincter is hypertonic, this can contribute to urinary retention.

b. **Muscle: Deep transverse perineal.**

> **Role**: This is partially covered by the superficial transverse perineal muscle, which we viewed in Figure 2.10. Similarly, it helps to provide stability within the pelvic floor, acting as central support for connected muscles. It also supports the expulsion of the last drops of urine at the end of urination. The deep transverse perineal includes the compressor urethrae, which is sometimes described as a separate muscle. The compressor urethrae is a group of fibers within this muscle, which help to support the external urethral sphincter with maintaining continence

by adding some compression to the urethra and pulling it back in the direction of the vagina.

Hypotonicity implication: Hypotonicity can contribute to incontinence and POP.

Hypertonicity implication: Hypertonicity can contribute to pelvic pain conditions including vaginismus.

c. **Muscle:** The perineal membrane isn't technically a muscle as it is constructed mainly from connective tissue that acts as a support for internal organs, creating a membrane that separates the most superficial and deep layers of the pelvic floor.

The muscles in this middle layer (the urogenital diaphragm) have some fast-twitch action but are typically in a tonic state of contraction, thus, utilizing the endurance capabilities of slow-twitch fibers.

Pelvic Diaphragm: The Pelvic Floor's Deepest Layer

The final layer of the pelvic floor is known as the pelvic diaphragm, which is the innermost layer, forming an elastic base (the actual floor) beneath the pelvic organs in the pelvic cavity. This isn't just a floor but technically also a few walls. The muscles that make up this layer can be seen in Figure 2.12.

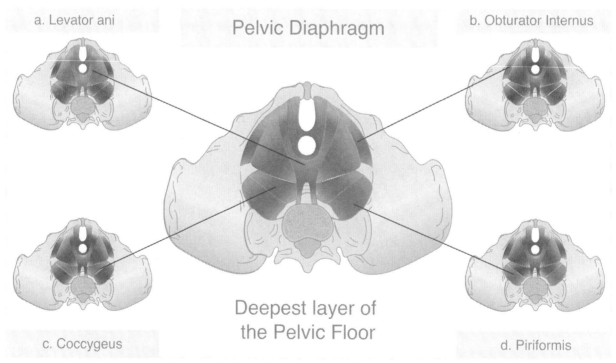

Figure 2.12: Pelvic floor deep layer—Pelvic diaphragm.

Being the deepest layer, the pelvic diaphragm is viewed from above, and highlighted in green in Figure

2.12. The levator ani is not an individual muscle but rather a group of muscles, which we will explore in more detail below, along with the other muscles that make up this layer.

a. **Muscle group:** Levator ani—This is a group of muscles, which you may have heard of, and is often referred to as the "hammock." Levator means "a muscle whose contraction causes the raising of a part of the body." These muscles can be considered the actual "floor" of the pelvis. They help with the stabilization of the organs that sit within the pelvis. The muscles that make up levator ani are shown in Figure 2.13.

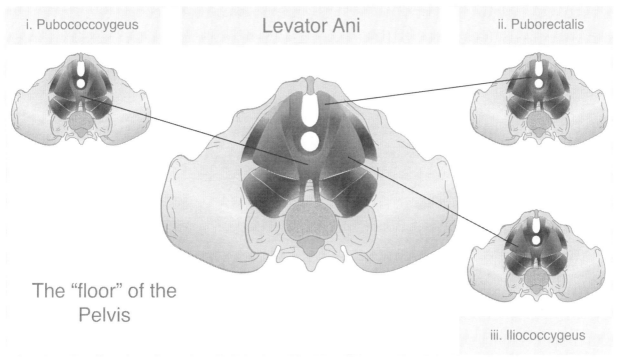

Figure 2.13: The levator ani group of muscles.

Figure 2.13 shows the three muscles that form the levator ani. They are:

i. **Muscle: Puboccoygeus.**

Role: The pubococcygeus is also known as the PC muscle and, like the bulbospongiosus, it plays an important role in orgasm. We will talk more about the PC muscle when we explore the origin of traditional pelvic floor exercises in the next section.

Hypotonicity implications: Hypotonicity in this muscle can contribute to incontinence (both urinary and fecal) and POP.

Hypertonicity implications: Hypertonicity can produce pain in the low belly, bladder, or perineum. This can also be accompanied by urgency/frequency or painful sex.

ii.   **Muscle: Puborectalis.**

Role: The puborectalis supports the external anal sphincter in maintaining fecal continence by creating a kink in the rectum (which we will review in the next chapter).

Hypotonicity implications: Hypotonicity can contribute to flatulence and fecal incontinence.

Hypertonicity implications: Same as puboccoygeus.

iii.   **Muscle: Iliococcygeus muscles.**

Role: Provide support to the puborectalis and pubococcygeus to ensure overall stabilization of the pelvic floor, and it has been cited as the actual "levator" that elevates the pelvic floor.

Hypotonicity implications: Hypotonicity in this muscle can contribute to POP.

Hypertonicity implications: Hypertonicity can cause deep vaginal, perineal, or rectal pain as well as pain before, during, or after defecation. It can also contribute to pain during sex.

The remaining muscles in this deep pelvic floor layer can be viewed more as "wall" muscles rather than "floor" muscles due to their orientation (side and back facing) when you sit/stand.

b.   **Muscle: Obturator internus (and externis).**

Role: Like piriformis, the obturator internus exists on both left and right sides. The internal portion covers the obturator foramen on each side (the hole in the hip bones, which we viewed in Figure 2.7), with the external portion attaching to the greater trochanter on the top of the femur bone. Its primary function is external rotation, extension, and abduction of the hip; however, it plays an important role in hip stabilization and normal pelvic floor muscle function.

Hypotonicity implications: Hypotonicity can destabilize the pelvis and cause hypermobility.

Hypertonicity implications: Hypertonicity can cause pain in the anus, coccyx, vulva, or vagina. Can also lead to referral pain on the back of the thighs (sometimes confused with hamstring issues). Can also contribute to generalized pelvic pain often with burning or aching.

c.   **Muscle: Coccygeus (also known as ischiococcygeus).**

Role: This muscle exists on both the right and left sides of the coccyx. Attaching to both the coccyx, the sacrum, and the ischial spine (above the sitting bones on the pelvis). In animals, this muscle is used to wag the tail. Our lack of a tail allows this muscle to instead play a supporting role within the pelvic floor.

Hypotonicity implications: Hypotonicity can have a destabilizing effect, contributing to POP.

Hypertonicity implications: Hypertonicity can produce pain toward the sacrum or buttocks. It can also produce pain on sitting or during defecation. It can also produce feelings of intestinal fullness and pressure around the anus/rectum.

d. **Muscle: Piriformis.**

Role: The piriformis exists on both the left and right sides and forms part of the back wall of the pelvic floor. It is primarily a deep hip external rotator (among other functions) and also provides some stability within the pelvis. The piriformis is constantly minimally contracted and attaches to the greater trochanter (the bony protrusion) on the top of the femur bone, thus participating with the obturator internus in strapping the pelvis to the legs. We will explore the role of the piriformis in relation to hip stability later in this chapter.

Hypotonicity implications: Hypotonicity of the piriformis can cause hypermobility around the hips, which can have a destabilizing impact on the pelvic floor.

Hypertonicity implications: Hypertonicity can cause pain in the sacrum or buttocks. Piriformis can also contribute to sciatic pain.

Even though the piriformis and obturator internus form part of the pelvic floor, they primarily assist in hip stability. Whereas the pelvic floor muscles provide a ring of support around the pelvic floor openings, piriformis, and obturator internus form a broader ring of support surrounding the pelvic floor muscles by strapping the pelvis to the legs as shown in Figure 2.14.

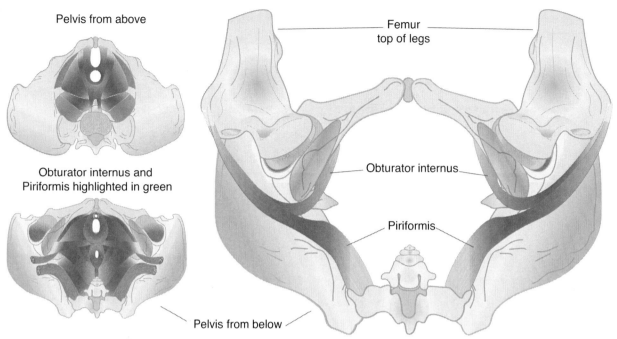

Figure 2.14: External ring of support for the pelvic floor.

The images on the left in Figure 2.14 show the piriformis and obturator internus from above and below, highlighted in green. The larger image to the right shows the pelvis from below with the femurs in place and the piriformis and obturator internus attaching to the outside of the femur (greater trochanter). If these muscles are dysfunctional or hypertonic, that can have a negative impact both on pelvic floor function and hip stability.

The Story Behind Kegel Exercises

Traditional pelvic floor exercises are known as Kegels. They are named after Dr. Arnold Kegel, the American gynecologist who identified the importance of exercising this part of the body. Dr. Kegel[10] observed that "six months after a well performed vaginal repair with construction of a tight, long vaginal canal, the tissues, especially the perineum, will again become thin and weak" and "everyone agrees that suitable exercises will improve the function and tone of weak stretched, atrophic muscles."

In particular, Dr. Kegel emphasized the importance of the pubococcygeus (PC). While working with cadavers (dead bodies), he discovered that this muscle was typically very atrophic (wasted away or hypotonic). Atrophic muscles are capable of limited function as we learned when we reviewed the length-tension relationship earlier in this chapter.

His studies led to the discovery that the PC (pubococcygeus) muscle was one of the most versatile in the body and he noted "After having been stretched over a wider range than any other skeletal muscle, the pubococcygeus can regain physiologic tension and, as we have demonstrated, it is able to recover its function after many years of disuse and partial atrophy."

Put simply, the PC muscle, if used, has the potential to recover and become stronger—it has the best length-tension potential in the body. Are you excited to hear this? I danced around the room when I first read it! This statement confirmed my belief that I could rebuild my pelvic floor strength. What Dr. Kegel uncovered in his studies is what I have subsequently experienced through my rehabilitation. If you put in the required effort to strengthen your pelvic floor and optimize muscle function, your life will improve in ways you could never have imagined.

Dr. Kegel devoted his life to exploring this delicate area. He conducted many studies and found that in many cases, women were unable to contract the PC muscle. In these cases, he recommended finding a muscle that the patient could contract, and then with consistent varied exercises over a period of time, the PC would be discovered and eventually strengthened.

The ultimate goal with pelvic floor strength training is to find and engage the PC muscle. Strengthening the PC has the added benefit of increasing the volume of tissue both in the PC and in the surrounding musculature. This is one reason why, in Part Two of this book, we will break the Kegel down into separate steps when beginning to enhance the mind-to-muscle connection. We will try to find the various muscles in the various layers and to see what is working and what is not. At some point, you *will* find and engage the PC.

Heightened awareness of the muscles in your pelvic floor and the ability to contract and relax them on demand should increase sensation in the area leading to an improved sex life. The level of muscle control you can attain can be quite dramatic. The ability to focus the center of contraction on specific muscles within your pelvic floor creates a subtler activation.

Think of it like the difference between being able to move your hand as a whole versus being able to move not just your hand but also each finger individually. A combination of gentle touch and focused awareness will be covered in the training program in Part Two of this book. Your empowerment is within your mind's grasp.

To Kegel or Not to Kegel, That is the Question

It is important that we address the long-running debate regarding the benefit of doing Kegels. If you have been googling to find out what you should do to help resolve your PFD, you will find conflicting and confusing information. The Kegel debate kicked off in 2010 when Katy Bowman, biomechanics expert and author of *Don't Just Sit There*, was interviewed for a fitness blog.

In the interview, Bowman stated, "Weak glutes + too many Kegels = PFD." Bowman became an overnight sensation with this controversial statement. Weak glutes definitely have an impact on PFD, and it should be clear from what you are learning about the connectedness of the body that pelvic floor exercises alone will not be sufficient to restore function.

Think about what we have learned about how muscles work. We know that the length-tension relationship should be optimized if we are to produce maximum strength. We also know that the symptoms of PFD are prevalent with both hypotonic and hypertonic muscles. If you can remember back to the exercise where you made a fist and then tried to contract that fist further, you were not able to. This would have the same impact as performing Kegels on an already contracted pelvic floor.

When performing the baseline tests in Part Two, we will assess both strength and flexibility. This will give an insight into your pelvic floor and how it is functioning. There are many studies[11] that conclude the symptoms of stress incontinence are improved by utilizing Kegels alone. It has also been scientifically proven that the only way to produce hypertrophy (increase in muscle fiber bulk and strength) is to perform maximum strength Kegels. Dr. Kegel himself suggested progressive resistance exercises would provide the most benefit.

Our goal with the pelvic floor, movement, and relaxation modules of the eight-phase program in Part Two of this book will be to rebalance the length-tension relationship in muscles throughout the body (including the glutes). This will involve strengthening hypotonic muscles, releasing hypertonic muscles, and getting all muscles doing their proper job. We will utilize many techniques both for relaxation, release, and strength building using progressive overload.

The Fundamentals of Building Strength

If you have been considering surgery as a treatment for PFD, the knowledge you've learned in this chapter should have clued you in to the fact that surgery is not likely to fix the issue with your pelvic floor muscle function. It seems that the key learnings from Dr. Kegel's research have been lost somewhere along the way.

Treating hypo- or hyper- tonic muscles with a scalpel or by implanting plastic mesh will not improve the length-tension relationship, nor will it restore biomechanical function, which is where all muscles throughout your body work in harmony. Surgery will, however, add scar tissue, which can contribute to conditions like POP due to the inflexibility of scar tissues, which interrupt normal load distribution. We will discuss this in the next chapter. In cases where surgery is absolutely required, you still need to work on muscle rehabilitation and scar tissue release following surgery.

In order to increase muscular strength, you need to work with the principles of strength training. These are:

- **Specificity**: You will get better at what you do (e.g., Kegels).
- **Reversibility**: If you stop doing what makes you strong, you will become weaker.
- **Overload**: You need to work to at least 60% of your capacity to gain strength.
- **Progression**: As your strength increases, you need to keep increasing your capacity if you want to continue seeing gains.

We will employ these principles in the eight-phase program using a graded exposure system where the level of difficulty increases as the phases progress. This approach will allow you to progress or regress depending on how your body is responding. You will learn more about this approach in Part Two.

The Pelvic Floor Muscles During Childbirth

Now that you have seen the pelvic floor muscles, you may be wondering what happens to them during childbirth. We know from Dr. Kegel's research that the PC muscle has the ability to stretch more than any other skeletal muscle before returning back to its normal resting length, and yet, during childbirth, this and other muscles in the pelvic floor can become injured resulting in dysfunction.

Labor is a long, slow process and it takes time for the muscles to expand to the required length to allow for a natural delivery. There is a natural reflexive action involved in the birthing process, which is known as the fetal ejection reflex[12]. With this reflex, a rise in adrenaline produces the contractions necessary to birth a child without the need to actively push, almost as though the body does the pushing for you.

This process happens as part of a symphony of hormonal changes, including a rise in oxytocin, which acts like a natural pain reliever while your body works to prepare your pelvic floor for birth. You could imagine that the fetal ejection reflex would have a similar feeling to defecation that happens through peristalsis (the wave-like contractions from the smooth muscle of the bowel that make your poops come out without you having to push).

Oxytocin is known as a "shy" hormone, requiring safe and familiar surroundings. According to Dr.

Michael Odent, a renowned French obstetrician and childbirth expert, simply being observed during birth can increase stress hormone levels (catecholamines), which can slow or stop labor. This is something to consider if you are planning a birth. Choose a facility where you feel comfortable, calm and safe.

In a true, natural birth, there are long pauses during the second stage of labor while the pelvic floor is gradually lengthening. It can even seem that contractions have stopped during this stage but that is not necessarily the case.

The biomechanical purpose of having three muscular layers in the pelvic floor comes into play during this second stage of labor. The layers of muscle (and connective tissue) slide along each other forming a funnel (similar to a telescope)[13] which is the passage through which the baby will travel. The deepest pelvic floor layer, the pelvic diaphragm (the actual floor), will lower and expand. As it does so, the urogenital diaphragm beneath it (the middle layer) also expands and lowers. Finally, the outermost pelvic floor layer (the superficial perineal layer) expands to allow the baby's head to crown.

Figure 2.15 shows the expansion of the most superficial perineal layer of pelvic floor muscles beneath the skin during the second stage of labor.

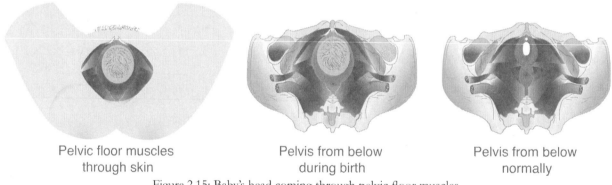

Pelvic floor muscles
through skin

Pelvis from below
during birth

Pelvis from below
normally

Figure 2.15: Baby's head coming through pelvic floor muscles.

The image on the left in Figure 2.15 shows the baby's head with the pelvic floor muscles exposed. The center image shows the pelvis from below with some of the superficial perineal layer of muscles highlighted. The image to the right shows these same muscles highlighted in their normal resting position.

We can assume that the extreme stretch and recovery of the PC muscle that Dr. Kegel discovered is designed by nature as it is one of the key muscles that needs to stretch during childbirth. Practicing prenatal yoga can help prepare your pelvic floor for this stage of delivery by encouraging both engagement/contraction and stretching/relaxation of the pelvic floor, helping to establish an optimal length-tension relationship.

Breathing techniques (pranayama) can also support this stage of labor. I believe that understanding how your pelvic floor is constructed, how it functions during a normal day, and how it expands during labor can make a real difference when it comes to giving birth, healing postpartum, and maintaining continence.

Of course, it is important to approach labor and birth with an open and flexible mind as births almost never go according to plan. Working with a good doula or midwife, and trusting their experience and judgment throughout the birthing process, should make for a more relaxed and positive birthing experience.

By now you should have a good understanding of basic muscle function and how that relates to your pelvic floor. In the next chapter, we will begin to explore relationships between the pelvic floor and other muscles as we reach out into the body to learn about the business of your body's movement.

Chapter Three:
The Business of Your Body's Movement

The business of your body's movement is somewhat complex. In this chapter, we will attempt to simplify this business using analogies that will help you to understand the management of pressure and tension. We will move further away from the pelvic floor as we do this, expanding on relationships between the pelvic floor and other muscle groups.

You will learn about breathing function and how it impacts the pelvic floor. This will help you to understand why we have included breathing modules in the eight-phase program. You will also learn about the function of your connective tissue and nervous system in relation to the business of your body's movement.

Even with the use of simplified analogies, there is a lot to digest in this chapter so, take your time going through it. Remember that you do not need to commit the information to memory as you can return to it for reference at any time.

The Pelvic Floor's Relationship to Other Muscles

Having touched briefly on muscle relationships in Chapter Two, I thought we should begin this chapter by exploring some key relationships between the pelvic floor and other muscles, starting with the breathing diaphragm.

There is an antagonistic relationship between the pelvic floor and the breathing diaphragm. When the breathing diaphragm is relaxing and doming upwards on exhalation, the pelvic floor is contracting and rising upwards. Likewise, when the breathing diaphragm contracts and flattens downwards on inhalation, the pelvic floor must relax and stretch due to increases in intra-abdominal pressure. This antagonistic relationship is not as straightforward as the biceps/triceps example but, if you can grasp this relationship, it is easier to understand the hydraulics of breathing.

To understand intra-abdominal pressure and the hydraulics of breathing, we must first explore the cavities of the body (torso) that are shown in Figure 3.1:

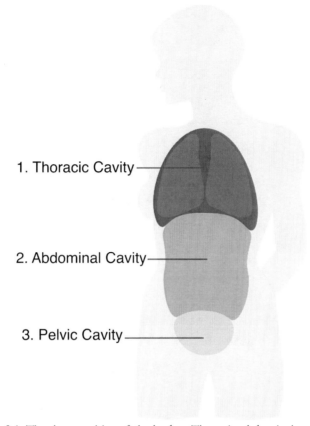

1. Thoracic Cavity

2. Abdominal Cavity

3. Pelvic Cavity

Figure 3.1: The three cavities of the body—Thoracic, abdominal, and pelvic.

Figure 3.1 labels these cavities as follows:

1. **The thoracic cavity**, which houses the heart and lungs.
2. **The abdominal cavity**, which houses the intestines, liver, stomach, and other organs.
3. **The pelvic cavity**, which houses the pelvic organs that we have already seen in Figure 2.8.

These cavities are airtight chambers surrounded by membranes (connective tissue). When we talk about intra-abdominal pressure, we are typically referring to the pressure in the "abdominopelvic cavity," which is a combination of the abdominal and pelvic cavities.

The diaphragm muscle sits between the thoracic cavity and abdominal cavity. It stretches across the base of the entire rib cage while the pelvic floor stretches across the base of the pelvic cavity. The abdominal muscles stretch across the front of the abdominal cavity and so they participate in the relationship between the pelvic floor and diaphragm.

You can see the abdominal muscles in Figure 3.2.

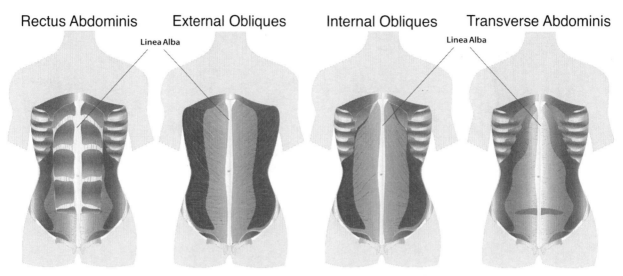

Figure 3.2: Muscles of the abdominals.

As you can see in Figure 3.2, the abdominal muscles exist on the left and right sides and are connected centrally by fascia (connective tissue). In order for muscles to generate force, they need to attach to something firm, such as bone. In the absence of a bone in the center of the abdominal cavity, the muscles are surrounded by a tougher connective tissue (similar to a tendon). This tendonous connective tissue (known as an aponeurosis) meets and overlaps, forming the linea alba, a tougher band of tissue down the center. Pregnancy can stretch this dense connective tissue resulting in abdominal separation known as diastasis recti (DR).

You may be surprised to realize that three of the abdominal muscles (internal/external obliques and transverse abdominis (TrA)) are on the sides of the abdominal cavity with only the rectus abdominis covering the central portion. Figure 3.3 shows how the TrA and obliques are layered at the side with the rectus abdominis in the center.

Figure 3.3 also highlights the difference in fascial layering above and below the arcuate line (which is highlighted with a green line). The external obliques fascia sits above the rectus abdominis above the arcuate line with the fascia from the internal obliques spitting and wrapping around the rectus abdominis.

The direction of muscle fibers in each of the abdominal muscles performs a specific movement of the trunk. The rectus abdominis flexes the trunk forward. The external oblique and internal obliques on opposite sides work together to bring the opposite shoulder to the opposite hip.

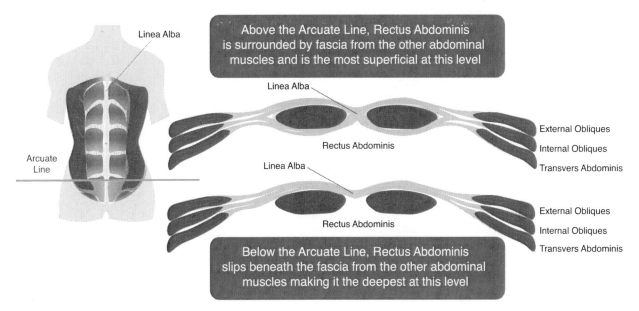

Linea Alba

Above the Arcuate Line, Rectus Abdominis is surrounded by fascia from the other abdominal muscles and is the most superficial at this level

Linea Alba

Rectus Abdominis

External Obliques

Internal Obliques

Transvers Abdominis

Arcuate Line

Linea Alba

Rectus Abdominis

External Obliques

Internal Obliques

Transvers Abdominis

Below the Arcuate Line, Rectus Abdominis slips beneath the fascia from the other abdominal muscles making it the deepest at this level

Figure 3.3: Cross-section of core, showing fascial connections above and below the arcuate line.

The internal obliques also perform lateral flexion, while the TrA compresses the abdominal cavity bringing the belly button closer to the spine. Core exercises, such as crunches, are performed in varying directions to stimulate these different abdominal fibers. Strengthening all core muscles can help to reduce DR. We will utilize a variety of exercises in the movement modules of the eight-phase training to strengthen the abdominal muscles.

As well as flexing the trunk, the core muscles form an external protection layer for the internal organs. If you place your hand on your belly while you breathe, you will feel it expand and contract. If you strongly contract your abdominal muscles when you take a deep inhalation, you will have less expansion of your abdominals and will, therefore, feel more downward pressure on your pelvic floor muscles.

The pelvic floor will need to expand more to make up for any lack of expansion in the abdominals. This action helps to highlight the relationship between the core, pelvic floor, and diaphragm. As you deepen your awareness and the subtlety of connection to your own body, you will begin to feel how these relationships are playing out in your specific case.

Understanding Intra-Abdominal Pressure

In order to understand intra-abdominal pressures, we first need to understand some basic physics. Pressure is a force that is pushing against something. If you have ever taken a flight, you may be familiar with the increased air pressure having an impact on your ears. This pressure pushes against your eardrums, which can "pop" while in flight. If you felt ear pain or discomfort before popping, you may have held your nose and closed your mouth while blowing hard. This counters the outside pressure on your eardrums by creating a higher inner pressure within the cavity of your ears, nose, and throat.

The issue with pressure is that it has to go somewhere, and your body is constantly adjusting to balance internal pressures within the boundaries of your organ's elasticity, in the same way that you can try to adjust your ear pressure in an airplane.

Imagine that your pelvic cavity is a vacuum-packed bag, sitting in your pelvic bowl with your elastic pelvic floor muscles at the base. The muscles should stretch to expand when you inhale, thus, distributing the downward force from the pressure increase. If the elastic base isn't flexible enough, the bag could spring a leak!

A University of Michigan study[14] found that a sudden hard cough can increase intra-abdominal pressure, resulting in stretching of healthy pelvic floor muscles by about 1 cm. This is an example of what happens with stress incontinence: the external pressure, coming from the breathing diaphragm and core muscles, adds to the internal pressure on your pelvic diaphragm. If urethral closure pressure (from the external urethral sphincter and pelvic floor) is less than the downward intra-abdominal pressure, this can result in urinary leakage.

Pressure will take the path of least resistance. If the pelvic floor is strong, for example, but there is weakness in the abdominal wall such as a diastasis recti or other herniation, the excess pressure can push out through that weak spot. This is also what causes symptomatic POP. You can read more about POP and its treatments in Part Three of this book.

If we can influence the balance of tension between the breathing diaphragm, the core, and the pelvic floor, we can learn to reduce those unwanted pressure leaks. The pelvic floor, breathing, movement, and relaxation modules of the eight-phase training in Part Two of this book, will teach you how to manage intra-abdominal pressure for this purpose.

The Hydraulics of Breathing

See Figure 3.4 to help you visualize the relationship between the pelvic diaphragm and the breathing diaphragm. The image on the left in Figure 3.4 shows the body at rest. The center image shows the chambers during inhalation, with the arrows showing the impact of increased pressure. As you can see, the diaphragm domes downwards as it contracts, causing the pelvic floor to relax and lengthen.

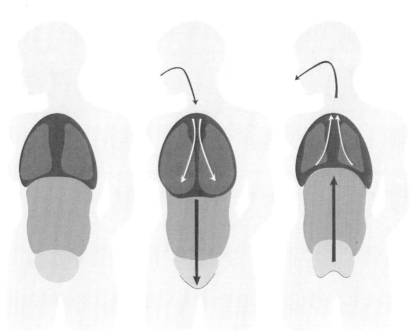

Figure 3.4: The hydraulics of breathing.

The image on the right in Figure 3.4 shows the chambers during exhalation, with the arrows showing the impact of decreased pressure. As you can see, the diaphragm domes upwards as it relaxes, while the pelvic floor contracts and raises[15]. This demonstrates the impact of breathing on the pelvic floor.

As the abdominopelvic chamber is airtight, inhalation causes the lungs to expand as the diaphragm muscle contracts downwards. This downward pressure pushes on the pelvic diaphragm causing it to stretch. Upon exhalation, pressure is reduced, and the pelvic diaphragm contracts and lifts upwards.

The following exercise will help you to feel the relationship between your pelvic floor and diaphragm.

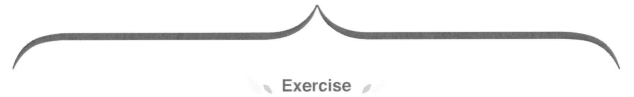

Exercise

breathing to feel the synergy between pelvic floor and diaphragm.

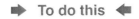

➡ To do this ⬅

1. Sit comfortably and close your eyes.
2. Bring your awareness to your pelvic floor and inhale.
3. Exhale, and sense the movement of your pelvic floor.

What you should find is that there is a slight downward pressure on inhalation and an uplifting motion on exhalation. This movement can be very subtle, particularly if there is stiffness in either the pelvic floor or the breathing diaphragm. Don't worry if you didn't feel any movement. We will utilize many breathing techniques in Part Two of this book to get everything moving again.

Functional Breathing

Before you practice the breathing techniques in the breathing modules of the eight-phase program, it is important to understand functional breathing. By understanding functional breathing, we are empowered to identify dysfunctional breathing patterns, which is important because they can impact your pelvic floor function.

I get so many questions about breathing. People ask about belly breathing, diaphragmatic breathing, nasal breathing, mouth breathing, and chest breathing. So many labels applied to the breath. In fact, there are only four different functional types of breathing and what differs with these breaths is the muscles used for the breathing motions. All breathing techniques will utilize these functional types of breathing in some shape or form. The four functional breaths are:

1. **Quiet inspiration**: Quiet inspiration is driven by the diaphragm contracting with a slight contribution from the small muscles between the ribs (external intercostals). When the diaphragm contracts, it domes downwards. The external intercostals, which stretch from the back of your ribcage all the way around to the sides, will shorten to contract, causing the ribcage to expand out to the sides, and the sternum (breastbone) to lift forward. This increases thoracic cavity volume, which, in turn, decreases the pressure within the lungs (governed by Boyle's law).

    The law of diffusion dictates that air will flow from areas of high pressure to low pressure so, the lower pressure created by the expanding rib cage will draw air into the lungs. This happens until the pressure within the lungs reaches equilibrium with the atmospheric pressure outside the body. This takes place outside of conscious control and is managed by your nervous system.

2. **Quiet expiration**: Quiet expiration uses no muscular control and is completely passive. Expiration is due to muscles recoiling to their resting length following contraction. The relaxation of muscles acts like a pump that expels the air. The decrease in thoracic cavity volume causes an increase in

pressure (Boyle's law at play again) within the lungs, which, in turn, creates low-pressure conditions that will trigger the next inhalation (due to the law of diffusion).

Quiet expiration depends on the recoil of muscles after inhalation, which highlights why it would be important to have an optimal length-tension relationship. If you have hypo- or hyper- tonic muscles at rest, breathing can become dysfunctional due to an inability to contract/recoil.

3. **Forced inspiration**: As well as utilizing the diaphragm and intercostals, forced inspiration will recruit accessory muscles to further increase thoracic cavity volume. Typically, that would include muscles around the upper chest, including the sternocleidomastoid (S.C.M.), the scalenes (a muscle group around the neck), and the pectorals (chest muscles). This helps to lift the rib cage from the top, thus allowing for a larger intake of air.

"Chest breathing" is a label sometimes applied to a dysfunctional breathing pattern, when the quiet inspiration utilizes these accessory muscles instead of the diaphragm and external intercostals. This would be common in people who have limited elasticity (ease of recoil) or limited compliance (the ability of the chest to expand).

4. **Forced expiration**: Unlike the passive exhalation that happens with quiet expiration, forced expiration will use muscles to depress the ribs, creating a more forceful pump to exhale the air. The abs (both internal/external obliques, rectus abdominis, and transversus abdominis) as well as the internal intercostals (which sit below the external intercostals), are typically recruited for forced expiration.

It is important to understand that forced expiration patterns are functional because believing that forced breathing patterns are dysfunctional could result in you trying to use quiet inhalation or exhalation when a forced pattern is needed.

Both quiet and forced breathing patterns happen automatically. For example, when you are sleeping, your body is using quiet inspiration/expiration to sustain your oxygen levels. If you go for a run, your body will automatically use forced inspiration/expiration to increase the volume of oxygen coming into your lungs to meet the increased oxygen demands.

You can work to improve elasticity and compliance using breathing exercises. This can lead to an increased lung capacity, which can improve breathing function. All breathing exercises utilize some form of forced breathing.

An example of a breathing exercise is the kapalabhati technique, which is sometimes called "belly breathing." With kapalabhati, the air is forcefully exhaled by strongly contracting the core, following which the core is relaxed which creates a strong inhalation. We will utilize the kapalabhati breathing technique in the breathing module in phase eight of the training.

Dysfunctional Breathing Patterns

Dysfunctional breathing patterns should be viewed from the perspective of the normal resting breath. If at rest, you need to perform a forced inhalation or exhalation to breathe, this is indicative of dysfunction, potentially from a lack of ribcage mobility or diaphragmatic stiffness (in the absence of asthma or some other lung pathology).

You may have heard that chest breathing or belly breathing are bad or dysfunctional. They are just labels that can refer to different breathing techniques. I would only consider breathing to be dysfunctional if, with the resting breath, forced inspiration is replacing quiet inspiration or forced expiration is replacing quiet expiration.

The following exercise will help you to see if your normal resting breath is utilizing quiet inspiration and expiration:

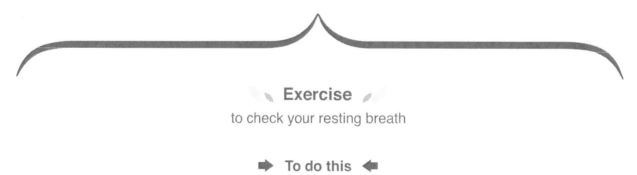

Exercise
to check your resting breath

➡ To do this ⬅

1. Sit squarely on a chair with your sitting bones beneath you.
2. Allow your shoulders to slump, depressing the ribcage, while allowing your head to hang (to take your upper chest muscles out of the equation), letting your belly relax (to take your abs out of the equation).
3. As you relax into the slumped position, just allow your breath to happen naturally without any conscious effort on your part.
4. Notice how you feel in this position.

The reason we are slouching forward for this exercise is to depress the ribcage taking the accessory muscles out of the equation and forcing the use of the diaphragm. If you felt like you couldn't get enough air in and had some feelings of panic, this is an indication that your normal resting breath may be utilizing forced inhalation and exhalation.

You can try the same exercise sitting up straight without slumping and notice if you still feel panicky. If you find your shoulders are lifting to help you breathe, this would be an indication of dysfunctional quiet inspiration using accessory muscles. Don't worry if you found your pattern is dysfunctional as we will utilize many breathing exercises in Part Two, which will get your ribcage and diaphragm moving again helping to restore functional breathing.

Stomach Vacuums and Hypopressive Exercises

Having explored the hydraulics of breathing and the mechanics of the functional breath, we can now delve a little deeper into one of the key breathing techniques used in the breathing modules of the eight-phase training—hypopressives. The stomach vacuum (hypopressive) is a side effect of the hydraulics of breathing. Practiced by yogis for millennia and by bodybuilders since the seventies, stomach vacuums have been used to enhance breathing, reduce waist size and improve aesthetics.

In the eighties, Marcel Caufriez, a Belgian doctor, realized the benefits of utilizing stomach vacuums to improve pelvic floor and core control. Spanish doctors Tamara Rial and Piti Pinsach worked along with Marcel Caufriez to create a fitness program known as hypopressive or low-pressure training, which can be utilized to complement Kegel exercises.

This style of training aims to achieve a stomach vacuum (apnea) in various positions. The word apnea actually means "cessation of breathing" but when we use the word in relation to hypopressives, we are referring to the breath-holding after exhalation, when the stomach vacuum is present.

With the breath held out, you make the motion of a forced inhalation, utilizing the diaphragm, intercostals, and accessory muscles to increase thoracic cavity volume without allowing air to flow into the lungs. This expansion of the ribcage forces the contents of the airtight intra-abdominal cavity to be drawn inwards and upwards, creating a stomach vacuum.

Some studies have shown a benefit to adding hypopressive training to traditional pelvic floor muscle training[16] while others[17] have shown it provides no additional improvement. I am very much of the opinion that we should treat the individual. The effectiveness of any treatment will be very much dependent on the root cause of your specific issue.

If you have restricted movement in your diaphragm or pelvic floor, this breathing technique can increase flexibility. It also has the added benefit of lifting the pelvic organs upwards, which can help to relieve the symptoms of POP while stimulating regeneration of connective tissues through this upward pulling motion (we will learn more about this regeneration in the next chapter).

When you begin your journey of empowerment and undertake these exercises, you will soon discover if this type of exercise is beneficial for you. You may actually enjoy the practice and choose to do these exercises just for fun.

As part of my own rehabilitation, I utilized a yogic breathing technique called *uddiyana kriya*. This is a form of hypopressive exercise, which I found to be beneficial. Subsequent to my rehabilitation, I participated in teacher training for hypopressives as I felt it was important to understand the system designed by Caufriez, Rial, and Pinsach. Rather than using that specific system, I have developed my own sequences based on my understanding of the rebalancing of tension throughout the body. These sequences are detailed in the breathing modules of Phases Five to Seven of the eight-phase training.

Dysfunctional breathing patterns can have a negative impact on pelvic floor function. Breath-holding, and failure to expand the diaphragm and belly when breathing can add unnecessary downward pressure, increasing the likelihood of dysfunction. This is why I believe yoga and hypopressives can have such a positive impact as both practices promote proper breathing techniques, which can improve the reflexive action that exists in the relationship between your core, pelvic diaphragm, and breathing diaphragm.

Many people struggle to achieve a stomach vacuum when they begin the training. The following exercise is a "trick" technique that will allow you to feel a slight stomach vacuum by creating a hypopressive apnea, even if you cannot create an apnea normally. This exercise is also helpful if you didn't feel the relationship between your pelvic floor and diaphragm in the earlier exercise, as you will most likely feel it here.

Exercise

"trick" to create a stomach vacuum (apnea)

➡ To do this ⬅

1. Exhale completely.

2. Close your mouth and hold your nose as shown in Figure 3.5.

3. Try to inhale.

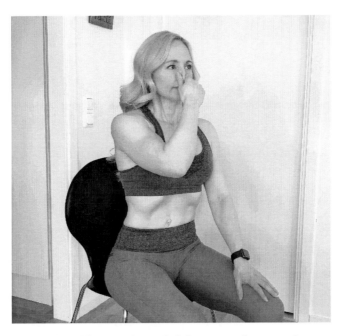

Figure 3.5: Breathing exercise to feel the apnea of a stomach vacuum.

When you hold your nose with your mouth closed and try to breathe into your empty lungs, as shown in Figure 3.5, the expansion of your lungs within the airtight intra-abdominal space should result in a slight stomach vacuum. The vacuum will draw your pelvic floor and core upwards as the diaphragm is drawn upwards into the empty space within the thoracic cavity. This is your apnea.

When you reach the breathing module in Phase Five of the eight-phase program, you can utilize this exercise to feel an apnea before you start. This can help you to feel the sensation of apnea before you begin your practice, which will enhance your potential for achieving a strong apnea.

The Relationship Between Muscle and Bone

By now, I hope you understand that the job of a muscle is to contract, and that the contraction of a muscle pulls on the bones to which it is connected, which creates movement, such as the movement of the ribcage for breathing. Taking this understanding a little further, I would like to explore the relationship between muscle and bone in a little more detail to help cement the knowledge you have gained so far within this book.

Bones are solid while muscles are like pieces of elastic, which attach to the bones through connective tissue structures (tendons). These elastics contract to move the bones, which, in turn, move the joints thus moving the body.

With breathing, the bones being moved are the ribs, which depress to pump the air out and expand to allow the air to rush in. If you look back to our example of the biceps in Figure 2.6, you will see that the biceps actually cross the elbow joint, connecting the upper arm to the forearm. When the biceps contracts (shortens), it pulls the forearm toward the upper arm moving the elbow joint. This demonstrates how muscles move bones. Throughout our bodies, we have many muscles that cross joints, which enable us to move our limbs and our bodies.

We have learned about one of the critical relationships that exists between muscles (antagonistic relationship), which was demonstrated in Figure 2.6 where we undertook an exercise that allowed us to feel the antagonistic relationship between the biceps and triceps.

You didn't need to consciously think about relaxing the triceps when contracting the biceps or vice versa because your nervous system does that for you in what is known as reciprocal inhibition[18]. The nervous system utilizes these relationships between muscles to enable smooth and fluid movement.

We have learned about the muscle's length-tension relationship giving us an understanding that hyper- or hypo- tonic muscles can have difficulty with contracting and relaxing and, therefore, can impact smooth movement, limiting the ROM that is achievable by a joint.

One such example of this limited ROM can sometimes be seen in the "muscle-bound" bodybuilder.

Bodybuilders gain substantial strength from lifting very heavy weights. They are truly "muscle-bound," which is obvious in the way their arms sit away from the sides of their bodies when they are relaxed. Their muscles are extremely strong and bulky, however, they can also become extremely inflexible. This inflexibility can result in dramatically restricted ROM.

If I were to put this restricted ROM into layman's terms, I would simply explain that sometimes extremely muscle-bound guys struggle to reach around to wipe their own bum, which is the butt of this bodybuilder meme shown in Figure 3.6.

It is known in pro-bodybuilding circles that the job of bottom wiping may need to be assigned to the loving girlfriend.

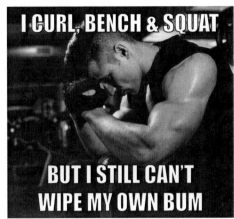

Figure 3.6: Bodybuilder can't wipe his bum meme.

The Impact of Hyper/Hypotonic Muscle on Bones

In order for muscles to operate efficiently, they need to maintain an optimal length-tension relationship. Muscles attach to bone and, therefore, if they are hypertonic while crossing a joint, they will pull the bone out of normal anatomical alignment, thus, limiting ROM.

These hypertonic muscles can change the position of the humerus, and prevent the shoulder from achieving its full ROM. The net result can be that the bodybuilder lacks sufficient ROM to reach behind to wipe his own bum. From this, we can start to understand how the length-tension relationship of a muscle can have an impact on the alignment of the connected bones.

Hypotonic muscles can also have a negative effect as lack of sufficient tension in a muscle can allow joints to be hypermobile, meaning they can move beyond their normal range, which increases injury risk.

We have already learned that the length-tension relationship is controlled by the central nervous system (CNS)—the body's electrical system, which turns muscle contraction *on* and *off*. If we were to put that hypertonic bodybuilder to sleep, we would be powering down this electrical system turning off all the *contract* switches. In that unconscious state, the likelihood is that the ROM for the bodybuilder to wipe his own bum could be achieved in that sedated state.

So why does he fail to achieve the necessary range in an awakened state? When he reaches around, his nervous system feels danger and contracts to protect the muscles and tendons from injury. If you are suffering from pelvic floor hypertonicity or a pelvic pain condition, your nervous system is also using the same protective response. However, this response can be unnecessarily protective. To understand why, we must first understand the role of the nervous system in the business of your body's movement.

The Management of Movement

I like to view movement as a way to communicate with your nervous system, just like your nervous system communicates with you by making you aware of sensations in the body. From birth to adulthood, we learn the movement patterns that allow us to crawl, stand, walk, run, etc. The brain, being the control center, sends the "intention to move" signals to the various parts of the body but the brain does not know the specific muscles. The learning of movement patterns is stored as reflexes at the spinal cord level.

Let's try a new analogy to understand the organization of movement. Imagine that your body is a company, and its business is movement. Your brain is the CEO. Your spinal cord is VP of operations. The tendons (connective tissue structures) are like the little offices. Each office has a department manager (Golgi tendon organ). Then you have your muscles, which are the employees in the business of your body's movement. Figure 3.7 is a visualization of this business.

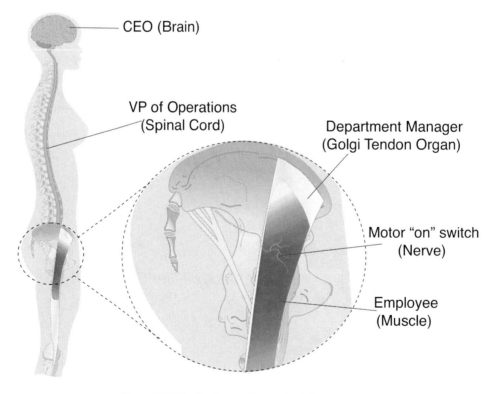

Figure 3.7: The business of your body's movement.

Figure 3.7 zooms in on a side view of the hip, highlighting a department manager (tendon organ), the muscle's motor *on* switch (nerve), and the employee (muscle). Whereas the overall business is run by the CEO, movement is more of a local operation. The CEO may set the direction for the company to move, but the actual movements are managed locally.

The body is an efficient organism. It consciously and subconsciously assesses the environment around you and learns based on what it experiences. New learnings will be saved as reflexive actions at the spinal cord level, and can be used again in the future. Deviations from normal movements (perturbations) are managed through these pre-programmed reactions and reflexes, helping to ensure the smooth and safe operation of the business. Your nervous system's primary function is to keep you safe, ensuring your survival, and that is what governs the reflexes at a local level.

Each muscle contraction adds tension as it pulls on its tendons. Department managers (tendon organs) are constantly monitoring the stretch of tendons and will react very quickly to stop a muscle contraction if there is any risk of tearing the tendon. They stop the muscle contraction by triggering reciprocal inhibition (making the antagonist muscle contract). Tendons heal more slowly than muscles so, department managers will always sacrifice a muscle to save a tendon.

Whereas the department managers (tendon organs) are monitoring the stretching of tendons, employees (muscles) are monitoring the stretching of muscle fibers. If an employee senses its fibers are stretching, it will contract to resist the stretch in an attempt to protect the stretching muscle tissue. This all happens very quickly as the signal does not have to travel far when it bounces through the reflex arc, which reaches from the muscle to the spinal cord and back

When you undertook the exercise of raising your hand in Chapter Two, you had·a chance to feel how the movement of your arm had a subtle impact on your lower extremities. This was due to the biomechanical distribution of tension that happens through this business of your body's movement. When one muscle contracts, it pulls on its tendons, which, in turn, pull on other muscles and tendons, all of which respond using the reflexes that are stored at the spinal cord level. This can be viewed as a bottom-up style of management, which is a thoughtless, fearless movement.

A good example of a pre-programmed reflexive action is the stumble reflex. When you trip and stumble, reflexes will manage the local distribution of tension through a sequence of contractions and muscular inhibitions. These happen within 50 to 60 milliseconds and prevent you from falling over (bottom-up control).

If you were depending on the CEO to send a conscious signal to prevent your fall, you would be waiting somewhere in the region of 120-180 milliseconds, which is enough time for you to topple. The latter would be considered top-down management of movements, which is less efficient.

The Pattern of Protective Responses

Patterns of movement, which are learned, are not always functional, such as the bodybuilder who can't wipe his bum. Dysfunctional patterns are common following infection or injury. Let's imagine you sprained your ankle when you stumbled; the injured muscle is an employee that can't come to work. Other employees will have to do extra work while that employee is out of action. You will likely develop a compensatory pattern of movement in the form of a limp while you are injured.

Oftentimes, pain will continue long after injured tissues have healed. The nervous system senses danger when injury is present. When the injury has healed, the pattern of movement that existed originally doesn't automatically return. The limp will remain in place unless you consciously and actively rehabilitate. In the case of your ankle sprain, this would mean that you would have to walk on that foot again without fear of further hurt. This can mean moving a little into the nervous system's pain signals.

The initial process of forcing yourself to walk on that foot is top-down management of movement, which happens in the early stages of rehab and helps to reinstate functional reflexes. Stiffness in tissues will decrease as you increase mobility by walking and doing exercises to restore function. This helps to rebalance the load of tension through your ankle, allowing employees to come back to work. This eventually reinstates the bottom-up management of movement and can help to alleviate persistent pain signals.

Rehabilitation involves re-teaching the department managers and employees to use functional reflexes. This process uses movement and relaxation exercises to communicate safety to the nervous system. This is a crucial understanding if you have been dealing with pelvic hypertonicity or pain.

In Part Two of this book, you will perform exercises based on this knowledge. These will help you communicate with your nervous system to overcome persistent pain while restoring functional movement patterns. This should contribute to a reduction of the symptoms of PFD while improving your quality of life.

Understanding Hip Mobility

Identifying the patterns within your own body will have a huge impact on your potential for rehabilitation.

This is particularly true in relation to hip mobility. There are many muscles involved in hip stability and mobility, and these can have a direct impact on pelvic floor function due to their impact on the hips. Before exploring these muscles and their functions, take a look at Figure 3.8, which shows the six movements that the hip makes.

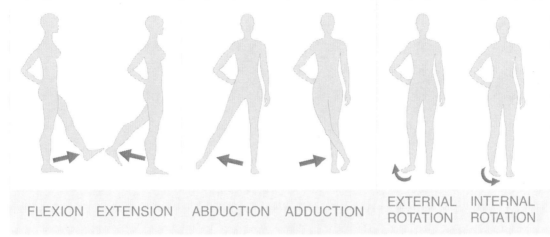

FLEXION   EXTENSION   ABDUCTION   ADDUCTION   EXTERNAL ROTATION   INTERNAL ROTATION

Figure 3.8: The movements of the hip.

Each image in Figure 3.8 shows a blue arrow indicating the path in which the leg moves with the associated hip movement. In the case of rotation, the leg remains in place but you see the rotation form of the foot, with external rotation pointing the toes out to the side, and internal rotation pointing the toes in toward the body.

We will perform exercises utilizing these hip movements in the training in Part Two of this book. You don't need to remember these movements and can refer back to this section in the future if needed.

The Muscles Supporting the Hips

The muscles that are connected to or crossing the pelvic girdle are shown from multiple viewpoints (Left, front, right, and back) in Figure 3.9, which starts with a right view, front view, left view, and then back view. The purpose of the image is to show the muscles from at least one angle in order that we can visualize where these muscles exist in space. Throughout the following pages, we will explore the function of a few key muscles that support the hips as they have a profound impact on pelvic floor function. We will strengthen and stretch these muscles in the Movement and Relaxation modules of the eight-phase training.

Note: The hamstrings on the back of the legs and the quads at the front of the legs have been omitted from this image, however, they do also play an important role in hip stability and pelvic floor function.

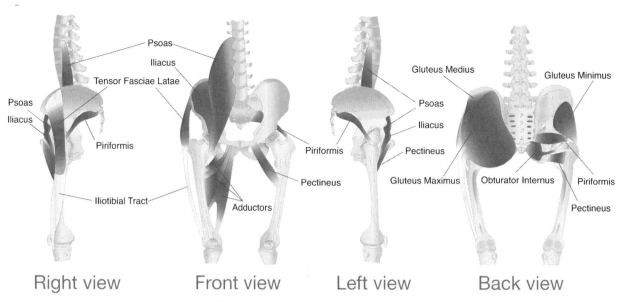

| Right view | Front view | Left view | Back view |

Figure 3.9: Muscles supporting the hip.

The Role of the Psoas

Let us first examine the role of the psoas as it has fascial connections to both the diaphragm and the pelvic floor. It is a poly-articular muscle, meaning it crosses more than one joint (multiple vertebrae, the sacrum, and the hips). The upper fibers of the psoas are connected with the breathing diaphragm through connective tissue structures and, thus, can potentially have some accessory role in breathing. The lower fibers participate with hip flexion and are connected at the base to the pelvic floor through connective tissue. If hypo- or hyper- tonic, the psoas can tilt the pelvis out of neutral alignment, which can impact pelvic floor function.

The psoas attaches to the spine, connecting to all vertebrae from T12 to L5. From there, it stretches across the front of the pelvic girdle, attaching to the top of the femur on the inside of the leg (the lesser trochanter). It also plays an important role in the stabilization of the spine. The psoas is a very deep muscle, which is primarily believed to be a hip flexor. However, its role in hip flexion is debated[19].

With flexion, you decrease the angle of a joint. Think about your body when you are lying down. Your skeleton is in a straight line so, your hip joint is at its anatomical zero. In order to sit up, you must decrease the angle between your leg and your body. This involves bringing the torso up so your skeleton is now bent at the hip with a 90° angle—your hip is flexed. Walking also involves hip flexion. When you take a step forward, the leg in front is connected to a flexed hip joint, and the leg behind is connected to an extended hip joint.

The psoas is a hip flexor; it contracts in order to help with hip flexion and stretches to allow you to extend at the hip. This muscle is pivotal to stabilization of the hip, which is directly related to the alignment of the body. Imagine what would happen if the psoas becomes hypertonic; it would restrict the ROM of the pelvis potentially tilting it out of neutral alignment. This can impair your ability to walk properly. Hypotonicity could contribute to hypermobility and instability, increasing the potential for injury.

When thinking about walking, you should consider that control of your legs starts all the way up at the top of the psoas (the twelfth thoracic vertebrae), which is just a little higher than your waist. When we begin to explore alignment and identification of your life pattern, you will see how your day-to-day habits and movement patterns can contribute to problems with this and many other muscles.

The Role of the Piriformis

You may recall that we have already discussed the piriformis as it forms part of the deepest layer of the pelvic floor (the pelvic diaphragm). In Figure 2.14, we viewed it from above and below, and could see how it helped to strap the pelvis to the legs (attaching to the greater trochanter on the outside of the leg). In Figure 3.9, you can see the piriformis from all four angles, which should give you an even better visualization of where this muscle exists in space.

The main function of the piriformis is external hip rotation. When you sit on the floor cross-legged, your hip joints are externally rotated. Rotation is not relevant to all joints in the body, but as the hip is a ball and socket joint, it can rotate around at multiple angles. Other functions for this muscle include abduction and extension (see Figure 3.8).

Abduction is movement away from the midline of the body (for example, when you spread your legs), while adduction is movement across the midline (for example, when you sit in a chair and cross your legs). Coach Eugene Tao taught me an easy way to remember the difference between abduction and adduction: "bad girls" (spreading the legs) = abduction, and "good girls" (closing the legs) = adduction (maybe that's a little too close to the taboo for comfort!).

The piriformis muscle runs quite close to the sciatic nerve so, it is sometimes attributed to sciatic nerve pain. Hypertonicity (known as piriformis syndrome) can contribute to pelvic pain. Hypo- and hypertonicity are believed to contribute to incontinence.

The Role of Obturator Internus

There are many other smaller muscles highlighted in the back view in Figure 3.9, which are mostly responsible for external hip rotation. One of these muscles is the obturator internus, which we have already viewed as part of the deepest layer of the pelvic floor (the pelvic diaphragm). The obturator internus (along with piriformis), straps the pelvic floor to the legs as was seen in Figure 2.14. In the back view in Figure 3.9, you can see that the obturator internus stretches from the front side of the pelvis to the femur (greater trochanter). You can imagine that if it is hyper- or hypo- tonic, it will contribute to hip instability, thus, increasing the likelihood of developing PFD.

Obturator Internus and Piriformis Combined—the External Ring of Support

The external ring of support provided by the obturator internus and piriformis can contribute to PFD if there is hypo- or hyper- tonicity. Hypotonicity can present in the form of protective tone, which can result in reduced ROM of the hips, directly impacting pelvic floor mobility. Hypotonicity can present as hypermobility around the hips and can have a destabilizing effect on the pelvic floor.

The Role of the Gluteus Muscles

The back view in Figure 3.9 shows the gluteus maximus and medius. These muscles play a pivotal role in walking and hip stabilization. Weak glutes can destabilize the pelvis, which will, in turn, have a knock-on effect on pelvic floor function (remember Katy Bowman's weak glutes + too many Kegels = PFD). The gluteus maximus has an antagonistic relationship with the psoas, so if one of these two muscles has hypo- or hyper- tonicity, the other will also have issues.

When I began my rehabilitation, I had a flat bum (unless I was wearing my heels) due to hypotonicity of the glutes. Much of my rehabilitation was focused on rebalancing the tension through my body while strengthening my glutes. I undertook exercises to retrain efficient movement patterns thus teaching my nervous system that it is safe to use these muscles through a good ROM. After all, exercises and movements can be considered effective methods to communicate with your nervous system.

The Role of the Adductors

The adductor muscles are part of a functional group of muscles on the inside of your leg. They are in a fascial pocket that directly connects to the pelvic floor and obturator internus. You can feel the adductor longus like a taut band on the inside of your leg, connecting to your pubic bone. Hypertonicity and tightness in the adductor group can pull on the pelvic floor so, it is important to maintain a good length-tension relationship.

The adductors are also protective in nature and can snap the legs closed in those suffering from vaginismus or dyspareunia. Learning to relax these muscles can help to reduce pelvic floor tension.

The Movement and Relaxation modules of the eight-phase training program work in synergy to help restore function throughout the body. For now, try to understand and visualize the muscles and how they interact. There are many more muscles that participate in hip stability, and we will work on getting them all doing their proper jobs in Part Two of this book.

Connectivity is Key

To get all your muscles doing their jobs, you need to understand how they are held together, and that is where your connective tissue system comes in. I believe it is one of the most important systems of the body, and, in this section, I will try to explain why it plays such a crucial role in the business of your body's movement.

The connective tissue network (your fascia) was recently identified as a "new" organ in the body named the interstitium[20]. It's not really new as it has always been there, but this recent study has revealed that the role of connective tissue is far more critical than previously believed. My rehabilitation was heavily focused on load distribution through connective tissues and viewing the body as a unity.

You can view connective tissue as the glue that holds your body together. Every muscle, bone, and organ in your body is floating in a unitary net. It is the connective tissue network that connects every cell in your body. Your muscles, nerves, veins, and organs are enclosed in a big bag of connective tissue. This bag has pockets for every muscle, organ, bone, etc.

All these bags are connected; much like a multidimensional string of sausages. It is your connective tissue that holds your shape and mechanically distributes tension throughout the entire system of the body. It is the pull on this sausage string that creates the symphony of contractions and co-contractions in the business of your body's movement.

Your connective tissue system includes a large variety of substances in the space between your cells, including a gluey snot-like substance known as ground substance. This helps to provide slipperiness between muscles to ensure fluid movement.

I was very privileged to have the opportunity to study the Anatomy Trains programs with Tom Myers, one of the thought leaders in the world of fascia. With over forty years of experience, his passion for understanding human movement coupled with his open-minded approach, have led to some amazing discoveries. Tom's teachings dramatically changed the way I viewed human movement, and, for me, they provided a crucial piece in the puzzle of my understanding of anatomy.

Traditional anatomy describes the body in a bits-and-pieces way, which fails to identify that the body is a unitary system. If we are to truly identify the underlying patterns of our PFD, we must understand this missing piece. Tom's hypothesis is that there are seven major tracks of connective tissue stretching from the head to the toes, providing a system of tensegrity (tension with integrity) for stabilization.

Tensegrity structures can be seen in architecture, for example with suspension bridges. Tensegrity structures include some parts that are compressive and others that are in tension, with the tension parts having some elasticity allowing them to recoil. In the case of the body, your bones are the compressive forces with muscles and connective tissues providing the tension (elasticity).

An example of a tensegrity structure is shown in Figure 3.10, which is a tensegrity model of the hips.

In Figure 3.10, the wooden rods represent the compressive structures (bones) with the black elastic strings representing the parts in tension (muscles/ connective tissues). Moving any part of this structure impacts the position of all other parts, highlighting the unity of the structure.

Tom discovered seven different tracks of connective tissue, which run through the entire body, providing stability, strain, tension, fixation, and resilience as well as supporting postural compensations. The connective tissue is a complex web that provides connectivity between different muscles and serves to communicate the power of muscle contractions thus enabling an even distribution of load when the body moves.

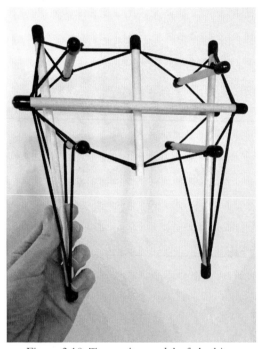

Figure 3.10: Tensegrity model of the hips.

You can view the connective tissue net as the mechanical system in which your body's electrical system (the nervous system) lives. The tendons (offices in which your department managers exist) that connect your muscles to your bones are part of this body of connective tissue.

This unitary system is formed just fifteen days after conception. Connective tissue has a different consistency to muscle tissue. Whereas muscle tissue has more elastic properties with fibers that run in the same direction, connective tissue has more plasticity and has fibers that form a double lattice.

The pattern of fibers in the connective tissue is dependent on your movement patterns. This is because movement causes cells and fluids within the connective tissue to become displaced. This displacement leaves behind a slimy trail that holds the memory of that movement. You could visualize that the connective tissue cells act like slugs moving through your body and creating these slimy collagen trails. Eventually, these trails contribute to the formation of the connective tissue fibers through which tension is distributed.

Sedentary lifestyles result in these fibers having a more tangled appearance, as the fluids that should be creating little tracks on which tension will travel are instead pooling and eventually creating adhesions, which will contribute to a dysfunctional distribution of load. Figure 3.11 attempts to highlight the difference in the organization of connective tissue fibers between a sedentary and active lifestyle.

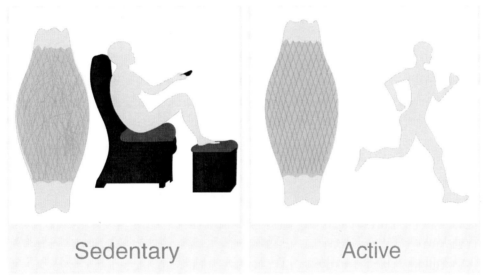

Figure 3.11: Connective tissue double lattice in sedentary vs active people.

You can see in the sedentary image of Figure 3.11, the fibers are disorganized, whereas the active fibers are in the double lattice pattern.

If you lead a sedentary life and suffer from PFD, you should consider becoming more active, even if you do not plan on working through the eight-phase program. Simply adding extra movement, such as a walk each day, can contribute to a more functional pattern of connective tissues.

If you are practicing yoga or Pilates, thinking you are only stretching your muscles, you should know that you cannot stretch your muscles without also stretching your connective tissue. Another important point is that stretching does not actually *lengthen* your muscles. It just provides a mechanism for you to communicate with your nervous system, which, in turn, can help with the release of protective tone, helping to restore optimal length-tension relationships and retraining the balance of tension throughout the body.

Stretching stimulates the movement of connective tissue cells and fluids, which can help with restoring functional patterns in connective tissue fibers.

Did you know that you can feel your connective tissue system six to ten times more than your muscular system? That heightened feeling can make it harder to relax when stretching. We will use yin yoga stretches in the relaxation modules of the eight-phase training program to help with reprogramming the pattern of tension in our connective tissues. It will be important to learn to relax as much as possible in the poses to optimize the effect of each stretch. You will learn to pay attention to what you feel, ensuring not to move from discomfort to pain as you practice.

The Ligaments of the Uterus

Of course, the connective tissue is not solely connected to muscles and bones. It also surrounds all your organs, including the pelvic organs. If you glance back at Figure 2.8, which shows the pelvic organs sitting in the pelvic bowl, you are looking at the typical bits-and-pieces type anatomy that is missing an important network of connective tissue structures—ligaments. These ligaments are a part of the multidimensional sausage string that provides support to the pelvic organs, and are collectively known as the ligaments of the uterus as shown in Figure 3.12.

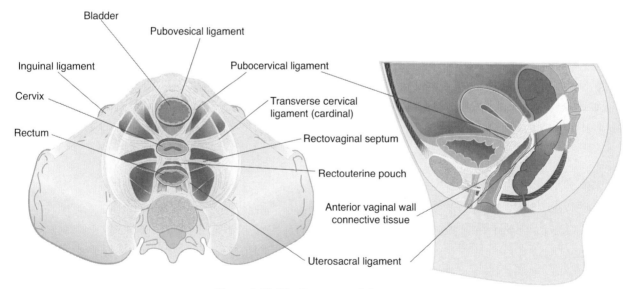

Figure 3.12: The ligaments of the uterus.

On the image on the left in Figure 3.12, you can see the ligaments of the uterus when viewing the pelvis from above. The image to the right shows the ligaments in the side profile with pelvic organs in place. These ligaments provide pivotal support around the pelvic organs. You can think of these ligaments like suspension cables that provide some stability while helping to distribute a load during movement.

You will notice that the cervix sits right in the center of this ligamentous structure. This is your center of gravity. A place deep in your body that provides stability and grounding. A hysterectomy, where the cervix is removed, can disturb the balance of tension through this pivotal point in the body. You can read more about the impact of hysterectomies in the POP treatment section of Chapter Eleven in Part Three of this book.

While Figure 3.12 shows the major ligaments of the uterus, you need to remember that they are just a small part of the unitary network of connective tissue. There are a lot more connective tissues in the pelvic area that are not shown, but this image should give you some idea of the importance of the ligaments of the uterus.

Pulling on the Sausage String

If you recall that your unitary connective tissue system is a multidimensional string of sausages, I want you to imagine what would happen if you pulled on one end of the sausage string. For example, if you raise your arm above your head. Due to its connectivity, it will impact all the sausages along the string in all directions. The degree of impact is greater the closer a body part is to the tissues being pulled. This helps to explain why you felt subtle movement in your legs in the exercise where you raised your arm above your head.

With everything being connected, when you pull from above, this will tug on the sausage string and lift things that are connected below. This is one of the reasons a hypopressive exercise results in a stomach vacuum (the diaphragm is pulling things upwards).

I believe hypopressives can help with prolapse because as well as enhancing the relationship between the pelvic floor and diaphragm, the upwards pulling can encourage your connective tissue *snails* to make supportive collagen tracks in an upward direction. I also like inversions such as headstands to help with prolapse as it also stimulates the movement of fluids.

However, connective tissues rehabilitate at a much slower rate than muscle tissues. Therefore, it really makes sense to focus primarily on muscular strength if you are suffering from prolapse while also practicing hypopressives and inversions consistently over a longer period to stimulate the connective tissue.

A weakened pelvic floor is believed to sit lower due to hypotonicity in the muscles, which makes sense, considering their resting length is longer (see Figure 2.4). The pelvic organs are connected to the pelvic floor through the connective tissue network, therefore, if it is sitting lower, it will pull the sausage string in a downward direction resulting in a change in the position of the organs. Over time, this pulling can contribute to a shift in the pelvic organs, potentially creating symptoms of POP.

I often hear POP referred to as organs "falling" or "slipping" out of their normal anatomical position. That was how my doctor described my prolapse to me (my bowel "falling" into my vagina). When you understand the form and function of the connective tissue, you will realize that the organs are being pulled by connective tissues or pushed by downward pressure rather than falling or slipping, especially in the earlier stages of POP. This goes a long way to explaining the dragging sensation that many women feel when they have POP.

Connective tissue adhesions and other scar tissues in the pelvic area can restrict mobility, which, in turn, can result in additional pulling. Scarring and adhesions can also contribute to the creation of a path of least resistance, as those tissues will not expand uniformly when under increased intra-abdominal pressure.

This is one reason myofascial release, visceral mobilization, and physical therapy can provide relief to the symptoms of POP. The therapist can release tension/adhesion/scarring in tissues, which had been contributing to the symptoms either through pulling or by reducing elasticity, resulting in exposure of a point of weakness. These therapeutic manipulations can encourage organs to return to their normal anatomical position.

Treating POP with surgery, particularly if the POP is mild or low grade, can be counterproductive as surgery introduces additional scar tissues without addressing the underlying imbalance in the distribution of tension. This could explain why the rate of POP recurrence, following initial repair surgery, can be as high as 59%[22].

A study[21] in August 2019 on the development of a biotensegrity-focused therapy for the treatment of POP found that the release of taut pelvic tissue improved pelvic organ positions while also reducing symptoms. This study highlights how important it is to understand the web of connectivity and to approach POP, as well as other PFDs, from a more therapeutic unitary approach.

I highly recommend you watch Anna Crowle on YouTube. She is one of the researchers responsible for this study. She explains this biotensegrity approach to the pelvic floor. What I hope to see in the coming years is a shift away from traditional bits-and-pieces thinking to a more unitary approach; not just with PFD but with all musculoskeletal conditions.

Maybe you are thinking after reading this chapter that there isn't much point in exercising your pelvic floor muscles and you should focus instead on getting everything stretched out. This would be inaccurate. Exercising muscle creates stress in the muscle, which stimulates growth and rehabilitation. Exercise also stimulates adaptation and rehabilitation in connective tissues (although connective tissues rehabilitate and adapt at a much slower pace than muscle tissue). We will discuss this in the next chapter.

When retraining your pelvic floor, rather than thinking that you are exercising specific muscles, I would like you to imagine that you are retraining movement patterns in your nervous system—working to get all body parts to do their proper job. When you approach your training in this way, you are tapping into more than just the pelvic floor by reaching out through the body to restore unitary function. This approach can make a dramatic difference, empowering you to return to activities that your PFD has prevented.

Hopefully, you now have a better understanding of the business of your body's movement, and a grasp of the interconnectedness of your bodily systems. This is fundamental knowledge if you are to retrain efficient and functional movement patterns to truly empower your flower. Part Two of this book is built upon these fundamental understandings.

With this knowledge at hand, we will move on to the next chapter where we will zoom out to see how your daily life can impact the business of your body's movement.

Chapter Four:
How Movement Patterns Create Your Shape

Having anatomically connected the dots, we must now zoom out to identify the link between patterns in the anatomical body and patterns in your day-to-day life. If we were to put our engineering caps back on, we could liken this to looking not just at the software program that we have created, but also, at how the user interacts with that program.

This chapter will help you to see how your daily movement patterns can impact the balance of tension in your body giving you much-needed information to ensure you can function more efficiently.

I focused very heavily on Human System Interfaces (HSI) when I worked as a software engineer. I had to consider the user's interactions and write the code for efficiency so the user could make as few clicks as possible to complete a given function. The "shortcut" is a great example of this.

Prior to the creation of desktop shortcuts, if a user wanted to open a software application (e.g.: Microsoft Word), they would click start, programs, Microsoft Office, and then Microsoft Word. That is four clicks to open the application. The creation of the shortcut allowed the user to double click. That was further improved by adding an icon to the toolbar, requiring a single click.

Of course, software and HSI have developed dramatically since I last worked in software engineering. The *one-click* shortcut is now the default. People would be quite frustrated if their smartphone required more than a single click to open an app. Humans like efficiency, as does nature, which has efficiency built-in.

In everything we do, we try to find the shortcut. We are looking for a quick fix that will remove our problems and challenges in an instant. With your body, there is no quick fix, but rather a consistent progression. As we begin to explore the links between body and life, I want you to see that each moment in your life, either contributes toward maintenance/repair or breakdown/destruction. Your choices dictate your direction.

Much of the information in this chapter is commonly known, however, it is not commonly connected. By identifying the links between your body and your daily life pattern, you are empowered to make the small changes needed to improve your pelvic health.

Understanding Muscle Build-up and Break-down

We previously zoomed in to see the building blocks of our skeletal muscles so, the next logical step is to understand muscle build-up and breakdown. This is particularly important if you need to build strength in your pelvic floor.

Let's imagine that our muscle fibers (myofibrils) are elastic threads. These threads are strands of muscle protein. All skeletal muscles are constantly synthesizing protein. This means that muscles are constantly either building up or breaking down.

To understand how this process of building up and breaking down relates to you, let's imagine you want to maintain the same bodily strength you have today. Maintenance of existing muscle strength and mass is known as muscle protein equilibrium. To achieve muscle protein equilibrium, you must continue to utilize your muscles in the usual way for you (stimulus), and you also need to provide your body with the relevant fuel (protein) to sustain that muscle mass.

If you wish to build stronger muscles and increase muscle mass, you must have a positive muscle protein balance. This involves increasing the stimulus (the strain you place on your muscles through movement and exercise) and increasing your intake of protein (through the food you eat).

Why protein? Because your body will digest protein into amino acids and use them to repair and strengthen muscles. To strengthen your muscles, you must have excess amino acids remaining, following muscle maintenance and repair. This is why bodybuilders consume lots of chicken and protein shakes. Increasing exercise without consuming sufficient protein could result in a negative muscle protein balance, which will result in protein synthesis breaking down your muscle instead of building it up.

Of course, I am once again oversimplifying a complex bodily mechanism, but I believe that this explanation is sufficient to provide the knowledge needed for you to improve the strength and mass of your muscles.

The Impact of Aging on Muscles

Another factor that impacts protein synthesis is aging. Aging is a natural organic breakdown (not due to disease) in which function decreases and fragility and vulnerability increase. Aging is inevitable for each and every one of us. Lifestyle and nutrition can play a huge role in slowing down age-related breakdown, and that is something we will strive to achieve as part of our empowerment.

A study[23] by the University of Texas found that protein synthesis diminishes with age. The study concluded that "ensuring adequate nutrition, including sources of high-quality protein, and promoting regular physical activity will remain among the frontline defenses against the onset of sarcopenia in older adults."

Sarcopenia is loss of muscle function and mass. The older you get, the more important it is to work to maintain your strength and muscle tone. This is demonstrated in Figure 4.1.

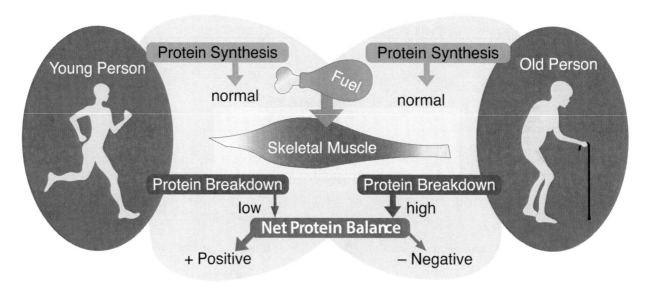

Figure 4.1: Impact of aging on protein synthesis.

On the left in Figure 4.1, the young person consumes a chicken leg as fuel and has a positive protein balance. On the right side, an elderly person consumes that same chicken leg but has a negative protein balance. This serves to show how the same fuel results in lower net protein balance in older people (where old is 65+). From this we can garner that the older you get, the harder it is to maintain protein equilibrium, and thus the more important it is that you work to continue to stimulate muscle growth while eating sufficient protein.

Understanding Muscle Atrophy

Sarcopenia or muscle atrophy is evident if you break your leg and have to wear a cast for a couple of months. When the cast is removed, your broken leg will be visibly smaller than your healthy leg. This is due to a negative muscle protein balance resulting in muscle breakdown. Even with continued healthy consumption of protein while in the cast, failure to stimulate the protein synthesis through exercise will result in muscle breakdown in the broken leg.

Exercise places tension and strain on muscles, which creates tiny traumas to the small threads of elastic muscle fiber (sarcomeres). Your body works to repair those threads and can even thicken these threads to ensure you have the strength to meet the demands you have placed on that muscle.

If you are wondering why the body would break down the muscle in the broken leg even though you are eating sufficient protein, the simple answer is supply and demand. If you do not demand the use of a muscle, your body will assume it is not needed and will take the valuable building blocks from that muscle to sustain other more useful muscles. It really is "use it or lose it" when it comes to your body.

The body strives to be efficient and will make sure to spend your protein resources where you need them most. From your body's perspective, that could mean building additional muscle across the back of your neck to support the weight of your head as you spend your days looking down at your phone. I'm sure from your perspective, you would rather your body spend your protein resources rebuilding your pelvic floor. In Part Two, you will learn how to communicate this message to your nervous system so it spends its protein resources wisely.

It takes time to build stronger muscles. You should also bear in mind that connective tissue regenerates at a much slower pace than muscle tissue. This means you will need to give yourself a lot of time if you want to make a sustainable change in your pelvic health. Your nervous system also needs to adapt and learn the new patterns of function. Consistency over a longer time will produce the best results, which is why the program in Part Two is an eight-phase program rather than an eight-week program.

Muscle Trauma from Childbirth

Not all muscle trauma comes from exercise. This is particularly true when it comes to the female pelvic floor. Childbirth can be very traumatic to the pelvic floor, with the potential for extreme stretching, tearing of muscles, and, in some cases, having the muscles cut with scissors (episiotomy).

With such extremes of trauma, a rehabilitation program is absolutely required to ensure recovery of normal muscle function following childbirth. Unfortunately, there is little postnatal support for rehabilitation of the pelvic floor—this is something I am determined to change.

I had very little support following the delivery of my first baby. When I complained about the pain in my coccyx, I had several doctors come and poke the bone. They all took the opportunity to view the stitches on my perineum and none of them commented on the quality of the repair (which I now know was suboptimal). My shameful predicament could have contributed to this, but even with my subsequent births, there was no effort to help with pelvic floor rehabilitation.

I went home from the hospital with a sheet of paper that explained some simple abdominal exercises but no mention of the pelvic floor. Following the birth of my third child, I was offered the spoken statement "do your Kegels." In my experience, it is not normal to be referred to a pelvic floor physiotherapist or other professional to help with restoring the function of your pelvic floor, unless you live in France as there it is standard practice.

When I had the surgery to repair the rectocele and perineum, I was prescribed painkillers and laxatives when leaving the hospital. I was told I could resume normal activities within a few weeks. At the follow-up consultation two weeks later, my surgeon confirmed that everything was healing nicely. I asked if there was anything, in particular, I needed to do following the surgery to aid repair.

The only suggestion was to buy pelvic dilators to gently expand the size of the vaginal opening as it was quite small following the repair. I was assured that there was no need for muscle rehabilitation. If it had been surgery to repair a muscle in my shoulder, I would have been sent for months of physiotherapy.

Even though my surgeon believed no post-surgery rehab was needed, I know that not to be the case. Pelvic floor physical therapy would have helped to restore function while increasing muscle mass in the area. By the time I had my mesh-removal surgery, I had empowered myself with the knowledge I am sharing in this book; knowledge that I subsequently used to successfully restore my continence and pelvic floor function.

Muscle Repair

The process of muscle repair utilizes satellite cells that jump to action following injury. These satellite cells multiply and surround the area of injury. They fuse together, attaching to the muscle fibers, and making them stronger. They can even form new muscle fibers. The process of repair has the potential to increase both the number and thickness of fibers thus increasing muscle mass and strength. Again, I am oversimplifying a complex process, but my goal is to give you a simple overview so, you know why you will work hard to rebuild strength.

The type of muscle injury/trauma can vary greatly from the microscopic tears that are common with exercise to more substantial tears that can prevent you from using your muscle. If you can visualize your muscle fibers as elastic threads, imagine what would happen if these threads were tangled. It would be much harder for them to uniformly stretch and contract than if all threads were neatly aligned. The same is true for muscle. Major tears can result in lots of scar tissue and crossed fibers, which can impede proper contraction.

For a muscle to function properly, the threads (fibers) should have some semblance of alignment with the direction of force that will be placed on that muscle. It can be easier for fibers to realign when the tear is natural, versus the tear that is inflicted using a scalpel or scissors. With all major tears, regaining full muscle function is difficult but not impossible. A combination of stretching, contraction, and massage can assist with the breakdown of scar tissue, and encourage the fibers to realign restoring somewhat normal function.

The Importance of Varied Training

We learned in the previous chapter that there are different muscle fiber types (slow twitch and fast twitch) and different contraction types (eccentric, concentric, and isometric). It is important to have varied training to stimulate the various fiber types, utilizing the different types of contractions from varying angles to ensure that all muscle fibers are stimulated. The exercises we will use will pull on the various tracks of connective tissues as we work to build strength and flexibility in all the different planes of movement.

To increase muscle mass, it is also important to increase the load applied to these muscles in order to stimulate growth. For example, with pelvic floor exercises, this would include performing maximal strength contractions in various positions.

By adopting this approach, we will move toward the goal of healthy muscle volume and tone (good length-tension relationship). Variation is key, why? My favorite example, which I believe highlights the need for variation, relates to my own body.

As a yoga instructor and practitioner of the Ashtanga yoga method for many years, I have undertaken a six-day-a-week practice of a sequence that includes sixty *chaturangas*. A chaturanga is a type of push-up.

There are also sixty downward-facing dogs and many iterations of jumping back and jumping through (where you take your weight in your hands jumping the legs backward or forward through your arms).

All of these movements involve pushing, where the hands are pressed against the floor. This consistent steady practice has resulted in me believing I had great upper body strength. When I practice handstands, I am pushing my entire body weight. I am visibly strong. However, when my son came home with a pull-up bar, I was shocked that I could only perform a single pull-up.

Why is this? Yoga is all push and no pull. My upper body has been trained to work very well in one direction. When I change the direction of stress, the strength is not there. It is not just the muscular strength, but the load balancing ability of the connective tissue that plays a role.

To build the strength to pull myself up, I needed to stress the muscles and connective tissue in the pull direction (which works the muscles of the back). The introduction of weight training with an emphasis on pulling has already begun to create the necessary adaptations within my body to increase pull strength. Push and pull strength are demonstrated in Figures 4.2 and 4.3 respectively.

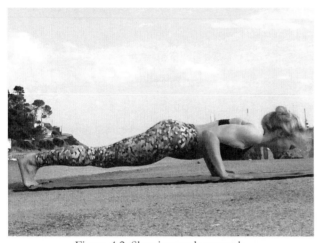
Figure 4.2: Showing push strength.

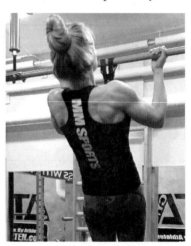
Figure 4.3: Showing pull strength.

In Figure 4.2, I am performing a chaturanga pose that trains push strength with a primary focus on the pecs. In Figure 4.3, I am performing a banded pull-up, which trains pull strength with a primary focus on back muscles. Although the primary focus with these movements isn't the same muscle group, both movements work a lot of the same muscles (e.g.: shoulder girdle, biceps, triceps, etc.). Balanced strength requires training with both movements.

How does this relate to the pelvic floor? Pelvic floor muscles must function with a great variation of stresses and pressures; from breathing to orgasm to childbirth. Stress is not just from movement (such as walking, running, and jumping) but also from lack of movement (e.g., extended sitting).

Stress incontinence highlights weakness under certain conditions. When I did that first pull-up on my son's new pull-up bar, I had an episode of stress incontinence (the equivalent of a "skeet pee"). This made me reassess my rehabilitation (I had been fully continent for a few months at that stage).

I added climbing to my weekly activities to stress my pelvic floor muscles in a new direction and was able to perform pull-ups without leakage.

If we stress the muscles from different angles under different loads, we can optimize the business of the body's movement. We can establish reflexive patterns that get all employees (muscles) to do their proper job, catering for a wide variety of functional movements. If all of your pelvic floor exercises are performed lying down, your pelvic floor will function well lying down but you may still have issues standing, twisting, reaching, jumping, etc.

In my opinion, the information covered so far in this chapter presents some critical information for those trying to rehabilitate the pelvic floor. This knowledge brings with it so much power when it comes to restoring strength and function. Soak up this knowledge and observe how you experience it firsthand through your own journey of empowerment.

The Pattern of Your Posture

Continuing in our theme of connecting the dots, we will now approach the muscles from yet another angle; by looking at the pattern of your posture. You may recall that each muscle can be viewed as an organ with muscle tissue, connective tissue, nerves, and blood vessels.

To achieve good blood flow and a nice clear nerve channel for the neurological signals to travel, the body must be in balance. A balanced healthy posture requires a good "neutral" position. When the body is neutral, the lines of tension are evenly balanced and minimal energy is needed. This is the wonderful efficiency of nature at play.

Unfortunately, the pattern created by everyday life isn't necessarily supportive of a healthy neutral position. Muscles do not act independently. They are just employees in the business of your body's movement. You can voluntarily control your muscles by, for example, deciding how you want to sit.

Let's say you want to cross your legs. Your brain (CEO) will send signals to the VP of operations to initiate the movement. The VP will send signals to the muscles (employees) that attach to the bones surrounding the joints on your legs (e.g., hip and knee joints). Muscles will contract to initiate the movement. Your connective tissue will mechanically distribute the load, which communicates to the department managers (tendon organs) who are monitoring tension as you make the movement.

Crossing your legs will alter your position in space, meanwhile, the distribution of mechanical tension through your connective tissue will stimulate additional reflexive contractions and co-contractions that will keep you balanced and smooth as you make the movement. These additional contractions occur simultaneously with your conscious intent to move. This is proprioceptive control.

It is this proprioceptive control that will introduce compensations if some of your muscles (employees) are not doing their proper job or are injured. These compensations can result in hypertonic muscle contractions (protective tone) that the department managers have initiated by inhibiting muscles that are placing excessive load on tendons. These compensations can become the default if the injury persists or if you fail to retrain a functional movement pattern following injury.

Over time, your connective tissue must adapt to support that pattern, even if it is dysfunctional. It mechanically balances load throughout your body and will create reinforcements (remember the collagen trails) to allow you to maintain your patterns. These reinforcements can accumulate over time, creating structural compensations to hold your shape. Figure 4.4 attempts to show this cycle of structural compensation.

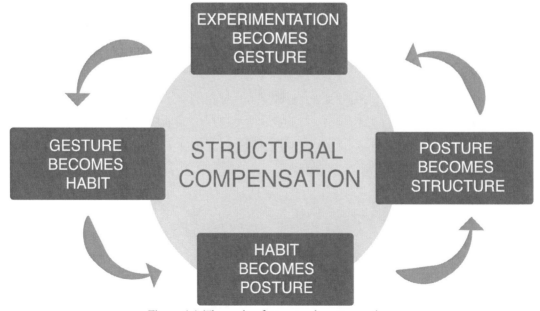

Figure 4.4: The cycle of structural compensation.

The cycle of structural compensation shown in Figure 4.4 leads to your movement patterns being held in place by your connective tissue. It starts with experimentation. You could visualize a baby first trying to perform a movement. Eventually, that movement becomes habitual due to the nervous system creating patterned reflexive responses to support it. The constant repetition of that habit will create the posture the child holds, and that posture will form their structure, which is held in place by their connective tissue, which will have adapted to support it.

In the case of the injured ankle, experimentation happens as your tissues are healing. You begin using the foot again. If you continue to limp instead of deliberately walking correctly, that limp can become a habit. Eventually, that habit becomes gesture, and your connective tissue will adapt to create supportive structures to support the limp.

Of course, it's not always an injury that creates a structural pattern. Sitting slumped for long periods or always crossing your legs can also create structural compensations. These movements are not a problem on their own. That is not what I am suggesting here. It is the constant repetition of these movements over a prolonged period that introduces dysfunctional compensations.

When you break down the pattern of your daily life from the perspective of posture, the goal is to identify the positions in which your body spends most of its time. Too much time spent in suboptimal positions that contribute to muscular compensations will stimulate your connective tissue system to create reinforcements, the accumulation of which will result in that form being held in place. Not only can this restrict ROM, but it can also leave you susceptible to injury and can prolong pain even after the injury has been resolved.

Text Neck—the Smartphone Posture

A good example of this type of structural compensation is looking down at your phone. Looking down at your phone in itself is not a problem but rather a normal part of human movement. However, if you spend the majority of your waking hours looking down like that, you could develop a condition known as forward head carriage or "text neck."

Tilting your head may seem trivial, however, if in the pattern of your daily life you spend many hours each day in that position you are communicating to your nervous system that this is your *normal* position. Adaptations will be made to help you stay in that position while expending minimal energy.

What began as experimentation (looking down at your phone), forms a habit that becomes your posture, which eventually produces structural reinforcements in your connective tissue system.

A recent study[24] by Dr. Ken Hansraj M.D. has shown that the increased degree of forward head carriage puts extreme pressures on the spine with a 60-degree angle resulting in 60 lbs (~27 kg). of pressure on the spine versus the 10 to 12 lbs (~5 kg). of pressure that exists when the spine is neutral. Figure 4.5 shows the varying degrees of pressure the further forward the head leans.

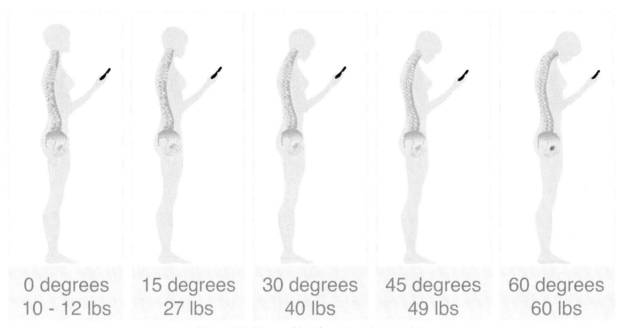

| 0 degrees | 15 degrees | 30 degrees | 45 degrees | 60 degrees |
| 10 - 12 lbs | 27 lbs | 40 lbs | 49 lbs | 60 lbs |

Figure 4.5: Forward head carriage (text neck).

Figure 4.5 shows how each additional 15-degrees of neck flexion increases the weight that is placed on the cervical spine in these positions. Persistent forward head carriage can result in a loss of the natural curvature of the neck. Unnecessary pressure due to "text neck" over time can alter the body's posture as it works hard to pull the head back into the neutral position.

While the bones of the neck are held in flexion, the postural muscles will be strongly engaged to support the weight. Remember that your muscles are in little bags of connective tissue that are part of the unitary net of fascia, so this additional tension around your neck will be translating into other parts of your body by pulling on the sausage string.

The business of your body's movement involves maintaining balance; therefore, the department managers (tendon organs) will sense the excess tension and will inhibit the excessively tense muscles. This, in turn, activates the contraction of antagonist muscles, effectively taking some employees out of work while others have to take the slack.

Some muscles will be locked in eccentric contraction (stretched and under strain), while other muscles will be concentrically contracted (contracted while under strain) and there may even be some other muscles that are completely inhibited and not participating at all, left to atrophy. In these scenarios, it becomes very difficult to maintain a balanced length-tension relationship throughout the body.

The Importance of Blood Flow

It is also important that we understand the impact excess tension can have on blood flow. If you recall that each muscle is an organ with blood vessels and nerves throughout. Think about what happens if a muscle is hypertonic.

Hypertonicity impedes the circulation of blood and other fluids, and can also impact nerve signals. As you can imagine, if your blood supply is restricted and neurological signaling is inhibited, you may experience many side effects including pain, numbness, tingling, or even muscle atrophy.

Sometimes, these tight muscles cause no symptoms. Other times, they may cause referral pain in another part of the body. Your muscles receive their fuel from your blood vessels. If your blood is not flowing efficiently, your muscles will starve and eventually atrophy (break down).

Physiotherapists often use manual therapy to release these constricted muscles and tissues. When your physiotherapist presses on a hypertonic muscle, they are using touch to communicate with your nervous system by changing the tension in the system. This sends a signal to release the contraction, which allows blood flow to return to the area, bringing with it the nutrients needed to rebuild and repair. By the time you get to the end of this book, you should see that empowerment comes when you find ways to communicate with your nervous system to help restore function.

It is important to note that *tight muscles* and pain sensations are just symptoms. Getting a massage or taking a pain killer is just treating the symptom. The root cause of the problem remains—in this case, forward head carriage from constantly looking down. When you discover an imbalance of tension in your body, you should always zoom out to find the root cause and then adjust the pattern of your daily life accordingly.

If you do not find and deal with the root cause of your issue, you will find yourself back in the physiotherapist's office again and again without a resolution. In the case of text neck, a simple change in the pattern of your daily life, like holding your phone at eye level or raising your computer's monitor to eye level, can prevent dysfunctional patterns from accumulating into structural compensations.

Working on changing your life pattern is critical to maintaining any improvements you have gained with the help of your physio through manual therapy, exercise, or stretching. This is particularly true when it comes to the pelvic floor.

The Net That Holds Your Shape

By now you should have a picture of how your body is using your connective tissues and muscles to keep your body aligned in order to maintain balance while expending minimal energy. The description of text neck should give you some clue as to the impact of your life pattern on your structure. You might even be worried that a lifetime of sitting slouched in your chair means you will be stuck in a hunched position for the rest of your days.

Thankfully, just as your physiotherapist can release muscular tension, your structural integrator can release structural compensations in your connective tissue.

When studying the Anatomy Trains programs by Tom Myers, a big focus is placed on understanding how connective tissue relates to structure. Tom Myers was a student of Dr. Ida Rolf who pioneered structural integration[25]. This is a system to correct postural alignment through myofascial manipulation—a technique known as "Rolfing." Rolfing involves a type of myofascial release that gently stretches the connective tissue, giving space for the muscles to move.

The Anatomy Trains programs detail the seven different tracks of connective tissue that run through the body, helping to distribute tension. These seven tracks reach from the top of your head to the soles of your feet. Each track crosses your hips distributing tensional loads throughout your body. We won't detail the tracks in this book; you can buy the *Anatomy Trains* book if you are interested in diving deeper.

The exercises detailed in Part Two of this book will utilize the Anatomy Trains tracks to retrain the specific lines of tension, allowing a more even and appropriate distribution of load during movement.

Fueling Your Connective Tissue

We have touched on fueling muscles with protein. We also need to fuel our connective tissue. If you move every muscle and joint in every direction every day of your life, you are more likely to maintain your agility and have healthy connective tissue. However, as with muscular health, movement alone is insufficient. Your connective tissue, like all bodily parts, cannot be built or maintained without fuel.

Bearing in mind that connective tissue creates lubrication for your muscles and joints, I would like you to do a small experiment (compliments of Dr. Shalini Bhat). Dissolve some sugar in water and then soak your hands in that solution. Let them dry and then try to rub them together. You will notice that they are sticky and don't move smoothly.

Now, wash your hands and dip them in some oil. Rub your hands together and you will notice that they slip and slide with ease. Dr. Bhat hypothesizes that fueling yourself with a diet that is high in sugars can cause your connective tissue to become sticky, preventing efficient slide and glide. On the other hand, she suggests that fueling yourself with a diet that is low in sugar while containing sufficient healthy fats should allow more efficient slide and glide.

Another point to note is that a major component of connective tissue is water. Dehydration can negatively affect your connective tissue (and your other bodily systems). This is another important dot to connect, particularly if you are limiting your fluid intake due to incontinence. Don't do that! Diet and hydration have an impact on your posture, which in turn has an impact on your pelvic floor so, eat well and stay hydrated.

Finding a Neutral Posture

We have learned that the human organism strives to find an equilibrium of balance while expending minimal energy, which requires a neutral posture. So, what is a *good* or *neutral* posture?

There are various definitions for posture types, and they are shown in Figure 4.6.

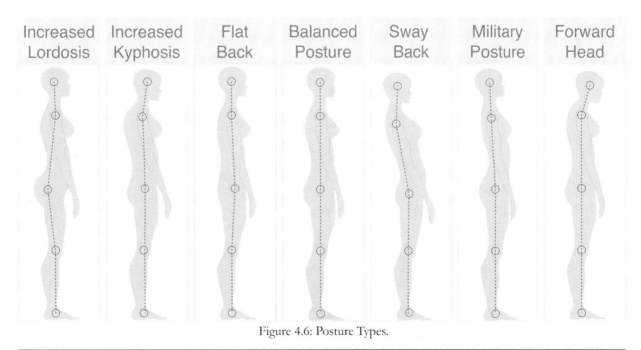

| Increased Lordosis | Increased Kyphosis | Flat Back | Balanced Posture | Sway Back | Military Posture | Forward Head |

Figure 4.6: Posture Types.

The posture types in Figure 4.6 show many different shapes and their associated postural names. Don't be tempted to pick yourself out of this line-up. I am showing these images only to highlight what you may have found when googling posture. The balanced posture image in the center is indeed a balanced posture. The remaining posture types emphasize misalignment of the spine only. However; a proper assessment of postural alignment should consider where all body parts are in relation to each other and in relation to the floor.

If you were to hang a plumb line (a string with a weight attached) from the center of your ear, the line should go through the center of your shoulder, hips, knees, and ankles as per the "Balanced posture" in Figure 4.6. You should consider this "balanced posture" as a guide rather than an absolute rule.

We are all shaped differently. Our muscles and bones are as uniquely shaped as our faces. This uniqueness has an impact on posture. The *perfect* posture for your bone structure is most likely aligned differently to the *perfect* posture for mine. The more important aspect with posture is symmetry as well as similar degrees in ROM and muscle-force production from left to right. We will never be completely balanced and symmetrical but it is good to at least try to move toward a balanced center.

Figure 4.7 highlights the front view of a "balanced posture" next to the side view and attempts to highlight that eyes, shoulders, hips, knees, and ankles should be level while the head should be centered between the shoulders, which should be centered over hips that are centered over knees and ankles.

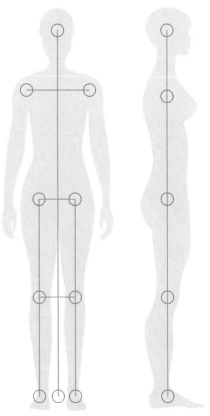

We will perform a simple self-assessment of alignment in Part Two of this book. This will give you some indication as to whether or not your posture is out of alignment. However, I highly recommend going to see a healthcare provider for a proper assessment. That could be a structural integrator, Rolfer, physical therapist, or chiropractor.

If misalignment is found, I would recommend a program of structural integration (involving twelve sessions of connective tissue release). If you do undertake such a program, you should make changes to the pattern of your daily life to allow you to adopt the new pattern in the longer term.

Figure 4.7: Neutral alignment.

Discovering Your Life Pattern

When we perform the self-assessments in Part Two of this book, you will attempt to identify the pattern of your life. To give some indication of how this is done, I will use the example of my life pattern when I started my career as a software engineer. This pattern is visualized in Figure 4.8.

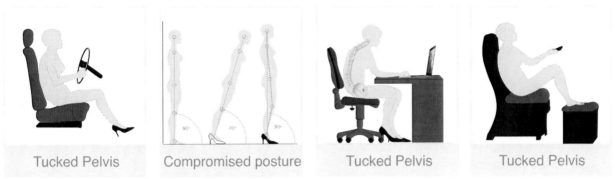

Tucked Pelvis   Compromised posture   Tucked Pelvis   Tucked Pelvis

Figure 4.8: My software engineering life pattern.

My Software Engineering Life Pattern

Each morning, I would wake up, climb out of bed, and get myself dressed. I would rush around getting the kids ready for school. This was typically quite a stressful endeavor as they liked to stay in bed. I would drag them from bed, forcing them to wash, brush their teeth, and eat their breakfast. We would load into the car and I would drive to drop them off at the relevant locations (crèche, school, etc.).

I would then drive to the office, parking as close to the door as possible. I didn't like walking far as I always wore high-heels (3 inches high) due to believing that I was too short... that and the fact that they gave me a bum (otherwise, it was flat). I brought my laptop to and from work every day so I would have the strap for my laptop bag over one shoulder. I would go straight to my desk on arrival to work and would spend most of my day sitting at my computer engrossed in whatever code I was writing.

My eyesight wasn't great so, very often, I would hunch forward toward my screen, allowing me to see more clearly. I often rested on my elbows while reading from the screen. I sat in a swivel chair but with a tucked pelvis rather than sitting on my sitting bones. I would eat lunch in the office canteen before returning to my desk for more work. My meals were not very colorful, and I was fond of chocolate during the afternoon break. I would struggle to finish work on time so, my mother would collect the kids from school and take them to sports, music, and other activities.

Eventually, I would leave the office—laptop over my shoulder. I would drive home, cook dinner for the kids, put them to bed, and then slouch on the sofa in front of the TV, exhausted. I would often go to bed a little too late, due to having arrived home late. I would struggle to rise with the alarm the following day. This pattern continued throughout the working week. Each of the images in Figure 4.8 shows how compromised my posture was, with a tucked pelvis being a major feature.

Analyzing the Pattern of Daily Life

When analyzing this pattern, we are looking for body positions that are held for long periods of time. I was spending almost 75% of my waking hours sitting with a tucked pelvis (posterior pelvic tilt). By tucking my pelvis and slouching for such long periods, I was creating a body position that would disturb the relationship between my breathing diaphragm and pelvic floor, impacting my breathing pattern. To demonstrate this, we will do a short exercise.

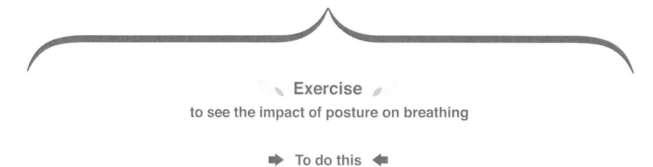

Exercise
to see the impact of posture on breathing

➡ **To do this** ⬅

1. Sit on a chair and tuck your pelvis under so you are sitting on your sacrum rather than your sitting bones.
2. Relax your body allowing your ribcage to depress.
3. Try to take a deep breath.

What do you notice? It's more difficult to breathe, right? Unlike the breathing exercise we performed in chapter three to check the resting breath, we are doing this with a tucked pelvis and little ability for the abdominal tissues to expand

With the tucked pelvis, we change the balance of intra-abdominal pressure due to the increased flexion of the spine. The tucked pelvis combined with the depressed rib cage makes it more difficult to perform quiet inspiration and expiration so, there is less movement of the diaphragm and ribcage. This results in having to use forced breaths. This isn't a *bad* position. You should be able to sit in all sorts of positions. It is the duration of time spent in this position, which creates compensations.

To inhale sufficient oxygen when sitting in this position, I was using forced inhalation and exhalation for most of my day. Not only was this creating additional tension around my neck and shoulders, but it was also reducing the function of my breathing diaphragm, which would have directly impacted the function of my pelvic floor.

Over the course of a typical day, you take around 20,000 breaths. I was taking almost half of my breaths in this position. That repetition would have been a constant communication to the nervous system creating a neurological mapping, which is a reflexive pattern that would serve to perpetuate dysfunction.

When I started to investigate the root cause of my PFD, and to explore my patterns of movement, I could see that with every breath in these sitting positions, I was repeating a dysfunctional pattern that was contributing to my issues. Maybe you are feeling a bit panicked now wondering if you are negatively impacting your pelvic floor with the way you sit. Let's do another exercise to ease your mind, where we will focus on finding an optimized posture for sitting.

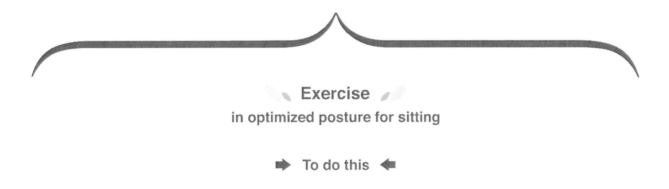

Exercise
in optimized posture for sitting

➡ To do this ⬅

1. Sit on a chair, making sure you are resting on your sitting bones.
2. Allow your body to rest against the back of the chair without pushing your back into the chair or trying to force yourself into a "military" upright position.
3. Relax your shoulders allowing your ribcage to depress slightly (almost as though you are allowing a slump in your upper back but without dropping your head and shoulders forward).
4. Allow your tongue to rest on the roof of your mouth with your teeth slightly apart (jaw resting) and your lips closed.
5. Allow inspiration and expiration to be quiet and through your nose without effort, while allowing your shoulders to remain relaxed.

If you have good breathing function, you should find it easy to breathe sitting in this position. If you struggled to breathe through your nose and maybe felt a bit panicked when breathing with your mouth closed, this could be indicative that you may be a mouth breather.

Your lungs are responsible for transporting oxygen to your blood. By ensuring you are breathing efficiently, you enhance this transport system. We need oxygen to burn the fuel that creates the energy (ATP) that moves our muscles. Optimizing our oxygen supply, therefore, will result in higher fuel availability for movement.

The breathing modules in the eight-phase program will train you to breathe through your nose, using your diaphragm to power your breathing. Functional breathing has the added benefit of calming your nervous system, which can help with stress management.

I hope you are beginning to see how everything is connected in this spectacular organism. At this point, you may already be seeing how the pattern of your own life is impacting your pelvic health.

Understanding the Impact of Pelvic Tilt

Another consideration is the impact of pelvic tilt on the organs and tissues within the pelvis. We looked at the ligaments of the uterus in Figure 3.12 and discussed how they were not only part of the multidimensional sausage string but also a key structure for distributing load within the pelvis.

Figure 4.9 attempts to show how the directional forces could be impacting the organs and tissues within the pelvis. Neutral pelvic alignment is considered to be when the anterior superior iliac spines (ASIS) and pubic symphysis are somewhat aligned, which is shown in the center image of Figure 4.9. In this neutral position, the bladder rests on the pubic symphysis. You can see how a posterior pelvic tilt (tilted backward giving a flat back) and anterior tilt (tilted forward giving a duck butt) can impact the positioning of the pelvic organs.

When holding the pelvis in either the posterior or anterior tilt, we are pulling on the tissues within the pelvis and changing the balance of tension through the ligaments of the uterus. We are also shifting the pelvic floor out of alignment with the breathing diaphragm, which changes the balance of intra-abdominal pressures which can exacerbate PFD.

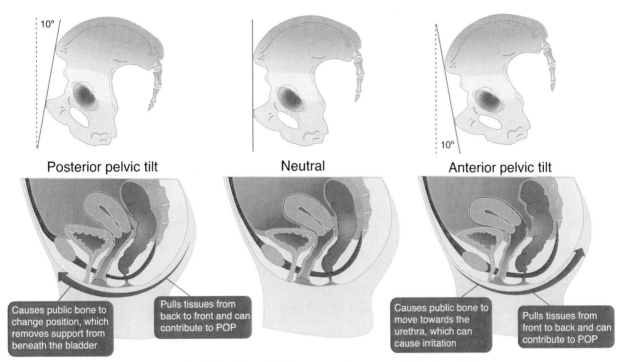

| Posterior pelvic tilt | Neutral | Anterior pelvic tilt |

Causes public bone to change position, which removes support from beneath the bladder

Pulls tissues from back to front and can contribute to POP

Causes public bone to move towards the urethra, which can cause irritation

Pulls tissues from front to back and can contribute to POP

Figure 4.9: Pelvic tilt and its impact on the organs within the pelvis.

Again, I have to emphasize that the pelvis should be able to move in these directions, so they are not "bad." However, if you hold non-neutral positions for the majority of your time, you are stimulating structural compensations within the pelvis and could be creating sufficient pull on the organs which, when combined with increased intra-abdominal pressures, can trigger the symptoms of POP.

A study[26] by Harbor University, California, found that "Women with advanced uterovaginal prolapse have less lumbar lordosis and a pelvic inlet that is oriented less vertically than women without prolapse." Lumbar lordosis refers to the curve in your low back. This curve is reduced or removed completely when you have a posterior pelvic tilt.

Another study[27] by the University of South Carolina found that "An abnormal change in spinal curvature, specifically, a loss of lumbar lordosis, appears to be a significant risk factor in the development of pelvic organ prolapse." This helps to highlight the impact of pelvic tilt on your pelvic health. You can find out more about POP and its treatments in Part Three of this book.

The ability to tilt the pelvis posteriorly and anteriorly is important and can be considered normal ROM, however, the pelvis should not always sit at the extremes and should instead spend the majority of its time in a neutral position. There are additional misalignments of the pelvis, which are possible, but I believe the information already provided should give a sufficient understanding, and I recommend seeing a structural integrator for a proper structural assessment if you are concerned about misalignment.

It is important to get a feeling for your own pelvic position. It is also good to understand what the different pelvic tilts feel like so, let's try an exercise in feeling your pelvic position from the front:

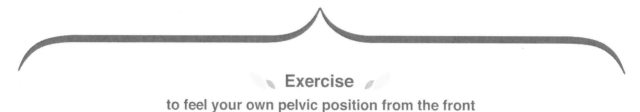

Exercise
to feel your own pelvic position from the front

➡ To do this ⬅

1. Stand up, find your ASIS projections and place your index fingers on them.
2. Tuck your pelvis under and notice that the space between your fingers gets slightly wider.
3. Now untuck your pelvis and tilt in the opposite direction. Notice that your fingers come a little closer together.

This separation and coming together of fingers can be quite subtle on the front so let's try an exercise to feel pelvic position from the back:

Exercise
to feel your own pelvic position from the back

➡ To do this ⬅

1. Reach your hands around and feel for your sitting bones. It may help if you bend forward slightly as this will help to expose them.
2. Put your fingers on your sitting bones.
3. Tuck your pelvis under and notice that the space between your fingers gets shorter.
4. Untuck your pelvis and tilt in the opposite direction (creating a duck butt). Notice that the space between your fingers gets wider.

These two exercises should help to highlight that there is a difference between these two extreme pelvic positions. You will most likely notice a greater difference when you have your fingers on your sitting bones. As you tuck your pelvis under to create a posterior pelvic tilt, your fingers come closer together. As you untuck into a *duck butt* by anteriorly tilting your pelvis, your fingers move away from each other. Now we will do another exercise to feel the pelvic floor when we are tilted.

Exercise
to feel the pelvic floor with a pelvic tilt

➡ To do this ⬅

1. Place your hand on your vulva (over clothes is fine), with the heel of your hand just below your pubic symphysis and your fingers reaching toward your anus.
2. Tuck your pelvis under into a posterior pelvic tilt. Can you feel how your pelvic muscles shorten with this motion?
3. Untuck your pelvis and move into an anterior pelvic tilt. Can you feel how your pelvic muscles lengthen with this motion?

We will undertake exercises in Part Two of this book, which will help you to create the necessary strength and flexibility around the hips to support a healthy neutral position, providing optimal support for your pelvic floor.

Your Hip Bones When Walking

We have reviewed static pelvic positions but, another important consideration is, what happens to the pelvis when walking.

As you walk, there is movement in the hip bones with each step you take. Walking pattern (gait) is very unique from person to person and it is heavily impacted by your posture. My tucked pelvis and weak glutes would have impacted the ROM of my hips, resulting in each step being a repetition of a compromised pattern that would have compounded dysfunctional reflexes and structural compensations.

When I began to train for my first marathon, I did so without first addressing my posture. I didn't even realize that I had a suboptimal posture. I just believed I looked great in my heels! The combination of my tucked pelvis and my constant walking in heels meant that when standing barefoot and straight, my whole body leaned forward. I didn't feel that I was leaning forward, and nor did anyone point it out.

This forward lean would have resulted in an imbalanced distribution of tension through my legs with each step I was taking. Figure 4.10 shows an example of load through the lower limb in a balanced posture versus a forward lean posture.

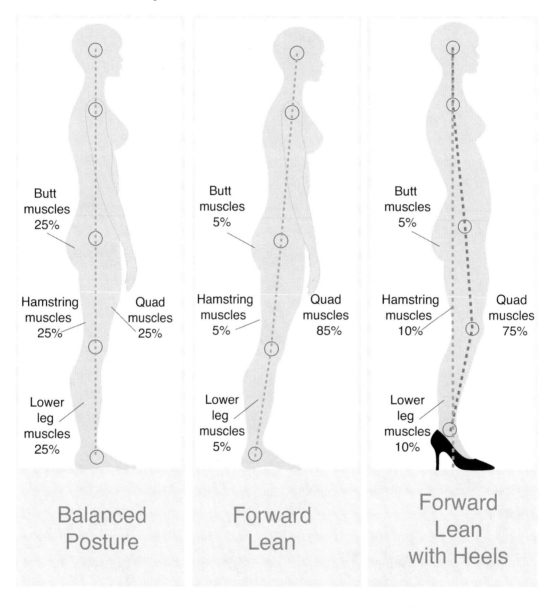

Figure 4.10: Balance of tension—Lower limb

Figure 4.10 shows a balanced posture, a forward lean posture, and a forward lean with heels. The percentages are there to give a visual representation of how load distribution could change in dysfunctional postural patterns, rather than being exact percentages. You should be able to see from this that there is a more extreme load placed on some tissues (the quads in this case) and less load on others (e.g., the butt muscles (glutes)).

This visual representation was inspired by another of my teachers, Dave O'Sullivan, physiotherapist for the English rugby team. I signed up for his mentorship program after hearing about his structured approach to rehabilitation. He uses progressive overload to reprogram the neurological mapping throughout the body in order to rebalance tension. This approach is very much aligned with the unified approach that I had taken when rehabilitating my own pelvic floor.

After running my first marathon, I had a knee injury, which resulted in quite a lot of pain. Finding a resolution to the knee pain was a struggle and during my search for a resolution, I visited numerous specialists including multiple physiotherapists and a knee surgeon. I was offered knee surgery (which I declined) and was given multiple cortisone injections into the knee in an attempt to resolve the issue.

All specialists looked at my knee in isolation. No one was zooming out to look at the structural pattern being held by my connective tissue, nor were they asking about the patterns of my life. No number of injections or surgeries would have made any difference. The only way to resolve my knee issues was to change the patterns that were creating the issue (which I did when rehabbing my pelvic floor).

Had my physio been following a more holistic approach, like that of Dave O'Sullivan, chances are that not only would my knee issue have resolved but my general posture, breathing, and pelvic floor would all have improved over the course of the treatments. You can see from reading this paragraph that there is a *lot* to consider when you start to review the pattern of your life!

The Impact of Heels on Posture

A contentious topic is the impact of wearing heels on posture and pelvic floor function. I was a heel-wearing girl for the first twenty years of my adult life. Not only did this contribute to a forward-leaning posture, but it also resulted in some of the ligaments in my feet shortening, causing my toes to curl (due to the toes gripping in my lovely stilettoes over many years). If you had looked at my pelvis from the side when I was wearing heels, it would have appeared to be neutral, even though I had a posterior pelvic tilt. If you want to see why that is, you can try the following exercise:

➡ To do this ⬅

1.   Stand up with your back against the wall and place one hand behind the small of your back and one on your stomach. Make sure your hips are stacked over your knees and knees over your ankles.

2.   Tuck your pelvis under (posterior pelvic tilt). You will notice that your low back will flatten.

3.   Now lean your weight forward so your body is coming away from the wall. You will feel the weight move more toward the front of your feet with lower limb tension moving more into your quads.

You will also notice that the curve is back in your lumbar spine and it appears that your pelvis is neutral even though you are holding a posterior pelvic tilt.

The pelvis appears to be neutral in relation to the floor. The spine appears to have the correct curvature so, no flat lower back, and yet still the glutes are not engaging (flat bum), and the knees and hips are stacked beyond the ankles. You might even notice that your ribcage has flared a bit to compensate for the forward-leaning (hello future "swayback" spinal posture!). This highlights the importance of assessing posture in relation to other body parts as well as their relationship to the floor.

Of course, a forward lean posture doesn't just impact the balance of tension in the lower body. You will also see compensations in the upper body. An example of the balance of tension in the core (including the diaphragm, abdominals, pelvic floor, low back, and gluteal muscles) with these compensations can be seen in Figure 4.11.

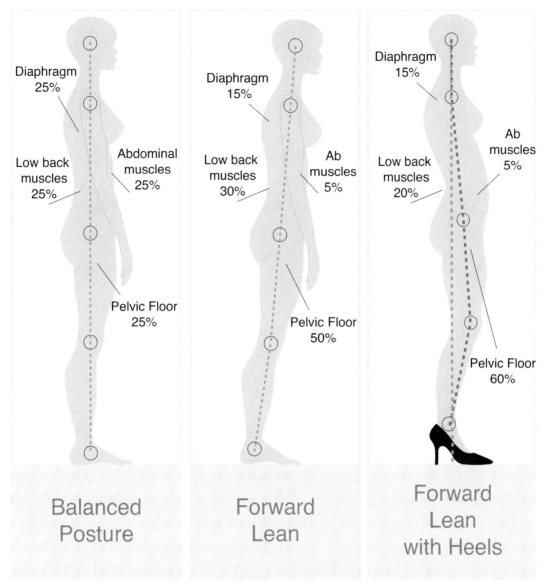

Figure 4.11: Balance of tension in the core.

Again, the percentages in Figure 4.11 are not precise. They serve to highlight how changing the balance of tension redistributes load in an imbalanced and dysfunctional way. In the forward lean examples, you will see that the pelvic floor is likely to take more load than with a normal balanced posture.

If we go back to the analogy of the business of your body's movement, Figure 4.10 and Figure 4.11 should help you to understand how the balance of tension is distributed through the connective tissue.

In these postures, you can imagine how some employees (muscles) are working extremely hard while others are on vacation. The department managers (tendon organs) may inhibit the contraction of certain muscles that are producing excessive load on tendons and this will further compound dysfunction.

You can also imagine how much more energy would be required in the forward lean and heel-wearing postures than with the neutral position. It is by no means simple, but, hopefully, you can see from these visualizations that you have the power to make big improvements with small, consistent changes (the simplest of which could be removing your heels!).

The pelvic floor, breathing, movement, and relaxation modules in the eight-phase program in Part Two of this book are designed to help retrain the balance of tension throughout the body to get all employees back to work.

It is important that you make changes to the pattern of your daily life as well as performing the eight-phase training. Part Three of this book offers symptom management and life strategies in Chapter Ten. These can be used in conjunction with the eight-phase training to help support positive improvements in your posture. Improving your posture and changing your life patterns will take time, but I believe it is time very well spent.

Consistency will be key if you are to make sustainable changes. It is critical that you realize that *you* are the one responsible for your patterns and so *you* will be responsible for changing them. It was only through taking responsibility for my own pelvic health that my situation dramatically improved.

We have now come to the end of this chapter and hopefully, you have a better understanding of the link between your daily movement patterns and your shape. With this knowledge at hand, we will proceed to the next chapter where we move our focus to understand the functions of the organs within the pelvis.

Chapter Five:
Emptying the Pelvic Bowl, and Orgasm!

If you are suffering from PFD, it is highly likely that your condition impacts the functions of the organs in the pelvis, namely urination, defecation, and sexual function. In this chapter, we will once again use simple analogies to explain these functions, which are governed by nervous system reflexes.

When it comes to urination, defecation, and sexual function, the nervous system communicates with you through sensations. When you feel the need to pee, the need to poop, or if you feel aroused, these are all communications from your nervous system.

If these bodily sensations go unnoticed or are ignored, it can be viewed as miscommunication between you and your nervous system. This can contribute to PFD, so it's really important to learn about the reflexives and to learn to both listen and respond to them.

I view the ability to listen and respond to these sensations as a superpower because it empowers you to regain control. In this chapter, I will attempt to guide you to understand these subtle reflexes. The symptom management and life strategies chapter in Part Three provides tips on how to use your superpowers to optimize function.

The Process of Urination

We will begin by exploring urination (also known as micturition or in layman's terms—going for a pee). The urinary system, like all other systems in the body, does not act independently. It is managed by the nervous system and interacts closely with the cardiovascular system. The urinary system is shown in Figure 5.1.

The main organs of the urinary system in Figure 5.1 are the kidneys, the ureters, the urinary bladder, the urethra, and both internal and external urethral sphincters. The brain and spinal column are also shown in Figure 5.1. The spinal column has been sectioned to show the T11 to S5 vertebrae with the nerves highlighted (parasympathetic in blue, sympathetic in green, and somatic in red). These are the nerves that control urinary function. (View color figures at empoweryourflower.com)

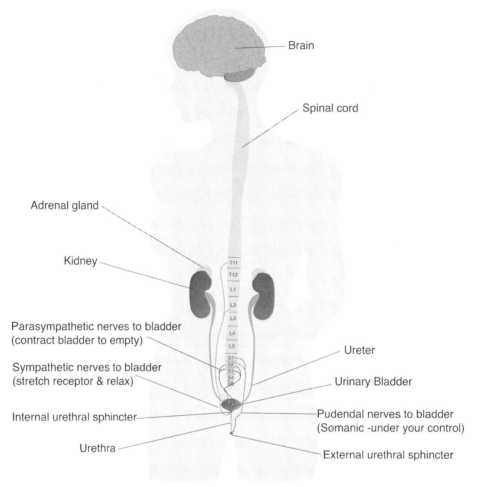

Figure 5.1: The urinary system.

Your kidneys are responsible for producing urine, which is a process that cleans toxins from the blood while helping to maintain balanced blood pressure. Toxins that have been removed from the blood are transported in the urine, through tubes called the ureters, to the bladder so you can pee them out.

Your bladder is a small bag that holds urine, and is constructed of smooth muscle known as the detrusor. The bladder acts like a balloon that expands while filling. The bladder rests on the pubic bone when the pelvis has a neutral pelvic tilt.

At the neck of the bladder, your internal urethral sphincter muscle holds the bladder closed. This muscle is also composed of smooth muscle fibers and so it is not under conscious control. Your urethra (pee pipe) is a small tube that leads from your bladder to the outside world. Your external urethral sphincter muscle, which we identified when looking at the urogenital diaphragm of the pelvic floor in Figure 2.11, is located at the end of your urethra and is responsible for holding the pee pipe closed.

The muscles within the pelvic floor form a funnel onto which the bladder sits. A normal bladder holds between 300 and 800 ml of urine and is typically emptied eight to ten times per day.

Throughout the process of bladder filling, the detrusor muscle remains relaxed while the internal and external sphincters remain contracted. The detrusor muscle has receptors that sense the level of stretch in the bladder. Figure 5.2 shows the urinary cycle.

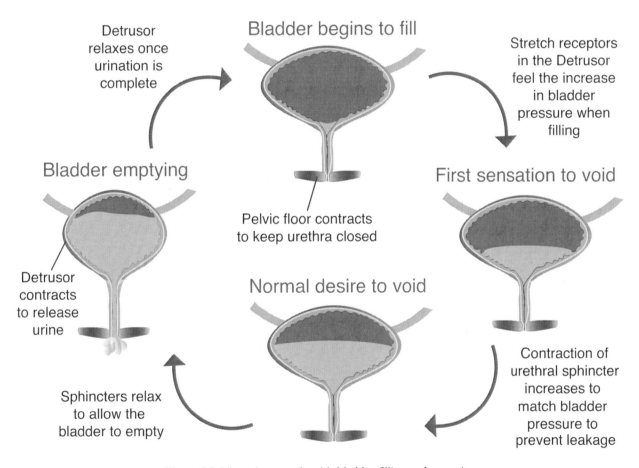

Figure 5.2: The urinary cycle with bladder filling and emptying.

Starting at the top-center image of Figure 5.2, the bladder is empty and the urethra is held closed by the external urethral sphincter of the pelvic floor. The first sensations to void are triggered when the bladder starts to fill. Normal desire to void happens when there is a reasonable volume of urine in the bladder (250–350 ml). The detrusor muscle contracts while the sphincters relax to allow emptying.

The amount of urine you produce depends on multiple factors including how much you move, eat, drink, and sweat. Your body is always striving to achieve an equilibrium in fluid balance. Measuring the volume of fluid you drink and pee is required when keeping a bladder diary (which we will explore in Part Three). However, you will not pee 100ml of urine for every 100ml you drink. The equilibrium your body strives to achieve is an overall balance of hydration in the entire body rather than a straight equation of liquid in equaling liquid out.

The Reflexes of Urination

During this normal cycle of urination, there are several reflexes that help to maintain continence. Pressure within the bladder increases as the volume of urine increases and this initiates the "guarding reflex."[28] This is a reflexive action that increases the strength of contraction of the external urethral sphincter to compensate for the increased pressure within the bladder, while at the same time contracting the internal urethral sphincter and relaxing the detrusor muscle to prevent urination.

This is a good example of the VP of operations (nervous system through your spinal cord), taking control of one of your voluntarily controlled muscles (the external urethral sphincter). When the bladder is full, the sensation of urgency to pee is increased. This is your nervous system communicating with you.

When you are ready to empty the bladder, you voluntarily relax the external urethral sphincter, while your nervous system relaxes the internal sphincter and contracts the detrusor muscle to empty the urine. This process is a complex neurological mechanism, which can easily be knocked out of sync.

If you consistently urinate before your bladder has filled (known as "just in case" or JIC peeing), you interrupt this reflexive mechanism and can introduce urinary dysfunction. By peeing when you don't need to, you are communicating to the nervous system that its sense of bladder fullness is incorrect. Your nervous system learns from this and will reprogram the bladder to signal a need to empty with much less urine.

JIC peeing is one example of ignoring your reflexes, which if consistently practiced can *reprogram* urinary reflexes into a dysfunctional pattern. Remember that your VP of operations learns and creates the pre-programmed instructions and reflexes that your muscles (and organs) will use. Problems with urinary function can manifest in a multitude of ways such as inability to release the flow of urine or an inability to hold urine in the bladder between voids.

A study at Cairo University[29] found that contraction of the external urethral sphincter prevents the internal urethral sphincter from relaxing thus activating the "voluntary inhibition reflex." This reflex is a way for you to voluntarily trigger the guarding reflex to prevent emptying (think of how you hold when there is no toilet nearby). When you hold the external sphincter closed for a few seconds, the detrusor relaxes.

You may think that contraction of the external urethral sphincter is a big thing, like squeezing a fist. I remember trying to "grip for dear life" to the contents of my bladder when I found myself incontinent. Maximum strength contractions are not needed for continence. Instead of gripping "for dear life," I would like you to use a visualization to help maintain continence.

Visualize your bladder like a balloon, with the base of the balloon (the hole into which you blow) being the urethra. When you blow up the balloon, you fill it with air and that creates substantial pressure. If you let go of the balloon after blowing it up, it would have enough pressure within to fly around the room. Now, I want you to imagine that your external urethral sphincter is the muscle that will hold this balloon closed. If you are gripping to your pelvic floor "for dear life," trying to prevent urine leakage, this would be the equivalent of trying to hold a balloon closed with a clenched fist. Not very efficient.

All that is needed is a small pinch of the balloon to hold the air inside. You don't have to squeeze as hard as you possibly can. Just a small pinch will do it.

When you think back to your life when you had continence, it is likely you won't remember having to create major pelvic floor contractions to hold your pee, and that is because you didn't. Remembering continence, and the sensation of pinching your urethra closed with your external urethral sphincter, will help you greatly when working to overcome incontinence. Your nervous system doesn't forget the reflexes that you once knew so, if you can remind it of the memory of that reflex, it can help with restoring continence.

Learning to sense and pinch the sphincter closed will trigger the guarding reflex, which can also help to relax the bladder and can be of huge benefit to those who suffer from urgency, an overactive bladder, or other bladder pain conditions. We will utilize this knowledge as a strategy to achieve continence in the symptom-management strategies in Chapter Ten in Part Three of this book.

Interrupting Your Reflexes = Reprogramming Your Reflexes

An important point to note is that interrupting your reflexes is reprogramming your reflexes. During the year and a half when I had the mesh sling beneath my urethra, I sat on the toilet for many hours every day relaxing my external urethral sphincter as this helped to relieve the pain. This was almost a bearing down on my pelvic floor. I was mimicking the act of urination as this "pretend peeing" was the only relief I could find from the symptoms of cystitis, which plagued my days.

I imagine that I felt relief due to the change in bladder pressure impacting the position of my urethra in relation to the mesh sling. During most of my time sitting on the toilet, I didn't actually need to pee.

If you have ever had cystitis, you will be familiar with that feeling of extreme urgency to urinate that results in just a few burning dribbles that can sting ferociously. You will be aware of the feeling of temporary relief when you eventually urinate fully. I would frequently empty a few drops while doing this pretend peeing and eventually I would feel a little relief.

Unfortunately, this repeated unnecessary pretend peeing resulted in a neurological reprogramming of my bladder reflexes. I had interrupted the normal neurological signals that are part of this complicated dance between the smooth detrusor muscle and the internal and external sphincters.

The detrusor muscle senses pressure to know when the bladder is empty, filling, and full (as shown in Figure 4.2). Let's use an analogy to show how this might work. We can imagine that the bladder is much like the cistern on your toilet. The detrusor sensor is like the float ball in the cistern. As the bladder fills, the detrusor senses the pressure communicating the level of urine to the brain, or in the case of the float ball, its rising is communicating fullness. Once it is full or almost full, the brain will send the signal to empty.

In the case of your toilet cistern, you are the brain that will decide to empty it. If you try to flush the cistern when the tank is empty, you will have difficulty, but once it is almost full, it can be flushed with ease (like a properly functioning bladder). Figure 5.3 shows the workings of a normal cistern.

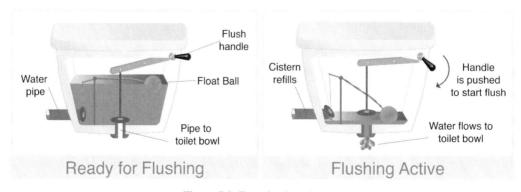

Figure 5.3: Functioning cistern.

The image on the left in Figure 5.3 shows a full cistern that is ready to flush. The float ball is a little like a stretch receptor in that its height indicates that the cistern is full. Notice how the float ball sinks to the bottom of the cistern when it is empty. This opens a valve that allows the cistern to refill.

Now, imagine what would happen if you forced the float ball to stay down at the base of the cistern. The cistern wouldn't ever get to fill as the valve that closes the water pipe would remain open. If you try to flush the toilet when the cistern is empty, it would flush only a weak stream that would be ineffective in clearing the contents of the toilet bowl.

This is similar to what happens with the bladder if you "pretend pee" or consistently urinate when you don't need to. You are forcing the external sphincter to relax opening the urethra to unnecessarily force urine out. This prevents the bladder from ever really filling. Your bladder's stretch receptors will become confused, associating a partially full bladder with a full bladder due to your early emptying (reprogramming of your reflexes).

If you (the person who flushes the toilet) are the toilet's brain, you would have to fix whatever is causing the float ball to sink if you want to use the toilet's normal flushing function. In my case, the "pretend peeing" was a workaround to ease the pain, which was a symptom of the root cause of my issue—the mesh sling.

My failure to allow my bladder to function normally, coupled with tissue damage caused by the mesh sling and its subsequent removal, contributed to the symptoms of mixed incontinence and overactive bladder, which I experienced following my sling removal surgery.

By understanding these interactions, I had the knowledge needed to relearn how to "hold" between visits to the bathroom. By understanding the pattern of my urinary function and listening to the subtle reflexes of my body, I was able to successfully reprogram my bladder function.

This ability to sense and understand the subtle reflexes involved in urination are like a superpower when dealing with incontinence. I used this superpower to help restore continence which dramatically improved my quality of life. You will learn how to do the same in Chapter Ten (Symptom Management and Life Strategies) in Part Three of this book.

Urine As an Indicator of Health

You should now understand the process of urination, but what is urine, and can it show us anything?

Urine is a stream of waste produced by your kidneys and, as such, acts as an indicator of health. Your kidneys filter your blood, removing toxins, waste, and water. By eliminating water from the blood, the kidneys help to regulate blood volume, which in turn has an impact on blood pressure. As such, urine is a tool to help you see what is going on inside your body.

Urine color is a good indicator of health. If it is clear in color, you may be drinking too much water. Drinking too much water can flush your system of vital nutrients and vitamins with the most extreme outcome being death from fatal water intoxication[30].

Pale yellow or straw-colored urine is considered normal and healthy. If it starts to become darker yellow, you may need to drink more water. Amber or honey-colored urine is an indication that you may be dehydrated. Some vitamin supplements (e.g., soluble Vitamin C) can also turn the urine a bright yellow color. Other medications can also impact the color of your urine. You can check with your healthcare provider if you have any concerns.

The food you eat can also impact the color of your urine. For example, eating beetroots or drinking beetroot juice can turn your urine a pinkish or red color. If you have pinkish-red urine without consuming anything with dark red coloring, or if your urine has a brownish tinge, that may be traces of blood, and you should seek medical advice.

Your kidneys also help to balance the pH of your urine. If you are suffering from cystitis, a low pH can contribute to the burning sensation when you pee. The lower the PH, the more acidic the urine. You should consider your diet carefully if suffering from cystitis. Many people suggest drinking cranberry juice. I definitely found this to provide some relief, although the results from scientific studies into the impact of cranberry juice on urinary infections have been somewhat inconclusive[31].

Some sources suggest that orange juice and lemon juice, although acidic, can increase the pH level in your urine making it more alkaline. I did not find this to be true in my case, but that may be due to other factors.

An alkaline diet is proven to result in a more alkaline PH[32] in urine, so it may be worth discussing what that entails with a nutritionist should you be suffering from cystitis. Diet is an important factor when trying to optimize pelvic health. This is further emphasized when we explore the next function taking place in the pelvic area—defecation.

The Reflexes of Defecation

Defecation (or, in layman's terms, going for a poop), like urination, relies on a complex neurological mechanism that controls the reflexes that induce bowel movements. The naming of these reflexes is more convoluted than those for the bladder.

With the bowel, we have the "intrinsic myenteric defecation reflex," which is responsible for the contractions (peristalsis) that move the poop (feces) through the last stretch of the rectum toward the anus. Let's call this the "I feel like I need to poop" reflex.

When the wave of contraction caused by this reflex reaches the anus, it signals the internal anal sphincter to relax. If the external sphincter also relaxes at this point, defecation can occur, however, without the second major reflex, the parasympathetic defecation reflex, voiding would be weak.

The parasympathetic defecation reflex quickly moves the contents of your bowel out of your body and into the toilet bowl and, therefore, I like to call it the "Oh shit" reflex. Contractions with this reflex come in waves similar to the "I feel like I need to poop" reflex but these contractions are much stronger and are responsible for pushing the poop out into the toilet.

If you have ever seen a wee baby doing a poop, when their face goes a bit red as they are squeezing out a big one, that is the "oh shit" reflex at play. I have heard some people say that a good poop is as good as an orgasm, which I expect is due to the strength of the "oh shit" reflex. As the external anal sphincter is under voluntary control, the "oh shit" reflex is most effective if you consciously decide to open your bowel.

The reflexes of defecation are another subtle signal from the nervous system, communicating to you that it is time to empty. If you don't listen to this reflex, you can interrupt the normal function of your defecation in the same way that urination is interrupted by not urinating when your nervous system tells you to do so. Ignoring these reflexes can weaken the "oh shit" reflex.

When you get the signal to poop, go to the bathroom and poop. If you don't have a poop signal, don't try to force yourself to poop. By listening to your body, you can use the automatic smooth muscle contractions to empty rather than voluntarily straining which can exacerbate the symptoms of POP. Learning to listen to and respond to the reflexes of defecation is another of your superpowers in your battle against PFD.

Fecal Incontinence and Anal Sex

Lack of control due to weakness of the external anal sphincter can result in fecal incontinence. External anal sphincter weakness can be caused by childbirth or other trauma. Since we are striving to break taboos, it would be foolish not to broach the subject of anal sex when we explore defecation. Maybe you know someone who has developed fecal incontinence from anal sex, which begs the question, does anal sex cause fecal incontinence? Not necessarily.

A good poop sausage and a penis are not so dramatically different in size. If you participate in anal sex because you like it and want to do it, your anal sphincter will be relaxed and welcoming. If you are doing it when you don't really want to, your anal sphincter will be contracted and fighting against the incoming penis, which can result in trauma.

A 2016 study[33] into anal intercourse and fecal incontinence showed that fecal incontinence rates in women were higher in those who reported having anal sex. They found a 2.5% increased risk of fecal incontinence connected to anal sex.

The decision to have anal sex is a very personal one. When making that choice, a good understanding of how your pelvic floor muscles work during defecation could prove useful. Figure 5.4 highlights the pelvic floor muscles relevant to defecation.

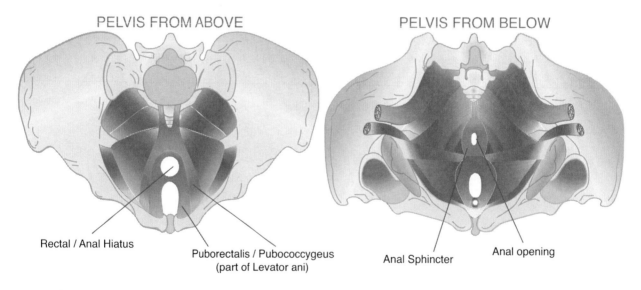

PELVIS FROM ABOVE

PELVIS FROM BELOW

Rectal / Anal Hiatus

Puborectalis / Pubococcygeus
(part of Levator ani)

Anal Sphincter

Anal opening

Figure 5.4: Pelvic floor muscles involved in defecation.

In the image on the left in Figure 5.4, we see the pelvis viewed from above with the puborectalis and pubococcygeus highlighted. In the image on the right, we are viewing the pelvis from below with the anal sphincter highlighted. The puborectalis muscle provides additional support to the anal sphincter by creating a kink in the rectum. The extra support provided by puborectalis, cordons off the exit when you are standing, sitting, walking, and running during the course of your day.

Figure 5.5 shows the anorectal angle and demonstrates how the rectal kink is removed when squatting.

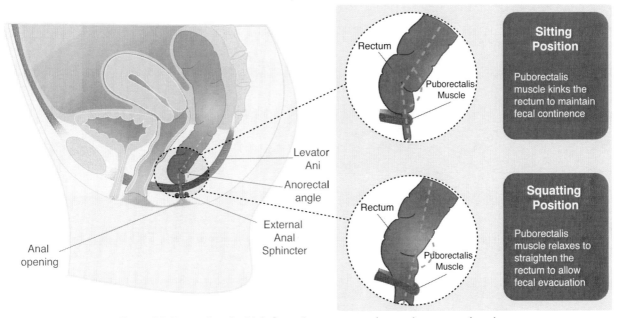

Figure 5.5: Removing the kink from the rectum to change the anorectal angle.

The two zoomed images to the right of Figure 5.5 show the anorectal angle in sitting and squatting positions. Squatting puts your knees higher than your hips, allowing your rectum to straighten out ensuring a speedy and blissful "oh shit" experience.

Have you seen the ad for the squatty-potty? If not, I would advise you to go online, find it and watch it immediately. It shows a unicorn on a toilet using the squatty-potty while producing rainbow-colored poop. It's funny and demonstrates this phenomenon quite nicely.

Knees higher than hips coupled with relaxation of the external anal sphincter enables optimal contraction strength of the smooth muscle of the bowels (the "oh shit" reflex) thus allowing complete emptying of the bowel. Figure 5.6 highlights the correct sitting position for pooping.

The image on the right in Figure 5.6 shows how sitting upright with a 90-degree angle at the hip keeps the kink in the rectum. By assuming more of a squat-like position with a 35-degree angle in the hips, the kink is removed.

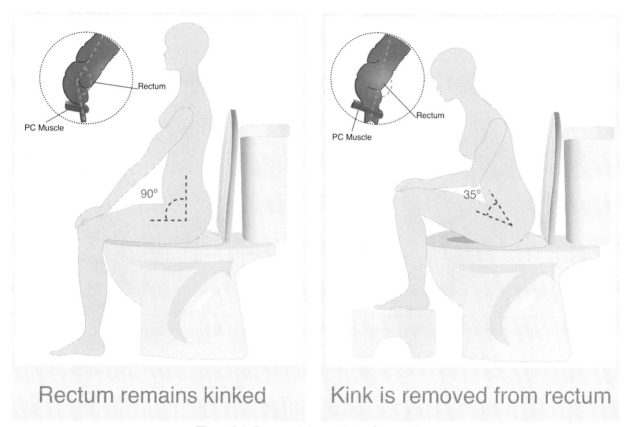

Rectum remains kinked   Kink is removed from rectum

Figure 5.6: Correct sitting position for pooping.

Notice that the spine is neutral when the kink is removed from the rectum and the lady is sitting straight (although slightly leaning forward). This also keeps gravity on your side. You could lean forward with your feet flat on the floor to get the 35-degree angle but then you will have less of a gravity assist so, I recommend elevating your feet.

If you can't find a small stool, use whatever is at hand (some thick books, a box, some yoga blocks, a bin on its side). You need to have your knees higher than your hips while allowing your pelvic floor to relax so you can empty. You can consider this one of the easiest corrections to your life pattern.

Coming back to the subject of anal sex; if it is something you are practicing, you need to bear this rectal kink in mind. Make sure you choose a position that gives this same ~35° angle at the hip to remove the rectal kink. This will help prevent unnecessary pressure against the puborectalis muscle and remember to use plenty of lubrication as the anal passage does not produce lubrication for sex like the vaginal passage.

The Impact of Constipation on the Pelvic Floor

With an understanding of removing the anal kink, let's continue our focus on defecation, more specifically constipation, which can have a very negative effect on pelvic floor health. Dry hard poop can cause straining, which increases intra-abdominal pressure. If you must strain every now and again, that isn't an issue. If you consistently strain when you poop, you can put unnecessary strain on your pelvic floor muscles and the ligaments of the uterus. This can exacerbate the symptoms of POP.

It is important to remember that straining is not always due to constipation. It can also be the result of diarrhea, an existing PFD, or incorrect posture when you poop (just imagine the effort it would take to push your poop past the kink in your rectum if you have a hypertonic puborectalis muscle).

If I look back to my own pelvic issues, I had a rectocele (downward pressure pushes the rectum toward the vaginal cavity) which makes it more difficult to empty the bowels. The rectocele was likely the result of a combination of damage from childbirth compounded by bad posture, incorrect toilet sitting position, and straining due to regular constipation from a poor diet.

It frequently felt like I had not completely emptied my bowels and I would often strain until I was blue in the face, trying to squeeze the last bits out. I had stopped listening to my reflexes and believed that I needed to always push to get the poop out. I didn't realize how very bad straining was for my pelvic health so, ensuring I didn't get constipated became an important focus for me.

It is difficult to resist the urge to strain so we will use strategies that tap into the relationship between the diaphragm and the pelvic floor to help prevent straining. These strategies involve making different sounds. The sound you make is a personal preference. Some people advise humming or mooing. When making sounds, you are slowing down and controlling exhalation, which creates balanced intra-abdominal pressure allowing the reflexive "oh shit" mechanism to function for emptying rather than bearing down.

Personally, I find singing to be the best method to prevent straining. The act of singing interrupts the natural respiratory movement of the diaphragm as singing causes your abdominal muscles to contract gently controlling the outflow of air. Dr. Michel Odent suggests that singing also helps during labor to open the vaginal passage for birth. I would imagine that would also prevent unnecessary pushing, allowing the fetal ejection reflex to work its magic.

Another benefit of singing is that it creates a distraction, which is useful if you are afraid to poop. Fear can prevent you from relaxing the anal sphincter. I typically swap the lyrics in a song to make it a song about pooping. Think "You've lost that pooping feeling" in place of "You've lost that loving feeling." This helps me to relax my anal sphincter as my focus is shifted to making up a new poop song. The combination of this distraction and controlled intra-abdominal pressure generally allows for a speedy and reflexive evacuation of poop.

Practice makes perfect. If you are eating a nutritious diet, you should have at least one chance to practice your poop song every day, improving both your pelvic floor health and your chances of succeeding at Poop Idol.

Making the Perfect Poop Sausage

Have you ever considered what your poop says about you? Just as your urine acts as a window to your health, your poop can also say a lot about your digestive health. You can think of your digestive system as a long pipe that transports fuel through your body. This pipe stretches from your mouth to your anus.

While studying biology at school, I was especially interested in digestion and have been fascinated by my poop ever since. The shape, size, color, consistency, and smell can change quite dramatically, depending on what I have eaten. It wasn't until I had surgery to repair my rectocele that I stumbled upon the Bristol stool scale which you can see in Figure 5.7.

Figure 5.7 shows the Bristol stool scale, which breaks poop into seven different types based on texture and consistency. It is used to help diagnose digestive issues. On this scale, Types 1 and 2 are considered to be severely or mildly constipated. Types 3 and 4 are considered normal. Type 5 indicates a lack of fiber in the diet. Types 6 and 7 are mild to severe diarrhea.

I am quite competitive so, after I discovered the Bristol stool scale, I challenged myself to make perfect poop

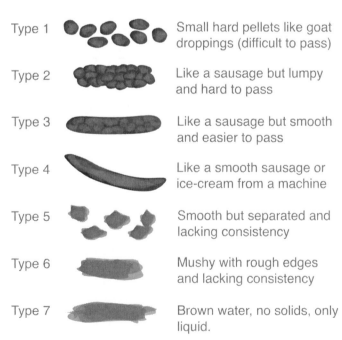

Figure 5.7: The Bristol stool scale.

every day. The next time you take a dump, have a look back at the scale in Figure 5.7 to see how your own poop measures up.

Perfect poop is a silky-smooth sausage with a soft and moist consistency that slips out without leaving a dirty anus. Not much wiping required, no feeling of incomplete voiding, and no straining.

If you find you have to use half a toilet roll to get clean when you wipe your bum, your external anal sphincter muscle might be weak. I had the pleasure of meeting Beate Carrière, author of *The Pelvic Floor*, who gave a tip to help improve anal sphincter tone and reduce wiping. She advised that, before wiping, you should perform ten contractions of the external anal sphincter with a full relaxation in between each contraction. You will learn how to do this in Part Two of this book. This technique should help to tighten things up, reducing the amount you need to wipe to get clean.

The Impact of Your Microbiome on Your Poop

Given the need to avoid constipation, it is important to consider contributing factors. One study[34] suggests that there is a higher prevalence of constipation among obese people compared to people of normal weight. If your weight is above the normal healthy range or your poop does not fall into the "normal" categories on the scale, you should explore your diet and the health of your microbiome.

The microbiome is a term used to describe the complex ecosystem of microbes (bacteria) that live in and on your body, the vast majority of which live in your gut. You also have microbes living on every inch of your skin. When you are born, you are inoculated by your mother's vaginal microbiome as you travel through the birth canal. This inoculation is part of a ritual where mothers pass on their immunity (and that of their ancestors).

Your immune system undergoes major development during the first two years of your life and continues to adapt until your death. Scientists have realized that the microbiome plays a major role in immunity and they are scrambling to understand more about the microbiome and its role in our survival[35]. Much of the research is being driven by a rise in antibiotic resistance[36] and the increase of diseases linked to diet[37], such as diabetes and obesity.

Your digestive tract is smothered in microbes. Your diet influences which microbes thrive, and which decline. Sometimes these microbes can attack you causing illness and disease. An example is the bacterium clostridium difficile, which causes severe diarrhea. Clostridium difficile, known as C-diff, is an infection of the lower intestinal tract. For many years, doctors have struggled to fight the C-diff infection with antibiotics. Many patients suffer repeated infections with some even leading to death.

Microbiome studies have led to an important therapy that involves implanting fecal matter (poop) from a healthy person into the rectum of patients with C-diff. Cure rates with this treatment show an astonishing 98% success. This treatment is known as FMT[38] or fecal microbiota transplantation. FMT was first performed in 1958 by a doctor named Ben Eiseman in Colorado.

The practice of FMT has become more commonplace. However, it is not without some hurdles. One C-diff patient[39] received an FMT donation from her sixteen-year-old daughter who was healthy but overweight. The FMT cured her C-diff but caused an unintentional and rapid weight gain of 34 lbs (~15 kg). She was placed on a medically supervised diet and exercise program but, despite her efforts, she continued to gain weight. This case led to a change in policy at hospitals performing FMT to only use poop from donors of normal weight.

This discovery also resulted in new studies[40] into how FMT may be used as a potential cure for obesity. I am explaining this as it highlights just how important your gut microbes are. A healthy microbiome can have a very positive effect on your life. These microbes play a huge role in digestion, body weight, metabolism, and the quality of your poop. Good quality poop means less straining.

Not all microbes are good microbes so it is imperative that we feed the good bacteria to keep them strong and healthy. In turn, these healthy microbes will play a role in keeping us healthy. In Chapter Three, we learned about muscle build-up and breakdown, and established that we need a diet that includes high-quality protein, is rich in healthy fats, and is low in sugar.

If we can supply our microbiome with a healthy diet, having the right balance in protein, fat, fiber, vitamins, and minerals, we are on course to produce beautiful poop sausages, helping to maximize our pelvic health with the added benefit of improved overall health.

What Is a Healthy Diet?

What does it even mean to have a healthy diet? Maybe you learned about the food pyramid at school. The idea of the food pyramid was to simplify the process of making healthy food choices. The food pyramid was first introduced in Sweden in the early seventies. It was a pyramid structure with five different shelves each containing a different food group. Fruit and vegetables sit on the bottom shelf, with grains, bread, potato, and rice on the shelf above. On top of that was dairy, then meat and fish. Fats and oils were on the second to last shelf with sugary treats on the top of the pyramid. The shelves get smaller as they rise to the top of the pyramid indicating that you should eat less of those foods on the higher shelves.

Even with the food pyramid, it isn't necessarily clear what a "healthy" choice is, which is could explain why 34% of adults and 15–20% of children and adolescents in the US are obese[41]. This is relevant to pelvic health because every one-point increase in BMI over 25 increases your chance of developing incontinence by 1%[42] so, maintaining a healthy weight plays an important role in continence.

A 2016 study[43] in the USA showed that the rate of obesity in men had plateaued by 2014, however, a significant linear trend was still prevalent in females with obesity hitting 40.4%.

With obesity in women being so prevalent, the diet trend is bigger than ever. There are many different diets and programs that have sprung to life in recent years. Some promote low fat, high carb, others promote high fat, low carb. There are diets to make us eat like hunter-gatherers, vegetarians, pescatarians, and vegan diets. There are even diets that involve only eating fruit that has fallen from a tree.

Documentaries that delve into corruption relating to the sugar, meat, dairy, and pharmaceutical industries have been released in recent years. All this information can lead to immense confusion, making it hard to decide who to trust about what to eat, although deciding what to eat may not be solely your choice.

It is believed that gut microbes can influence our food choices and even our mood. A study in 2014 showed that "Gut bacteria directly stimulate afferent neurons (signals traveling back to the brain) of the enteric nervous system to send signals to the brain via the vagus nerve."[44] The enteric nervous system is part of the CNS that governs the gastrointestinal tract. These microbes could be sending messages that influence your food choices, leading some scientists to suggest that your gut microbes may act like a second brain[45]. This information may help you to think twice (using your actual brain) before putting that sugary treat in your mouth.

In the months following my mesh implantation, I was desperate to make my body heal. I needed to find a way to alleviate the harsh symptoms that plagued my day. I met US-based author Dr. Alejandro Junger and followed his "Clean" diet to help restore my body's natural ability to heal. His program prompted me to pay more attention to my eating habits and their impact on my overall health. Clean eating made a big difference to my bowel function and helped me to eliminate diet as a potential cause of the issues emanating from the implanted mesh.

Monitoring Input and Output

By paying attention to what you consume, and monitoring the waste that leaves your body, you gain valuable insights into your health. A food diary allows you to monitor your input. For the food diary, you can use an online tool like My Fitness Pal or just do it the old-fashioned way with a simple notepad and pen.

If you eat something that provokes a reaction (such as abdominal cramping, excessive gas, or really smelly poops), you can make decisions on whether or not to eliminate that food. For example, I can eat cruciferous vegetables like broccoli and brussels sprouts in reasonable quantities, but if I eat an excess of these vegetables, I will get crampy in my tummy and produce the most foul-smelling gas. I use this information to guide me when I am deciding what to eat.

We won't be using a food diary when we explore symptom management and life strategies in Part Three of this book, but you should know that it may be beneficial for you to track your intake, particularly if you are working to lower your BMI. Monitoring how your body physically and mentally reacts to the foods that you eat can prove useful. If you choose to keep a food diary, you can also observe and record your body's reactions in the minutes and hours after eating. Look at your poop to see where it lands on the Bristol stool scale. All of this information will help to gage if your diet is right for you. The creation of a specific diet plan is outside the scope of this book, but I will cover some basic nutritional advice in the Life Strategies section of Chapter Ten in Part Three.

Taking a Break from Food

Sometimes you may need to take a break from eating by undertaking a fast. You may have heard of fasting, alternate-day fasting, or time-restricted feeding. Fasting periods have long since been practiced by different cultures. When you fast, you give your body's digestive system a chance to rest, helping to balance cholesterol and insulin levels. Fasting can also trigger the production of growth hormone, which increases muscle protein synthesis. Fasting is not something you should just jump into blindly. It is best to check with your healthcare provider or a nutritionist before beginning a fast to verify that there are no contraindications based on your current health.

The Importance of Vitamin Balance

When we discuss diet, we are usually talking in terms of macronutrients (known as macros). Macros provide the fuel (energy) for movement and repair. There are three main categories of macro: proteins, carbs, and fats. It is also important that we consider the micronutrient balance. Micronutrients are vitamins and minerals that should be provided by our food intake (such as Vitamin C or zinc). If your diet isn't providing sufficient micronutrients, supplementation may be required. I have been a walking science experiment for some years and have my bloods regularly checked to ensure I have an optimal balance of nutrients.

When I began my rehabilitation, I visited my General practitioner (GP) for a blood check. My blood results showed low iron, B12, and Vitamin D. Scandinavian daylight does not provide sufficient UVB to make Vitamin D through the skin so, it's common for Swedes to supplement. I would always recommend blood testing before adding any supplements to your diet.

Supplements can be expensive and there is no need to take them if you don't actually need them. By ensuring you have sufficient nutrients in your body, you maximize the availability of the necessary building blocks for repair, which should improve your overall capacity for healing.

Ideally, you should receive the necessary vitamins and minerals from food but sometimes you may need to pop a pill. I added a supplement with a combination of B vitamins along with Vitamin D (plus K2 to help with Vitamin D absorption), Iron, Vitamin C, and iodine (from kelp). I had my bloods retested two months after beginning supplementation and my mineral levels had normalized. I recommend you have your bloods tested both before and after adding supplements to your diet to ensure your vitamin and mineral levels have normalized.

So, we are done with urination, defecation, diet, and nutrition. That leaves us with one remaining function to explore within the female pelvic region, sexual function.

What's Involved in Sexual Function?

Sexual function is by no means straightforward. In fact, it is rather complex. Typically, sexual function involves desire, arousal, stimulation (be it clitoral, vaginal, or both), and orgasm (climax). Sexual function includes both voluntary and involuntary functions of the sex organs, body, senses, mind, and nervous system. It can be a solo act involving masturbation or copulation with another person. Maybe future studies will show that our microbes also play a role; time will tell.

Your Hormones During Orgasm

When you climax, your body simultaneously releases the powerful hormone oxytocin which has a strong pain-relieving effect (that's right, a headache is not a good excuse for skipping sex). Oxytocin, known as the love hormone, gives us that warm and fuzzy feeling that makes us want to snuggle after sex. Interestingly, oxytocin is also released in large doses during labor to help ease painful contractions.

Your Pelvic Floor During Orgasm

Most pelvic floor muscles play a role in orgasm, however; the primary muscles responsible for creating the strong delightful contractions are the bulbocavernosus (connected to the clitoris), the ischiocavernosus (which covers the crus of the clitoris and assists the bulbocavernosus), and the pubococcygeus (PC muscle).

Figure 5.8 shows female sexual anatomy in three different zoomed images.

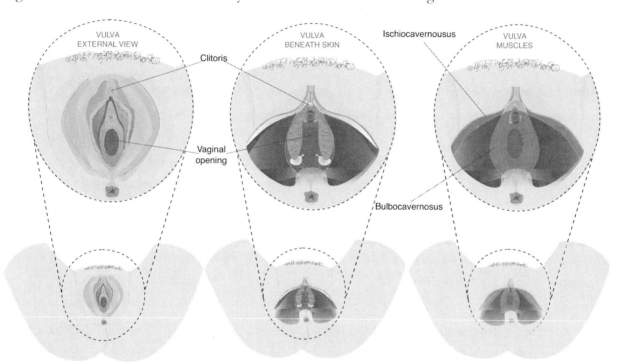

Figure 5.8: Female sexual anatomy.

The image on the left in Figure 5.8 shows the external vulva zoomed. The center image shows the clitoris and glans beneath the skin, while the image on the right shows the pelvic floor muscles that are primarily involved in orgasm. The PC muscle cannot be seen in these images as it is part of the levator ani at the deepest layer of the pelvic floor, which we viewed in Figure 2.13.

The pelvic floor muscles simultaneously contract and relax during orgasm, creating waves of pleasurable sensation that pulsate throughout the body. With all orgasms, the contractions will involve most muscles in the pelvic floor.

If you have experienced orgasm through clitoral stimulation alone, your bulbocavernosus is the primary contracting muscle. If you have experienced orgasm through penetration alone, the pubococcygeus (PC muscle) is believed to be the primary contracting muscle.

The Impact of Pelvic Floor Strength on Sexual Function

The bulbocavernosus and PC muscles can both be strengthened by Kegel exercises. A study[46] by the University of Pampa in Brazil found that women with stronger pelvic floor muscles showed higher scores for desire, excitement, and orgasm. If you are suffering from some form of PFD, it can have a very negative impact on your libido, which, in turn, has a knock-on effect on your sexual function and thus your quality of life.

I found myself pregnant a few weeks after losing my virginity at the age of sixteen. We were young and didn't really know what we were doing. I actually didn't reach orgasm the few times I had intercourse before finding out I was pregnant. The birth wreaked havoc with my pelvic floor so what I thought were amazing orgasms through the course of my adult life were in fact quite subtle. Sex was lovely but by no means earth-shattering.

Following the insertion of my mesh sling, it was almost impossible to have sex. When I did try, it was very painful, which inhibited any possibility of a climax. To add insult to injury, vaginal penetration would increase the sensation of irritation around my bladder.

Following sex, the ensuing pain would result in me sitting on the toilet, sometimes for hours on end. Relaxing the external urethral sphincter was the only relief I could find from the sensation of cystitis.

The good news is that following my mesh sling removal surgery and my subsequent rehabilitation, I was able to restore the function of my pelvic floor. I remained celibate for almost one and a half years following the surgery, simply enjoying my own company and recreating the subtle connection between my mind and body. I used this "down-time" to regain both my pelvic floor strength and control.

When I stepped back onto the dating scene, I met a lovely Italian guy. After a few dates, I decided it was time to try out my rehabilitated lady parts. I can't say he did any special bedroom gymnastics, but for the first time in my life; I experienced what can only be described as an earth-shattering, mind-blowing orgasm. I was amazed. Shocked! Awestruck!

I thought this Italian guy was some class of magician. A magic man sent to rock my world. The following day, he told me that he wasn't over his ex so, we didn't see each other again. I was left to dream of the amazing orgasms that I might never experience again. It was almost six months before my next sexual encounter, with a lovely Swedish guy. To my absolute amazement, I had another marvelous orgasm and with it came an epiphany—the earth was shaking because of me; It was me!

By unearthing the patterns that created dysfunction and taking the steps to restore function, I resolved my pelvic floor issues and restored optimal length-tension within my pelvic floor muscles. In knowing that I was responsible for these spectacular orgasms, I also knew I needed to write this book.

Not only can women heal, following extreme pelvic floor trauma, but we can empower ourselves to have the most amazing orgasms possible. The ability to empower yourself to fully enjoy sex can be seen as one of your superpowers.

The Science Behind Orgasm

I have explained throughout the previous chapters how I connected the dots to identify possible root causes of my pelvic floor issues. Even with this knowledge, I was surprised by some of the studies I found when doing research for this book. There are studies that show men (90%) are more likely to experience orgasm through intercourse than women (50%)[47,48]. Another study found that only 21–30%[49] of women reported having an orgasm through penetration alone without any clitoral stimulation.

Having learned about the female sex organs, which we viewed in Figure 5.8, this made sense to me. The clitoris is like the head of the male penis, holding the bulk of nerves that sense sexual stimulation. For me, the clitoris is like an *on* switch. I can have an external orgasm by just flicking that switch. I can have a combined external and internal orgasm by flicking the *on* switch (stimulating the clitoris) prior to or during penetration, but I cannot have an internal orgasm on its own without first flicking the *on* switch. If you are a guy reading this… don't forget the *on* switch (clitoris) if you want to pleasure a woman. If you are a woman that likes to please other women, I expect you already know.

Another study[50] found that "a woman's history of vaginal orgasm is discernible from her walk." They used a sample of healthy Belgian women, half of whom historically experienced orgasm through intercourse and the other half who experienced orgasm through clitoral stimulation. They had these women walk in front of a group of trained sexologists to see if they could infer the woman's orgasmic history by observing only her gait (walking pattern). The result was astounding with the sexologist correctly identifying women's orgasm type with 81.25% accuracy! How did the sexologists make the assessment? By analyzing if the gait was fluid, energetic, sensual, free, and without flaccid or locked muscles.

Orgasms depend on muscular contractions. If you think about hypo- and hyper- tonicity, you can imagine how weakness or tightness can impact the quality of those contractions and thus your orgasms.

Some hypertonic conditions (such as vaginismus or dyspareunia) can even prevent penetration or make it painful to perform clitoral stimulation. These conditions are most often caused by the nervous system creating a protective tone in the form of hypertonicity or muscle spasms. The relaxation modules in the eight-phase training in Part Two focus on releasing hypertonicity, while the symptom management and life strategies chapter in Part Three offers tips on dealing with these conditions.

We have learned which muscles are primarily responsible for the different types of orgasm. In the pelvic floor assessments in Part Two of this book, we will break our pelvic floor exercise down to focus on contracting different parts of the pelvic floor. This will help to assess which pelvic floor "employees" (muscles) are doing their job.

The combination of modules in the eight-phase training (pelvic floor, breathing, movement, relaxation, and mind/meditation) in Part Two, combined with the symptom management and life strategies in Part Three should help to improve the function of your pelvic floor muscles and the overall balance of tension through the whole body. This, in turn, should contribute to an improvement in the quality and strength of your orgasms.

The Impact of Diet on Sexual Function

Another consideration is the impact your diet can have on your sexual function. Almost everyone is familiar with aphrodisiacs, these are foods that are rumored to increase libido (sex drive). Oysters, dark chocolate, and avocados all feature on the list of libido-boosting foods. I'll leave it for you to decide if aphrodisiac foods really work (trial and error).

What I would like to focus on is the joining of yet another dot in our web of connectivity. Hormones play a major role in sex and orgasm. Hormones don't just magically appear. They are manufactured by the body. As you have learned, the body cannot create something from nothing. It needs fuel, and that fuel is the food you eat.

Hormones are manufactured from amino acids (proteins/polypeptides—water-soluble) or lipids (steroids—fat-soluble) which are essential building blocks to life. Amino acids can only be absorbed from the food you ingest. Lipids (e.g., cholesterol) are both ingested and produced by your liver (note: your liver uses fats, sugars, and proteins that you have ingested to make cholesterol[51]).

So, what are hormones? Hormones are chemicals produced in the endocrine glands, shown in Figure 5.9.

Figure 5.9 shows the hypothalamus, the pineal gland, the pituitary gland, the thyroid, the thymus, pancreas, adrenal glands, and ovaries. These endocrine glands produce and distribute hormones that regulate bodily processes such as metabolism, sleep, immunity, growth, reproduction, mood, and sexual function.

Hormones are chemicals used to communicate messages throughout your body. They travel in the bloodstream, delivering messages to your organs and cells.

As I mentioned earlier, when you climax, oxytocin is released in high doses[52], and since your body uses the food you eat to produce this hormone, failure to eat nutritional foods can have a ripple effect on the quality of your hormones, which can impact the quality of your orgasms, which can impact the quality of your life.

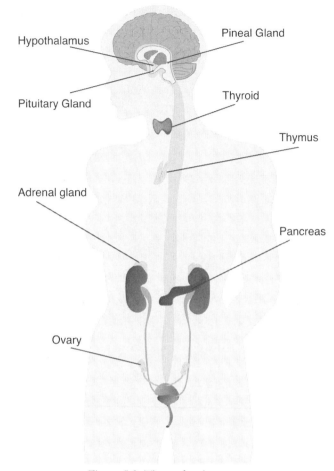

Figure 5.9: The endocrine system.

Basic nutritional advice is provided in Part Three of this book. However, if you are experiencing symptoms of hormonal imbalances (such as menstrual issues, vaginal dryness, breast tenderness, etc.) you should speak with your healthcare provider or nutritionist to see if a change in diet could be needed to promote healthy hormone levels.

That completes our overview of the functions of the pelvic organs. We covered a lot of information, so this may be a good time to take a short breather, allowing the knowledge to sink in before you continue reading. In the next chapter, we will begin to explore the connection between mind and muscle.

Chapter Six:
Connecting Your Mind to Your Muscles

Hopefully, you now understand the importance of taking a more holistic approach to your pelvic health. Empowerment is not just physical. We have discussed at length the different systems and functions of the body. We have discussed the life pattern and the effect of our choices, but we have not explored the role of the mind.

This short chapter should give you some valuable insights into the connection between mind and muscle and will present the theory behind some of the methods we will use in the pelvic floor and mind/meditation modules of the eight-phase training in Part Two.

I like to live in the land of logic as my analytical mind is very content when subjects make sense. When we begin to delve into the mind, things become complex and make a lot less sense. The crazy maze of fat and chemicals that make up your brain can baffle even the brightest of sparks.

The brain is believed to be the home to your consciousness, which brings with it so much subjectivity. Drawing the line between reality and fact, or imagination and fiction, can be challenging. I will do my best to convey my beliefs, experiences, and understandings in this chapter. I will attempt to highlight connections between science and beliefs, so we can make connections without getting lost in this complex maze of possibilities.

The mind's role in orgasm

In the previous chapter, we learned about the physical aspects of orgasm. We will begin this chapter by discussing the mind's role in sex and orgasm. Let's start with a question: can the complexity of the connection between the brain and female sex organs be clearly mapped out in a brain scan? The answer is yes! Neuroscientists began working on the creation of a comprehensive brain map in 1962[53]. Imaging technology has bounded forth since those early days allowing them to make good progress with the brain map.

Mapping highlights how sensory areas of the brain are linked to various body parts. In order to map the female sex organs, those organs must be stimulated while the brain is being scanned. It wasn't until 2011 that the clitoris, vagina, and cervix were mapped on the sensory cortex[54].

The study was carried out by Barry Komisaruk and his team at Rutgers University. They found that the clitoris, cervix, and vagina activate separate and distinct areas of the brain consistent with the different nerves that connect to these sex organs. Komisaruk suggests that these "different routes of entry to the brain are undoubtedly of significance."

If you have experienced both clitoral and vaginal orgasm or a combination of the two, you will know that they can feel subtly different. These different routes of entry might help you to understand the subtle difference in the orgasmic euphoria.

Although this study was aimed at mapping the female sex organs to the brain's sensory areas, there was another observation that is of interest. Kayt Sukel, the author of *Dirty Minds*, participated in this study and wrote about her experience[55]. Sukel's brain was scanned by a functional magnetic resonance imaging (fMRI) scanner. She was asked to physically perform a few simple exercises and subsequently, she was asked to imagine performing these same exercises. Following this, she was required to stimulate herself to orgasm.

In one of Sukel's article's[56] entitled "Sex on the brain: Orgasms unlock altered consciousness," she explains that Komisaruk's previous studies had found increased activity in the prefrontal cortex during the course of orgasm. Sukel's physical and imagined exercises activated the same locations within her brain, however, there was heightened activity when imagining the exercises in comparison to physically performing them. The prefrontal cortex is considered to be involved in many aspects of human consciousness and this study led some researchers to believe that consciousness was somehow altered by orgasm.

A researcher, Janniko Georgiadis from the University of Groningen, performed similar experiments[57] but found that part of this same brain region "switched off" during orgasm. Sukel interviewed Georgiadis who suggested that this "switching off" could indicate the person "letting go" to achieve orgasm. Georgiadis said, "I don't think orgasm turns off consciousness, but it changes it"[58].

How or why orgasm changes consciousness is unclear, but what is clear is that there is a connection. In the eight-phase program, we will explore exercises in the pelvic floor modules that help to enhance the mind-to-muscle connection, and meditations in the mind/meditation modules that will help us to relax and let go. This combination helped me to increase the strength of my orgasms and I hope it will also help you.

Does the Vagina Have a Consciousness?

So maybe you are now wondering if the vagina has a consciousness. Naomi Wolf, New York Times best-selling author of *Vagina—a new biography*, asks that very question. Naomi had a "thought-provoking, revelatory experience" that led her to delve deeper into neuroscience and physiology to find answers. Naomi offered that "the vagina is the gateway to a woman's happiness and to her creative life."

She delved into the differences between East and West exploring Tao and Tantra. Her book was subject to some pretty harsh criticism following the book's release[59], however, that did not stop it from flying off the shelves.

If you were to ask me that same question; does the vagina have a consciousness? My answer would be no. If you would instead ask me if I can utilize my consciousness and the power of my mind to change my pelvic floor and vagina, I would say a definite yes. It was for this reason that I was very interested in the difference between prefrontal cortex response for physical versus imagined exercises.

Using Thought to Create Physical Change

A year after my initial repair surgery, while I was still suffering from the mesh in my body, I stumbled upon an article in the Daily Mail Online[60]. The article was entitled "Scientists discover just IMAGINING exercising can make you stronger, tone your muscles, and delay or stop muscle atrophy."

That was a very bold and sensational headline. In Chapter Three, we learned that muscles do not act independently. They are just employees in the business of your body's movement. We also learned about how muscle is built up or broken down through protein synthesis. This is all quite logical and relatively easy to understand. Then we come to this chapter where we discuss the mind, we are sucker-punched with the revelation that we can flex our mind to strengthen our muscles.

The article in question referenced a scientific study[61] from Ohio University. The study did not focus on pelvic floor strength but on wrist flexor strength. Three groups participated.

Group one underwent wrist immobilization for four weeks to induce atrophy. Group two underwent immobilization but performed mental imagery of strong muscle contractions five days per week.

Group three was used for control. The subjects were tested at the beginning of the study (baseline), at the end of four weeks (post), and one week following the end (recovery).

Group one showed a loss in muscle strength of 45% after four weeks, whereas group two showed only a 24% loss in muscle strength. That's around 50% less muscle loss for the people who imagined exercising their wrist flexor. Group two also recovered faster than group one. The control group showed no change. The study concluded that neurological mechanisms substantially contribute to disuse-induced muscle weakness and that you can attenuate loss in strength by regularly activating those brain regions.

What does that mean? If you imagine strong contractions in a muscle you are unable to use, it will break down (atrophy) at a slower pace. From this, we could deduce that to "think ourselves stronger" can be of benefit in a program of rehabilitation.

If we relate this to the business of our body's movement, you might expect that imagining the exercise is still sending a communication to the employees (muscles) and so the employees are alert for return to work. It should also be abundantly clear that we cannot rely solely on imagined contractions to build strength, but it is definitely a tool that we should utilize.

Mind-to-muscle Connection

Another consideration when exploring the mind-to-muscle connection is that of awareness. If you are consciously aware of the muscle you want to strengthen, you can imagine contracting it. This would "light up" the part of your brain associated with that particular muscle (like the wrist flexor).

The studies that mapped the different sex organs to the brain utilized touch to make the connection between the clitoris, vagina, cervix, and brain prior to performing the imagined exercises.

If you have never strongly contracted your PC muscle, do you think you would be able to activate the right brain location by imagining a strong contraction of that muscle? I expect not, as you would not be consciously aware of it. This was one of the reasons Dr. Kegel suggested finding a pelvic floor muscle a woman could contract. If you can reach one of the employees in the area and add sufficient load to it, the pull on your connective tissue would help to distribute the load to other local muscles, eventually recruiting the PC muscle to participate in contraction.

As a yoga teacher, I use touch to bring awareness if a student has a muscle that needs to be contracted.

An example would be in warrior pose, which is shown in Figure 6.1.

In warrior pose, a strong contraction of the quads on the back leg is required. I always cue this activation verbally, but I frequently find that students cannot create the mind-to-muscle connection to perform the contraction. All it takes is for me to gently touch the quads with my finger. This brings sufficient awareness for the student to create the contraction.

For the purpose of rehabilitation, we will utilize touch to enhance the awareness of muscles within the pelvic floor to aid in the development of a stronger mind-muscle connection. Once you have awareness of these

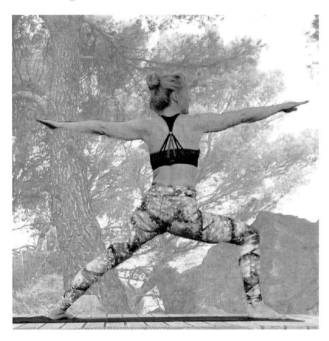

Figure 6.1: Warrior pose in yoga.

muscles and have begun to work on strengthening them, we can include a meditation where we imagine the strong lift and squeeze.

I believe that this approach was pivotal to my rehabilitation, particularly in the early days when my physical muscle contractions felt weak. I also used this approach to train myself to hold my pee, following the removal of the mesh. I meditated and imagined that I was bursting for a pee while imagining the sensation of holding it (like I was able to do when I was a kid). This is similar to the "remembering continence" strategy that I suggested in Chapter Five when discussing the balloon analogy in relation to holding your pee.

Your nervous system retains information on all your patterns, even the old ones. If you can remember continence and the sensation of continence in your body, you can interrupt your incontinence episodes with that memory to help regain your continence by guiding your nervous system to shift back to the older more functional pattern.

There have been no scientific studies to prove this method works, and I have no actual proof that it contributed to eliminating my incontinence, aside from the fact that I did it and I am now fully continent. This technique has also helped some of my coaching clients. It is completely up to you whether you take a combined approach of touch and imagined contractions, or the remembering continence strategy, which will be detailed in Parts Two and Three.

We have come to the end of this short chapter. You may be feeling a little shocked that we will use imagined contractions to help on our journey of empowerment. To me, this is just dipping the toe into the deep waters of the mind. In the next chapter, we are going to dive right in, reaching the depths of the mind, for it is in these depths that true empowerment can be found.

Chapter Seven:
Empowering Your Mind to Heal

We have reached the final chapter of Part One of this book. Whereas the earlier chapters were very much involved in the physical, this chapter steps into the world of thoughts. You will learn in this chapter that your thoughts, although mental and not physical, can have a massive bearing on what happens in your body.

Did you know that your nervous system cannot tell the difference between thoughts and reality? You may have felt this if you have ever dwelled on a frightening thought only to notice your heart racing and the feeling of panic setting in.

What you think can greatly impact what manifests in your body. This is particularly true for tension and pain. Your thoughts represent a crucial mechanism for communicating with your nervous system and, in this chapter, we will work to identify patterns of thought and explore some techniques to help to change these patterns.

Identifying the Pattern of Your Thoughts

Identifying the pattern of your thoughts is by no means straightforward or easy to do. It requires an ability to zoom out, detaching a little from the hustle and bustle of your mind. I will do my best to guide you based on my own experience.

Prior to having my initial repair surgery in 2013, I was seeing a psychologist to work through some of the deeply buried emotional trauma that I mentioned in the first pages of this book. This trauma impacted my thoughts, weighing me down. Therapy presented me with an opportunity to talk through traumatic life situations and experiences. The sessions with my therapist helped me to trace back through my life and to see that I was still carrying my past like a negative weight at the back of my mind.

As I mentioned earlier, I was attempting to heal psychological wounds while the physical wounds from my surgery were healing. It was during this process that I realized that, as well as having a life pattern, I also had thought patterns.

When the relationship with my Swedish boyfriend ended soon after having the mesh implanted in 2014, I was beside myself with shock. I felt like I had awoken from a lifelong sleep. I called all my friends to tell them that I was awake. They just laughed and said I sounded crazy, and yes, it still sounds bat-shit-crazy today.

I wrote an article[62] about my experience which was published on tinybuddha.com, a "self-help" blog site. For me, this was a turning point in my life when I became aware of the movement of my mind. Even though I felt more alive than ever before, I was also feeling the panicked waves of desperation that are typical following sudden heartbreak. I used my breathing as a tool to find a deeper connection to my body. This helped to slow my thoughts down.

With each breath, my body became calmer and my awareness heightened. I felt very alive and very bright, as though the light in my brain was permanently switched on. I had so many trains of thought that ran constantly through my mind. My breathing exercises seemed to slow each train of thought. It felt as though I was existing in a calm centered space. I no longer felt the need to speak with my therapist.

It was from this calm center that I was able to see that each thought train followed a particular pattern. Depending on the initial thought, I could almost predict where that individual train of thought would lead. I could see the pattern of my thoughts.

I had come across an article[63] by Daniel Amen M.D., a world-renowned psychiatrist who specializes in brain disorders. I signed up to his website, mybrainfitlife.com. This is a website that promotes brain health and offers brain training, meditation, and other therapies to help eliminate negative thoughts. I listened to his words. He said, "You cannot stop your thoughts, you cannot change your thoughts, but you can change how you react to your thoughts." Maybe this is common sense, but for me, hearing these words led to another epiphany.

I had been watching my constant thought trains and trying to understand their patterns. It was quite comical to watch how my brain was working. I could see my patterns and how they triggered my reactions but was unable to stop myself from reacting, leading me to believe there was nothing I could do to create change. However, Dr. Amen's words made me realize that even though I could not stop the thought train, I could change my reactions, and with that, everything changed.

Doing "The Work" on Your Thought Trains

One of the therapies offered on mybrainfitlife.com was "ANT therapy" (ANT = automatic negative thoughts). ANT therapy involves simply questioning your thoughts. I say "simply" because you are required to ask just four simple questions in relation to each negative thought. You are then asked to turn the thought around a few different ways.

The therapy is based on Byron Katie's *The work*[64] and can be viewed as a simple form of cognitive behavioral therapy (CBT). I had been sitting for some months, watching the pattern of my thoughts before starting this therapy. I could see where my thoughts would lead, and I could sense what my reaction would be, but prior to trying ANT therapy, I could not change my reactions.

Taking control of my breath was slowing my thought trains somewhat, but they still moved extremely fast. Having to apply questions to the thoughts required me to stop the thought train momentarily. You can't move on to the next station if you have to stop the train.

When you ask these questions, you have to view that negative thought from multiple angles while noting how the thought makes you feel. Think about what sort of emotions typically accompany negative thoughts: anger, annoyance, irritation, despair… the list goes on. You then ask yourself how you would feel if you didn't feel the negative emotion associated with that thought, which reveals emotions like joy, happiness, contentment, etc.

When you take the time to stop and view your negative thoughts from a different perspective, they do not seem so real anymore. After running through the ANT process a few times, I began to feel more positive. I was so impressed that I bought Byron Katie's book, *Loving what is*, and read it cover to cover. Your world can change when you start to view things from a new perspective.

An Example of ANT Therapy

Let's use a very simple example of this ANT therapy. First, some background; I am both organized and structured. In my home, I have two mottos; 1) A place for everything and everything in its place, and 2) If you want to keep the place clean, you have to keep cleaning it. These mottos were my daily mantras from the age of eighteen.

My friends call me Monica (from *Friends*). My kids claim that I have O.C.D. as in over cleaning disorder.

This in itself isn't necessarily a problem, however, in certain situations, my over-cleaning disorder would manifest in irrational negative thoughts.

For this example, let's say someone decided to help empty my dishwasher. Following this very kind assistance, I would open my kitchen drawer to see that the knives, forks, and spoons were no longer neatly stacked in the way I place them (all facing the same direction and fitting neatly on top of each other like in Figure 7.1).

Rather than the neat appearance of cutlery in Figure 7.1, I would find the cutlery just fired in willy-nilly, albeit to the correct compartment in the drawer.

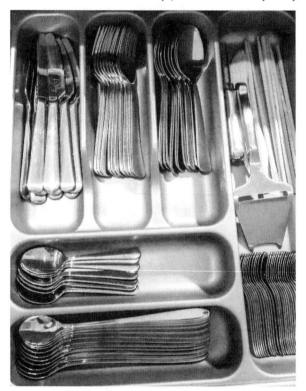

My blood would boil. I would think; "UGHHHH, why the f*@k bother helping me if you are not going to do it properly?!" You can see how dumb this thought is, right? Well, I couldn't. That is, until I did the work on this thought.

The result of doing the work on this thought changed my perspective. Now, when I open my drawer and see a mess of upside-down spoons, knives, and forks, I think to myself, "Someone loved me enough to help." This may not sound significant but I can tell you that identifying and changing this negative thought pattern had an extremely profound effect on my life.

Figure 7.1: My kitchen drawer.

Changing my perspective changed my life. My kids really noticed the change. They referred to the "old" me as "The Female Hulk" and the new me as "Peace-out Mammy" (yes, they think I have turned into some sort of yoga-loving hippy full of love and light).

Why is this relevant to pelvic health? You might be thinking this is another subject deserving to be covered in a different book but, yet again, there is a major dot here that needs to be connected. If we miss this dot, we miss out on true empowerment. I will explain but, first, we come back to some logic.

From the Brain to the Central Nervous System

Your brain is an organ, consisting mostly of gray matter that is formed from billions of nerve cells (neurons). At roughly the size of two clenched fists, weighing around 1.5 kilos, your brain pretty much looks like a walnut.

Your brain has two halves, which are referred to as hemispheres. The left hemisphere controls the right side of your body and the right hemisphere controls the left side of your body as visualized in Figure 7.2.

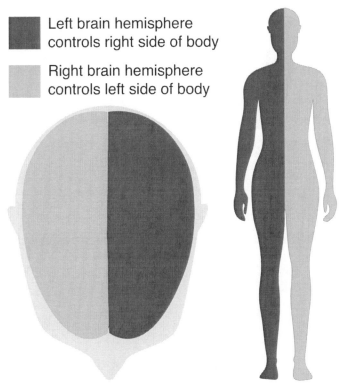

Figure 7.2: The brain's hemispheric control.

Figure 7.2 highlights the left side of the brain and the right side of the body in pink to show hemispheric control. Likewise, the right side of the brain and the left side of the body are highlighted in purple. Speech and creativity are controlled by the left side, with logic and reasoning controlled by the right. If we put back on our engineering hats, we could imagine that the brain is like a computer.

Part of the brain acts like the computer processor, making decisions, and executing tasks. Part of our brain acts like a hard disk, storing information for later use (long-term memory). Part of the brain acts like your computer's random access memory (RAM), storing information that needs to be quickly accessed for the currently running tasks (think short-term memory). Your spinal cord stems from the root of your brain. Your brain and spinal cord together are collectively known as the central nervous system (CNS).

Imagine that your spinal cord is the cable that connects your computer to the internet. Let's imagine that this single internet cable branches out to reach the servers and other computers that make up the internet. The peripheral nervous system consists of branches that stem from the spinal cord reaching out to the extremities of your limbs, just like the branches of cables reaching out to other computers on the internet.

With this analogy, we can imagine that the communication involved in sending an email to a person on the internet is like the communication happening in your body when you go to shake someone's hand. You send the mail (signal to shake hands) from your computer (brain—CNS), it travels through the internet cable in your house (Spinal cord—CNS) before finding its way through a branch of cables (peripheral nervous system) to reach the computer of the person you want to receive it (actual handshake).

This is an over-simplification but hopefully, it gives you some clue as to the flow of communication that happens internally. With this basic understanding, we can take a closer look at the peripheral nervous system to see why ANT therapy is relevant to pelvic health and rehabilitation.

Fight or Flight Versus Rest and Digest

When we talked about the business of your body's movement, we talked about the brain sending "intent to move" signals, which initiated muscular movements. These signals travel through the first branch of the peripheral nervous system (somatic nerves). These are the nerves' branches that allow you to voluntarily control muscles.

The second branch comprises the autonomic nervous system, which has the nerves used for involuntary control (controlling breathing, heart beating, digestion, urination, defecation, etc.).

Your autonomic nervous system breaks into two further branches. I believe that by now, most people have heard of these branches, or at the very least of their functions. The first branch is known as the sympathetic nervous system (SNS). The SNS is responsible for the "fight or flight" response. This is the nervous system that would kick in when you are being chased by a saber-toothed tiger. The second branch is known as the parasympathetic nervous system (PNS). The PNS is responsible for the body's "rest and digest" response. It is responsible for the calm state when relaxing in the shade of a tree before the saber-toothed tiger approaches.

If we use our computer analogy, we can imagine that our brain is a computer and the autonomic nervous system is the Windows operating system. In this scenario, rest or digest mode is like Windows running in standard mode. You will have access to the full processing power of your PC and can run many tasks simultaneously. All of your hardware drivers (control software) will be running and you can complete your computing tasks with ease.

Fight or flight, on the other hand, can be compared to Windows running in safe mode. Safe mode disables many functions, features, and drivers. The operating system is still "alive" but it is difficult to complete tasks. Your computer's operating system operates either in standard mode OR in safe mode. In the same way, your autonomic nervous system operates either in "fight or flight" mode (SNS) OR in "rest and digest" mode (PNS).

While running in PNS mode, there is a good blood supply to the gut and digestive organs. The immune system is stimulated, and the body can direct energy to functions like digestion and repair.

In comparison, the SNS is the system that keeps you alive under stress. The adrenal glands produce cortisol (a stress hormone) and blood supply is diverted away from the gut, which slows digestion. Blood pressure is increased, and the immune system is suppressed. Blood sugar levels are also increased to provide a fast energy source, so you can make a quick getaway (it's that damn tiger again!).

Does this mean that you should avoid using your SNS at all costs? No. A body functioning optimally, needs to switch between the two systems regularly, creating balance. Problems can arise if either the SNS or PNS are dominant.

This is why ANT therapy is relevant. If your nervous system is out of balance, due to constant negative thinking, you will have sympathetic dominance. This will impact your defecation, urination, and sexual function, as well as your body's ability to effectively repair.

Your SNS is active when you orgasm. The SNS is also responsible for contracting the internal urethral sphincter as part of the guarding reflex, which we discussed in Chapter Four, which prevents urine from leaving the bladder.

The PNS, on the other hand, is responsible for contracting the detrusor muscle to empty the bladder.

The dance between SNS and PNS should be rhythmic and balanced. Figure 7.3 shows some of the functions of the SNS and PNS.

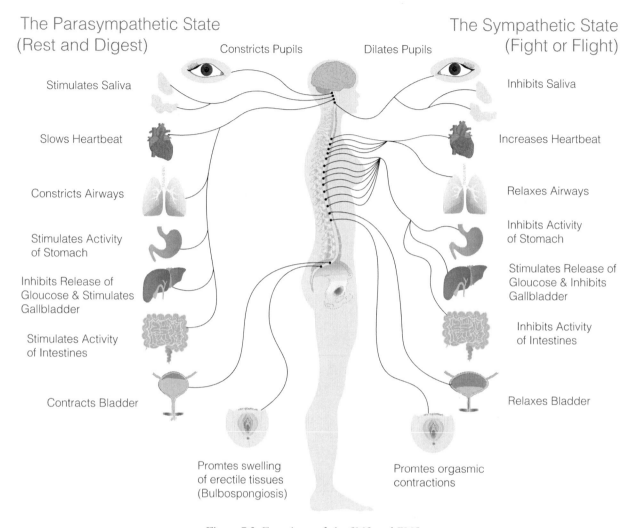

The Parasympathetic State (Rest and Digest)

Constricts Pupils
Stimulates Saliva
Slows Heartbeat
Constricts Airways
Stimulates Activity of Stomach
Inhibits Release of Gloucose & Stimulates Gallbladder
Stimulates Activity of Intestines
Contracts Bladder
Promtes swelling of erectile tissues (Bulbospongiosis)

The Sympathetic State (Fight or Flight)

Dilates Pupils
Inhibits Saliva
Increases Heartbeat
Relaxes Airways
Inhibits Activity of Stomach
Stimulates Release of Gloucose & Inhibits Gallbladder
Inhibits Activity of Intestines
Relaxes Bladder
Promtes orgasmic contractions

Figure 7.3: Functions of the SNS and PNS.

Figure 7.3 shows at which level of the spinal column the various PNS and SNS nerve fibers branch out to the relevant organs.

The Flip-flop Between SNS and PNS

If we think of the hunter-gatherer, who had to deal with that saber-toothed tiger, we could imagine how the SNS and PNS helped ensure her survival. After eating a meal, her system would be at rest, activating her PNS. When the PNS is active, her system is in an anabolic state, meaning that it can utilize the body's smallest molecules as building blocks for repair and regeneration.

After a while, the hunter-gatherer would start to feel hungry and she would have to go looking for food. This would involve getting up and foraging around or hunting an animal. This would mean a lot of dynamic movement, which stresses the muscles and joints. This is physical stress. If she struggled to find food, this could also lead to worry, i.e., emotional stress.

Stress (whether it be physical, emotional, or chemical (from medications for example)) activates the SNS, preparing the body to fight against attack. When the SNS is active, your system is in a catabolic state, meaning it can break body parts back down into the smallest molecules that can subsequently be utilized as fuel for defense (think running from the saber-toothed tiger).

Remember; the body is an organism whose primary goal is to survive. The hunter-gatherer will move until she finds her next meal, after which, she will sit down, eat, and rest. This flip/flopping between the PNS and SNS sustains life.

The Impact of SNS or PNS Dominance

So, what causes an imbalance? There is no simple answer, but I will try to provide one by first focusing on the PNS.

Imagine (in pre-covid times) that you have an easy job that allows you to work from home. You can do your shopping online, having your food delivered to your door. You relax in front of the TV after work. You don't have to walk far—from your bed to your desk, to your kitchen, or your living room. On an average day, your walk between 600 and 1000 steps. There is no financial stress, as your salary is greater than your expenses. You are not moving much so your body does not suffer physical stress. It is very likely that your system could become PNS dominant. You might experience an extreme lack of energy, tiredness, stiffness in your muscles and joints, headaches, profuse sweating, and digestive issues.

On the other hand, let's imagine that you have a high-pressure job and have to travel to work every day by car. You sit in traffic for an hour before arriving at the office. You grab a coffee and a sandwich to eat at your desk while you deal with the first emails of your day. You play squash or do some other exercise at lunchtime (as you know the importance of exercise) and eat lunch back at your desk while working. You work late but find time to go for a run when you get home. You manage to clock up over 10,000 steps per day. In this scenario, you would be under emotional and physical stress. It is possible that your system could become SNS dominant and that you would suffer symptoms like restlessness, anxiety, fatigue, reduced libido, short temper, insomnia, and digestive issues.

Balance is absolutely required in order to maintain good health. SNS dominance is a catabolic state that can hinder repair. PNS dominance would likely not stress your tissues enough to promote healing, and as we all know after spending lots of time in isolation due to Covid, the PNS life would probably also result in emotional stress. Rehabilitation from PFD requires a healthy balance between SNS and PNS, and we will strive to find that balance through our training in Part Two and the symptom management and life strategies in Part Three.

If we go back to my newly awakened self in 2014, was I stressed? Hell, yes. I was experiencing waves of panic rush through my body. Some days, I felt like jumping out of my own skin. While going through that really stressful time, I gave extra attention to the reduction of stress by practicing yoga, meditation, and breathing to help calm my nervous system. I continually brought myself back to my "calm place," which is the rested state. This is what we will aim to achieve while working toward empowerment.

Flipping and flopping between extremes of SNS and PNS is not ideal. Better to "meet yourself in the middle," gently floating between SNS and PNS. One of the meditations on mybrainfitlife.com was the Kirtan Kriya, a kundalini meditation, which Dr. Amen had explained is used as a treatment for Alzheimer's patients[65]. The meditation takes only twelve minutes per day and has been proven to improve memory in studies of people with subjective cognitive decline. We will perform the Kirtan Kriya in the Mind & Meditation module in Phase Five of the eight-phase training.

Kirtan Kriya is like exercise for the brain. I believe that a combination of this simple daily meditation coupled with doing the ANT therapy on negative thoughts dramatically reduces the extreme swings between SNS and PNS. This enabled me to take one of the biggest steps in my rehabilitation— changing my mind.

If in your mind, you are constantly riding negative thought trains, your nervous system will be on high alert, and, over time, your body will start to break down. Sometimes we don't see that we are SNS dominant as the stresses are so small that we don't immediately see the accumulated impact. Like the messy cutlery drawer. An accumulation of small stresses will have an impact over time, just like the accumulation that occurs in your body if your life pattern creates structural compensations.

The Self-created Nature of Suffering

I had an epiphany when doing the analysis of my thoughts. I realized that my suffering was self-created. People are oftentimes up in arms when I say this, and maybe you are too. Let me explain starting with the simplest example—the kitchen drawer. The sleeping version of me would open the drawer, see that things were not correctly placed, and... board the thought train:

First Stop

"UGHHHH, why the f*@k bother helping me if you are not going to do it properly?!"

Emotion: Anger.

Second Stop

"She has been in my house often enough to know where things go."

Emotion: Irritation.

Third Stop

"She did this deliberately."

Emotion: Rage.

Fourth stop

"F*@king bitch. How would she like it if I did this in her house?"

Emotion: Disgust.

...and from here, the train runs back to the first stop doing a "++" on the emotion each time around the block.

Does this little train of thought seem even vaguely familiar to you? (Maybe not in relation to cutlery!) I think it is even a bit stressful to read. After doing the work of ANT therapy on this thought, the train takes a different route. Let's jump on board:

First Stop

"OMG, someone loved me enough to help."

Emotion: Appreciation, gratitude, joy, delight, love.

Second Stop

"How very kind. I hope I can help someone today."

Emotion: Excitement, anticipation.

The train ends here.

Back to my statement about suffering being self-created; can you see how I was creating this suffering myself? When I saw it, I sat with a thick A4 notepad and started to write down every negative life experience. I broke each experience down into statements and for each statement, I performed the ANT therapy.

I realized while doing this that for most of the negative situations, I had found someone to "blame." Someone outside of myself who, in my mind, was responsible. Like my eldest son's father for not supporting me when I was pregnant or Irish Catholic society for making me feel that I was dirty and impure.

Even though I had talked through these situations with my therapist, I still carried them. Then, I had yet another realization. By placing blame outside of myself, I was also placing my power outside of myself. I had taken responsibility for bringing my three children into the world but had blamed others for the hardship that I faced when raising them alone.

Before long, I didn't have to do the work on these statements. I just wrote my experience of the situation, how I felt about that situation, and looked for my responsibility in that situation.

Then I noticed something quite profound. When reliving those situations in my mind, I could feel the stress of those situations in my body. I observed the areas where I held this tension (mostly around my shoulders and hips). These physical sensations in the body that were subtly taking place while I relived the negative situation allowed me to see the pattern of emotional stress in my body.

The tension you hold during stressful situations can stay with you over an extended period if you continue to think about that stressful situation, particularly if you relive the emotions when you think about it. This tension is a muscular contraction, which pulls on the multidimensional sausage string.

If you overload your body with physical tension from emotional stress, that could trigger some inhibition that will change the balance of tension in your body leading to dysfunction.

This process of doing ANT therapy and releasing tension is also critical if you are suffering from chronic pain conditions. What you think about your pain will impact how the pain manifests in your body. If you believe your pain to have a sinister cause, this communicates danger to the nervous system, which can trigger an excessive protective tone and an increase in pain level.

This does not mean that your pain is not real. Pain is very real and is designed to make you sit up and take notice. It is one of the strongest communication methods your nervous system can use to get a message through to you.

The nervous system's main goal is ensuring your survival so, it will protect you by giving you pain or even strong emotions to prevent you from doing things that could bring you harm. This is great if you are in actual danger, however, conditions involving chronic pain often exist when the danger is no longer there. Chronic pain can be the result of miscommunication. Lingering negative thought patterns can contribute to this by adding additional tension.

Hopefully, you are beginning to see how the journey of empowerment can teach you to optimize the communication between you and your nervous system to avoid unnecessary pain and dysfunction. The relaxation and mind/meditation modules of the eight-phase training are designed to help release these pent-up tensions from your body and mind.

Changing the Pattern of Emotional Stress

During stressful situations, our SNS is active, with the body adapting in a protective way, often closing the heart and creating a protective layer of tension around our delicate organs. Yoga teaches us that there are seven energy centers within the body, known as chakras. There is no scientific data to validate the chakra system, but I believe that these chakras were identified due to the manner in which different emotions manifest in the physical body.

If you've ever had a "gut feeling," that would be viewed as the third chakra known as manipura. A more scientific way to view your "gut feeling" would be to explain that your body instinctively responds to an external stimulus with a visceral reaction, which results in a physical response to the emotion.

If you can learn to listen to the subtle language of your body as it reacts to situations, you can take some control over these reactions, creating a more calm and centered self. The ability to do this is yet another superpower in your arsenal against PFD.

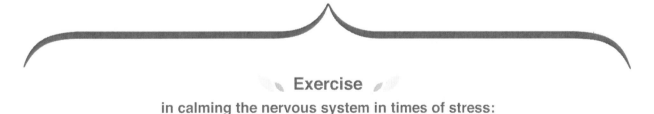

Exercise
in calming the nervous system in times of stress:

Instead of getting lost in reaction, try this the next time you are in a stressful situation.

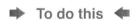

➡ To do this ⬅

1. Bring your awareness to your body.
2. Notice the beat of your heart and notice if you are sweating.

3. Notice where you are holding tension in the body and try to relax in that area.

4. Notice if your breathing is deep or shallow and wherever you are in your breath cycle, exhale the air out.

5. Take a deep inhalation for a count of four, and exhale slowly for a count of eight.

6. Repeat the deep inhalation and slow exhalation for a further six to ten calming breath cycles while continuing to relax your body (one breath cycle is an inhalation plus the subsequent exhalation).

Taking control of your breath in this way, where you inhale deeply for a count of four and exhale slowly for a count of eight, will help to calm your nervous system by "faking" parasympathetic reflexes, triggering a "rest and digest" response. This helps to lower your heart rate and reduces the perceived stress level. This exercise really helps *in the moment*.

Noticing how your body is reacting in times of stress can also help you to identify when you are under stress but haven't noticed, for example when thinking about a past negative experience. Past negative experiences are kept alive when you allow the same thought patterns to run rampant in your mind while allowing the subtle visceral responses to those thoughts to continue in the established pattern of tension in your body.

Reclaiming Your Power by Taking Responsibility

A lot of the experiences that had caused my negative thought patterns involved abuse—physical, emotional, and sexual. Abusers are completely to blame for the abuse that they inflict. When we carry the thoughts and emotions from past abuse into our present moment, we keep those abuses alive.

The abuse has stopped but we are still living it. This is such a disempowering state in which to exist. When you begin to work on breaking the patterns of your thoughts and changing the established physical pattern of stress, it will be fruitless if you don't come to the realization that your suffering is unconsciously self-created.

That's not to say that you are to blame for the abuses you have experienced in your life, not at all. It is to say that without taking responsibility *for your suffering* (not for the abuse), without owning your suffering, you cannot change it.

To own your suffering is to acknowledge that what you think creates the emotions that you feel. When you take responsibility for your thoughts, you empower yourself to change them. Instead of thinking, "He has ruined my life" and feeling miserable, you could think, "He hasn't ruined my life" and feel positive about the future. He can only ruin your life if you give him the power to do so by continuing with the negative thoughts that make you live out the abuse long after it has ended.

When you do the ANT therapy, you are prompted to question how you feel when thinking those negative thoughts, versus how you would feel if you didn't have that thought. Taking responsibility for your own suffering gives you the power to experience new emotions in place of the original stress-producing emotions. You have the power to create a pause and to be there for that past self who still lives in those thoughts.

This gives you the opportunity to change the direction in which your thought trains travel, and empowers you to end your own suffering by bringing yourself back into the present moment.

Removing the Mental Blocks

One of the biggest mental blocks when trying to let go of your suffering comes from not feeling able to let go of the blame. This is particularly relevant if you are one of the unfortunate women who have undergone mesh surgery resulting in complications.

It is really difficult to accept that the surgeon for whom you had deep respect and trust could implant a permanent device without making you aware of the associated dangers. There is a feeling of dismay when you realize that your trusted surgeon still uses mesh knowing the harm it has done to you. Knowing that there is huge controversy around the clinical trials that brought the device to market. When you find out that the device leaves one in every ten women having to deal with life-altering complications, the anger can be overwhelming.

If you are one of the women who is now confined to a wheelchair or who has lost her bladder or bowel, left to live with a stoma, your current reality is far from a bed of roses. The negativity that overshadows a once happy life is like a storm cloud that follows you around.

I realized something critical when dealing with my complete incontinence, following mesh removal—the bitterness I felt toward my surgeon was not impacting his life, it was impacting mine. It was taking valuable energy away from the mammoth task of healing.

The thoughts that created the negative emotions were causing me to hold more tension in my hips. I needed to find a way to move beyond this anger. To take my power back and to use that power for healing.

I tried to understand things from his perspective, by putting myself in his shoes, but hard as I tried, I could not imagine how he could continue to use mesh, knowing how much harm it had inflicted.

My surgeon is still implanting this dangerous device in unsuspecting women every day. I can't change his mind about mesh. I can't change the mind of the other surgeons. It's not that surgeons are bad people. I brought myself back to that first appointment where he had suggested the surgery. This guy wasn't trying to hurt me. He was trying to make my life better. He truly believed in the device he was implanting.

Medical professionals choose their profession to help people, and many believe that mesh helps people. If we are to go by the data—it helps nine out of every ten women implanted. With millions of women receiving the implants, that leaves hundreds of thousands in shatters. How not to feel bitter about this level of hurt?

I needed to find empathy. Then, I realized, we have all caused hurt at some point in our lives. Calling someone a name or pulling someone's hair at school, breaking someone's heart. Some hurt is physical, some emotional, but each one of us knows what it is to hurt another. I used that knowledge to help me find empathy.

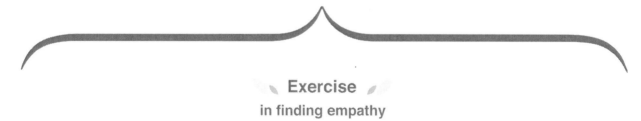

Exercise
in finding empathy

Try the following exercises to help you find empathy with someone who has caused you pain:

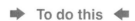

➡ To do this ⬅

1.   Think of any situation in your life where you hurt someone, even if unintentionally. This will remind you that you know what it is to cause hurt.

2. Remember back to the situation where someone caused you pain.

3. Imagine that you are that person who has caused the pain, thinking about how their life must be. Imagine how it must feel to do their job or participate in their relationships.

4. Utilize the memory of that situation where you caused pain to someone else, and see yourself in the person who has caused you pain.

If you know what it is to cause hurt to someone else, you can see yourself in the person who has caused hurt to you because we are all human. Inflicting pain on another is part of the human condition. In seeing yourself in the other person, some small level of empathy can be found.

When I undertook this exercise in relation to my surgeon, I could see he wanted to help women, which is why he was doing those surgeries. I could relate to his desire to help others as I too have this desire, which is why I am writing this book.

He wasn't strong enough to take responsibility for the harm he had caused. He wasn't strong enough to change his mind about implanting plastic in women. He will stop using mesh only when it is banned, or when his superiors tell him so. He is weak. I could see the human in him, and the human in me. This is where I found empathy, and with that empathy, I was able to let go.

I decided to stop looking back in anger and, instead, to turn my eyes forward, and to use my current energy for my own empowerment. I let go; not just of the bitterness toward my surgeon for causing me to hurt, but to all the hurts in my life. I let go of a lifetime of negative experiences and with that, my suffering disappeared.

Without the weight of my suffering, I am strong. With my strength, I have put pen to paper in an effort to educate women. I can't convince my surgeon he should not continue to use mesh in surgery, but I can convince women that they can empower themselves to heal without going under the knife.

Empowered by the Seed of Human Potential

Letting go of those negative experiences that were the cause of my suffering opened the door to something new. Allowing myself to have empathy allowed me to see myself in everyone I met and that fundamentally changed something.

By seeing myself in others, I almost felt as though I was looking at the seed of human potential. I was witnessing how that potential was playing out in the surrounding environment. In seeing that you have the potential to be a "bad" person, you can also see your potential to do "good." Then, your eyes are open to view the world differently. When you can see the ways that you create your own suffering, you empower yourself to end it.

The journey of empowerment is a journey of deep introspection. A journey that allows you to face your hurt, your frustration, and your bitterness, and to drop those emotions, giving you vital energy for healing.

We each hold the power to create the life we are living. In order to create the life we want, we need to approach our difficulties with a positive mindset. Nothing can be managed that isn't measured. We need to identify where we are now by creating a baseline, and to decide where we want to be by setting goals. With goals in hand, we need to create a plan that moves us from here to there. We need to truly empower ourselves. True empowerment comes when you take the journey within. When you find your own seed of potential, you have come to the root of empowerment, and from there, you can blossom.

The Science Behind the Seed of Human Potential

Was that too airy-fairy for you? I did say that I would try to stick to the world of logic rather than getting lost in the maze that is the complexity of the mind so, let's put our engineering caps back on to explore the science behind our potential.

Our genes predispose us to act in a particular way or develop a certain illness. This predisposition is just a potential. The images we see, what we believe, our experiences, who we listen to, the food we eat, the air we breathe, the stress we are under, the chemicals we are exposed to, our microbiome, and many other things play a role in how our genes are expressed. If you believe your genes make you fixed and predetermined, you are wrong.

If you break everyone and everything down to their smallest elements, you would find the basic building blocks of our universe: atoms—composed of three elementary particles; protons (+), neutrons, and electrons (-). Protons and neutrons bind together to form the nucleus at the center of the atom. The electrons orbit the nucleus. Almost 100% of the atom is filled with space.

This space is not barren, it is filled with quantum fluctuations; little fields of potential energy that appear and disappear spontaneously. Brian Cox and Jeff Forshaw, quantum physicists and authors of

The Quantum Universe describe these quantum fluctuations as particles and antiparticles that appear out of nothing before disappearing again[66].

I like to imagine these quantum fluctuations are like little sparkles of energy that pop in and out of your field of existence. I like to believe that human consciousness lives in that sparkly fluctuating space within the atoms, and that we are somehow all connected to all things at all times, on this very basic sparkly level. For making that nonsensical charlatan statement, Neal deGrasse Tyson, you are welcome to come and slap my wrists.

Of course, the field of quantum biology is getting started now so these quantum fluctuations in relation to human (and animal) biology have just begun to be explored. A great book on the subject is *Life on the Edge* written by Jim Al-Khalili and Johnjoe McFadden. That's the rabbit hole that I am currently exploring, and I expect that many unknowns will be revealed in the years to come.

Coming back to what is already known; atoms are either positively or negatively charged. The human body consists of six main atom types, which attract each other and bond together to form amino acids. These amino acids bond together to form a long strand of DNA, which contains your unique genetic code. This DNA code is your unique pattern for life. This code is used to build the very proteins that are the building blocks for your cells that form your muscles and bones. So how is this pattern relevant to your pelvic health?

The genetic code held within your DNA is a pattern filled with possibilities, but they are just that—possibilities. In the previous chapter, we reviewed the link between our biology and our life. We know that our bodies are constantly building up and breaking down. This process involves millions of chemical reactions that are constantly occurring. Our hormones, which impact how we feel emotionally, are the result of chemical reactions. For example, oxytocin and serotonin, which can make us feel great, and the stress hormone cortisol, which can make us feel uneasy.

Interactions with other people involve emotions, which are chemically based. We are constantly surrounded by an external environment filled with people, sounds, images, and smells that influence how we feel. If you are aware of this influence, you can see how it affects your life pattern.

When you see your life pattern, you can change it. When you can grasp this fundamental understanding, you will see that you are not predetermined. You have the power to influence your environment. **The seed of your human potential is that you have the power to change.**

Even if your entire life up to this very moment has consisted of negative emotions, abusive situations, illness, nutrient-poor diet, and terrible life patterns, you hold within you the potential to change. I needed to change, and that is exactly what I did.

Reprogramming Your Thought Patterns

I am not a neuroscientist, nor a psychiatrist, or psychologist. I needed to change my mind, but I didn't know how. It was the wise words of Dr. Amen that resonated with me: "You cannot stop your thoughts, you cannot change your thoughts, but you can change how you react to your thoughts." The thought trains that had lingered in the back of my mind over the course of my life were no longer running, but what about the tracks on which they traveled?

I believe that neural pathways are learned chemical patterns that are like train tracks that run through the brain. It is on these tracks that our "thought trains" travel. These tracks didn't magically appear one day. They were created through learning. From birth to the present moment, you have been learning.

Your childhood brain is like a sponge that soaks up information, making it easy for you to be conditioned by your family, friends, and society. This conditioning teaches you to behave a particular way, conforming to social norms, and helping to ensure your survival. Your genes (DNA) predispose you to possible behaviors, but these behaviors will only manifest if the environment in your life stimulates them.

Can you unlearn something? In my opinion; not easily. Particularly when you have practiced that learning every day for forty years, like my negative thinking. If you always think a certain way, you will continue to think in that way, unless something changes.

The adult brain is not set in stone. It is malleable due to neuroplasticity. This means that you can form new neural connections in response to new situations or stimuli. The challenge is that oftentimes; the situation or stimuli is old or is triggering an old thought pattern like the kitchen drawer response. If presented with that same situation, I would react in the same way unless I consciously choose to react differently. So how did I change my reaction?

1. Breath
2. Awareness
3. Observation.

These tools create the space to zoom out allowing you to see things from a new perspective. Luckily, my "over cleaning disorder" was quite extreme. This presented me with very many situations (environmental stimulus) that could trigger the "kitchen drawer" reaction.

Laying New Tracks in Your Mind

In yoga, we are told that it takes forty days to break a habit, ninety days to gain a new habit, in 120 days you are the habit, and at 1000 days, you are the master of it. This is based on ancient yogic teachings.

A study[67] by researchers at University College London concluded that health professionals should advise patients to adopt habit-forming actions to promote long-term behavior changes. They cited one study that found new habit formation could be achieved "on average around 66 days after the first daily performance."[68] However, they noted that "Working effort-fully on a new behavior for 2–3 months" gave the best chance of "making the behavior become 'second nature'."

The decision to change your mind, like an epiphany, happens instantly. Making the change permanent requires repetition over many instances. Permanently changing the "kitchen drawer" reaction took very little time, possibly due to the very frequent triggers. Before long, I could see the reaction before reacting.

The effort it took to choose a new reaction felt enormous at first. As though I was physically lifting 220 lbs (~100 kg) train tracks and laying them by hand. Each time I pushed down the new pathway, I felt a little stronger and the tracks a little lighter. I knew that change was required, it just took some time for my chemistry to catch up.

Eventually, the new pathway became my default. I expect the old pathway is still there, as I still have the memory of it, but there has been a definite change in direction with this and many other negative thought patterns. Overall, I have changed my mind about very many things, and this has resulted in less extreme reactions and a much happier existence.

Empowering Your Flower

Why is this relevant to empowering your flower? Not only because questioning your thoughts can help to bring your autonomic nervous system into a more balanced state, or because you will sleep better and have better digestion, or because changing your mind will help your body to heal and become stronger, or because building stronger muscles and adopting healthier life choices involve the same principles, or even because of the increased quality of life that will be the result of this change of mind. It is important because **I need you to change your mind.**

With one in three women experiencing some form of PFD in her lifetime, and with mesh surgery being offered as the first line of treatment, **we need to collectively change our minds**.

Regardless of your gender, race, or creed, you are living in a world that has a corrupt view over the female genitalia—where the vulva and vagina remain shrouded in taboo. We have all been subjected to conditioning that has passed on negative attitudes and beliefs about female sex organs and sexuality. It's been the accumulation of antipathy over millennia.

If enough people can change their minds and speak openly about these PFDs, it will help those who are currently suffering in silence. It will help to expose the dangers of mesh implants, empowering women to say no. The minds that change and voices that amplify these hidden issues will result in an emergence of something more—an accumulation that will result in the global empowerment of the female flower for generations to come.

Together we can and will make a difference.

Part two

Empower Your Flower
Nourish, develop, blossom and grow

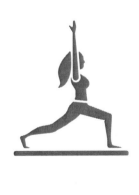

Overview of Part Two

By now you have joined the dots in the complex web of connectivity, which underlies your patterns and you realize that there are patterns at every turn.

As we begin with Part Two, we leave the theory behind and start the practical aspects of empowering the whole woman. Part Two shares the assessments, provides guidance on goal setting, and details the eight-phase training plan. The knowledge you have gained reading Part One provides the foundation and reasoning for the eight-phase training. It can be helpful to read through Part Two once before beginning the assessments. There are two chapters in Part Two:

Chapter Eight: Measuring your baseline

Chapter Eight takes you through the process of performing the baseline assessments, and guides you in setting goals and selecting the right phase for your pelvic floor. If this is a phase other than phase one, you should spend one week on each earlier phase before commencing your selected phase. This will ensure that your body and mind are also ready for the selected phase.

You can refer to this chapter to repeat the assessments when you reach the goal milestones at the predefined points in the training. These milestones align with the perceived level of difficulty of the training.

Chapter Nine: Eight-Phase Training Plan

Chapter Nine details the full eight-phase training program, stepping through the phases one at a time and detailing the modules for each phase, including the pelvic floor, breathing, movement, relaxation, and mind/meditation.

At the end of each phase, there is a progress checkpoint where you can reassess your progress. This checkpoint helps you to decide if you should progress, continue on your current phase, or regress. You will most likely spend multiple weeks on your selected phase as change in the body takes time and requires repetition.

In Part Three of this book, you will find the symptom management and life strategies chapter that can supplement the eight-phase training, as well as information on the different PFDs, including the medical and surgical treatments offered. You will also find details on the various healthcare professionals and therapists that you may call upon to support your rehabilitation.

Chapter Eight:
Measuring Your Baseline

Before we begin, I would like to issue a disclaimer; The information in this book should by no means be considered a substitute for the advice, guidance, and treatment of qualified medical professionals. This book provides information and details of exercises and activities that were used in my own rehabilitation, but you may require something different. All matters pertaining to your physical, emotional, and mental health should be supervised by a healthcare professional.

There are many conditions not covered in this book, which can impact the pelvic floor, such as interstitial cystitis (IC), endometriosis, fibromyalgia, Ehlers-Danlos syndrome (EDS), pelvic congestion syndrome, and polycystic ovary syndrome (PCOS). Other physiological, neurological, and mental conditions can also have a dramatic impact on your pelvic health, resulting in symptoms similar to those of PFD.

Some of the exercises in this book may not be suitable for you and can flare other conditions. I advise that you always work with a health professional to ensure any movement, relaxation exercise, symptom-management strategy, or lifestyle modification is right for you.

With all of that said, I want to emphasize that **you must take full responsibility for your own pelvic floor health**. Your pelvic floor physiotherapist will not perform your pelvic floor exercises for you. Your structural integrator will not change your daily movement patterns. Healthcare professionals and therapists help by offering guidance and treatment, but responsibility remains with you. Above all, I would like you to listen to your body and learn to adapt any practice you undertake based on what your body communicates.

It is important to find experts and specialists that you can trust, and for them to do an excellent job with the treatment that they provide. Whether that treatment is conservative or invasive; just remember that rehabilitation remains your responsibility. By taking responsibility, you empower yourself to make the changes needed.

The Search for a Root Cause

The root cause of PFD is not so easy to pinpoint, as there are so many factors that can impact your pelvic floor. You have learned in Part One that the body is complex, as is the mind. When you throw day-to-day living into the mix, there are endless possibilities that can impact your pelvic floor health.

The purpose of the eight-phase program for PFD set out in this book is to empower you to take control where you can, eliminating as many contributing factors as possible in order to improve your current situation, and thus improving your quality of life. You can review the program with your healthcare provider to ensure it is right for you.

When it comes to the risk factors for developing PFD, there are some over which we have *no control* such as:

1. **Aging**: Figure 4.1 showed how aging impacts our rate of protein synthesis. This natural drop in protein synthesis is a risk factor for developing PFD. This may contribute to the development of urinary incontinence, which affects almost 50% of women aged sixty-five and older[69,70]. We cannot stop ourselves from aging, but we can learn how to care for our bodies to limit the impact aging can have. I believe the exercises and activities in this part of the book will help limit the effects of aging.

2. **Hormone changes**: hormonal changes, particularly around menopause, can cause atrophy of vaginal tissues, which negatively impacts pelvic floor function. One study[71] found that 38% of post-menopausal women show symptoms of vaginal atrophy. We cannot stop the hormonal changes that are common with menopause, but we can try to stimulate the body to continue maintaining our tissues and to manage or reduce our symptoms. I believe the exercises and activities in this part of the book will help limit the effects of hormone changes.

And some over which we have some control:

3. **Childbirth**: Childbirth, whether natural or by cesarean section, increases the risk of developing PFD, due to excess strain on the pelvic floor, and trauma from tearing or episiotomies. Births never go according to plan but having a plan and being prepared for rehabilitation following birth, can help to limit the impact of childbirth. I believe the eight-phase training will help restore pelvic floor control following childbirth. *Note*: It is important to seek guidance from your healthcare provider before commencing any new exercise regime after birth.

4. **Obesity**: Your risk for developing PFD increases by 1% for every BMI point increase over twenty-five[72]. Managing your weight can help to reduce this risk. A combination of diet and exercise can help you maintain a healthy BMI. The diet and weight loss tips in Chapter Nine provide some

guidance but you should consider working with a nutritionist if you need to restore a healthy BMI.

5. **High impact sports**: Gymnastics, trampolining, running, and other high-impact sports place a lot of stress on the pelvic floor and as a result, 41% of female athletes experience the symptoms of stress incontinence[73]. You can reduce this risk by learning to manage intra-abdominal pressures and maintaining good pelvic floor health if you do undertake these sports. The eight-phase training shares the steps I used to reduce this risk.

And some risks are completely *within your control* such as:

6. **Smoking**: Smoking is a risk factor for PFD. One Norwegian study found that those who smoked twenty or more cigarettes per day were at a greater risk of developing urinary incontinence[74]. If you are a smoker who suffers from PFD, you should consider quitting. Not only will this help your pelvic floor, but it will also be beneficial for your overall health.

We can take certain steps to mitigate against many of these risks but most cannot be eliminated completely.

When it comes to pelvic floor surgeries, they also increase the risks of developing additional PFD symptoms, even when performed as a treatment for the condition. One study showed a ~30% risk that reoperation will be required following a single surgery for POP[75]. Every surgery adds scar tissue. Scar tissue does not have the same elasticity or tensegrity as normal tissues which can contribute to prolapse symptoms, something to consider if you are exploring surgery as a treatment option.

Regardless of where you find yourself, you can make changes to reduce or eliminate your symptoms. I urge you to try all possible measures to avoid surgery. If you conclude that surgery is your only option, I urge you to avoid surgery that uses any form of mesh. There are natural alternatives to mesh, which provide equal results with fewer complications[76]. These are detailed in Part Three of this book. **Mesh ruins lives, period**.

Do not let risk factors induce fear. Risk is just a potential. We are always moving either toward function or dysfunction. By empowering your flower, you have the potential to influence the direction in which you move, no matter your current status. Do not judge or criticize yourself when reviewing the results of your baseline assessments. Do not consider where you are right now to be *bad*. It simply is *what is*. A measure of what is real for you right now.

Before we begin the practical aspects of empowerment, I would like to explain that the eight-phase program detailed in this book covers the exercises and activities that I undertook in my own rehabilitation. It includes different styles of yoga, weight training, breathing exercises, relaxation exercises, and meditations. You might flick through the pages and immediately know that some of the exercises therein are not for you. For example, you may have no desire to ever stand on your head… that's OK. You can still undertake your own journey of empowerment while skipping the movements that are not right for your body. Seek the guidance of your healthcare professional before you begin.

The Road to Rehabilitation

When I initially documented my rehabilitation program, I wrote it up as a monthly plan with a breakdown week by week. When I reviewed this plan, I realized that my own recovery did not follow a weekly or monthly structure. It was more intuitive, based on me listening to the subtle messages from my body and adjusting my actions accordingly.

For this reason, the program is detailed in phases rather than weeks or months. Each module within each phase has a success metric defined, and at the end of each phase, there is a checkpoint to help you decide if you should progress or regress.

For me, rehabilitation did not happen in a short time following a straight line. I expect it will be the same for you. Figure 8.1 highlights the difference between the plan you may want and the actual path to empowerment, which is long and paved with obstacles.

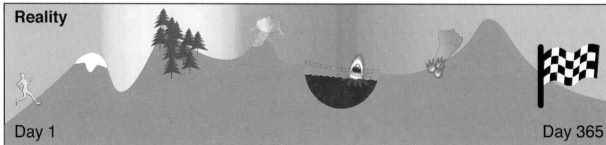

Figure 8.1: The journey to empowerment.

As you can see from Figure 8.1, the journey to empowerment is not a straight path. It is a long and treacherous path that leads to empowerment. It can often feel like you take two steps forward and one back. You are also not in the same place in your journey as me, or the person beside you. We are all working with a unique body in a unique environment with our own unique challenges.

When learning about the fundamentals of strength building in Chapter Two, I explained that this is a graded exposure system with the decision to *progress, continue at the same level, OR regress*, depending on how your body is responding. You can move as quickly or as slowly as your body allows. Using a phased, graded exposure approach makes it easy for you to regress if a new phase feels too difficult, allowing you to work within the confines of your own body. You will find out more about the levels of difficulty later in this chapter when we review the program structure.

The Importance of Showing Up

If you have ever practiced a regular physical activity, such as yoga or a team sport, you will be familiar with the feeling of having great energy for practice some days and no energy for practice on others. In yoga, we accept that feeling and know that showing up on the mat is what is important. Determination, dedication, and discipline will be needed.

I am asking you to show up for yourself each day and to remember that many small steps will result in an accumulation that will improve the quality of your life. Do a little, often, and you will succeed.

Establishing Your Starting Position

Before beginning any journey, you need to establish two things: your starting position and your destination. With that information, you can plan your journey. In the case of the journey to empower your flower, your current position will be established by performing several assessments. Your destination will be defined through goal-setting exercises.

Whereas it is unlikely that we can definitively identify the root cause of our issues through the assessments, we should be able to identify contributing factors. Our plan will eliminate or reduce as many contributing factors as possible while fitting in with normal daily life.

When setting goals, the approach will identify what is important for you from a quality-of-life perspective. Rather than setting a broad goal such as "eliminate incontinence," your goals should be to do things that your PFD is currently preventing such as "pick up my three-year-old without leaking" or "dance for an hour at my sister's wedding without feeling prolapse symptoms" or "have sex on my honeymoon without pain."

Once you have completed the assessments and goal-setting exercise, you will be guided on how to select your starting phase for training. Each phase is made up of five modules for the following topics: the pelvic floor, breathing, movement, relaxation, and mind/meditation, which you will work on concurrently.

The next section will provide more detail on how the eight-phase program modules are structured.

Program Overview and Structure

One of the most important aspects of any graded exposure system is the ability to both progress and regress. With the eight-phase program, the phases have been grouped by the perceived level of difficulty. Any increase in difficulty is aligned with progress milestones. You will be guided to set goals that align with each of these progress milestones. When you reach a progress milestone, you will repeat your baseline assessment to assess if you are ready to move to the next difficulty level. The levels of difficulty are shown in Figure 8.2.

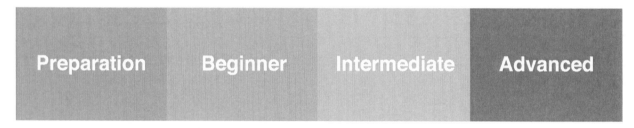

Figure 8.2: Levels of difficulty for the eight-phase program.

These levels in Figure 8.2 have been color-coded and are described below:

1. **Preparation**: Color-coded blue, this level could be considered ground zero. For example, this level is useful if you have lost the connection between your brain and your pelvic floor or if you are not used to physical activity. The purpose of this level is to prepare your body for active movement and activity and to begin the process of rebalancing tension through the body.

2. **Beginner**: Color-coded green, this level builds on the preparation level with exercises that are designed to build isolated strength using both push and pull exercises while accessing all planes of movement. There are three phases in this level. If you have never been physically active, this level may feel quite challenging. You may need to regress to spend more time at the preparation level if you find this level is too difficult.

3. **Intermediate**: Color-coded in orange, this level assumes a reasonable level of strength has been established at the beginner level. Onto this foundational strength, balance and functional movement are added to fire up co-contractions. Bodyweight is used to distribute load and tension into your

tissues. This level has two phases and teaches coordination between muscle groups, which will prepare your body for the more dynamic movements of the advanced level. You can regress to the beginner level if you feel you lack the strength for this level of training.

4. **Advanced**: Color-coded in red, this level assumes you are strong and that good load distribution through your body has been established. Onto this, we add directional forces and explosive movements to our pelvic floor training such as jumping, push and pull exercises. These exercises can feel substantially harder than those at the intermediate level. If you feel you lack the strength and coordination, you can spend more time at the intermediate level. When you have successfully completed the advanced level, you should have achieved all the goals you set for yourself, and will be in great shape to set new goals such as taking up a sport or just maintaining your optimized health.

Goals are set to coincide with the progress milestones which are marked in Figure 8.3.

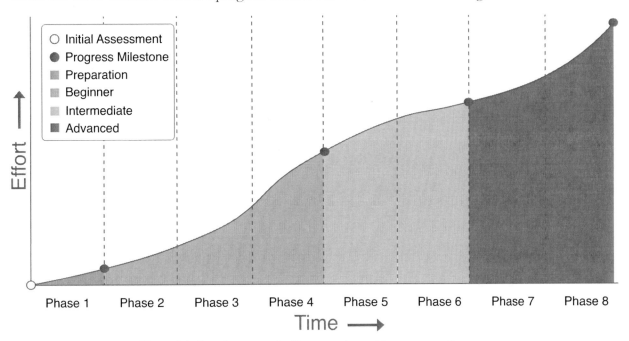

Figure 8.3: Development of effort over time with progress milestones.

Figure 8.3 plots effort on the Y-axis and time on the X-axis of the graph. The colored bars show the progressive increase in effort over time. The progress milestones are marked with a purple dot between each difficulty level. You will be guided on how to set your goals in line with these milestones.

When you reach each progress milestone, you will repeat your baseline assessments to review your progress. The level of effort and the amount of time it will take to complete the phases shown will be very much dependent on your own unique situation.

Table 8.1 lists the exercises that will be performed for each module and phase in the eight-phase training.

Eight-Phase Modules	Prep	Beginner			Intermediate		Advanced	
	Phase 1	Phase 2	Phase 3	Phase 4	Phase 5	Phase 6	Phase 7	Phase 8
Pelvic Floor	Kegel Breakdown	Full Kegel	Endurance Kegel	Speed Kegel	Co-Contract	Maximize Strength	Standing Rotations	Functional Training
Breathing	Nasal Breathing	Breath Strengthening	Breath Remapping	Nadi Shodhana	Basic Hypopressive Exercise	Intermediate Hypopressive Sequence	Advanced Hypopressive Sequence	Kapalabhati Breathing
Movement	Yoga Preparation	Yoga Basics	Core Re-tensioning	Rebalancing Yoga	Bandha Strength Yoga	Max Kegel Yoga	Ball Routine	Dynamic Power Yoga
Relaxation	Restorative Yoga	Yin Yoga Forward Folds	Yin Yoga Backward Bending	Yin Yoga Twists & Lateral Movement	Yin Yoga Hip Opening	Yin Yoga Pelvic Floor	Yin Yoga Happy Hips	Yin Yoga All Body
Mind & Meditation	Yoga Nidra	Flex your mind to flex your muscles	ANT therapy	Conquer your fear	Kirtan Kriya	Self Affirmations	Journaling	Blossoming Goddess

Table 8.1: Eight-phase modules.

The exercises shown in Table 8.1 will be detailed in Chapter Nine. The goal of this training is to rebalance both mind and body to increase your quality of life. Repetition is required to create change.

In addition to the eight-phase training, I would strongly recommend that you review Chapter Ten in Part Three, which provides information on symptom management and life strategies. The information in that chapter is specific to the symptoms of your PFD. For example, if you suffer from vaginismus, you will find information on how to use dilators. If you suffer from an overactive bladder, you will find information on bladder retraining. Not only will the strategies in Chapter Ten complement your training, but they will also increase your chances of success in your battle with PFD.

The Importance of Practicing a "Pelvic-floor-first" Approach

If you have PFD, it is important that you put your pelvic floor first with any physical training as to do otherwise could exacerbate your PFD. The focus of the eight-phase training is to use a pelvic-floor-first approach and, as such, the exercises in the breathing, movement, relaxation, and mind/meditation modules align with the pelvic floor module for each phase. Figure 8.4 is a visual representation of the progression of training with the pelvic floor modules.

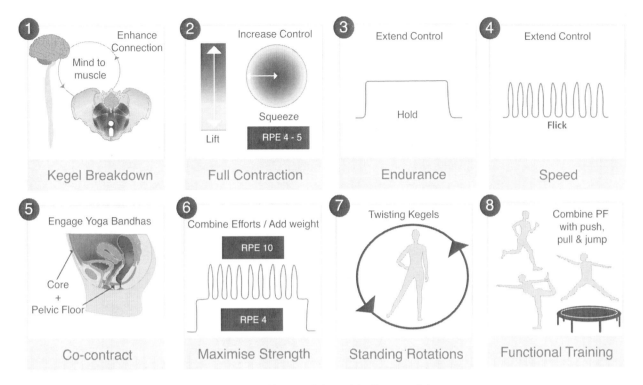

Figure 8.4: Phases of the pelvic floor module.

Figure 8.4 shows how the pelvic floor training progresses through the phases to support your return to an active lifestyle. This is pelvic floor strength training that should move you beyond the need to perform endless repetitions of Kegels.

If you are suffering from a non-relaxing variety of pelvic floor dysfunction (NR-PFD) such as chronic pelvic pain syndrome (CPPS), vaginismus, levator ani syndrome (LAS), or some other condition of hypertonicity, you *should not* undertake pelvic floor strength training (unless advised to do so by your healthcare provider). Instead, you will focus on reverse Kegels, which is a technique that teaches pelvic floor relaxation. Reverse Kegels are detailed in the Phase One pelvic floor module.

The breathing, movement, relaxation, and Mind/Meditation modules are designed to align with the pelvic floor training in each phase. These modules are relevant for both PFD and NR-PFD. However, if practicing NR-PFD, the movement module exercises will always be performed without actively contracting the pelvic floor. You will be reminded of this in each movement module.

For both PFD and NR-PFD, the goal of pelvic floor training is that you establish a balanced length-tension relationship through the pelvic floor and in relation to other muscle groups. This will ensure that the balance of tension and intra-abdominal pressures can be managed, and you can turn your focus to living an amazing life, where you use Kegels/reverse Kegels only when your body tells you they are needed.

The Importance of Consistency

You have seen how the program modules are structured, and I have emphasized the importance of consistency. To maintain consistency, you need to practice exercises regularly. If you were to practice just once per week, it would take an eternity to see progress. If you practice every day, you are more likely to see results. To help with consistency, I propose you follow a schedule like that shown in Table 8.2.

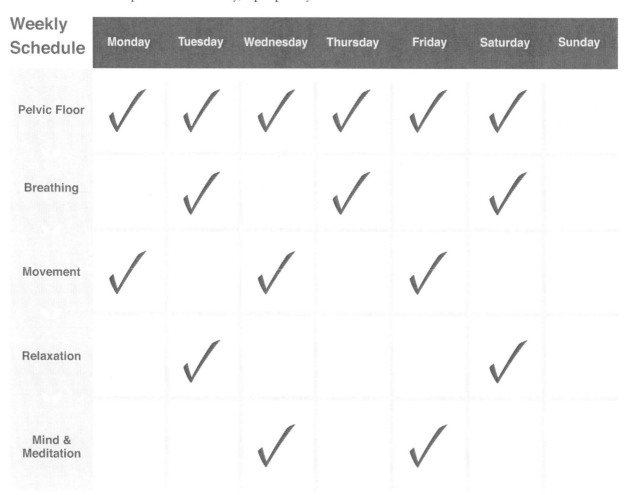

Weekly Schedule	Monday	Tuesday	Wednesday	Thursday	Friday	Saturday	Sunday
Pelvic Floor	✓	✓	✓	✓	✓	✓	
Breathing		✓		✓		✓	
Movement	✓		✓		✓		
Relaxation		✓				✓	
Mind & Meditation			✓		✓		

Table 8.2: Suggested weekly schedule.

As you can see from Table 8.2, I am suggesting that you practice your pelvic floor exercises six days per week, with breathing and movement exercises on three days, and, lastly, relaxation and mind/meditation exercises twice per week. If you suffer from NR-PFD, swap the frequency of the Movement and Relaxation modules (so it would be relaxation three times per week and movement twice). Each pelvic floor exercise session will take approximately five minutes to perform. The breathing, movement, and relaxation sessions will take an average of twenty-five minutes.

You should adapt the suggested schedule to fit within your normal week and it is OK to practice sessions together. For example, on Tuesday, you could practice the pelvic floor exercises, followed immediately by the breathing and relaxation exercises.

Success Comes With Consistent Steady Practice

Remember that success comes with consistent steady practice. You are working to create habits that will accumulate to create positive changes in your quality of life. Habits are formed by consistent repetition over time. Remember, it takes forty days to break an old habit, ninety days to gain a new habit, 120 days to become the habit, and 1000 days, to be the master of it.

You should practice a given phase until you feel it is habitual and your body has accumulated change from the practice. At the end of each phase, you will reach a checkpoint where you can review your progress against the success metric for each module. This will help you when deciding if you should progress to the next phase, remain on the current phase, or regress to an earlier phase.

When you reach a progress milestone, where you are moving to an increased level of difficulty, you can repeat the baseline assessments to reassess your status before deciding to progress. If you have not reached your goal for that level of difficulty or feel that you are not ready to take on a more difficult practice, you can take some extra time at your existing level. My coaching clients are great at listening to their bodies and I have seen many clients intuitively reintroduce an earlier exercise when they feel their body needs it.

Each exercise that you learn in the eight-phase training and the strategies that you adopt from Chapter Ten can be considered tools in your toolbox that you can utilize to manage or improve your PFD. These tools, once learned, will be with you for a lifetime.

You can continue to cycle through the phases until you have achieved the changes you were hoping for. You can always return to the program if you develop new symptoms or set a new goal that requires an increased level of activity if you feel that is needed.

It is important to remember that change happens slowly over time. It took me eighteen months to eliminate my incontinence after mesh removal. I had a few months symptom-free before my son brought home the pull-up bar that prompted me to work on building pelvic floor strength when pulling.

Change happened for me because I was consistent. If at any stage I felt that I had pushed ahead too soon or experienced a relapse in symptoms, I would regress to the previous stage and resume from there. The path from dysfunction to function is never a smooth straight line.

You should find an *accountability buddy* to help you to stay on track. If you don't have a partner or friend who can fulfill this role, just join the community at theflowerempowered.com or join our Facebook Support Group where you will find lots of support and encouragement. You can also ask me questions in these communities, and I will do my best to answer.

I have mentioned rehabilitation many times in the previous chapters. Rehabilitation assumes prior trauma or injury. However, you may well be reading this book from the standpoint of prevention or maintenance. For prevention and maintenance, you can perform the assessments and run through the relevant level of the program as desired.

Practical Activities

Before we begin with our assessments, you will need to be comfortable with your vulva and you need to understand how to properly perform the pelvic floor exercises. For this reason, we will begin with the following practical activities:

Activity 1: getting to know your vulva.
Activity 2: learning the steps to complete a pelvic floor exercise (Kegel).

You can perform Activity 2 directly after Activity 1 as you will be nice and relaxed and in a comfortable position to begin the steps to perform a pelvic floor exercise. I suggest waiting a day or two before proceeding with the assessments. This should ensure that you are rested and gives you some breathing space to get comfortable with performing these activities before undertaking the assessments.

Activity 1: Getting to Know Your Vulva

With this activity, you will get to know your vulva. It is imperative that you become intimately familiar with how your vulva looks and feels.

You will need a mirror, one that is big enough to allow you to explore the full glory of your female flower. I use the Tysnes mirror from IKEA shown in Figure 8.5.

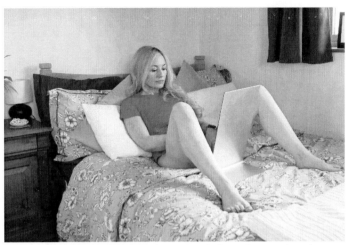

Figure 8.5: Tysnes mirror from IKEA for vulvar exploration.

As you can see in Figure 8.5, the mirror stands by itself which keeps the hands free for exploration. Good lighting will allow you to see every detail as you become familiar with your shape and form. Daylight is best but you can use a lamp or the torch on your smartphone for extra illumination if needed.

It is really important that you feel safe, relaxed, and comfortable when you are building a relationship with your genitalia. Negative emotions can trigger a stress response so, try to "set the scene" to bring yourself to a relaxed and positive state before you begin. This may include playing calming background music and placing soft pillows behind your back as I have in Figure 8.5.

The activity begins with exploration. The purpose of the activity is for you to become comfortable with looking at and exploring your vulva. You don't have to measure anything as you perform this activity, just try to find some love and acceptance for your female flower.

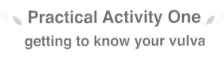

Practical Activity One
getting to know your vulva

➡ **Activity Steps** ⬅

1. Find a place in your home in which you can be completely comfortable and undisturbed.

2.   Take a few moments to relax before you begin to look. This is particularly important if you are feeling stressed about your PFD.

3.   Remove your underwear and lie back on the pillows.

4.   Close your eyes and think of your favorite place in the world. A place where you feel most at peace. Imagine that feeling of peace.

5.   Allow contentment to fill you.

6.   Take a deep inhalation for a count of four and follow that with a long slow exhalation for a count of eight (one breath cycle).

7.   Perform at least ten of these calming breath cycles. Breathing deeply and calmly has a soothing effect and can help to bring you into "rest and digest" mode.

8.   If you have low self-esteem, it can be helpful to repeat a positive mantra in your mind before you begin your exploration. My mantra is, "I embrace this wonderful body and the person I am." If this speaks to you, use it, otherwise, choose your own words to promote self-acceptance and self-love.

9.   When you feel completely relaxed, place your mirror in front of your flower and gaze at it with as much love as you can find in your heart.

10.   Using Figure 1.3 put on your engineering cap as you identify all the different parts of your vulva to get familiar with them.

Gazing at your vulva with as much love as you can find in your heart may sound airy-fairy and a little less like an engineer's view, but this is an important step toward changing negative beliefs if you have them. The idea is to swap negative emotions for positive ones.

These intimate moments, gazing at your vulva, form part of your relationship with yourself—the most important relationship in your life. You should know every crease and fold. Knowledge is power. The awareness of your physical form allows you to notice when anything changes, and this is paramount to maintaining your pelvic health.

The purpose of the "Getting to know your vulva" exercise is two-fold. Firstly, you should become familiar with it in order that you can notice changes. Problems often come with physical changes so noticing these changes may help you to catch issues early.

Secondly, you should use the activity as an opportunity to see the beauty of your flower. Remember that acceptance is key. You can only ever progress from where you are to where you can be. The first step should always be to see where you are. What is real for you right now at this very moment?

Maybe there is a lot of hair or just a little. Notice the color of your hair. Does it match the hair on your head or is it different? Maybe your hair is already turning gray or has begun falling out (common with menopause). Maybe you have very exaggerated labia minora or maybe they are small. The distance between the urethra, vaginal opening, and anus varies from person to person. Notice the unique features of your vulva. Notice any scarring, stretch marks, or discoloration. Notice if you have freckles or a birthmark. Notice and accept whatever you see. Accept it, embrace it, and love it!

Now that you have completed the exercise of looking down and becoming familiar with how everything looks, we will move on to the next activity—learning the steps to perform a pelvic floor exercise. The steps detailed in this activity will be used when you perform your assessments as well as when you perform your pelvic floor exercises so, you should use this activity as a learning exercise. The combination of all steps simultaneously performed equals a full Kegel.

Activity 2: Learning the Steps to Complete a Pelvic Floor Exercise (Kegel)

In this activity, you will learn how to properly perform a pelvic floor exercise. Knowing how to perform pelvic floor exercises correctly is important if we are to restore function. Before proceeding with the exercise, I would like to explain my approach to these exercises.

As discussed in Part One, pelvic floor exercises are known as Kegels because they are named after the doctor who identified the importance of exercising these muscles. Kegel exercises have traditionally been taught as a "squeeze and lift" of your pelvic floor muscles while relaxing the rest of the body and breathing normally.

In Chapter Two, you learned that there are different layers within the pelvic floor with each layer having multiple muscles. The traditional approach to creating a pelvic floor contraction is the equivalent of being able to move your hand as a whole rather than having motor control over each of your fingers. In yoga, we take a different approach to pelvic floor exercises and it is the yoga approach that I use.

In yoga, a pelvic floor contraction is viewed as an energetic lock known as *mula bandha* or "root lock." The purpose of the energetic lock is to support movement and control the internal flow of energy, which in biomechanical terms can be equated to controlling the pressure within the body's internal chambers (intra-abdominal pressure).

One of my favorite yoga teachers, Kino MacGregor, taught me how to properly activate mula bandha by building my pelvic floor contraction from six different elements. Unfortunately, I had already been implanted with mesh when she first explained this method to me, and I cried quietly to myself during that class, devastated that I had not learned this technique before the mesh had been implanted as that could have saved me a whole lot of pain.

Upon evaluation of the elements to create mula bandha, I realized that each element was activating different muscles within the pelvic floor. The combination of these six elements equals a single traditional Kegel exercise. The benefit of breaking the exercise down into these different elements is that we get to see which muscles (employees) within the pelvic floor are doing a proper job, while also getting a feeling for which employees are out on vacation.

Each element focuses on squeezing and lifting a specific area of the pelvic floor. We should try to bring our awareness and the center of contraction to the area on which we are focusing, while at the same time relaxing all other muscles and breathing normally. This is an important point as the contraction of the core, glutes, hip flexors, quads, or hamstrings will detract from the effect of performing these exercises in the early phases of training.

In yoga, we perform mula bandha with a co-contraction of the abdominals, which is known as *uddiyana bandha*. We will incorporate concurrent contraction of the core as part of the intermediate phase of training. For now, I would like you to simply focus on isolation exercises where the focus is solely on contracting your pelvic floor muscles.

Preparing for the Activity

Now that you understand the reasoning behind my approach to pelvic floor exercises, we will *run* through the *steps* to perform the activity. The instructions for the activity will detail the elements involved in creating a full pelvic floor muscle contraction.

The purpose of breaking the exercise down into these elements is two-fold. Firstly, to give you an insight into which parts of your pelvic floor are working, and, secondly, to enhance the mind-to-muscle connection between your brain and the different parts of your pelvic floor.

You will perform these steps reclined on pillows as per the previous activity. It can be useful to read through the activity steps before attempting the elements. You should perform this activity even if you have a hypertonic pelvic floor as it will give you valuable information needed when making your baseline assessments. Make sure to relax your body throughout the activity and do not hold your breath.

Practical Activity Two
Learning the steps to complete a pelvic floor exercise (Kegel)

➡ **Activity Steps** ⬅

Element 1: Draw front to back (pubic bone to tailbone)—Focus on bringing your pubic bone at the front and your tail bone at the back toward each other while lifting those muscles upward.

Element 2: Draw sitting bones toward each other (left ischium to right ischium)—Focus on bringing your left and right sitting bones toward each other while lifting those muscles upward.

Element 3: Close the urethral sphincter (hold your pee)—Focus on squeezing and lifting your external urethral sphincter. To put this more simply, pretend you are holding in your pee. You could also visualize trying to pick up a sesame seed with your urethral sphincter, or visualize pinching a balloon closed. You should feel the center of contraction on the front part of your pelvic floor as you do this.

Element 4: Close the anal sphincter (hold in a fart)—Focus the center of contraction on your anal sphincter with a squeeze and lift motion as though you are holding in a fart. Make sure not to squeeze your butt cheeks when you do this element. You could visualize trying to pick up a pea with your anal sphincter while keeping the center of contraction on the back part of your pelvic floor.

Element 5: Squeeze and lift your perineum (space between vagina and anus)—Focus on squeezing and lifting the space between your vagina and anus. This can be difficult if you've undergone an episiotomy or perineal repair surgery. It can be helpful to visualize sitting on a ball and imagine lifting your perineum away from the ball.

Element 6: Close and lift the vaginal opening (up toward the belly button)—Focus on closing the entry to your vagina while lifting the inside of your vagina upwards toward your belly button. For the lifting motion, try to feel a little higher up in your vagina when you lift (about 2 to 3 cm inside). There are lots of visualizations to help with this part. My favorite one is to imagine drinking a milkshake with your vagina, and sucking it up to your belly button.

Element 7: Simultaneously perform Elements 1 through 6—The combination of all six elements is classically known as a Kegel exercise. We will call this a Full Kegel, which is used in the pelvic floor module of Phase Two. If the combined exercise feels difficult at first, try to perform one element at a time, layering on the additional elements until you achieve a full Kegel. This is something that becomes easier as you increase awareness enhancing the mind-to-muscle connection.

Now that you have completed these two activities, you should have the knowledge needed to proceed with the assessments.

Assessments

In the upcoming pages, we will work through the assessments that are used for the initial baseline and progress milestones. The output of these assessments will be utilized to help you set goals and to select the relevant phase of training.

Assessment forms and tables are presented in this book. However, I suggest you download the Assessment PDF booklet from <u>empoweryourflower.com</u>. The PDF booklet is an editable document that can be completed digitally and saved to your computer. Alternatively, you can print the booklet for completion by hand.

The assessments in this stage include:
1. **Symptom Assessment**: Establishing your current status
2. **Symptom Flower**: Exploring what those symptoms prevent you from doing.
3. **Setting F-SMART Goals**: Mapping the road to success
4. **Pelvic Floor Assessment**: A detailed pelvic floor assessment in six stages:
    Stage 1: Visual assessment—where you watch the contractions.
    Stage 2: External touch—where you feel the contractions externally.
    Stage 3: Internal touch—where you feel the contractions internally.
    Stage 4: Endurance assessment—testing an endurance hold.
    Stage 5: Speed assessment—testing "quick flick" contractions.

Stage 6: Flexibility assessment—testing for tone and pain levels.

5. **Postural Assessment**: How do you stack up?
6. **Life Pattern Assessment**: What makes your shape?
7. **Mind Assessment**: Do you have balance in your mind?

You will use the information gathered in these assessments to set goals, select the relevant phase of training, and to help choose symptom management strategies from Chapter Ten.

Symptom Assessment—Establishing Your Current Status

If you are suffering from urinary incontinence or fecal incontinence, you can complete the Sandvik test to assess the severity of your incontinence. These tests can be found at theflowerempowered.com.

Urinary incontinence test: https://theflowerempowered.com/sandvik-test/
Fecal incontinence test: https://theflowerempowered.com/fecal-incontinence-severity-test/

Remember that you cannot manage what you do not measure, and the symptom assessment gives you a way to measure your symptoms. You will use this assessment sheet when selecting strategies for symptom management in Chapter Ten. You will use the symtpom management form shown in Figure 8.6 to track your symptoms.

Figure 8.6 is completed by checking the boxes against the symptoms you have for each condition (if they are relevant to you) and selecting the quality of life (QoL) impact for each condition. 1 is low impact and 10 is the highest impact. The symptom assessment can be shared with your healthcare professionals.

You can review definitions of the different types of incontinence and POP in Part Three of this book, however, you should not self-diagnose. It is best that you get an actual diagnosis from your doctor or pelvic floor physical therapist rather than self-diagnosing. The symptoms of PFD could relate to other conditions so potentially sinister causes should always be ruled out.

The names of some types of incontinence are interchangeable, such as overactive bladder (OAB) and urgency, which can both be experienced with or without urinary leakage. There are also other forms of incontinence, which are not listed on this assessment form, such as functional or reflex incontinence (neurogenic bladder). You can read more about those on theflowerempowered.com.

Symptom Assessment

Urinary Symptoms
Check all that apply

☐ Overactive Bladder / Urgency

☐ Stress Incontinence

☐ Mixed Incontinence

☐ Urinary Retention

☐ Self Catheterization required

Leakage Frequency
Select one (with urinary incontinence)

○ Never

○ Less than once per month

○ 1 to several times per month

○ 1 to several times per week

○ Every day and/or night

Leakage Volume
Select one (with urinary incontinence)

○ A few drops

○ A little

○ More

Quality of life (QoL) impact
With 1 being low impact and 10 being highest impact

1	2	3	4	5	6	7	8	9	10
○	○	○	○	○	○	○	○	○	○

Fecal symptoms
Check all that apply

☐ Uncontrollable Flatulence

☐ Fecal Incontinence

☐ Chronic Constipation

Leakage Frequency
Select one (with fecal incontinence)

○ Never

○ Less than once per month

○ 1 to several times per month

○ 1 to several times per week

○ Every day and/or night

Leakage Volume
Select one (with fecal incontinence)

○ Regular Skid-marks

○ A little

○ More

Quality of life (QoL) impact
With 1 being low impact and 10 being highest impact

1	2	3	4	5	6	7	8	9	10
○	○	○	○	○	○	○	○	○	○

POP Symptoms
Check all that apply

☐ Heaviness in vagina

☐ Dragging sensation

☐ "Golf ball" sensation

☐ Bulge from Vagina

☐ Back Pain

☐ Other (list below)

QoL impact
With 1 being low impact and 10 being highest impact

1 ○
2 ○
3 ○
4 ○
5 ○
6 ○
7 ○
8 ○
9 ○
10 ○

Pelvic Pain Symptoms
Check all that apply

☐ Chronic Pelvic Pain

☐ Vaginismus

☐ Bladder pain / spasms

☐ Anal Pain / spasms

☐ Painful sex / Dyspareunia

☐ Other (list below)

QoL impact
With 1 being low impact and 10 being highest impact

1 ○
2 ○
3 ○
4 ○
5 ○
6 ○
7 ○
8 ○
9 ○
10 ○

Figure 8.6: Symptom assessment sheet.

If you are suffering from POP, you should be aware that there are multiple types, which are measured using the POP-Q grading system that is shown in Figure 8.7.

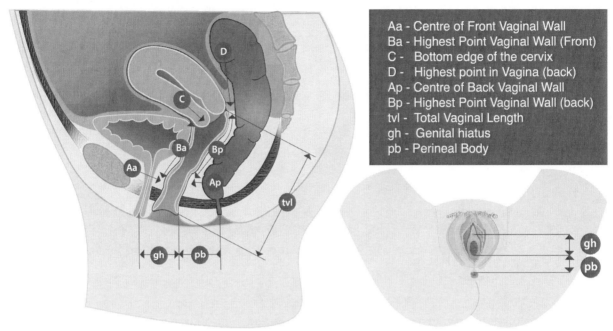

Figure 8.7: The POP-Q measuring system.

Figure 8.7 highlights different points of measurements with these measurements being used to grade the prolapse. The list to the right of Figure 8.7 details what the various letter codes are measuring. The measurement of POP grade should be performed by a gynecologist or pelvic floor physical therapist. Once again, you should not try to self-diagnose your grade.

Should you feel your symptoms getting worse at any time, you should *stop* and refrain from doing the movement that is triggering your symptoms. This advice relates to any form of training or increased loading (such as lifting heavy things at work).

If you are following the program in this book and experience an increase in symptoms, this could indicate that the exercises are not suitable. You should always train under the guidance of your healthcare provider or pelvic floor physical therapist (PT) and consult with them should symptoms persist or if new symptoms arise.

You must learn to listen and respond to the subtle language of your body, a body that is constantly changing and adapting to the loads which you place on it. Remember that your pelvic floor health is *your responsibility.*

Symptom Flower: Exploring What those Symptoms Prevent You from Doing

Look at your symptom assessment and ask yourself the question, "What are these symptoms preventing me from doing?". In May 2015, following mesh-removal surgery, mixed incontinence was by far my most irritating and embarrassing symptom. On many occasions, my whole bladder would just empty and there was nothing I could do to stop it. I lived just 400 meters from the local shopping mall. I would use the bathroom before leaving home and again in the mall.

Carrying the groceries back to the apartment would make me leak with every step. I couldn't understand where all the urine was coming from. I drank much less than normal and yet I was like a leaking cistern. It was horrible.

If I had asked myself, "What is this symptom preventing me from doing?" I would have responded, "Everything!" Therefore, I have created the symptom flower as it will help you to break this question down by the different aspects of your life.

The symptom flower exercise involves identifying how your most life-impacting symptoms relate to the different aspects of your life. Symptoms can have both positive or negative implications on different parts of your life. Capture the positive or negative impact of your most life-impacting symptoms and this should help to guide you on where to focus your goals when undertaking the goal-setting exercise.

We will assess your symptoms in relation to:

1. **Mind**: Your mind and thought patterns.
2. **Life**: Your lifestyle and life patterns.
3. **Pelvic floor**: Your pelvic floor muscles.
4. **Body**: Your body alignment and strength/weakness.
5. **Society**: The society in which you live.

As an example, I have included my symptom flower from May 2015, following mesh removal, which is shown in Figure 8.8.

You can see in Figure 8.8 how I completed the symptom flower activity by adding my most impactful symptom in the center of the flower and adding the impact of that symptom in the boxes for mind, life, pelvic floor, body, and society. I have shared this to show you how I interpreted the impact of my symptoms.

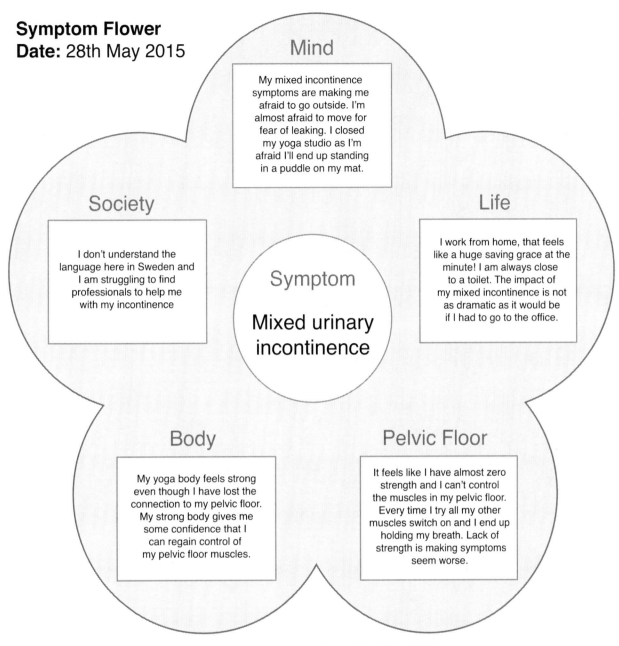

Symptom Flower
Date: 28th May 2015

Mind

My mixed incontinence symptoms are making me afraid to go outside. I'm almost afraid to move for fear of leaking. I closed my yoga studio as I'm afraid I'll end up standing in a puddle on my mat.

Society

I don't understand the language here in Sweden and I am struggling to find professionals to help me with my incontinence

Symptom

Mixed urinary incontinence

Life

I work from home, that feels like a huge saving grace at the minute! I am always close to a toilet. The impact of my mixed incontinence is not as dramatic as it would be if I had to go to the office.

Body

My yoga body feels strong even though I have lost the connection to my pelvic floor. My strong body gives me some confidence that I can regain control of my pelvic floor muscles.

Pelvic Floor

It feels like I have almost zero strength and I can't control the muscles in my pelvic floor. Every time I try all my other muscles switch on and I end up holding my breath. Lack of strength is making symptoms seem worse.

Figure 8.8: My symptom flower from May 2015.

Below are a few additional examples to give you some inspiration when completing your own symptom flower. Remember that these areas of life can relate to your symptoms in both positive and negative ways. They can even be neutral.

Society—The Society in Which You Live

For the society example, let's assume the symptom is incontinence. If you live in a society where it is taboo to talk about urinary dysfunction, this could prevent you from asking for help. You may feel embarrassed and alone, which could leave you suffering in silence, so in relation to the society in which you live, the symptom would be preventing you from seeking help.

Mind — Your Mind and Thought Patterns

For the mind example, let's also assume the symptom is incontinence. If you are positive in your thinking and have a "can-do" attitude, this can help you to stick to your goals and give you the power to believe that you can achieve them. In relation to your mind, therefore, your symptom may not be having a negative impact as you feel empowered to do something about it.

Perform the following activity to complete the symptom flower assessment.

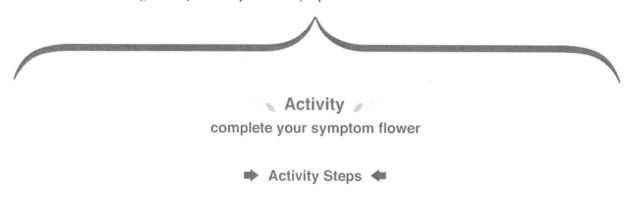

Activity
complete your symptom flower

➡ Activity Steps ⬅

1. Find a quiet place where you can complete the symptom flower uninterrupted.
2. Use the blank symptom flower form (Figure 8.9) to complete the exercise. Take your time while considering how the symptoms are impacting the different parts of your life.

Figure 8.9 shows the blank symptom flower. You will also find a blank symptom flower on page 2 of the assessment booklet. You will use your completed symptom flower assessment when setting goals for the program.

When I reviewed my symptom flower in May 2015, it became clear to me that my mixed incontinence was preventing me from living an active life. It was stopping me from going outside, and from teaching yoga without the fear of creating a puddle on my mat. This was negatively impacting my QoL and needed to change. It was also having a financial impact as I had closed my yoga studio due to fear of leaking while teaching.

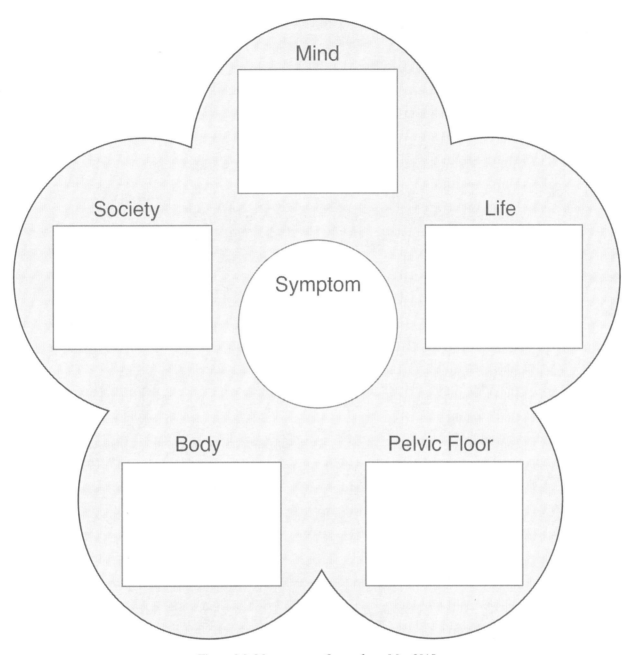

Figure 8.8: My symptom flower from May 2015.

Setting F-SMART Goals—Mapping the Road to Success

In business, we set goals that are SMART—**S**pecific, **M**easurable, **A**chievable, **R**ealistic, and **T**imely. When working with the pelvic floor, we need to set F-Smart goals. Maybe you are thinking "**F**ucking SMART goals," but, no... we need to have an end goal that is **F**unctional. *Functional* means it involves physical movement or activity.

Your goals should relate to a functional activity that your symptoms prevent you from doing. This will be something you wish to do again once you have alleviated or improved your symptoms, thus achieving an improved QoL. To help with this, look at your symptom flower to see what your current symptoms are preventing you from doing that you could do before.

In my case, I set myself the goal: *To teach a yoga class without leaking*. This goal is **F**unctional— involving physical movement or activity. It is **S**pecific—that I should teach a class without leaking. It is **M**easurable—In that, I was able to measure success by performing the physical activity without my symptoms (leaking). I believed my goal to be **A**chievable, even though at the time of setting the goal, it seemed momentous. The goal was something my current symptoms had been preventing me from doing, which I had previously been able to do.

I also believed my goal to be **R**ealistic. Had I set a goal of lifting a 10 kg weight with my vagina, that would have been very unrealistic!

To make it **T**imely, I had to put my engineering cap back on. I was very unsure how long it would take to reach my goal. I decided to break it down into smaller steps. To do this, I had to reverse engineer my goal. Figure 8.10 shows how I went about this reverse engineering.

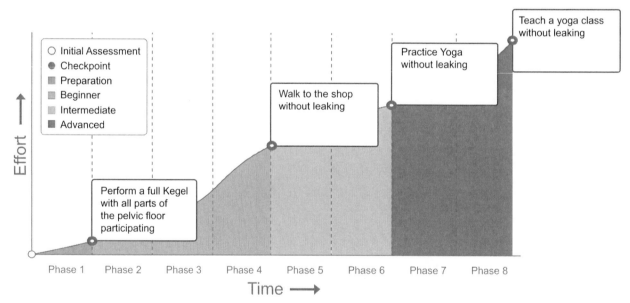

Figure 8.10: Reverse engineering my goal in 2015.

In Figure 8.10, I started by setting my end goal, *to teach a yoga class without leaking*, and then worked backward. If my end goal was to teach a yoga class without leaking, I would first need to be able to practice yoga without leaking. If I wanted to practice yoga without leaking, I would first need to be able to walk without leaking. If I wanted to be able to walk without leaking, I would need all my pelvic floor muscles to do their job when performing a full Kegel.

Remember, it takes forty days to create a habit. We will take advantage of that. Your end goal could take months or even years, but by breaking it down into multiple smaller achievable steps, you give yourself the chance to taste success sooner, which should propel you forward, helping you motivate yourself.

An Activity in Setting Your Goals

When you read through your symptom flower, consider which aspects of your life are most impacted by your symptoms. We will work on all aspects of your life in the program, but maybe there is an area that needs a little more focus. This symptom flower should help to determine where you should focus.

Goal-setting tip: you should choose a functional goal, which is something you used to be able to do that your symptoms are now preventing. If you used to run 10 km without leaking and you can no longer do that, your goal could be to get back to running 10 km without leaking. If you have never run 10 km, you shouldn't set that as a goal now, but you can subsequently make it a goal once you have achieved success with the empowerment program.

You will use the blank goal-setting reverse engineering graph in the assessment booklet on page 3 to set your goals. This is shown in Figure 8.11.

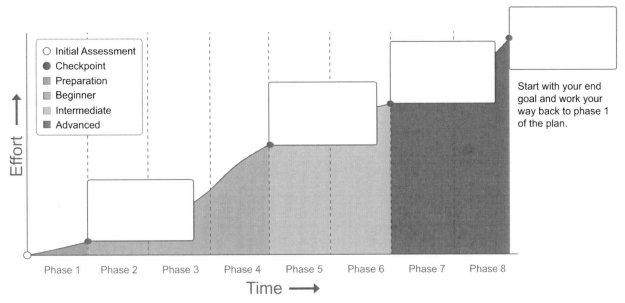

Figure 8.11: Blank goal-setting form for reverse engineering your goals.

As you can see in Figure 8.11, the goals are at the progress milestones at the end of each level of difficulty in the program. The activity steps below detail how to reverse engineer your goals.

Activity
Setting F-SMART Goals

➡ Activity Steps ⬅

1. **Identify your F-SMART end goal**: Your F-SMART end goal should be physically dynamic as you will strive to achieve it at the end of the advanced level. As an example, you could set the goal to run 10 km without leaking. Write your F-SMART goal in the furthest goal box from the left.

2. **Reverse engineer the previous step**: What do you need to be able to do before you can achieve that end goal? You will strive to achieve this goal at the end of the intermediate training so it should be reasonably challenging physically and/or mentally. As an example, if you want to be able to run 10 km without leaking, you will first need to be able to run 1 km without leaking. Bear in mind that this goal is at the intermediate level where you have been working on functional movement and co-contractions. You need to be physically fit to achieve this goal in preparation for the advanced level training. Write your goal in the third box from the left.

3. **Reverse engineer the previous step**: What do you need to be able to do before you can achieve the third goal? You will be striving to achieve this goal at the end of the beginner level so this should be something that fits well with the isolated exercises at this stage of the program. As an example, if you want to run 1 km without leaking, you will first need to be able to walk without leaking. Bear in mind that this goal is at the end of the beginner level where you have been working on isolated strength. You will need to be ready for the intermediate phase which is more physically demanding. Write your goal in the second box from the left.

4. **Reverse engineer the previous step**: What do you need to be able to do before you can achieve your second goal? As an example, if you want to walk without leaking, you will first need to be able to perform a proper pelvic floor exercise with all your pelvic floor muscles doing their job. You will be striving to achieve this goal at the

end of the preparation stage of the program. Bear in mind that this goal is generally a quicker win as it is at the end of the preparation phase which is simply preparing the body for active movement. Write that goal in the first box on the left.

It took just *two weeks* for me to reach my first goal of performing a full pelvic floor exercise with all muscles doing their jobs. Even though my pelvic floor was still weak, this success gave me the confidence and encouragement to continue my journey. I also found a workaround that would allow me to teach yoga again before fully regaining continence—I began teaching stand-up paddleboard (SUP) yoga. Teaching yoga on a paddleboard would often mean teaching with wet feet so, I was less worried about having a puddle on my mat!

Having completed your goal-setting exercise, you may be worried about having to figure out which phase of the training you should begin with. You don't have to figure it all out for yourself. The pelvic floor assessment in the next section will explain how you should select the correct phase of training for you to begin with. No matter where you find yourself, know that you can progress if you commit to giving yourself the grace of time to do so.

Remember that the most important relationship in your life is the one you have with yourself. Be prepared to nurture that relationship and to become intimately familiar with your female flower and how it relates to your life.

Consistent, slow, and steady progress will improve your chance of long-term success. Trying to push from zero to hero could leave you feeling defeated quickly. If you tend to give up easily, be aware of this and ask your accountability buddy to encourage you to stay on track.

Pelvic Floor Assessments—A Detailed Pelvic Floor Assessment in Six Stages

The pelvic floor assessments are quite detailed and require that you are comfortable with your vulva and understand how to perform pelvic floor exercises. Please make sure you have completed the practical activities in this chapter before you attempt to perform the pelvic floor assessments. Ideally, you will have completed the activities a few times, ensuring you are comfortable and familiar with them.

While we continue with this process of gathering data using the assessments, keep an open mind.

The information we are gathering is intended as a measurement of your current status. The first time you complete the assessment, it is establishing your baseline (where you are now). We will select the phase of training by reviewing the results of that baseline assessment. The training should then help you to reach your goals (where you want to be).

You can only manage what you measure, and although you can repeat the assessments at any time, I suggest you do it when you reach the progress milestones at the end of each difficulty level. You can then compare your new results to your baseline to see your progress.

If you are working with a healthcare professional, let them know you are undertaking these assessments and goal-setting exercises before starting. They are familiar with your specific body and will know if there are any exercises in the program that are not right for you. Remember that you are ultimately responsible for your pelvic health and as such, it is imperative that you are intimately aware of the current state of your pelvic floor.

You may be aware that there are various biofeedback devices that can be used to assess pelvic floor strength. I will provide details on these devices in Part Three, however, you should not use them yet as they often register co-contractions of other muscles. False-positive readings can leave you with a false sense of security and could potentially prevent you from reaching your goals; therefore, we will use manual assessments for this program using free biofeedback (your vision and touch). The steps used to perform manual assessments will be utilized in the first phase of training until you have gained good pelvic floor muscle control. You should be able to effectively isolate the different parts of your pelvic floor to perform the six elements of a Kegel without recruiting other muscles (such as abdominals and glutes).

When you perform the pelvic floor assessment, you need to score your contractions from 1 to 10 for each element of the exercise. The score is a combination of the pelvic floor's ability to both contract and lift. A contraction is the shortening of the muscle. The lift is the pulling upwards and inwards of the pelvic floor. The results are given using the following scale:

1. No contraction and no lift.
2. Very weak contraction with no lift.
3. Weak contraction with no lift.
4. Weak contraction with weak lift.
5. Moderate contraction weak lift.
6. Moderate contraction moderate lift.
7. Good contraction moderate lift.
8. Good contraction strong lift.
9. Strong contraction moderate lift.
10. Strong contraction strong lift.

To help visualize this scoring, imagine you are drinking a milkshake with your vagina, and take a look at Figure 8.12.

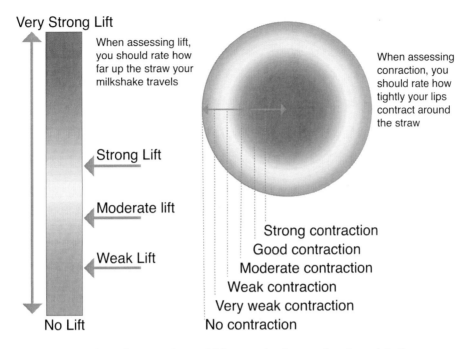

Figure 8.12: Visualization of contraction and lift strength when performing pelvic floor assessments.

Lift is visualized in the image on the left in Figure 8.12, where the level of lift would be how far up the straw the milkshake travels. A strong lift would bring the milkshake to the top of the straw (which would be your finger being pulled upwards when in your vagina in the assessment). The image on the right in Figure 8.12, visualizes how tightly your lips wrap around the straw, where a strong contraction would have the lips closing around the straw (which is a strong squeeze of your finger in the assessment).

The pelvic floor assessment will be performed in six stages:

Stage 1: Visual Assessment—where you watch the contractions.

Stage 2: External touch—where you feel the contractions externally.

Stage 3: Internal touch—where you feel the contractions internally.

Stage 4: Endurance Assessment—testing an endurance hold.

Stage 5: Speed Assessment—testing "quick flick" contractions.

Stage 6: Flexibility Assessment—testing for tone and pain levels.

You will record your results on page 4 of the assessment booklet, which is the form shown in Figure 8.13.

Visual Assessment

Exercise Elements	Score: No contraction (no lift) 1	Very weak contraction (no lift) 2	Weak contraction (no lift) 3	Weak contraction (weak lift) 4	Moderate contraction (weak lift) 5	Moderate contraction (moderate lift) 6	Good contraction (moderate lift) 7	Good contraction (good lift) 8	Strong contraction (good lift) 9	Strong contraction (strong lift) 10
1. Draw front to back										
2. Draw sitting bones together										
3. Hold in pee										
4. Hold in poop										
5. Lift perineum										
6. Close vaginal opening & lift										
7. Perform 1 - 6 simultaneously										

External Touch Assessment

Exercise Elements	Score: No contraction (no lift) 1	Very weak contraction (no lift) 2	Weak contraction (no lift) 3	Weak contraction (weak lift) 4	Moderate contraction (weak lift) 5	Moderate contraction (moderate lift) 6	Good contraction (moderate lift) 7	Good contraction (good lift) 8	Strong contraction (good lift) 9	Strong contraction (strong lift) 10
1. Draw front to back										
2. Draw sitting bones together										
3. Hold in pee										
4. Hold in poop										
5. Lift perineum										
6. Close vaginal opening & lift										
7. Perform 1 - 6 simultaneously										

Internal Touch Assessment

Exercise Elements	Score: No contraction (no lift) 1	Very weak contraction (no lift) 2	Weak contraction (no lift) 3	Weak contraction (weak lift) 4	Moderate contraction (weak lift) 5	Moderate contraction (moderate lift) 6	Good contraction (moderate lift) 7	Good contraction (good lift) 8	Strong contraction (good lift) 9	Strong contraction (strong lift) 10
1. Draw front to back										
2. Draw sitting bones together										
3. Hold in pee										
4. Hold in poop										
5. Lift perineum										
6. Close vaginal opening & lift										
7. Perform 1 - 6 simultaneously										

Endurance Kegel - slow twitch	Time (seconds)
Perform step 7 and hold for as long as possible	

Speed Kegel - fast twit	No. of contractions
Perform step 7 repeatedly for 30 seconds	

Figure 8.13: Pelvic floor assessment sheet

You can see that Figure 8.13 utilizes the Kegel elements that we learned in practical activity number two earlier in this chapter. The six stages of the pelvic floor assessment are detailed below:

Stage 1: Visual Assessment—Where You Watch the Contractions

Stage 1 is a visual pelvic floor assessment that you score based on what you see in the mirror. By scoring the different areas of the pelvic floor separately, we can help to identify if there are specific areas that are unresponsive. It may be that you have a strong contraction on the anal sphincter muscle and a weakness contracting the front of your pelvic floor.

It can also be that you bear down when trying to do these exercises, which can contribute to symptoms of stress incontinence. By doing this first visual assessment, you will get to see if your pelvic floor is moving away from the mirror (lifting = correct) or toward the mirror (bearing down = incorrect).

The results will be unique to you and will act both as a measure of progress and as a guide to where you should focus your efforts. You should make sure to wash your hands and have lubrication available if you need it.

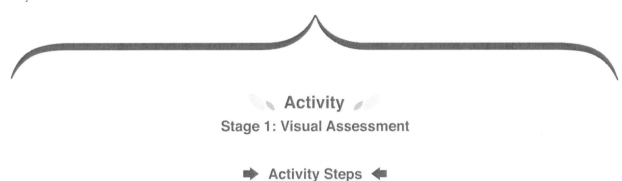

Activity
Stage 1: Visual Assessment

➡ Activity Steps ⬅

1.   Remove your underwear and prop yourself up on some pillows.
2.   Spread your legs and place the mirror in front of you so you can get a good view of your vulva.
3.   Perform ten calming breath cycles, where you count to four on the inhalation and eight on the exhalation. These breath cycles will help to relax your nervous system.
4.   Perform each element of the Kegel exercise while paying attention to the points below:
    a.   Relax your body and breathe normally.
    b.   Focus the center of your contraction on the area being contracted.
    c.   Try to lift the area being contacted while you are contracting.
    d.   Notice if your pelvic floor moves toward the mirror instead of away from the

mirror as this will indicate you are bearing down.

    e.   Notice if you are raising your eyebrows or making faces as you do your pelvic floor exercises as that would indicate that you are co-contracting those muscles along with your pelvic floor. The goal is to contract only your pelvic floor muscles while relaxing everything else.

5.   Record your scores in the visual assessment table.

Stage 2: External Touch—Where You Feel the Contractions Externally

Stage 2 is an external touch assessment. Sometimes the scores for this assessment may be better than the visual assessment due to the external touch bringing awareness to the area being contracted (enhancing the mind-to-muscle connection).

In Chapter Six, we learned that touch was used when mapping the pelvic organs to the brain. Touch helps to strengthen the mind-to-muscle connection as it helps to bring your awareness to the specific area you are trying to contract (which is a form of biofeedback). Remember this when performing the assessment. Bring awareness of your touch to that part of your pelvic floor in an attempt to enhance your contraction.

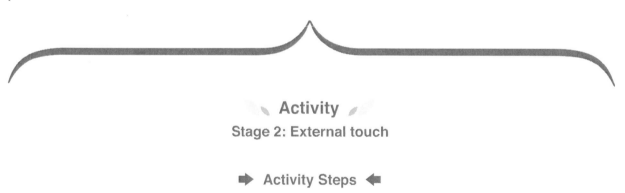

⭢ Activity ⭦
Stage 2: External touch

➡ Activity Steps ⬅

1.   Place your fingers over the area being contracted.

2.   Perform each element of the Kegel exercise up to element six while paying attention to the points below:

    a.   Relax your body and breathe normally.

    b.   Focus the center of your contraction on the area being contracted.

    c.   Try to lift the area being contracted while you are contracting.

3.   For element seven (full Kegel), place the heel of the hand that you write with just below

your pubic bone close to your clitoris. Allow your hand to relax on your vulva with your middle finger reaching back toward the tailbone.

4.   Record your scores in the external touch assessment table.

It is important to notice if your pelvic floor moves away from the touch of your hand or if you feel your pelvic floor is pressing into your hand as you contract. If you feel your pelvic floor pressing toward your hand, this is an indication that you are bearing down instead of lifting. If you find that you are unable to perform a contraction without bearing down, speak with your healthcare provider.

Stage 3: Internal Touch—Where You Feel the Contractions Internally

Stage 3 is an internal touch assessment. You will perform the same seven elements but instead of externally touching the area being contracted, you will place one or two fingers into your vagina while making the assessments.

If you suffer from vaginismus or another pain condition and are unable to put your finger in your vagina, you can use the scores from your external touch assessment for helping to select the level of training later in this chapter.

Please also be aware that an inability to perform the internal assessments due to pain is a clear sign that you should see a pelvic floor PT. You can find one from the specialist directory.

If you are proceeding with the internal touch assessment, your scores will be based on how much your pelvic floor squeezes and lifts your finger(s). You may need some lubricant if you suffer from vaginal dryness. I don't like to put anything on my skin that I wouldn't eat (as skin is permeable) so, I prefer to use organic cold-pressed coconut oil when I need lubrication. Remember to wash your hands before you begin, and again when finished.

➡ Activity Steps ◀

1.   Using a natural lubricant if needed (cold-pressed coconut oil), insert one or two fingers into your vagina.

2.   Perform each element of the Kegel exercise while paying attention to the points below:

    a.   Relax your body and breathe normally.

    b.   Focus the center of your contraction on the area being contracted.

    c.   Try to lift the area being contacted while you are contracting.

3.   Notice if your pelvic floor is pushing your finger out of your vagina or gripping it and pulling it upwards and inwards. If you feel that your vagina is trying to push your fingers out when you contract, this is an indication that you are bearing down.

4.   Record your scores in the internal touch assessment table.

The scores with the internal tests may be quite low if you have weakness around your perineum or in the deeper layers of the pelvic floor. Don't worry if you have low scores. You will work over the coming weeks and months to improve the function of your pelvic floor, and you should see these scores improve over time with consistent steady practice.

Stage 4: Endurance Assessment—Testing an Endurance Hold

Stage 4 is a pelvic floor endurance test, the purpose of which is to assess the function of the slow-twitch fibers of your pelvic floor. For this, you will perform a timed full Kegel. You can use your smartphone or a stopwatch to time the contraction, recording your result. The objective is to hold the contraction for as long as possible.

Activity
Stage 4: Endurance Assessment

➡ Activity Steps ⬅

1. Get your timer ready.
2. Start the timer at the same time as you begin your full Kegel while paying attention to the points below:
    a. Your contraction should be the strongest you can produce without co-contracting other muscles (such as glutes or core)
    b. Maintain a normal breathing rate while you hold the contraction.
3. Continue to hold your contraction for as long as you can.
4. Stop the timer when the strength of your contraction is significantly diminished.
5. Record the time in seconds for which you could hold your contraction in the endurance assessment table.

When I started my rehabilitation, I tended to lift my ribcage and tense my shoulders when trying the endurance hold. If you are doing this, stop, relax and try again. A true endurance contraction can be performed in a calm and centered state without co-contractions. Endurance takes time to build. I was shocked at how weak my contractions were when I first started. Practice makes perfect so know that you can increase your endurance in time with consistent steady practice.

Stage 5: Speed Assessment—Testing "Quick Flick" Contractions

Stage 5 is a pelvic floor speed assessment, the purpose of which is to assess the function of the fast-twitch fibers of your pelvic floor. You will need a stopwatch for this or use the stopwatch function on your smartphone.

Rather than trying to hold a full Kegel as you did in the endurance test, you will try to produce your strongest contraction, followed by complete relaxation, followed by contraction, then relaxation, etc., counting the number of contractions you can perform within a thirty-second period. The objective is to perform as many strong contractions as you possibly can in thirty seconds. Do this without panicking or using other parts of your body to assist you.

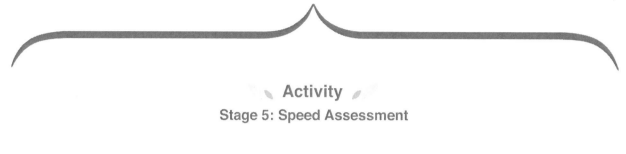

Activity
Stage 5: Speed Assessment

➡ Activity Steps ⬅

1. Put thirty seconds on your stopwatch and prepare to start.
2. Start the stopwatch at the same time as you begin your full Kegel while paying attention to the points below:
    a. You should contract as fast and hard as possible and then relax completely.
    b. Count each contraction.
    c. Repeat the strong contraction and relaxation in a "pulsed" way. Contract, relax, contract, relax, contract, relax etc.
    d. Maintain a normal breathing rate while you perform the exercise.
    e. Make sure not to co-contract other muscles while performing the exercise.
    f. Stop after thirty seconds.
3. Record the number of contractions you achieved in the speed assessment table.

You may have noticed that your pulse rate slowed toward the end and that you weren't able to achieve the same strength of contraction in the final seconds. This is normal when starting out. With consistent steady practice, you will be able to increase the number of pulses you can perform. I like to call these speed contractions quick flicks.

Ideally, you can achieve your strongest contraction and a complete relaxation with each quick flick. Training your pelvic floor to react strongly and quickly can help with the management of sudden changes in intra-abdominal pressure, which can help to reduce leaking due to stress incontinence. You will practice quick flicks in different positions during Phase 4 to increase the challenge.

Selecting your Pelvic Floor Training Module

Having completed your pelvic floor strength assessments, you can now choose which phase of training your pelvic floor is ready for. If your score dictates a phase other than phase 1, you should spend one week at each earlier phase until you arrive at the phase that your score has indicated. This ensures that your body and mind will also be ready for your selected phase.

Use the list below to select the training phase that aligns with your pelvic floor strength score from element 7 of your internal pelvic floor assessment (or the external pelvic floor assessment if the internal assessment was inaccessible for you):

1. If you scored **1 or 2**: You should focus on Preparation level training—Phase 1
2. If you scored **3 or 4**: You should focus on Beginner level training—Phase 2
3. If you scored **5 to 7**: You should focus on Intermediate level training—Phase 5
4. If you scored **8 to 10**: You should focus on Advanced level training—Phase 7

Regardless of which level has been identified here, make sure to begin with phase one and take one week practicing each phase until you reach the selected level.

Note: If you are suffering from NR-PFD, you will skip the pelvic floor strength training and replace it with the reverse Kegels module, which is detailed in the Phase 1 pelvic floor module. You will use the reverse Kegels module for all phases of training while working on the modules from the phase you selected from the list above.

The training is designed on the basic principles of *specificity* (you get better at what you do), *progressive overload* (to gain strength, you need to increase your load over time), and *reversibility* (if you stop increasing/maintaining strength, it will decrease). The system uses graded exposure, with each level of difficulty increasing the physical demands.

The exercises in the breathing, movement, relaxation, and mind/meditation modules are designed to match with the pelvic floor phase that you have selected. Of course, you can mix and match as you please, just make sure that **your pelvic floor comes first** regardless of what training modules you choose to do, and avoid exercises that trigger your symptoms.

Stage 6: Flexibility Assessment—Testing For Tone and Pain Levels

We will move on to an assessment of pelvic floor tone and pain levels. The purpose of the flexibility assessment is two-fold. Firstly, we are assessing the tone of the pelvic floor, looking for potentially hypertonic muscles. Secondly, we are assessing the pain levels within the pelvic floor muscles.

Before you begin, you should understand what to expect. The tissue on the inside of the vagina can feel lumpy and bumpy due to its many creases. It can also feel smooth. An average vagina is 3 or 4 inches deep and can expand by 200% during sex and childbirth[77]. Like a sock, your vagina isn't very big, until you put your foot in it (don't try to put your foot in your vagina). Your vagina is not your pelvic floor muscles. The vagina is a passage from the outside to the cervix (the opening into the womb).

It is important that you become familiar with how the inside of your vagina feels and understand how the vagina changes during the monthly cycle. Noticeable changes in types of mucus and cervical position are typical during the cycle. I tell you this not because I want you to check the position of your cervix but because I do not want you to panic if you happen to feel it. Figure 8.14 shows the change in cervical position during the menstrual cycle.

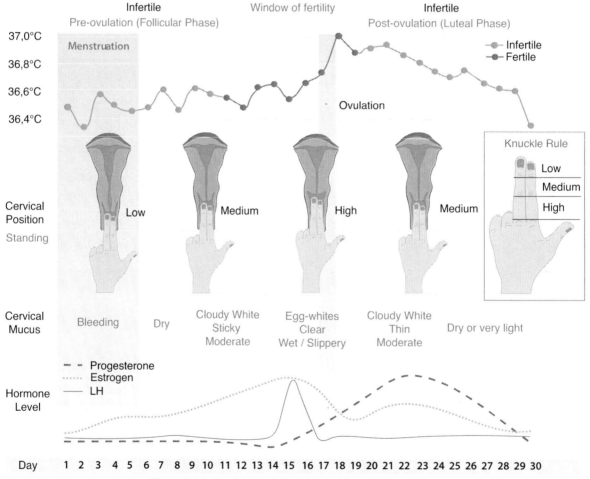

Figure 8.14: Cervical position changes during menstruation.

At the top of Figure 8.14, you can see an example of the basal body temperature variation during a normal cycle. Below that, you will see the fingers in the vagina showing the cervical position during the different phases of the cycle. Details on cervical mucus and hormone level are also shared in this figure.

I was frightened when I first felt my cervix as I thought my womb was prolapsing. Some prudent research and my fears were alleviated. As you can see from Figure 8.14, just before, during, and after menstruation, the cervix can sit much lower than normal. If you are trying to get pregnant using natural methods for family planning, then you may already be familiar with all of these measures.

Your body is constantly changing and adjusting to the pattern of your life. Awareness enables you to see progress and notice changes. Noticing changes may help catch potential issues or illnesses early. The Natural cycles app makes it easy to record the basal body temperature and allows you to track details such as mucus, cervical position, etc.

Assessing pelvic floor tone is typically performed by a pelvic floor physiotherapist. Unless you are a trained physiotherapist or manual therapist, you may not know what hypo- or hyper- tonic vaginal muscles feel like. I have devised a system, based on a well-known method used by chefs to check the cook on a steak. This is not an absolute measurement, but rather a way for you to gage and track flexibility.

Chefs assess how well a steak is cooked by how it feels. The softer the steak is to the touch, the less cooked it is, with a rare steak being softest and a very well-done steak being really hard. Steak is a muscle and so I figured the same system could be used when assessing muscle tone.

The method, shown in Figure 8.15 involves feeling the base of the thumb while holding the hand in one of five positions. Try each of the five positions:

1. Hand open and relaxed.
2. Thumb and index finger touching.
3. Thumb and middle finger touching.
4. Thumb and ring finger touching.
5. Thumb and pinky finger touching.

Relax your hand when you press the base of your thumb.

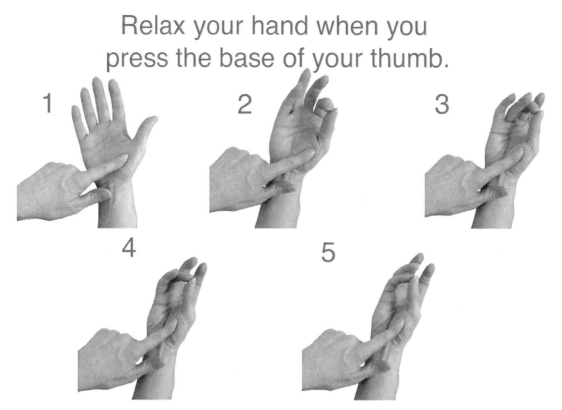

Figure 8.15: Flexibility assessment guide.

You will notice that the base of your thumb feels progressively firmer as you move from relaxed open hand to pinky finger touching thumb as shown in Figure 8.15.

When performing this assessment, you will compare how firm your pelvic floor feels in comparison to how the base of your thumb feels. Your score is simply a score from one to five where one is softest and five is firmest. Pain scores will be recorded assuming a scale where one is no pain and five is very painful. Press gently, as though you are checking the ripeness of a piece of fruit. If you are unable to put your finger in your vagina, you can feel externally from 3 pm to 9 pm and note the scores for both flexibility and pain. You should also make sure that you are assessed by a pelvic floor physiotherapist.

For the assessment, you will view the vulva as a clock as shown in Figure 8.16, which overlays the vulva with a clock where the clitoris is at 12 o'clock and the anus at 6 o'clock You will find this flexibility assessment clock on page 5 of the assessment booklet.

As always, wash your hands before you begin. I suggest you perform this assessment after your pelvic floor speed test as you will already be lying down with your mirror and lubricant (if needed) close at hand.

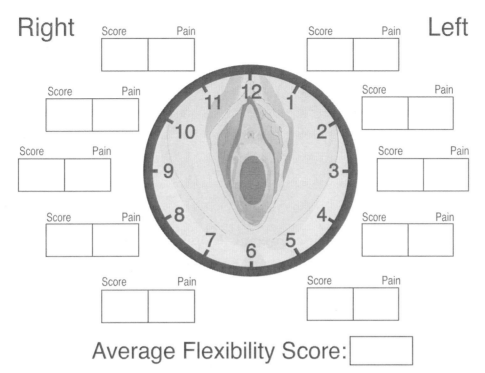

Right | Left

Score | Pain (×8 pairs of boxes arranged around the clock)

Average Flexibility Score:

Figure 8.16: Flexibility assessment vulva clock.

Activity
Stage 6: Flexibility Assessment

➡ Activity Steps ⬅

1. Lubricate your fingers with coconut oil or another type of lubricant.

2. Relax your pelvic floor completely and rest your head back as you prepare to begin.

3. Insert your finger into the vagina and, using gentle pressure similar to the pressure to check the ripeness of fruit, perform the following steps:

4. Feel the tissues under your finger beginning at noon on the clock. Note that your urethra and bladder are located in the noon direction and so this can feel a little more sensitive.

5. Keep your head relaxed back on the pillows and your pelvic floor relaxed as you move around the clock.

6. Note down your flexibility and pain score at each hour marker on the clock face in

Figure 8.16.

7.   When you reach 6 pm on the vulva clock, you are feeling the tissues of your perineum, pressing toward the rectum. Sometimes the perineal tissues will feel a little firmer (particularly if you have a thick perineal area).

8.   Continue around the clock until you have gone full circle.

9.   Record your scores on the relevant position in the flexibility assessment vulva clock.

Having completed your clock, calculate your **average flexibility assessment score**. To do this, sum your flexibility scores (by adding them together) and divide by twelve (the number of scores). Add your average flexibility score in the relevant box.

Remember that this *is your* baseline. You can't do it wrong. This is simply a method to assess how your pelvic floor muscles feel. By measuring with the same method each time, you have a useful comparison. If you notice anything unusual or if it feels painful to make this assessment, make an appointment with your pelvic floor PT.

We are going to use your average flexibility assessment score as a guide to identifying the potential hypertonicity of your pelvic floor. Hypertonic muscles are less likely to react to exercises and so we will need to focus on releasing tension around those muscles before adding in a lot of exercise. It's not that exercise is "bad" in this instance, it will just be less effective, and we want to be time-efficient.

When we talk about stretching the pelvic floor, we are not stretching the vagina. Stretching is a mechanism by which you can communicate with your nervous system by encouraging the release of muscular tension and protective tone, thus it plays an important role in the business of your body's movement.

There are many different types of stretching:

1.   **Active (static) stretching**: with active stretching, you assume a position that stretches some muscles, and you hold this position by tapping into the relationship with that muscle's antagonists. Yoga involves a lot of active stretching and will be a major part of the movement module.

2.   **Passive stretching**: with passive stretching, you assume a position that creates a stretch in your tissues, but you do not actively use muscles to hold you there. Yin yoga involves passive stretching. With yin yoga, the focus is on relaxing into your body's tension for three to five minutes. The target

is typically to stretch the connective tissue (fascia) as well as the muscles held in the fascial pockets. Yin yoga is a major part of the relaxation module.

3. **Isometric stretching**: With isometric stretching, you stretch a muscle while adding resistance. An example of this is stretching while hanging on a pull-up bar with weight hanging around your waist as shown in Figure 8.17. Don't worry, this exercise is not part of the eight-phase program. For me, this was part of my bodybuilding journey, which I undertook in 2019. I am sure you can tell by the look of my face in the mirror that this was not easy (I hung for over one minute with 22 lbs (~10 kg) around my waist).

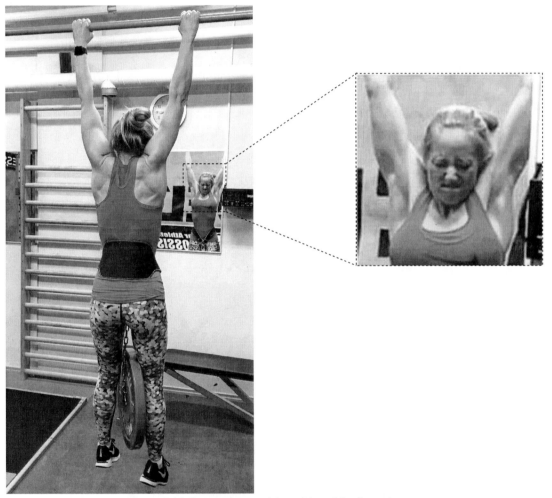

Figure 8.17: Isometric stretching with weight for resistance.

4. **Facilitated stretching (PNF)**: with facilitated stretching (e.g., PNF stands for proprioceptive neuromuscular facilitation), active or passive stretching is combined with some form of resistance (isometric stretching/counter contraction) to trigger additional relaxation of the muscle being stretched. This type of stretching utilizes the business of your body's movement by stimulating the department managers (Golgi tendon organs) to inhibit employees (muscles), making them relax

more as the antagonist engages. This is believed to increase the strength of muscle fibers closer to the tendon (where muscle connects to bone) thus increasing muscle stability. We will use this technique in the movement module, and as a symptom management strategy in Chapter Ten.

We will also utilize yoga stretches to move the bones onto which the pelvic floor is connected in order to ask the nervous system to release hypertonicity.

Confirming if You Should Work on Pelvic Floor Strength or Relaxation

The goal of pelvic floor training is to improve the length-tension relationship of the muscle tissues. For a hypotonic pelvic floor (weak), this will require pelvic floor strength training. For a hypotonic pelvic floor (tight), this will require pelvic floor relaxation exercises (reverse Kegels). We will use the pelvic floor flexibility assessment to confirm the type of pelvic floor training you should begin with.

If your average flexibility score was one to three, you will work on pelvic floor strength at your chosen phase. If your average flexibility score was four or five, you should replace the pelvic floor exercises from the relevant phase of your program with the reverse Kegels exercises in phase one of the training in Chapter Nine. You should also ensure to have your pelvic floor checked by a pelvic floor physiotherapist.

As you get better at strengthening/relaxing your pelvic floor, you should notice that it responds more efficiently when performing your pelvic floor assessment. This would be a good indication of an improved length-tension relationship within the pelvic floor.

That completes the pelvic floor assessments. We can now progress with our assessments of posture and life patterns.

Postural Assessment—How Do You Stack Up?

Assessment of posture is an art and proper body reading takes years to perfect. We are not attempting to make a full postural assessment, but rather to capture a snapshot of your current posture and to perform a basic alignment assessment.

You will need two photos: front-facing and side-facing. You can have someone help you take the photos, or you can take a short video and make screen captures from that video. The following instructions assume you are taking screen captures from a video on your smartphone.

Activity

Taking Photos or Video for Assessment

➡ Activity Steps ⬅

1. Make sure the room is brightly lit and that you place your smartphone with your front camera facing you in a position that is far enough away to get your head and feet in the shot.

2. Set the phone up either on a tripod or balanced in some way using books or other objects. I didn't own a tripod until very recently so, I have always improvised with whatever was to hand.

3. Make sure that the placement of your smartphone allows you to see your whole body from head to feet (which you will see as you are using the front-facing camera).

4. Capture your images using the following steps:

   a. Strip to your underwear and set the video recording.

   b. Stand with feet hip-distance apart with your body relaxed.

   c. Take five or six long deep breaths before turning sideways.

   d. Take five or six more long deep breaths.

   e. Stop the video recording.

Before getting dressed, you should check your video to ensure that you are in frame. You can do a retake if something is amiss.

Each time you repeat this assessment, make sure to take these photos at the same time of day, in similar lighting, with your camera in the same position, and wear the same underwear. This helps you to see differences that are not due to light, clothing, etc.

You can perform the assessment using:

a. **A printed photo:** Print out the image and use a ruler and pen to draw the relevant dots/lines. If you are using the digital assessment booklet, you can upload the photos into the booklet before printing, and then draw dots/lines on the printed version, or

b. **A digital photo**: Use any computer program that will allow you to draw straight lines. I used Microsoft Word for this purpose, but you can use any application that you have available to you. You can then upload the photos with dots/lines into the digital assessment booklet.

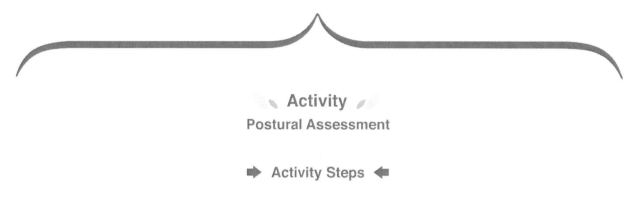

Activity
Postural Assessment

➡ **Activity Steps** ⬅

1.   Draw small circles on your images as per Figure 8.18 below.

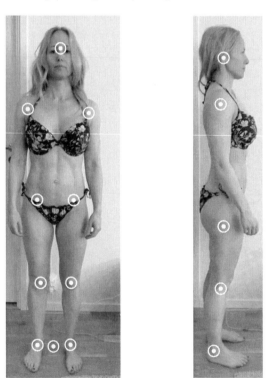

Figure 8.18: Posture assessment—Step 1.

The circles in Figure 8.18 mark the ankles, knees, hips, shoulders, and forehead between the eyes on the front-facing image. They mark the ankle, knee, hip, shoulder, and ear on the side-facing image.

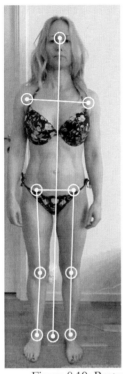
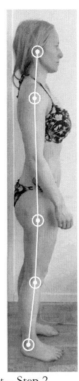

2. Connect these "dots" by drawing lines on your images as per Figure 8.19.

The lines in Figure 8.19 connect the ankles to knees to hips. The line from the forehead to the floor, left hip to right hip, and left shoulder to right shoulder on the front-facing image. The line connects ankle to knee to hip to shoulder to ear on the side-facing image.

Figure 8.19: Posture assessment—Step 2.

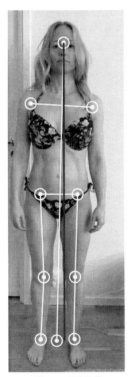
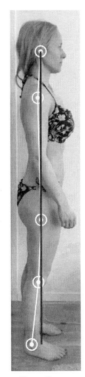

3. Lastly, draw a plumb line from the midpoint between the eyes to the floor between the feet on the front-facing image and from the ear to the floor on the side-facing image as per Figure 8.20.

This blue line, as shown in Figure 8.20, helps to highlight where the joints (circled) are in relation to this plumb line.

Figure 8.20: Posture assessment—Step 3.

Upon completion of this exercise, you have a snapshot of your current posture. This is a very simplistic posture analysis, which can help you to see misalignments, and it gives you a snapshot so, you can monitor changes as you progress through the program.

If you look at my completed assessment photos in Figure 8.20, you can see that I have some small misalignments. If you can see minor misalignments like this in your assessment, you can review the posture adaptations section of Chapter Ten (Symptom Management and Life Strategies), which includes suggested exercises and strategies to support the work you are doing through the eight-phase program.

If you find major misalignments in your assessment, you can work with an alignment specialist, such as a structural integrator, to have your alignment properly assessed and adjusted.

A typical structural integration program consists of twelve sessions, which are designed to assess and adjust the whole body. The structural integrator uses a massage technique that focuses on releasing connective tissue adhesions and getting the layers of connective tissue to slide and glide more efficiently. This can make a substantial difference to how your body feels due to the release of tension that happens with the treatment.

I underwent a program of structural integration, and, following my first session, which involved myofascial release throughout the body, my shoulders felt so free, it was amazing. I had not realized how much tension I carried in my shoulders. Since then, I have focused attention on relaxing my shoulders, particularly when working. I have used the posture adaptation strategies in Chapter Ten to help change my patterns while trying to maintain the adjustments made by the structural integrator.

It is important to know that structural integration sessions make adjustments to your connective tissue, however, failure to adjust the pattern of your daily life will allow your connective tissue to return to its normal adaptation.

With your posture assessment complete, we will now proceed with the life pattern assessment to identify the positions in which you spend the majority of your time (for example, sitting with a tucked pelvis). The only way to make a sustained change in your posture, following structural integration work, is to make a sustained change to your life pattern.

Life Pattern Assessment—What Makes Your Shape?

You might be wondering how you can know what to change with your life pattern. We will now conduct the life pattern assessment to see what sustains your shape. You will be guided on how to use this information in Chapter Ten when reviewing the Symptom Management and Life Strategies. This should help you to gage what changes should be undertaken.

Given that most people work five days per week, we will assess your life pattern by focusing on an average working day. This is not an exact science. The idea is to understand your movement pattern for a normal day thus gaining an understanding of the major contributors to the creation of your shape.

For example, if you spend most of your day sitting in the same position, this will likely be reflected in reduced hip mobility. With this knowledge to hand, you can make a conscious effort to vary your sitting position throughout the day which will improve your patterns over time, and this will be reflected in your posture and should contribute to increased hip mobility.

You may remember the example of my software engineering life pattern, which we viewed in Figure 4.8. I spent most of my day sitting with a tucked pelvis. Whether driving, sitting at the office, or slouching at home on the sofa. I always walked in heels. It is blatantly obvious that I was spending too much of my time sitting (with my pelvis tucked). It was easy to see when viewing Figure 4.8 that my pattern needed to change.

Figure 8.21 shows my life pattern assessment for a typical working day during that period of my life as a software engineer.

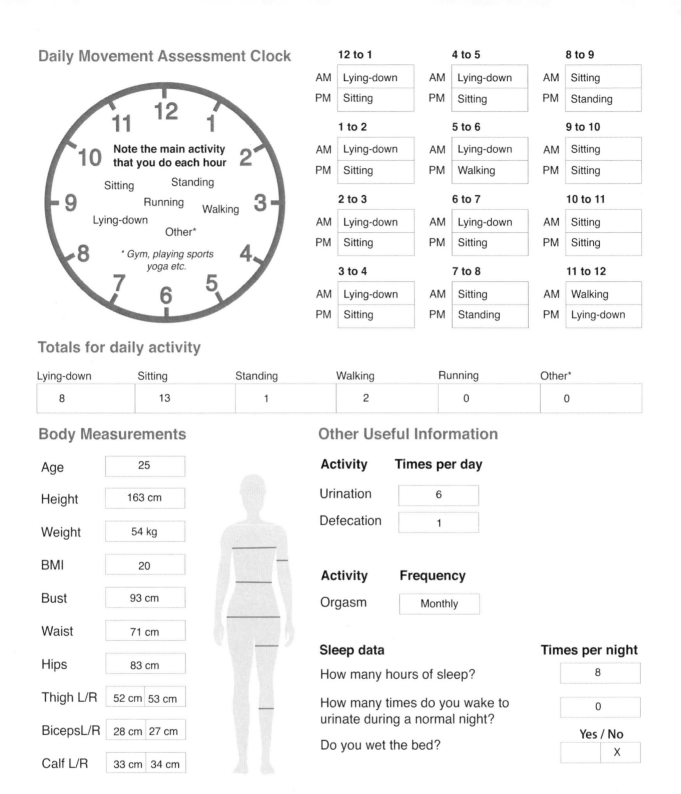

Daily Movement Assessment Clock

Note the main activity that you do each hour

Sitting · Standing · Running · Walking · Lying-down · Other*

* Gym, playing sports yoga etc.

	12 to 1		4 to 5		8 to 9
AM	Lying-down	AM	Lying-down	AM	Sitting
PM	Sitting	PM	Sitting	PM	Standing

	1 to 2		5 to 6		9 to 10
AM	Lying-down	AM	Lying-down	AM	Sitting
PM	Sitting	PM	Walking	PM	Sitting

	2 to 3		6 to 7		10 to 11
AM	Lying-down	AM	Lying-down	AM	Sitting
PM	Sitting	PM	Sitting	PM	Sitting

	3 to 4		7 to 8		11 to 12
AM	Lying-down	AM	Sitting	AM	Walking
PM	Sitting	PM	Standing	PM	Lying-down

Totals for daily activity

Lying-down	Sitting	Standing	Walking	Running	Other*
8	13	1	2	0	0

Body Measurements

Age	25
Height	163 cm
Weight	54 kg
BMI	20
Bust	93 cm
Waist	71 cm
Hips	83 cm
Thigh L/R	52 cm / 53 cm
Biceps L/R	28 cm / 27 cm
Calf L/R	33 cm / 34 cm

Other Useful Information

Activity	Times per day
Urination	6
Defecation	1

Activity	Frequency
Orgasm	Monthly

Sleep data

	Times per night
How many hours of sleep?	8
How many times do you wake to urinate during a normal night?	0
Do you wet the bed?	Yes / No — X

Figure 8.21: Completed life pattern assessment from software engineering days.

204

As you can see in Figure 8.21, I spent thirteen hours per day sitting. That is 75% of my waking hours. At that time (circa. 2001), when I realized that I was not moving sufficiently, I signed up to do my first marathon. That was the start of an exceptionally long journey into fitness. My current daily life pattern is highly active. Not only do I exercise for at least one hour per day, but I also walk at least 10 k steps every day, and I alternate time at my desk between sitting and standing (thanks to my adjustable desk).

Assess Your Life Pattern

Having seen the example from my software engineering days, you will perform your own daily life pattern analysis. You will then utilize this assessment in the self care section of Chapter Ten when choosing which exercises and strategies to implement. The changes you implement should have a positive impact on your posture.

You will need to use the form shown in Figure 8.22 for this activity. You will find a blank version of this form on page 7 of the assessment booklet. The PDF version is editable with a drop-down for the daily activity times, making it easier for you to complete.

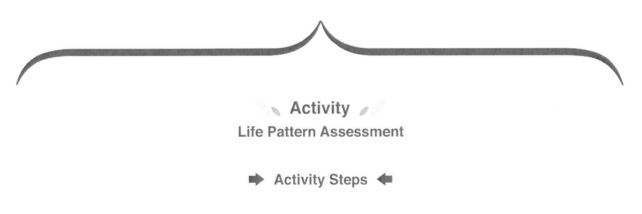

Activity
Life Pattern Assessment

➡ **Activity Steps** ⬅

1.   Fill in all the values.
2.   Count the number of hours for each activity and add it to the "Totals" box for hourly activities.

The outcome of this exercise will provide you with an overview of the level of activity you have over a normal day.

Daily Movement Assessment Clock

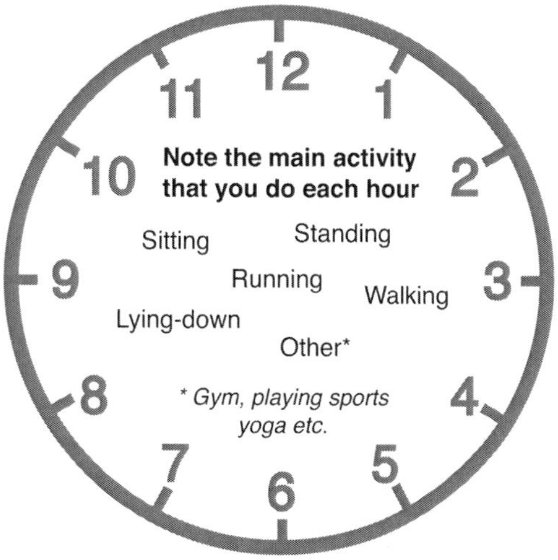

Note the main activity that you do each hour

Sitting
Standing
Running
Walking
Lying-down
Other*

* Gym, playing sports yoga etc.

	12 to 1		4 to 5		8 to 9
AM		AM		AM	
PM		PM		PM	

	1 to 2		5 to 6		9 to 10
AM		AM		AM	
PM		PM		PM	

	2 to 3		6 to 7		10 to 11
AM		AM		AM	
PM		PM		PM	

	3 to 4		7 to 8		11 to 12
AM		AM		AM	
PM		PM		PM	

Totals for daily activity

Lying-down	Sitting	Standing	Walking	Running	Other*

Body Measurements

Age

Height

Weight

BMI

Bust

Waist

Hips

Thigh L/R

Biceps L/R

Calf L/R

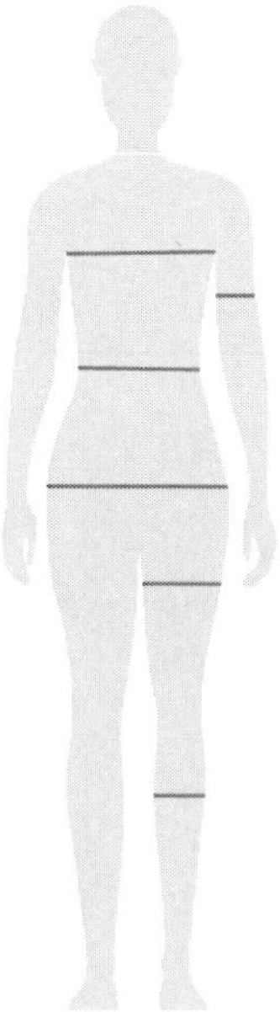

Other Useful Information

Activity	Times per day
Urination	
Defecation	

Activity	Frequency
Orgasm	

Sleep data

How many hours of sleep?

How many times do you wake to urinate during a normal night?

Do you wet the bed?

Times per night

Yes / No

Figure 8.22: Blank life pattern assessment form.

As you can see from Figure 8.22, the activities listed include sitting, standing, walking, running, lying down, and other. If you exercise once or more per week, or perform some other activity on a daily basis, you should include this as "other."

Along with your daily life pattern, I would like you to record your body measurements and some basic info on your urination, defecation, and frequency of orgasms. As you review your progress at the progress milestones, these values could change and so it is worth taking note for tracking purposes (remember you cannot manage what you don't measure!).

When you are reviewing the self-care section in Chapter Ten, this assessment can help you to choose the exercises and strategies you should implement to support your empowerment. That completes your life pattern assessment, leaving one remaining assessment for the mind.

Mind Assessment—Do You Have Balance in Your Mind?

The final assessment is a brain health assessment. The purpose of the assessment is to get a snapshot of the state of your mind. This is important as what you think can impact what manifests in your body. Your mental health can negatively impact your pelvic floor so, identifying and addressing any imbalances in the mind can support your empowerment.

The assessment is available free of charge on mybrainfitlife.com, compliments of Dr. Daniel Amen. Don't worry, you are not obliged to subscribe to the website in order to get your results, although I do highly recommend* this site as I benefited greatly from using it during my own empowerment journey.
* I have no affiliation to Dr. AMEN or Amen Clinics, Inc.

When I first performed the assessment, it showed I had a lot of anxiety and was out of balance. I used ANT therapy, meditation, and journaling to help rebalance my mind and made great improvements in my mental health and general outlook on life. The mind/meditation modules include these activities and more to help you find balance if needed. Figure 8.23 shows my recent brain health results, which scores brain health, sleep, memory, executive function, inner peace, mood, and flexible thinking. This test categorizes your brain health into one of sixteen possible types. When you have completed the assessment, take a screenshot or print your results.

If your results indicate a low score for any of the categories, the exercises in the mind/meditation module should help to bring things back in balance. When you review the self-care section of Chapter Ten, you will use the results of this exercise to help you select additional strategies to support your

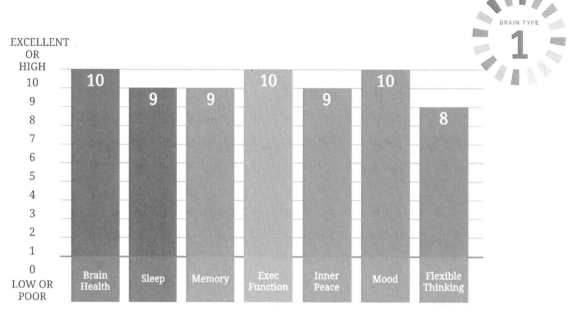

Figure 8.23: Brain health results.

empowerment. When you retake the assessment upon reaching the progress milestones, you can compare your new results to your baseline which will allow you to see your progress. That completes the final assessment.

Preparing to Begin Your Eight-Phase Training

The assessments are now complete, and your training phase has been chosen. The eight phases of training are detailed in Chapter Nine. Before beginning with training, I suggest you read through both Chapter Nine and Chapter Ten. These chapters provide full details of the eight-phase training and the symptom management and life strategies.

You will need your completed assessments to help you select relevant strategies and activities from Chapter Ten to support your empowerment. You can review the plan and strategies with your healthcare provider before you begin training.

When you create your weekly schedule at the beginning of the next chapter, make sure that it easily fits within a normal week. As you work through the training, please remember that each body is unique. You should listen to your body as you practice whilst avoiding movements that trigger your symptoms.

Remember that empowerment is a marathon and not a sprint. Give yourself the grace of time to improve and make sure you are consistent with your efforts. *Good luck*!

Chapter Nine:
Eight-Phase Training Program

In the previous chapter, you have completed your assessments and selected the phase of training to begin your empowerment program. This chapter details the entire eight-phase training program from Phase 1 (preparation level) to Phase 8 (advanced level). You should read through the training plan and fully read Chapter Ten before you begin your training.

Within each phase, you will find the modules for that phase. These are pelvic floor, breathing, movement, relaxation, and mind/meditation. Each module outlines an objective, a success metric, expected session duration, equipment needed, additional notes, and step-by-step instructions to perform the exercise(s). Pictures are provided for many of the physical exercises, and you can download yoga sequence sheets from empoweryourflower.com for all yoga flows. These can be placed at the top of your mat to guide you as you practice.

Remember that consistency is required to achieve your goals. Before you begin training, you will create a weekly schedule. In the first phase, you will practice your pelvic floor exercises six days per week with breathing and movement exercises on 3 days, and lastly, relaxation and mind/meditation exercises twice per week. If you suffer from NR-PFD, swap the frequency of movement and relaxation phases (so relaxation three times per week and movement twice).

Phase Checkpoints and Progress Milestones

At the end of each phase, you will find a phase checkpoint. This is a checklist that helps you to assess your progress against the success metrics for each module in that phase. The phase checkpoint can be reviewed at the end of each week to help you decide if you should continue at your current phase of training or progress/regress to an earlier or later phase.

At the end of phases one, four, six, and eight, you will reach a progress milestone, which will be highlighted in the phase checkpoint. This is a prompt for you to retake your initial assessments and check against your original goal. Of course, you can retake the initial assessments at any time but doing them weekly would be the equivalent of stepping on the scale every day when you are trying to lose weight... it's more likely to dishearten you than to encourage you to continue. Change in the body requires both time and consistency so, I advise that you wait for the progress milestones to retake assessments.

Adding Symptom Management and Life Strategies

This eight-phase training includes pelvic floor, breathing, movement, relaxation, and mind/meditation exercises. Combining these exercises is a more holistic approach to your empowerment. This will help to ensure your success. In addition to this, you should review the symptom management and life strategies in Chapter Ten. When reading Chapter Ten, you will be prompted in each section to use your assessments to help you decide if any of the exercises, tips, and strategies listed there could be helpful for you. You can choose what to add based on your specific symptoms.

Unlike the structured schedule for our eight-phase training, the symptom management and life strategies are not on a specific schedule but rather to be applied as needed. Please read through Chapter Ten and choose just one or two things to implement, to begin with. If you try to do everything at once, you may overwhelm yourself. Remember that you are taking the grace of time to empower yourself.

Cautionary Note Before You Begin Training

You should review your training plan with your healthcare professional before you begin training to ensure that it is right for you. Additionally, if you have recently given birth or undergone pelvic surgery, please get the all-clear from your pelvic floor specialist or doctor before doing any physical exercises.

Preparing Your Weekly Schedule

You can use the blank schedule in Table 9.1 to plan your weekly schedule. The pelvic floor sessions should take five to ten minutes and can be combined with other training modules to make the program more time-efficient.

If you choose to combine movement and relaxation sessions when completing your schedule, I suggest that, if your practice is scheduled in the morning, practice relaxation first followed by movement. This will ensure you end your practice energized to face the day. If practicing in the evening, practice movement first followed by relaxation. This will ensure you end your practice relaxed and ready for sleep.

Weekly Schedule	Monday	Tuesday	Wednesday	Thursday	Friday	Saturday	Sunday
Pelvic Floor							
Breathing							
Movement							
Relaxation							
Mind & Meditation							

Table 9.1: Blank weekly schedule.

It can be useful to print out your weekly schedule and put it somewhere visible (fridge door) or create events in your calendar to remind you. You can also share your schedule with your accountability buddy to help keep you on track. A blank weekly schedule can be downloaded from empoweryourflower.com.

Beginning Your Training

Once the schedule is complete and you have read through the remainder of the book, come back to this point to begin your training. This section details each phase and all its modules, beginning with Phase One. Skip to the phase you are on and read through the module details before each practice. You will be repeating the various modules on the days you have defined in your schedule (e.g., pelvic floor module exercises will be repeated six days per week). Repetition creates patterns and your mind, body, and nervous system will learn from those patterns.

For the yoga sequences (all movement and relaxation modules and the advanced breathing modules), you can download sequence sheets, which you can print to help guide you through your practice. You should print them out before you start training so, you have them to hand and place the relevant sheet at the top of your mat before you practice. You also have the option of purchasing a video version of the eight-phase training if you would prefer a guided practice. A link to the video course can be found at empoweryourflower.com.

You will find as the weeks pass that the repetition of these sequences will be committed to memory so you can eventually flow through them without having to look at the sequence sheet. The time it takes for each practice will be longer when you begin, but once your practice is established, you will get through the session in the alloted 25 or 30 minutes.

You should also check what equipment is needed for each phase and have the equipment to hand before you begin your training. This will help ensure your success.

Listen to your body as you go through the training. Bear in mind that any program to strengthen the body will create muscle aches and tiredness so, make sure to take a rest day if you feel you need it. The choice to progress or regress is very much dependent on how your body feels. If in doubt at any point, consult with your healthcare provider. Enjoy your training!

Eight-Phase Training Program
The training section begins here. It covers phases one through eight and the associated phase checkpoints and progress milestones.

If your assessment had dictated a starting phase other than phase one, please spend one week at each phase from phase one to your selected phase before you proceed with your selected phase. This will ensure that your body and mind are also read for your selected phase.

Phase 1
Preparation Level

Welcome to Phase 1 of the eight-phase training program. This is the only phase at the preparation level. The exercise modules are highlighted in Figure 9.1.1.

Eight-Phase Modules	Prep	Beginner			Intermediate		Advanced	
	Phase 1	Phase 2	Phase 3	Phase 4	Phase 5	Phase 6	Phase 7	Phase 8
Pelvic Floor	Kegel Breakdown	Full Kegel	Endurance Kegel	Speed Kegel	Co-Contract	Maximize Strength	Standing Rotations	Functional Training
Breathing	Nasal Breathing	Breath Strengthening	Breath Remapping	Nadi Shodhana	Basic Hypopressive Exercise	Intermediate Hypopressive Sequence	Advanced Hypopressive Sequence	Kapalabhati Breathing
Movement	Yoga Preparation	Yoga Basics	Core Re-tensioning	Rebalancing Yoga	Bandha Strength Yoga	Max Kegel Yoga	Ball Routine	Dynamic Power Yoga
Relaxation	Restorative Yoga	Yin Yoga Forward Folds	Yin Yoga Backward Bending	Yin Yoga Twists & Lateral Movement	Yin Yoga Hip Opening	Yin Yoga Pelvic Floor	Yin Yoga Happy Hips	Yin Yoga All Body
Mind & Meditation	Yoga Nidra	Flex your mind to flex your muscles	ANT therapy	Conquer your fear	Kirtan Kriya	Self Affirmations	Journaling	Blossoming Goddess

Figure 9.1.1: Phase 1 training—Preparation level.

The Phase 1 module's exercises highlighted in blue in Figure 9.1.1, help to prepare the body for a regular movement practice. The preparation level is designed for those who have little to no strength and minimal tone in the pelvic floor muscles. If you don't regularly exercise and live a sedentary life, this could be a good starting point, even if your pelvic floor is a little stronger.

This phase builds the foundation for the movement practices in the subsequent phases. The movement modules offer a system of graded exposure that progressively loads your tissues as the training advances.

Additional to the modules listed in Figure 9.1.1, you will find the pelvic floor module for reverse Kegels in this phase. You should use the reverse Kegels module in place of the pelvic floor module at all phases of training if your assessment highlighted that you needed to work on relaxation instead of strengthening.

Phase 1
Modules

 ### Pelvic Floor

Kegel Breakdown or Reverse Kegels

Breathing
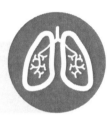

Nasal Breathing

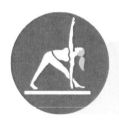 ### Movement

Yoga Preparation

Relaxation
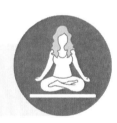

Restorative Yoga

 ### Mind & Meditation

Yoga Nidra

Phase 1: Pelvic Floor Module
Kegel Breakdown (Strength)

Objective

The objective of the pelvic floor training in this phase is to strengthen the connection between your brain and the various muscles of your pelvic floor. As you strengthen this connection, you will start to gain more control of these muscles. You should feel you have similar strength with each of the elements of the pelvic floor exercise.

Success Metric

Success is achieved when you can perform a controlled gentle squeeze of a finger inserted in the vagina, giving a score of at least three on the strength scale. This is the equivalent of a weak contraction with no lift. *Note*: You don't have to squeeze your finger hard; you just need to sustain a gentle controlled contraction for a count of five, while breathing with your body relaxed.

Additional Notes

At this phase of training, your pelvic floor is weak so, you should adapt other activities so as not to place unnecessary strain on your pelvic floor. Try to avoid heavy lifting. Ask for help if you have small children or need to carry groceries. Do not perform strong core exercises where you lift both legs. Running in this stage pelvic floor rehabilitation is not advisable.

Kegel Breakdown Instructions

In Chapter Eight, during practical activity number two, you learned the seven elements of a Kegel exercise; where the first six focus on the contraction of specific parts of your pelvic floor, and the seventh creates a full pelvic floor contraction. For this pelvic floor training module, you are going to practice performing these seven elements.

In order to enhance the connection between your brain and your pelvic floor, you will use touch to bring your awareness to the area being contracted (which is a form of biofeedback). This will require that you set up for the exercise in the same way as for the practical activity, making sure you will not be disturbed, having clean hands, and using some lubrication if needed.

You will practice the pelvic floor training six days per week. When you begin this training, you should perform these Kegels lying back on pillows as you did for the two practical activities at the start of

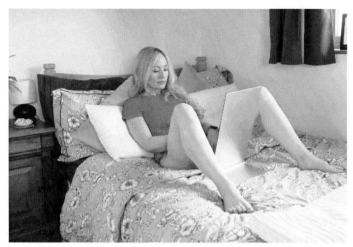

Figure 9.1.2: Using touch to enhance the mind-to-muscle connection within the pelvic floor.

By using pillows behind your back as shown in Figure 9.1.2, you should have sufficient support to reach your pelvic floor while remaining relaxed. The use of the mirror is optional, although it can help to ensure you are focusing on the right area for contraction.

Steps to Perform This Kegel Breakdown Exercise:

1. Get yourself into a comfortable starting position.
2. Perform ten calming breath cycles, inhaling for a count of four and exhaling slowly for eight.
3. Starting with element one of the seven elements, place your finger on the area being contracted, and exhale as you perform your first contraction. Try to maintain the contraction as you exhale. If you find it difficult to achieve a contraction, touching the area should help to enhance the mind-to-muscle connection.
4. Keep the rest of your body relaxed as you perform the contraction.
5. Perform each element while touching the area being contracted until you come to the seventh element where you perform a full contraction.
6. Place the heel of your hand on the clitoris and reach your fingers back toward the anus, applying very gentle pressure. When you contract, you are trying to sense the entire pelvic floor. This completes one set.
7. Repeat the seven elements (one set) three times.

As you continue to perform the exercises, you should find that the connection between your mind and your pelvic floor is enhanced and this should come with increased control. Consistency is key.

Once you feel that you are achieving contraction of all parts of your pelvic floor, you no longer need to use touch to enhance your mind-to-muscle connection and can switch to performing the exercises fully clothed while alternating your position each day as shown in Figures 9.1.3.a and 9.1.3.b.

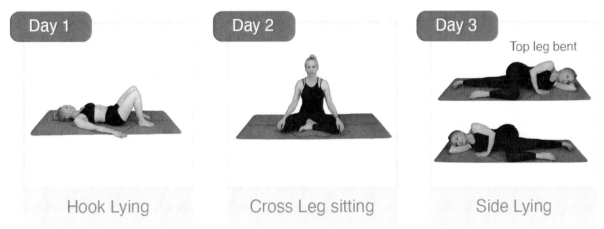

Figure 9.1.3.a: Positions to perform pelvic floor exercises.

You will perform 3 sets in each position shown in Figures 9.1.3.a and 9.1.3.b.:

Day 1: *Hook lying*—Lie on your back with your knees bent, resting your arms alongside your body. Perform three sets of the pelvic floor exercises in this position.

Day 2: *Cross leg sitting*—Sit cross-legged on your mat, with hands resting on your knees. If you collapse in your low back when sitting cross-legged, you should elevate your hips using a blanket as shown in Figure 9.1.4. Perform three sets of the pelvic floor exercises in this position.

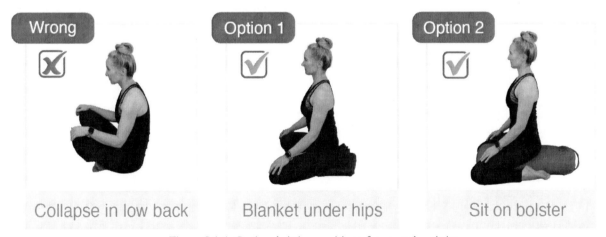

Figure 9.1.4: Optional sitting positions for cross-leg sitting.

Day 3: *Side-lying*—Lie on your side and bend your top knee at a 90-degree angle. Perform the exercises in this position on both left and right sides. Complete three sets of the pelvic floor exercises on each side.

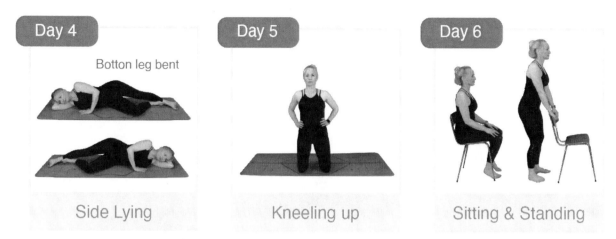

Figure 9.1.3.b: Positions to perform pelvic floor exercises.

Day 4: *Side-lying*—Lie on your side and bend your bottom knee at a 90-degree angle. Perform the exercises in this position on both the left and right sides. Complete three sets of the pelvic floor exercises on each side.

Day 5: *Kneeling up*—Kneel up with knees under hips and feet in line with knees. You can place a blanket under your knees if needed. Complete three sets of the pelvic floor exercises in this position.

Day 6: *Sitting & standing*—Sit relaxed in a chair, hands resting on your knees. Perform two sets of the pelvic floor exercises in this position, then stand with a gentle bend in both the knees and the hips, resting your hands on the chair. Perform the final set in the standing position.

You may find that it is harder to feel the different parts of your pelvic floor as you change position, particularly when kneeling up and standing. Consistent steady practice will help. You can also practice reverse Kegels at any point in the training if you would like to take a break from strengthening. Relaxation exercises are also helpful to those who are working to increase strength.

That concludes the pelvic floor strength module for Phase 1. The next section covers the reverse Kegels module. **If your assessments showed you needed to work on pelvic floor relaxation**, you should practice the reverse Kegels exercises in place of the pelvic floor module for all phases of training as shown in Figure 9.1.5.

You can see in Figure 9.1.5 that the reverse Kegels exercise will replace the pelvic floor exercise at all levels of the eight-phase training. We learned the importance of an optimal resting length, which was visualized in Figure 2.4. We learned that hypertonic muscles are not necessarily strong muscles. By encouraging the release of tension in your pelvic floor, you are also enhancing the potential for your pelvic floor to return to balanced strength, regaining the ability to contract and relax when needed.

Eight-Phase Modules	Prep	Beginner			Intermediate		Advanced	
	Phase 1	Phase 2	Phase 3	Phase 4	Phase 5	Phase 6	Phase 7	Phase 8
Pelvic Floor	Reverse Kegels							
	If your focus is relaxation, you should only practice Reverse Kegels (Phase 1 Pelivc Floor Module)							
Breathing	Nasal Breathing	Breath Strengthening	Breath Remapping	Nadi Shodhana	Basic Hypopressive Exercise	Intermediate Hypopressive Sequence	Advanced Hypopressive Sequence	Kapalabhati Breathing
Movement	Yoga Preparation	Yoga Basics	Core Retensioning	Rebalancing Yoga	Bandha Strength Yoga	Max Kegel Yoga	Ball Routine	Dynamic Power Yoga
Relaxation	Restorative Yoga	Yin Yoga Forward Folds	Yin Yoga Backward Bending	Yin Yoga Twists & Lateral Movement	Yin Yoga Hip Opening	Yin Yoga Pelvic Floor	Yin Yoga Happy Hips	Yin Yoga All Body
Mind & Meditation	Yoga Nidra	Flex your mind to flex your muscles	ANT therapy	Conquer your fear	Kirtan Kriya	Self Affirmations	Journaling	Blossoming Goddess

Figure 9.1.5: Practice reverse Kegels exercise at all phases for pelvic floor relaxation.

Phase 1: Pelvic Floor Module

Reverse Kegels (Relaxation)

Objective

The objective of the reverse Kegels module is to down-train the pelvic floor to reduce pelvic tension and hypertonicity. As you learn to relax your pelvic floor, you should find that pelvic pain and tension are reduced. If your assessment defined that you should practice reverse Kegels in place of strengthening, you should use reverse Kegels for your pelvic floor training sessions (phases 1 through 8), unless advised to do otherwise by your healthcare provider.

Success Metric

Success is achieved when you can relax your pelvic floor fully in all of the positions specified and no longer feel the symptoms of hypertonicity.

Additional Notes

If you suffer from hypertonicity, it is of benefit to have a full assessment from a pelvic floor PT. They can confirm if any additional treatment is needed to help induce relaxation. It can be helpful to practice a pelvic floor release using a therapy ball (or something softer like a sock) prior to performing reverse Kegels. This involves sitting cross-legged, placing the ball under your perineum, and relaxing on the ball for a minute before performing reverse Kegels. You can use visualization to enhance this relaxation, imagining that the ball is a strawberry, and your pelvic floor is chocolate. Visualize the chocolate melting over the strawberry as you sit on the ball to help you relax.

Reverse Kegel Instructions

When you begin, the reverse Kegels will be performed in the same position as practical activity two from Chapter Eight, which is shown in Figure 9.1.2. You will start by performing each element of a Kegel exercise focusing on relaxation instead of contraction.

Steps to Perform the Reverse Kegel Exercise:

1. Get yourself into a comfortable starting position.
2. Perform ten calming breath cycles, inhaling for a count of four and exhaling slowly for eight.
3. Starting with element one of the seven elements, place your finger on the area being relaxed and inhale as you focus on allowing your breath to increase intra-abdominal pressure, expanding your pelvic floor. Your tummy and pelvic floor should be relaxed allowing expansion throughout the inhalation. *Note*: You should not *bear down* here or push your pelvic floor outwards. Simply *let go* allowing the intra-abdominal pressure to expand your pelvic floor naturally.
4. Exhale while continuing to relax and let go.
5. Perform each element while touching the area being relaxed until you come to the seventh element where you will perform relaxation focusing on the entire pelvic floor.
6. Place the heel of your hand on the clitoris and reach your fingers back towards your anus, applying gentle pressure.
7. Perform the seventh element relaxing the entire pelvic floor on each inhale, maintaining the relaxation on each exhale, continuing for ten breath cycles. This completes one set.
8. Repeat the seven elements (one set) three times.

Once you feel you are achieving relaxation of all parts of your pelvic floor, you no longer need to use touch to enhance your mind-to-muscle connection. You should switch to performing these exercises in alternating positions as demonstrated in Figures 9.1.3.a and 9.13.b. Changing the positions is an important step since the pelvic floor naturally holds more tension in upright and standing positions, so learning to relax in these positions will reduce pelvic tension throughout your normal days.

If you have dysfunctional breathing patterns with limited diaphragmatic/rib cage flexibility, the exercises in the breathing modules will help you to make improvements, which should increase your potential for relaxing your pelvic floor. If you are focusing on pelvic floor relaxation, you should relax your pelvic floor in all movement sessions. If you find that any poses in the training trigger hypertonicity for you, remove them from your practice, listen to your body, and adapt accordingly.

As you continue to work through the program performing these relaxation exercises, you should find that your ability to relax your pelvic floor increases. Consistency really is key. It is so important not to give up on yourself as you go through this process. If you believe in your ability to empower your flower then amazing things can happen. That concludes the reverse Kegels instructions. You will practice your pelvic floor exercises on the days specified in your schedule.

Final Words for Phase One Pelvic Floor Module

Before moving on to the Phase 1 breathing module, I would like to offer some additional words. The goal of both strengthening and relaxation is to optimize the length-tension relationship within the pelvic floor muscles.

For those working on strength, you will eventually feel your pelvic floor tone is improving. At the end of each week when you reach the phase checkpoint, you can check the success metric for this phase. This is done by performing a controlled gentle squeeze of a finger inserted in the vagina, and giving a score of at least three on the strength scale. This is the equivalent of a weak contraction with no lift. Verifying this success metric can help you to decide if you should move forward to the next phase.

For those working on relaxation, you will eventually feel that your pelvic floor is relaxing. However, reverse Kegels have less of an impact on hypertonicity than the strengthening exercises do on hypotonicity. For this reason, you will continue to practice reverse Kegels for the entire duration of the eight-phase program. When you practice the exercises in the breathing, movement, and relaxation modules, you should do so with reverse Kegels (so always allowing an expansion on inhalation). It is the combination of your reverse Kegels and the breathing, movement, and relaxation modules that will help you to achieve your empowerment.

Phase 1: Breathing Module

Nasal Breathing

Objective

The objective of the breathing module in Phase 1 is to work on nasal breathing to ensure you are using the diaphragm for breathing rather than using accessory muscles around the neck, upper chest, and back. This can help to eliminate dysfunctional breathing patterns while also improving the relationship between the diaphragm and pelvic floor.

Success Metric

Success is achieved when you can breathe through your nose while keeping your neck, shoulders, and upper back relaxed, which ensures you are using your diaphragm to power your breathing.

Additional Notes

If you have a dysfunctional breathing pattern, where you use accessory muscles for *quiet inspiration*, you may find the exercises difficult to begin with. If you feel a little panicked when you slouch, you should sit up and perform a few calming breath cycles before trying again. It is important to remember that slouching is neither good nor bad.

When you slouch, your ribcage is depressed, and your accessory muscles are relaxed, allowing your breath to expand the ribs out to the sides and to the back. The ability to depress your ribcage, as happens when you slouch, is considered normal ROM.

It can take time to reprogram your breathing function but with consistent steady practice, you can make substantial improvements. For mouth breathers, you should also consider mouth taping during sleep, which is explained in the self-care section of Chapter Ten (symptom management and life strategies).

Nasal Breathing Instructions

For this exercise, you will focus on nasal breathing in a slouched position. You will practice this breathing exercise every second day. You may choose to practice this breathing exercise any time you are sitting relaxed during your day. This is an automated breathing practice where you relax into the slouched position and allow your body to breathe for you rather than forcing the inhalation/exhalation. Breathing is only through the nose; your mouth remains closed throughout.

I usually practice when I sit in my office chair as that is the chair that I use most (if I am not sitting on my ball or standing at my desk).

Steps to Perform the Nasal Breathing Exercise

1. Sit squarely on your sitting bones with your back resting gently against the back of the chair and your feet flat on the floor. If your feet don't reach the floor, use a small step as demonstrated in

Figure 9.1.6. Make sure that you are not pushing your back into the chair, just relax and resist the urge to sit in a military upright posture.

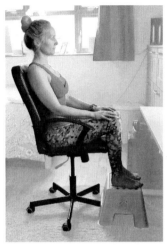

Figure 9.1.6: Sitting relaxed in a chair.

2. Close your mouth keeping your lips together with your teeth slightly apart, tongue resting on the roof of your mouth behind your front teeth.
3. Allow the inhalation to happen gently through your nose while relaxing your shoulders and chest. Your breath should be quiet and soft, automated not forced. Stay in this position for a few breaths.
4. Let your arms rest between your legs and allow yourself to slouch as shown in Figure 9.1.7, which demonstrates how you can let go of the upper part of your torso, including your arms and shoulders. You should also let your head rest forward, and relax your abdominals. This will gently depress the rib cage.

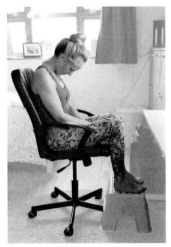

Figure 9.1.7: Slouching in a chair.

5. From this slouched position, allow your body to breathe through your nose. Your breathing should be quiet, not forced, and you should feel calm and relaxed. Breathing in this slouched

position takes your accessory muscles out of the equation making the diaphragm work harder.

6. Make sure to keep the rest of your body relaxed as you perform the exercise.

7. Breathe in this position for twenty breath cycles.

Practicing this nasal breathing exercise should help to restore functional breathing; more specifically, quiet inspiration, and expiration (which we learned about in Chapter Three).

That completes the breathing module for Phase 1. You should practice this at least twice per week, or more often if you feel your breathing is dysfunctional.

Phase 1: Movement Module
Yoga Preparation

Objective

The objective of the movement module in Phase 1 is to prepare your body for beginning a regular yoga practice. If you have never practiced yoga and begin immediately with a strong practice, you are at a higher risk of injury, particularly around your joints (wrists, ankles, knees, elbows, shoulders, hips, and spine). This gentle practice will prepare your body to safely perform basic yoga poses with a reduced risk of injury.

Success Metric

Success is achieved when you move through the sequence with ease and can comfortably perform a downward-facing dog, one of the most basic yoga poses. You don't have to have straight legs or heels on the floor, but you should be able to lengthen your spine and breathe in the downward-facing dog.

Additional Notes

This preparatory practice gives you the opportunity to get more familiar with your body. You will begin to enhance the mind-to-muscle connection throughout your body, bringing focus to muscles you may not currently be aware of. Be patient with your body as it slowly learns to gently move beyond its current limits.

In some positions, you may need to use blocks to *raise the floor*, depending on your flexibility, as shown in Figure 9.1.8. As you can see, the bocks provide a point of stability, which can allow you to practice poses even if you lack the flexibility for full expression.

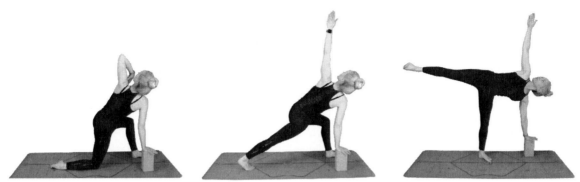

Figure 9.1.8: Examples of raising the floor in yoga using a block.

The sequence will take approximately twenty-five minutes including a five-minute relaxation at the end. You can download the sequence sheet for this yoga preparation sequence (Figure 9.1.9) from empoweryourflower.com and place it at the front of your mat when practicing.

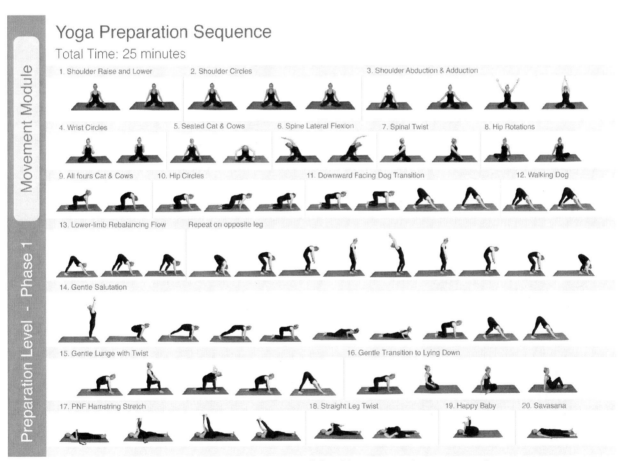

Figure 9.1.9: Phase 1—Movement module—Yoga preparation sequence sheet.

You can read the instructions and steps beforehand, and follow the poses on the printed copy of Figure 9.1.9 when you are practicing. This will help you to learn the sequence and eventually you will be able to practice it without looking at the sheet. Repeated practice creates change in the body.

Yoga Preparation Instructions

For this exercise, you will need a yoga mat. If you collapse in your lower back when sitting cross-legged, you should prop yourself up on a small towel or blanket in order to bring your pelvis into a neutral position (which was demonstrated in Figure 9.1.4). If you are unable to sit comfortably in a cross-legged position, even with the aid of a blanket or towel, you have the option to sit up on a bolster or to kneel across a bolster (also demonstrated in Figure 9.1.4).

You should practice this yoga preparation sequence at least three days per week if you are working on pelvic floor strength, or twice per week if you are working on pelvic floor relaxation. If you are working on pelvic floor relaxation, remember to relax your pelvic floor on each inhalation.

Steps to Perform the Yoga Preparation Sequence

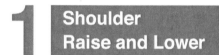

Shoulder Raise and Lower

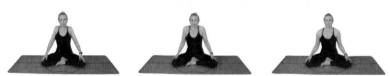

Figure 9.1.9.1: Shoulder raise and lower.

1. From a comfortable seated position, bring your awareness to your breath. Notice if it's deep or if it's shallow as you allow your shoulders to relax and you feel the weight of your body gently pressing into your sitting bones.
2. Perform five calming breath cycles (inhalation four, exhalation eight) as you allow your body to relax in this seated position.
3. Inhale bringing your shoulders up toward your ears and then exhale as you let them fall back down.
4. Repeat three times.

Shoulder Circles

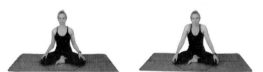

Figure 9.1.9.2: Shoulder circles.

1. Begin to roll your shoulders forward starting with small circles. *Note*: You are spreading your

shoulder blades away from each other as you do forward rolls.

2. Gradually exaggerate the movement until you are making big circles, as though you are massaging your own back with your shoulder blades.

3. Continue for three breath cycles.

4. Begin to roll your shoulders backward starting with small circles. *Note*: You are bringing your shoulder blades toward each other as you do backward rolls.

5. Gradually exaggerate the movement until you are making big circles, as though you are massaging your own back with your shoulder blades.

6. Continue for three breath cycles.

3 Shoulder Abduction & Adduction

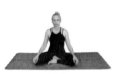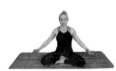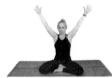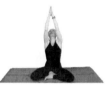

Figure 9.1.9.3: Shoulder abduction & adduction.

1. Inhale as you bring energy into your arms raising them overhead, bringing your palms to touch as you look up toward your thumbs.

2. Exhale as you bring your arms back down.

3. Repeat for three breath cycles (inhalation + exhalation).

4 Wrist Circles

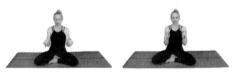

Figure 9.1.9.4: Wrist circles.

1. Begin to make small inward circles with your wrists for a count of five.

2. Change direction making outward circles for a count of five.

3. Shake your wrists out when you are finished making circles.

5 Seated Cat & Cows

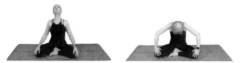

Figure 9.1.9.5: Seated cat & cows.

1. Place your hands on your knees and inhale as you begin cat and cow breaths where you round the spine forward all the way from the tailbone to the top of your neck.
2. Round your spine backward as you exhale, looking down toward your belly button.
3. Perform five of these cat/cow breath cycles. *Note*: The goal is to flex and extend your spine (in the sagittal plane).

6 Spine Lateral Flexion

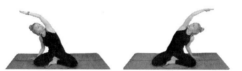

Figure 9.1.9.6: Spine lateral flexion.

1. Place your left hand on the floor beside you and inhale while lifting your right hand over your head and pressing your right sitting bone into the floor.
2. With each inhalation imagine you are lifting your ribcage away from your hips. With each exhalation, reach further away. Feel the stretch through the right side of your body from your sitting bone to your fingertips. *Note*: The goal is to move your spine sideways (in the frontal plane).
3. Perform five breath cycles in this position.
4. Come back to center and take the position on the opposite side for five breath cycles before returning to a neutral position.

7 Spinal Twist

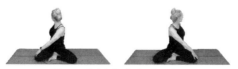

Figure 9.1.9.7: Spinal twist.

1. Bring your right hand onto your left leg and your left hand behind your back as you inhale to lengthen your spine and exhale to twist. *Note*: Don't pull with your hands to twist. Use the strength of your core and back muscles to create the twist. The goal is to rotate the spine (in the transverse plane).

2. Perform five breath cycles before returning to the center and taking the position on the opposite side.

8 Hip Rotations

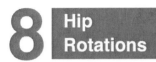

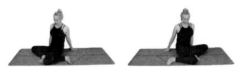

Figure 9.1.9.8: Hip rotations.

1. Release your legs from the cross-legged position taking a deer pose where you have both legs turned to the right at a 45-degree angle with your hands resting on the floor behind your back.

2. Rotating from the hips, shift your legs to the left and then to the right.

3. Repeat this five times (both left and right).

9 All-Fours Cat & Cows

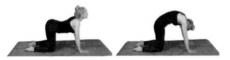

Figure 9.1.9.9: All-fours cat & cows.

1. Come to an all-fours position, making sure to stack shoulders over elbows, elbows over wrists. Your fingers should be spread nice and wide with your index fingers pointing forward. Make sure that your knees are beneath your hips and that your ankles are in line with your knees.

2. Inhale as you begin to perform some cat and cow breaths flexing and extending the spine. *Note*: You should find your spine has extra mobility in this position versus the seated cat-cow position as your hips are now free to move.

3. Focus on moving your spine from your tailbone all the way to the top of your neck for five breath cycles while pressing your mid-hand and fingertips into the mat.

4. Return to a neutral all-fours position.

10 Hip Circles

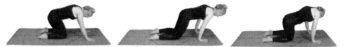

Figure 9.1.9.10: Hip circles.

1. Begin to make small circles with your hips moving toward the right and then the left.
2. Exaggerate the movement until you are making wide circles that will see you moving backward and forward on all-fours. *Note*: When you are forward with your shoulders beyond your wrists, press into the knuckles and fingertips. When you are backward with your shoulders behind your wrists, press into the heel of your hand.
3. Continue for a count of five.
4. Make the circles in the opposite direction; again, starting small before exaggerating the movement.

11 Downward Facing Dog Transition

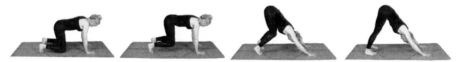

Figure 9.1.9.11: Downward-facing dog transition.

1. Return to a neutral all-fours position, turning out your toes (by putting the base of your toes on the floor).
2. Gently press into your hands, keeping pressure evenly balanced in your hands and allowing your shoulder blades to come away from each other.
3. Lift your knees off the mat so your knees are in line with your heels.
4. Press into your mid-hand and shift your hips up, keeping your knees bent and resting your tummy on your lap. *Note*: The goal of this exercise is to maintain a long straight spine while preparing yourself for a gentle downward-facing dog.
5. Straighten your legs to come to your first downward-facing dog. *Note*: Hands should be shoulder-distance apart, feet hip-distance. The spine should be elongated. Legs should only be straight if your spine is long and straight. When you have sufficient length in your hamstrings, your heels will reach the floor. Don't push to get the heels down. With time and consistent practice, it will happen.

12 | Walking Dog

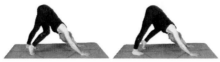

Figure 9.1.9.12: Walking dog.

1. Begin to walk the dog by straightening and bending one leg at a time as though you are walking on the spot.

13 | Lower-limb Rebalancing Flow

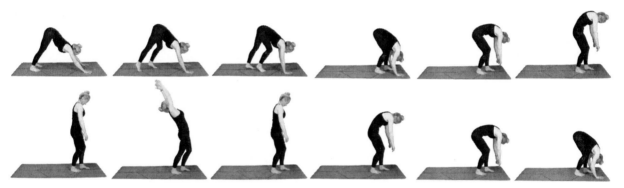

Figure 9.1.9.13: Lower limb rebalancing flow.

1. Inhale and look forward between your hands and prepare to walk your feet forward.

2. Exhale and take small steps to walk your feet closer to your hands while keeping your knees bent and gazing at the space between your hands.

3. Walk forward until your right foot is between your hands. Your feet should be hip-distance apart with the big toe of your left foot in line with your right heel. Keep your knees bent and let your upper body and head hang forward with your tummy resting on your lap.

4. Take an inhalation and exhalation in this position.

5. Inhale as you press into the midfoot, using the strength of your legs to press yourself up. The upper body remains hanging forward and you uncurl your spine one vertebrae at a time. Your knees remain softly bent.

6. Once you have uncurled all the way to your neck, your head will be neutral.

7. As you finish your inhalation, bring your hands over your head, and look up toward your hands while sending your hips forward. This creates a mini backbend. You can straighten the back leg in

this position but keep the front knee bent.

8. Exhale as you roll back down, curling one vertebra at a time (in the same way as you came up). Allow your head and arms to hang, soft bend in both knees, and weight shifting toward your heels.

9. Once your hands reach the floor, inhale, and bring your left foot forward beside your right foot and exhale as you step your right foot back, so your right foot is in line with your left heel, feet still hip-distance apart.

10. Inhale and repeat Steps 4–9 to take the flow on the opposite side.

14 Gentle Salutation

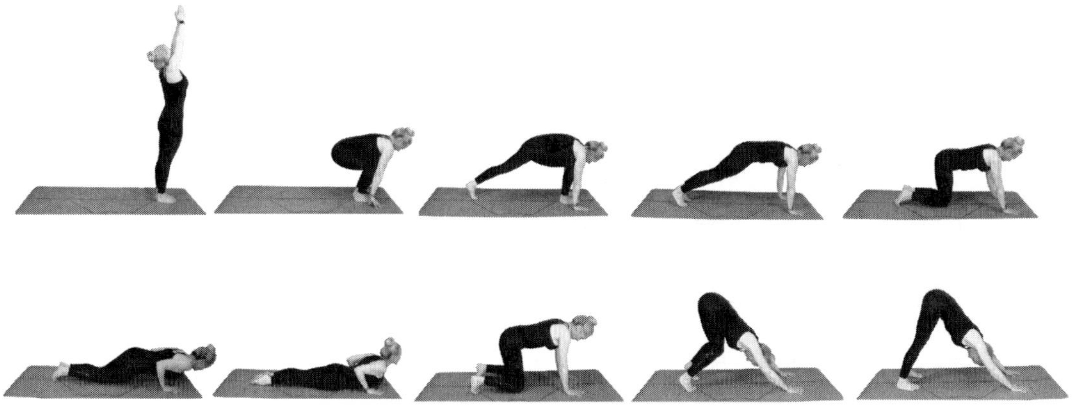

Figure 9.1.9.14: Gentle salutation.

1. Bring both feet together and inhale as you reach your arms over your head.

2. Exhale, pivoting from the hip and folding forward, placing your hands on the floor with your tummy resting on your bent knees. *Note*: Bend your knees as much as you need to allow the heel of your hand to reach the floor.

3. Inhale as you step back your right leg, then your left leg, coming to plank position.

4. Exhale and drop your knees as you bend your elbows, lowering your body all the way to the floor. *Note*: Keep the weight in the heel of your hand as you lower your upper body down to the floor.

5. Inhale and press into the heel of your hand as you lift your chest slightly, keeping the elbows bent and close to the body (*cobra pose*). Gaze forward using the hands for balance. The lift comes from muscles along the spinal column.

6. Exhale as you press through the mid-hand to push yourself back to a neutral all-fours position.

7. Inhale as you turn out your toes and lift your knees from the floor pressing your hips upwards coming to a gentle downward-facing dog, exhaling here.

15 Gentle Lunge with Twist

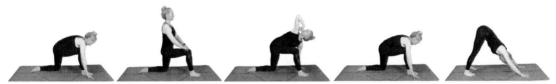

Figure 9.1.9.15: Gentle lunge with twist.

1. Inhale looking forward between your hands and exhale as you step your right foot forward, dropping your left knee to the floor.

2. Inhale and use the strength of your legs to come up to a low lunge, resting your hands on your right knee for balance.

3. Exhale placing your left hand on the floor. Inhale and place your right hand on your right shoulder, twisting your body and pointing your elbow up toward the ceiling. Take three breath cycles here. *Note*: You have the option to raise the floor using a yoga block if you do not have sufficient flexibility to twist while reaching the floor as demonstrated in Figure 9.1.8.

4. Exhale while taking both hands back to the floor, stepping the right leg back, and returning to the downward-facing dog.

5. Repeat Steps 1 to 4 on the opposite side, finishing in your downward-facing dog.

16 Gentle Transition to Lying Down

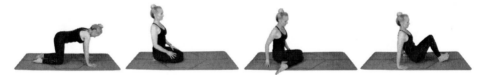

Figure 9.1.9.16: Transition to lying down.

1. Exhale, dropping your knees before sitting back onto your heels.

2. Bringing your hips to the floor on one side as you inhale and swing your legs around in front of you.

3. Exhale and lie down.

17 PNF Hamstring Stretch

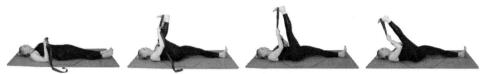

Figure 9.1.9.17: PNF hamstring stretch.

Note: You will need a strap for this position, which is facilitated (PNF) stretching of your hamstrings.

1. Create a loop at the end of the strap, bend your right knee, and put the loop around your right foot.
2. **Active Stretch**: Straighten your leg as you pull the strap to bring your leg as close to you as it will come. Take note of where your leg is in relation to your body.
3. Relax your leg in this position for a count of five.
4. **Counter Contraction**: Flex your foot and kick into the strap for a count of five. *Note*: When you kick into the strap, it should be as though you are trying to bring your leg back down to the floor. You should feel your hamstrings engage as you resist by pulling the strap.
5. **Active Stretch**: Relax your leg and pull the strap to bring your leg closer.
6. Repeat this active stretch/counter contraction cycle (Steps 2–5) three more times. You should notice that your leg has come closer than it was at the beginning of the exercise.
7. Place the strap to one side and hug your knee toward your chest, performing a full breath cycle here.
8. Repeat Steps 1 to 7 on the opposite side.

18 Straight Leg Twist

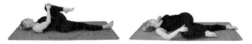

Figure 9.1.9.18: Straight leg twist.

1. Straighten your right leg while hugging your left knee and drop your left knee over to the right side for a spinal twist. Keep your shoulders on the ground. *Note*: You should relax completely in this twisting position. If you feel your shoulders lifting, you can place a blanket or bolster beneath your knees to raise the floor.
2. Perform five breath cycles in this twisted position.
3. Inhale to come back to the center and exhale, taking the twist on the opposite side.

19 Happy Baby

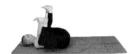

Figure 9.1.9.19: Happy baby (husband or lover).

1. Inhale as you bend your knees, taking your feet in your hands for a happy baby pose (or happy husband as I like to call it, or happy lover if your partner is female). *Note*: You should open your legs while keeping your knees bent around 90 degrees.
2. Simultaneously kick into your hands and you pull on your feet. Try to keep your whole spine on the floor (all the way to the sacrum). You can rock a little here if that feels good.

20 Savasana

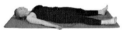

Figure 9.1.9.20: Savasana.

1. Release your feet and take your *savasana* (final resting pose), close your eyes, and let go of all effort
2. Relax in this position for five minutes.

That completes the yoga preparation sequence. This gentle yoga practice prepares your body for a more active life. Even if you are active, it can be good to take a step back to this type of gentle practice while you work on improving your pelvic floor function. This can help to ensure you are not overloading and exacerbating your issues with a more rigorous activity level. This practice is also beneficial to those who are working on pelvic floor relaxation. Practice with compassion and remember to listen to your body.

Phase 1: Relaxation Module

Restorative Yoga

Objective

The objective of the relaxation module in Phase 1 is to support your body in complete relaxation.

You will practice restorative yoga, which encourages complete relaxation with the support of bolsters, cushions, blankets, and other props. We focus on relaxation first, to drop excess tension, before we begin the focus on rebalancing tension in the next phase of training.

Success Metric

Success is achieved when you can completely relax your entire body in each of the positions.

Additional Notes

You can improvise with props, according to what you have available. For example, you could perform these poses on your bed instead of lying on your yoga mat. You can use a bunched-up quilt as a bolster and your pillows as additional props. Practicing in a dimly lit room with soft relaxing music in the background can make it easier to relax in the poses.

You can download the sequence sheet for this restorative yoga sequence (Figure 9.1.10) from empoweryourflower.com and place it at the front of your mat when practicing.

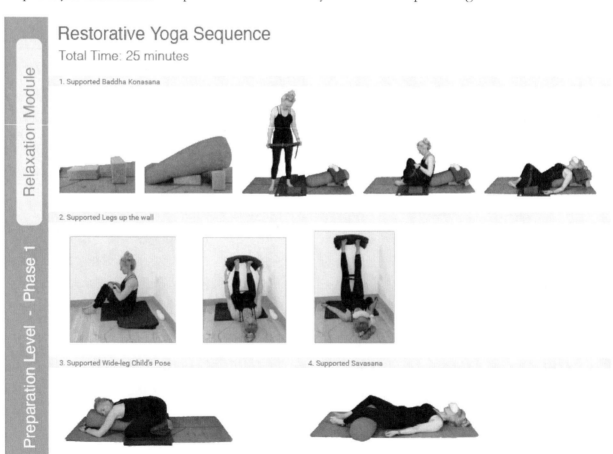

Figure 9.1.10: Phase 1—Relaxation module—Restorative yoga sequence sheet.

You should read the instructions and steps beforehand and follow the poses on the printed copy of Figure 9.1.10 when you are practicing. This will help you to learn the sequence and eventually you will be able to practice it without looking at the sheet.

Restorative Yoga Instructions

You will practice four restorative yoga poses in this sequence. The practice will take twenty-five minutes, including time for setup, and transition time between poses. Make sure to move slowly and calmly between poses, and allow yourself to find the very depths of potential relaxation.

You will need a bolster or some pillows, a yoga blanket, and a wall; the headboard/wall behind your bed could also work. An eye pillow is a really nice addition, even if the room is dimly lit, as the weight over the eyes can stimulate a deeper relaxation.

Steps to Perform This Restorative Yoga Sequence

1 Supported Baddha Konasana

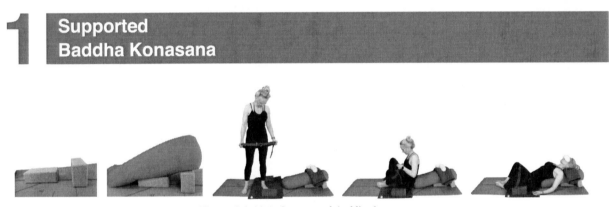

Figure 9.1.10.1: Supported *baddha konasana*.

Note: You will use two yoga blocks, a bolster, a strap, and an eye pillow for this position.

1. Start by setting up your blocks with one lying flat on its broad long side and the other on its narrow long side.
2. Place the bolster on these blocks.
3. Loop your strap and bring it around your thighs.
4. Sit with your backside against the bolster and adjust the strap around your thighs so it allows your legs to open as much as is comfortable. For additional support/comfort, you can place blocks beneath your knees, a blanket behind your head, and an eye pillow over your eyes.
5. Allow your arms to relax with your forearm resting on the floor, palms facing up.
6. Relax in this position for five minutes.

2 Supported Legs up the wall

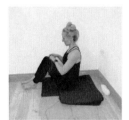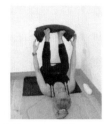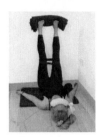

Figure 9.1.10.2: Supported legs up the wall.

Note: You will need two blankets, a strap, and an eye pillow for this position. You need sufficient wall space to extend your legs.

1. To set up, place your mat with a folded blanket against the wall.
2. Have a second blanket (one with a decent amount of weight) folded for placement on feet.
3. Loop your strap and bring it up around your thighs, sitting your hips close to the wall
4. Lie on your side with your backside against the wall and twist around so that your back rests on your yoga mat, your bum resting on the wall.
5. Bend your knees and place your folded blanket on your feet. You can tighten the strap around your legs if they are wider than hip-distance apart.
6. Extend your legs while balancing the blanket on your feet. The blanket and strap help to support you so you can relax your legs in this position. You can also place a boster or blanket on your tummy for extra support if needed.
7. Rest your arms by your side and use an eye pillow
8. Relax in this position for three minutes.

3 Supported Wide-leg Child's Pose

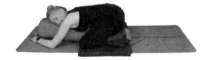

Figure 9.1.10.3: Supported wide-leg child's pose.

Note: You will need two blankets and a bolster for this position.

1. Kneel on the blanket, spreading your knees so they are mat width apart while your toes are touching.
2. Place the second blanket between your sitting bones and your heels and place the bolster between your legs.

3. Lie forward on the bolster, placing your right cheek on the bolster.

4. Relax with your right cheek on the bolster for two-and-a-half minutes before switching to the left cheek and relaxing for a further two-and-a-half minutes.

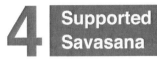
Supported Savasana

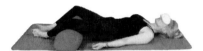

Figure 9.1.10.4: Supported savasana.

Note: You will need a bolster and eye pillow for this pose and can optionally cover yourself with a blanket.

1. Place the bolster beneath your knees and lie down with the eye pillow covering your eyes.

2. Relax in this position for five minutes.

That completes the restorative yoga sequence. This restorative yoga practice can be beneficial if you struggle to relax and carry a lot of excess tension in your shoulders, hips or pelvic floor. The mind and meditation module that follows will also be helpful with reducing tension and stress, and nicely complements this restorative practice.

Phase 1: Mind & Meditation Module
Yoga Nidra

Objective
The objective of the Mind & Mediation module in Phase 1 is to teach you to find and release tension from your body. This relaxing meditation can help immensely if you suffer from a pain condition such as CPPS, vaginismus, or other conditions of hypertonicity. It can also be used to help you to fall asleep if you suffer from insomnia.

Success Metric
Success is achieved when you can completely relax your entire body for the duration of the meditation.

Additional Notes
Yoga Nidra is a meditation where you perform a complete body scan, relaxing the various body parts as

you progress. It will help you to identify where you hold tension and will guide you to bring relaxation to those areas. This is an advantageous meditation for those suffering from pelvic pain conditions.

Yoga Nidra Instructions

For this exercise, you meditate through a full body scan, relaxing body parts as you go. Particular focus is given to the relaxation of the pelvis, which is not typical with yoga nidra, but important for you as you work to overcome your PFD. The meditation takes twenty five minutes, and you will practice this meditation twice per week, or more frequently if desired.

Steps to Perform This Yoga Nidra Meditation

Access the meditation audio on empoweryourflower.com, and find a quiet place where you can meditate undisturbed for twenty minutes. I recommend taking a savasana pose for this meditation, however, many people like to do this meditation from a comfortable cross-legged seated position because they fall asleep when lying down. It is perfectly OK to fall asleep during this meditation, after all, your body is relaxed during sleep. If you opt to do a seated version, I recommend you use a meditation cushion under your backside and have some support behind your back. This can be a wall or a meditation chair.

Once you have practiced this meditation multiple times, you will have learned the steps and can practice them in your mind as you meditate in silence without the audio if desired.

That completes the Mind & Meditation module and brings us to the end of the Phase 1 training modules. You will perform the exercises from this module on the days specified in your weekly schedule.

At the end of each week, if you feel that you may be ready to progress to the next phase of training, you can perform the phase checkpoint review using Figure 9.1.11. This checks your progress against the success metric for each exercise and helps you to decide if you should proceed to the next phase of training. You can download a blank version of this form from empoweryourflower.com.

Phase 1 Checkpoint Review

Phase Start Date:_____

Checkpoint Date:_____

Pelvic Floor Module	Success

Strength: Success is achieved when you can perform a controlled gentle squeeze of a finger inserted in the vagina giving a score of at least 3 on the strength scale. This is the equivalent of a weak contraction with no lift. Note: You don't have to squeeze your finger hard; you just need to sustain a gentle controlled contraction for the count of five, while breathing with your body relaxed.

Yes ☐
No ☐

Relaxation: Success is achieved when you can relax your pelvic floor fully in all the positions specified and no longer feel the symptoms of hypertonicity. Note: Reverse Kegels can help to release pelvic tension, however, you will continue to practice the reverse Kegels module through the entire program and so if you do not achieve success with the pelvic floor relaxation at this phase, this should not prevent you from proceeding to the next phase of training.

Yes ☐
No ☐

Breathing Module - Nasal Breathing	Success

Success is achieved when you can breathe through your nose while keeping your neck, shoulders and upper back relaxed, which ensures you are using your diaphragm to power your breathing.

Yes ☐
No ☐

Movement Module - Yoga Preparation Sequence	Success

Success is achieved when you move through the sequence with ease and can comfortably perform a downward-facing dog, one of the most basic yoga poses. You don't have to have straight legs or heels on the floor, but you should be able to lengthen your spine and breathe in the downward-facing dog.

Yes ☐
No ☐

Relaxation Module - Restorative Yoga Sequence	Success

Success is achieved when you can completely relax your entire body in each of the positions.

Yes ☐
No ☐

Mind & Meditation Module - Yoga Nidra Body Scanning Mediation	Success

Success is achieved when you can completely relax your entire body for the duration of the meditation.

Yes ☐
No ☐

Phase 1 Checkpoint Review	Success

Have you achieved the success objectives and do you feel that you are ready to proceed to the next phase of training?

Yes ☐
No ☐

If no, please continue at the preparation level until you are ready to proceed.

If yes, this is also the end of the Preparation difficulty level. You should retake your assessments to measure your progress after completing the preparation level.

Progress Milestone Review - Preparation Level	Success

Have you already achieved your preparation level goal?

Yes ☐

If no, you have the option to repeat the preparation phase until you feel ready to proceed.

No ☐

If yes, proceed to Phase 2. Make sure to update your schedule. Good Luck!

Figure 9.1.11: Phase 1 Checkpoint review form.

As this is the end of the preparation level of training, you will be prompted in Figure 9.1.11 (Phase 1—Checkpoint Review) to repeat your initial assessments if you feel you are ready to progress. This is the first point at which you will be checking against the goals you have set for the program. Bear in mind that the preparation phase is intended to prepare your body for a movement practice. Your first goal should have been something that was achievable within a short time. If you have not achieved the goal, you can repeat the preparation phase again or if you feel ready, proceed with the beginner level.

Phase 2
Beginner Level

Welcome to Phase 2 of the eight-phase training program. This is the first phase at the beginner level, which is slightly more difficult than the preparation level. There are three phases in this level, which you should master before proceeding to the intermediate level. The following section details the Phase 2 training modules that are highlighted in Figure 9.2.1.

Eight-Phase Modules	Prep	Beginner			Intermediate		Advanced	
	Phase 1	Phase 2	Phase 3	Phase 4	Phase 5	Phase 6	Phase 7	Phase 8
Pelvic Floor	Kegel Breakdown	Full Kegel	Endurance Kegel	Speed Kegel	Co-Contract	Maximize Strength	Standing Rotations	Functional Training
Breathing	Nasal Breathing	Breath Strengthening	Breath Remapping	Nadi Shodhana	Basic Hypopressive Exercise	Intermediate Hypopressive Sequence	Advanced Hypopressive Sequence	Kapalabhati Breathing
Movement	Yoga Preparation	Yoga Basics	Core Re-tensioning	Rebalancing Yoga	Bandha Strength Yoga	Max Kegel Yoga	Ball Routine	Dynamic Power Yoga
Relaxation	Restorative Yoga	Yin Yoga Forward Folds	Yin Yoga Backward Bending	Yin Yoga Twists & Lateral Movement	Yin Yoga Hip Opening	Yin Yoga Pelvic Floor	Yin Yoga Happy Hips	Yin Yoga All Body
Mind & Meditation	Yoga Nidra	Flex your mind to flex your muscles	ANT therapy	Conquer your fear	Kirtan Kriya	Self Affirmations	Journaling	Blossoming Goddess

Figure 9.2.1: Beginner Level—Phase 2.

The exercises and activities for the Phase 2 modules, highlighted in green in Figure 9.2.1, are intended to build upon the foundational strength that you created during Phase 1. Beginning in this phase, you will work on full pelvic floor contractions if you are working on pelvic floor strength. We will work to strengthen the breathing muscles while increasing the intensity of our movement in all planes. We will enhance pelvic floor relaxation through our yin yoga practice and will utilize meditation to increase our potential for pelvic floor rehabilitation.

Remember, if your goal is pelvic floor relaxation, you will work on the reverse Kegels activity for all phases of training. It is detailed in Phase 1 pelvic floor module. The frequency of practice can change as you progress through the training so, make sure to read through all modules for Phase 2 and update your weekly schedule accordingly.

Phase 2
Modules

Pelvic Floor
Full Kegel

Breathing
Breath Strengthening
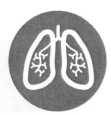

Movement
Yoga Basics

Relaxation
Yin Yoga Forward Folds
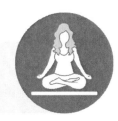

Mind & Meditation
Flex Your Mind to Flex Your Muscles

Phase 2: Pelvic Floor Module

Full Kegel

Having completed Phase 1, you should have a good connection between your brain and all parts of your pelvic floor. This is a solid foundation from which you can build. Good job!

Objective

The objective of the pelvic floor training module in Phase 2 is to increase the strength of your full pelvic floor contraction with a special focus on achieving some lift.

Success Metric

Success is achieved when you can perform a controlled squeeze of a finger inserted in the vagina, giving a score of four on the strength scale. This is the equivalent of a weak contraction with weak lift. You should be able to maintain this contraction with weak lift for a count of five while breathing calmly and having your body relaxed.

Additional Notes

It can be good to schedule a specific time in your day to perform these exercises as consistency will have a huge bearing on your results.

Full Kegel Instructions

For this exercise, you will focus on performing full pelvic floor contractions. You will continue to practice six days per week while alternating your position each day as per Phase 1 (Figures 9.1.3 a & b):

Day 1: Hook lying.
Day 2: Cross leg sitting.
Day 3: Side-lying (top leg bent).
Day 4: Side-lying (bottom leg bent).
Day 5: Kneeling up.
Day 6: Sitting & standing.

You should start to notice that contracting in these positions feels stronger than during Phase 1.

Steps to Perform the Full Kegel Exercise

1. Take the correct starting position for your practice (which alternates depending on the day, according to Figures 9.1.3 a & b).

2. Perform ten calming breath cycles, inhaling for a count of four, and exhaling slowly for a count of eight.

3. On your next exhalation, perform your full pelvic floor contraction, holding the contraction for the complete exhalation. Make sure to keep the rest of your body relaxed as you perform the exercise.

4. Relax your pelvic floor as you inhale.

5. Repeat for twenty full breath cycles.

You may find that your contractions become weaker as you go through your twenty breath cycles. Don't worry, as the weeks pass, you should find that your full Kegel feels more solid with the strength sustained to the end of your practice. Any shakiness or hesitation should be diminishing as time passes. Remember that we are working toward good pelvic floor function where we don't have to perform endless rounds of pelvic floor exercises so, stick with it now and lay a solid foundation for your empowerment. That completes the pelvic floor module (strength) for this phase.

Phase 2: Breathing Module
Breath Strengthening

Having completed Phase 1, you should be nasal breathing with good mobility of the diaphragm. You have laid the groundwork for functional breathing. Great work!

Objective

The objective of the breathing module in Phase 2 is to train the muscles involved in breathing to increase their strength, which can have a positive impact on your lung capacity. You will need a balloon or a straw for this exercise.

With this phase of breath training, your diaphragm must work extra hard on the inhalation to fill the lungs. The depressed position of the rib cage and the inhibition of the upper chest muscles in this slumped position, will encourage more expansion through the sides and back of the rib cage, helping to increase mobility

This exercise also begins to teach the management of intra-abdominal pressure, producing resistance during the exhalation phase. If you are working on pelvic floor strength with this training program, you will need to contract the pelvic floor and use a balanced contraction of the abdominal muscles to control the forced exhalation. This will feel much harder with the ribcage depressed. If you are working on pelvic floor relaxation, this exercise can help to expand the pelvic floor.

Success Metric

Success is achieved when you can inhale sufficiently and perform the exercise of filling the balloon without the feeling of exhaustion; all the while maintaining balanced intra-abdominal pressure.

Additional Notes

If you suffer from POP, you should use a straw rather than a balloon for this exercise, and avoid the exercise if you feel pressure bearing down on your prolapse. Once you have learned to master the control of your intra-abdominal pressure, during the exhalation, you can switch from a straw to a balloon. You should not feel excessive downward pressure during this exercise, and should be able to feel an upward lift of your pelvic floor as you contract it upon exhalation.

This exercise can feel difficult if your diaphragm is weak or your rib cage is stiff. You can poke a small hole at the end of your balloon to make it a little easier. As you get stronger, you can progress to a balloon without a hole.

Breath-strengthening Instructions

For this exercise, your inhalation should happen automatically (powered by your diaphragm), with air coming solely through the nose. You will practice this breathing exercise every second day.

Steps to Perform the Breath-strengthening Exercise

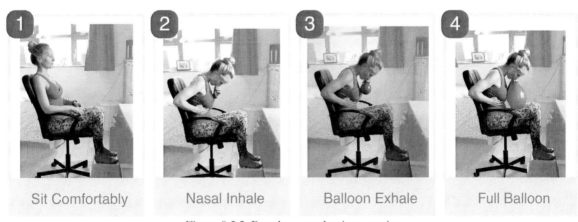

1	2	3	4
Sit Comfortably	Nasal Inhale	Balloon Exhale	Full Balloon

Figure 9.2.2: Breath-strengthening exercise.

1. Get yourself into a comfortable seated position, sitting squarely on your sitting bones with your back resting gently against the back of the chair. Make sure that you are not pushing your back into the chair. Close your mouth, keeping your lips together with your teeth slightly apart, tongue resting on the roof of your mouth behind your front teeth. Inhale gently through your nose while relaxing your shoulders and chest. Your breath should be quiet and soft. Take a few breaths here.

2. Slouch into a relaxed position, placing one hand on your lower ribs and the other holding the balloon or straw to your mouth. Allow an inhalation to happen through your nose, allowing that breath to reach into the sides of your rib cage. You should feel your rib cage expanding against your hand throughout this inhalation.

3. Exhale, blowing the air into the balloon/straw, while at the same time, contracting your pelvic floor and drawing it upwards. This may feel exceedingly difficult at first. It is important not to panic when you practice this breathing exercise. *Note*: You should feel your abs contract as you are exhaling as this is a forced exhalation.

4. Repeat for ten breath cycles or until you have blown up the balloon. Eventually, it will only require one or two exhalations to fill the balloon.

That completes the breath-strengthening practice. You will perform the exercises from this module on the days specified in your weekly schedule. If you found these breathing exercises to be difficult, don't give up. Consistency with your practice will strengthen your breathing muscles and increase your lung capacity. Stick with it.

 # Phase 2: Movement Module

Yoga Basics

Having completed Phase 1, your body should be familiar with the gentle practice of preparatory yoga, which should have enhanced the communication in the business of your body's movement. This is a nice foundation from which you can progress. Well done!

Objective

The objective of the movement module in Phase 2 is to increase both the pace of practice and the ability of your tissues to balance tension. This is achieved through flowing yoga poses that help to bias co-contractions of muscles in the lower and upper limbs. By improving the balance of tension in these peripheral tissues, you help to ensure the excess load is not being dumped into your core or pelvic floor. The sequence will take approximately twenty-five minutes, including the final rest.

Success Metric

Success is achieved when you can comfortably move through the sequence. It should be easy for you to complete the session within 25 minutes without getting out of breath.

Additional Notes

The exercises in this section are a progression from the preparation phase. The load through your limbs (arms and legs) will be increased to help you to tap into the business of your body's movement to reprogram your balance of tension. Feel free to refer back to Part One where the balance of tension was explained using Figures 4.10 and 4.11.

You can download the sequence sheet for this yoga basics sequence (Figure 9.2.3) from empoweryourflower.com and place it at the front of your mat when practicing.

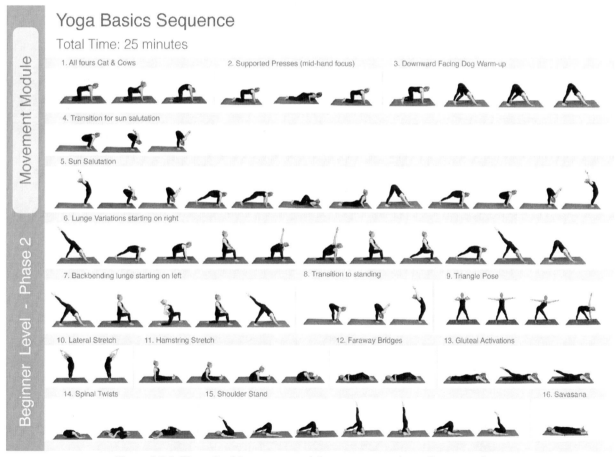

Figure 9.2.3: Phase 2—Movement module yoga preparation—Sequence sheet.

You can read the instructions and steps beforehand, and follow the poses on the printed copy of Figure 9.2.3 when you are practicing. This will help you to learn the sequence and eventually you will be able to practice it without looking at the sheet. Repeated practice creates change in the body.

Yoga Basics Instructions

These exercises will be practiced on a mat. You may need blocks for extra support, depending on your flexibility. You should practice this Yoga Basics sequence at least three days per week if you are working on pelvic floor strength, or twice per week if you are working on pelvic floor relaxation. If you are working on pelvic floor relaxation, remember to relax your pelvic floor on each inhalation

Steps to Perform the Yoga Basics Sequence

1 **All-Fours Cat & Cows**

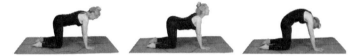

Figure 9.2.3.1: Movement module—Yoga Basics—All-fours cat & cows.

1. Starting in an all-fours position, perform five cat and cow breath cycles to warm up your spine.

2 **Supported Presses (mid-hand focus)**

Figure 9.2.3.2: Movement module—Yoga Basics—Supported presses.

1. From a neutral all-fours position, perform four push-ups (keeping knees down).
2. Exhale while lowering your chest toward the floor, taking the weight into the heels of your hands.
3. Inhale while pressing up through the mid-hand, to come back up to all-fours.
4. Repeat Steps 1 and 2 three times.

3 **Downward Facing Dog Warm-up**

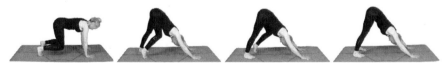

Figure 9.2.3.3: Movement module—Yoga Basics—Downward-facing dog warm up.

1. Inhale as you turn out your toes, and press yourself into a walking dog for a count of five, before returning to stillness in downward-facing dog.

2. Remain in the downward-facing dog pose for five breath cycles, making sure to keep a long spine and bending your knees as much as you need to.

4 Transition for Sun Salutation

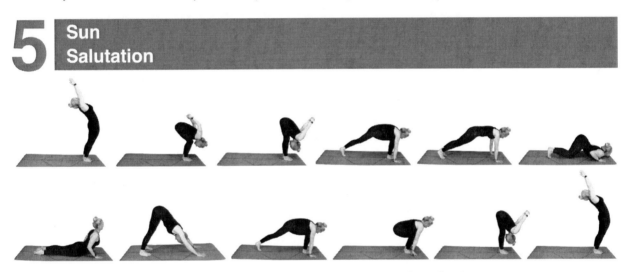

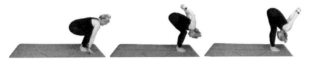

Figure 9.2.3.4: Movement module—Yoga Basics—Transition for sun salutation.

1. Inhale as you look forward between your hands, step the right foot and then the left foot forward, keeping both knees bent as you do so.
2. Exhale as you reach your hands behind your back, interlock your fingers, straighten your legs, and bow your head forward as you reach your arms straight out behind you.

5 Sun Salutation

Figure 9.2.3.5: Movement module—Yoga Basics—Sun salutation.

1. Inhale as you release your hands, bend your knees, and press through the midfoot to a standing backbend, reach your arms overhead. Your legs should be straight, with your hips shifting forward.
2. Exhale as you bow forward, bend your knees, reach your hands behind you, interlock your fingers, straighten your legs, and bow your head forward as you reach your arms straight out behind you.
3. Inhale, bending your knees as much as you need to allow you to place your hands on the floor beside your feet.
4. Exhale as you step back with the left leg, and then the right leg, coming to a plank position and inhale here. *Note*: Make sure to spread your shoulder blades by pressing into the floor in plank position. This will ensure you are engaging the right muscles on the back side of your body rather than collapsing in the back.

5. Exhale as you drop your knees, chest, and chin to the floor, gazing forward.

6. Inhale as you shift your body forward, bringing your hips to the floor and keeping your elbows close to your body, press into the heel of your hand while lifting your chest from the floor for cobra pose. *Note*: As you gain strength in your back muscles, you will be able to lift your chest higher as demonstrated.

7. Exhale as you press through the mid-hand, turning out your toes, and coming to the downward-facing dog. Take three breaths here.

8. Inhale looking forward between your hands and step with your right foot, followed by your left.

9. Exhale as you bend your knees, reach your hands behind you, interlock your fingers, straighten your legs, and bow your head forward while straightening your arms out behind you.

10. Repeat Steps 1 to 7, stepping back with the left leg instead of the right, and **finish the sun salutation in your downward-facing dog.**

6 Lunge Variations Starting on Right

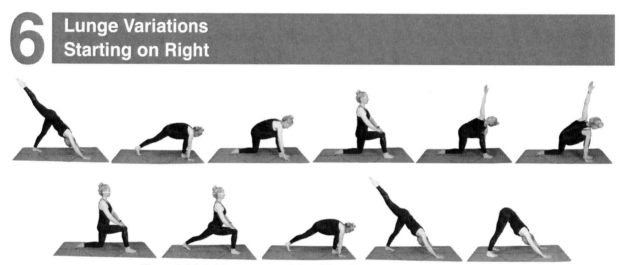

Figure 9.2.3.6: Movement module—Yoga Basics—Lunge variations.

1. From your downward-facing dog, inhale as you lift your right leg high in the air behind you. *Note*: Make sure to keep your hips parallel rather than opening the hips. Your leg should be in line with your body/arms.

2. Exhale as you shift your gaze forward between your hands, stepping your right foot forward. *Note*: If your foot doesn't come all the way between your hands, help it forward.

3. Inhale as you drop your back knee, and bring your body up resting your hands on your legs.

4. Exhale as you release your left hand to the floor. Place your right hand on your shoulder, inhaling as you twist your body, and shift your gaze upwards. If you feel balanced and your elbow is pointed straight up to the ceiling, release your right hand, and extend it toward the ceiling. Perform three breath cycles in this twisted position.

5. Exhale, turning your gaze to the floor, and place your right hand outside your right foot.

6. Inhale as you place your left hand on your left shoulder, twisting, and pointing your left elbow up toward the ceiling. If you feel balanced and your elbow is pointed straight upwards, release your left hand, and extend it toward the ceiling. Perform three breath cycles in this reverse twisted position.

7. Exhale, looking toward your feet, and lowering your left hand back to the floor.

8. Inhale as you come back up to your lunge, resting your hands on your knees. If you feel balanced, turn out your back toes and press them into the floor, lifting your knee from the floor. Perform three breath cycles here, adjusting to the feeling of balancing with the back knee lifted.

9. Turn your gaze to the floor, and place your hands on the floor as you exhale.

10. Inhale, releasing the right leg from between your feet and extending it back for a three-legged dog, and exhale, lower the leg back to a downward-facing dog.

11. Repeat Steps 1 to 10 on the left side.

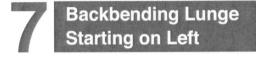
Backbending Lunge
Starting on Left

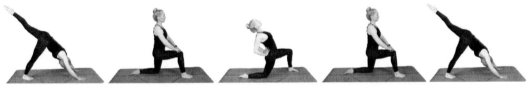

Figure 9.2.3.7: Movement module—Yoga Basics—Back-bending lunge.

1. Inhale as you raise your left leg for a three-legged dog.

2. Exhale as you step the left leg forward.

3. Inhale as you drop your back knee, bringing the upper body up, and supporting yourself by placing your hands on your left knee and exhale here.

4. Release your hands from your knee and place them on your low back, inhaling as you shift your hips forward, lifting your ribcage upwards and gazing toward the ceiling, making a small backbend. *Note*: Resist the temptation to drop your head all the way back, opting instead to elongate your neck as you gaze upwards. Perform three breath cycles here.

5. Inhale as you return to a neutral position, placing hands on your left knee.

6. Exhale, bringing your hands to the floor, and inhale, raising the left leg back to the three-legged dog, and exhale, lowering the leg into downward-facing dog.

7. Repeat Steps 1 to 6 on the right side.

8 Transition to Standing

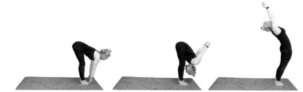

Figure 9.2.3.8: Movement module—Yoga Basics—Transition to standing.

1. From the downward-facing dog, step your right leg forward, followed by your left. Lengthen your spine, and inhale as you gaze forward.
2. Exhale as you reach your hands behind your back, interlocking your fingers, straightening your legs, and bowing your head forward as you reach your arms straight out behind you.
3. Inhale, releasing your hands and coming up with soft knees, reaching the hands overhead for a gentle backbend.
4. Exhale lowering your arms, standing in a neutral position at the top of your mat (*tadasana*), and inhale in preparation for triangle pose.

9 Triangle Pose

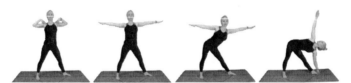

Figure 9.2.3.9: Movement module—Yoga Basics—Triangle pose.

1. Exhale as you take a big step back with your right foot in preparation for *trikonasana* (triangle pose).
2. Inhale as you bring your hands to touch your shoulders, pointing your elbows toward the front and back of your mat in line with your shoulders. Release your hands and simultaneously extend from fingertips on the right hand to fingertips on the left hand.
3. Exhale as you reach your left fingertips forward as far as you can, while sending your hips toward the back of your mat. *Note*: Keep a neutral spine rather than bending at the waist.
4. When you cannot reach your hips back any further, turn your palms to face forward and, while maintaining a neutral torso, rotate your arms so that your left arm is reaching toward your left leg and your right arm is reaching up toward the ceiling. Try to engage the left side of your body while lengthening the right side of your body throughout this movement. If you are very flexible, you can exhale to look at your toes, grab your big toe with peace-sign fingers before inhaling to look up

toward the ceiling. Alternatively, you can raise the floor using a block if needed.

5. Perform five breath cycles in this position and on your final exhalation, turn your gaze toward your toes and press into your feet, using the strength of your legs to bring your body back up.

6. Pivot on your feet to face the opposite side of your mat and repeat the pose on the left side following Steps 3 to 5 before stepping to tadasana in the center of your mat.

10 Lateral Stretch

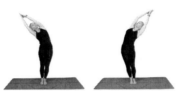

Figure 9.2.3.10: Movement module—Yoga Basics—Lateral stretch.

1. Inhale, bringing your arms overhead. *Note*: Try to cover your ears with your upper arms while lifting your rib cage away from your hips to keep your spine long.

2. Exhale, sending your hips to the right as you reach your hands over to the left. You should feel a deep stretch all the way from the ankle on the right to the fingertips on the right.

3. Perform three breath cycles in this position, lengthening the spine on the inhalation and reaching a little further on the exhalation.

4. Return to the center and repeat on the opposite side, giving maximum focus to shifting the hips to the side.

11 Hamstring Stretch

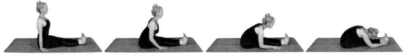

Figure 9.2.3.11: Movement module—Yoga Basics—Hamstring stretch.

1. Come to a seated position on the floor and extend both legs in preparation for *dandasana* (staff pose).

2. Place your hands on the floor beside your hips, lengthen your spine, tuck your chin, engage your quads, and gaze toward your toes. Your heels may lift from the floor slightly due to the engaged quads. Perform three breath cycles here.

3. Inhale as you lengthen your spine, preparing for a forward fold.

4. Exhale to fold forward for a hamstring stretch. *Note*: Maintain a long spine, and resist the temptation

to round your upper back. The goal is not to grab the feet but instead to stretch the hamstrings. Use the engagement of your quads combined with a drawing in of the low belly to bring yourself forward. Don't pull yourself forward using your hands. Only if your stomach reaches your lap should you grab your feet and relax your head on your legs.

5. Perform five breath cycles here.

12 Faraway Bridges

Figure 9.2.3.12: Movement module—Yoga Basics—Faraway bridges.

1. Lay flat on your back and bend your knees slightly, placing your feet flat on the mat.
2. Inhale as you press through the midfoot to lift your hips about 1 inch (2.5 cm) from the mat. *Note*: You should feel a co-contraction at the top of your calf and bottom of your hamstring with some glute activation. Hold the lift for a count of five before lowering.
3. Repeat three times.

13 Gluteal Activations

Figure 9.2.3.13: Movement module—Yoga Basics—Gluteal activations.

1. Turn to lie face down resting your head on the backs of your hands.
2. Relax your left leg and engage your right leg, reach your right toes away from your body as you press the right hip into the floor while lifting the leg for a count of three. *Note*: You should feel the right glute muscles engaging.
3. Lower the leg and repeat twice more on this side before taking the pose on the opposite side.
4. Flex the right foot and externally rotate the leg at the hip so that the inside of the foot is facing the floor.
5. Relax the left leg and lift the right leg, keeping the hip rotated while making sure both hips remain on the mat throughout, lifting the foot as high as possible for a count of three
6. Lower the leg and repeat this twice more before taking the position on the opposite side.
7. Place the palms of your hands under your shoulders and press through the mid-hand, pushing yourself up on all-fours before resting in child's pose. Take a few breaths here if needed.

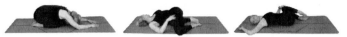

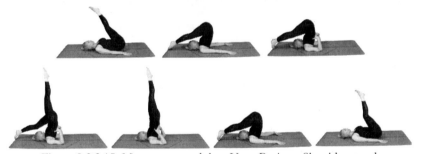

Figure 9.2.3.14: Movement module—Yoga Basics—Spinal twists.

1. From child's pose, come to sitting on the mat and swing your legs around in front of you before lying down.

2. Hug your knees into your chest and lift your hips, shifting them a little to the left.

3. Keep your shoulders relaxed on the mat and drop your knees over to the right side, taking a spinal twist while gazing over to the left. Perform five breath cycles here, relaxing as much as you can in your entire body during these breaths.

4. Inhale, bringing your head back to the center, then bring your knees back to the center before repeating Steps 2 to 3 to perform the twist on the opposite side.

15 Shoulder Stand

Figure 9.2.3.15: Movement module—Yoga Basics—Shoulder stand.

1. Straighten your legs and place your hands along the side of your body, pressing them into the floor as you bring your legs up over your head. Bring your feet to touch the floor for *halasana* (plough pose) in preparation for shoulder stand. *Note*: Place a bolster behind your head for your feet to rest on if they do not reach the floor. Your weight rests on your shoulders, and not on your neck.

2. Only if your feet reach the floor (or the bolster) should you release your palms from the floor, bending at the elbow and supporting your back with your hands. *Note*: Try to keep your elbows in line with your shoulders as you do this.

3. If your hands make good contact with your back, you can release one foot (or both together) from the floor, raising them up above your body for shoulder stand. Make sure that the weight is resting in the shoulders and on the back of the arms and not on your neck. If you feel pressure in your

neck, regress to the previous step (e.g., keep your palms on the floor and your feet on the bolster). *Note*: During your menstrual cycle, keep your hips on the floor, opting for the very first pose in this sequence where you just raise your legs up, pressing your hands into the floor.

4. Relax in your shoulder stand for ten breath cycles.

5. Lower your feet behind your head to the floor (or bolster) while keeping your hands supported on your back.

6. Release your hands from your back, reaching them out and pressing them into the floor as your roll down one vertebra at a time. *Note*: Only release your hands from your back when your feet are resting on the floor (or bolster).

16 Savasana

Figure 9.2.3.16: Movement module—Yoga Basics—Savasana.

1. Finish the practice by relaxing in savasana pose for five minutes.

That completes our Yoga Basics practice. You will perform the exercises from this module on the days specified in your weekly schedule. If you are new to yoga, this sequence may feel difficult at first, and you may find it takes longer to go through the sequence than the expected twenty-five minutes. This will change as you get used to the practice. Your tissues are learning to adapt to movements in all planes (directions). Within a couple of weeks of steady practice, it will become much easier, more fluid, and time-efficient. Remember that you always have the option to come to child's pose to take a short rest during the sequence if you need it.

Phase 2: Relaxation Module

Yin Yoga Forward Folds

Having completed Phase 1, you should be well practiced at completely relaxing your body in various restorative positions. This is a fantastic achievement!

Objective

The objective of the relaxation module in Phase 2 is to perform yin poses that help to rebalance the length-tension relationships, with a specific focus on the back side of the body and the pelvic floor. Yin poses are held for between three and five minutes. Yin, unlike restorative, is relaxation into the discomfort of the tension within your own body. In my opinion, this is a valuable way to communicate with your nervous system.

You will assume various positions (*asanas*) where you must relax all of your muscles while allowing your connective tissue to slowly release. Muscle stretches quickly like elastic while connective tissue stretches slowly like plastic.

In Chapter Three, we explored the double lattice pattern of connective tissue (Figure 3.11) and learned about the connective tissue cells (slugs) and their collagen trails. Relaxing in yin yoga creates directional pull that encourages fluids to move, helping to realign tissue patterns, which can contribute to an overall improvement of tensional balance in the body.

When relaxing in yin poses, it is important that you work within your body's own tension. I like to say, "Relax into your own discomfort" as it often feels uncomfortable in the poses; however, **you should never move from discomfort to pain**. The border between discomfort and pain is your edge. Pay close attention to your edge as you practice. You should not feel pain when you practice yin. Pay attention to your joints when you practice, you should not feel pain in or around your joints.

Each yin pose focuses on stretching a specific area. How the pose looks for you could be quite different from how it looks for someone else, as the pattern of tension in your body is unique to you. Rather than focusing on how it *looks*, focus on how it *feels*.

You should be completely relaxed when practicing yin. It can help to search for the gap between your thought trains when you practice. There is stillness in that gap, and you can find peace in that stillness.

Success Metric

Success is achieved when you can relax into your own body's pattern of tension, meeting the very edge of your discomfort without moving into pain. The restorative yoga and yoga nidra in Phase 1 should have prepared you for success with your yin practice.

Additional Notes

You can use lots of props, such as bolsters, blocks, and blankets to support you when practicing yin. Make sure not to push or pull your way into any of the poses. For seated poses, if you collapse in the low back—as shown on the left image in Figure 9.2.4—or if you have excessive pull on your hamstrings when sitting with the legs extended, you can place a blanket underneath your sitting bones. This helps to neutralize your pelvis. An additional blanket underneath your knees helps to reduce the pull on your hamstrings (as shown on the right image in Figure 9.2.4).

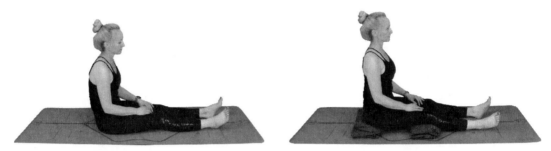

Figure 9.2.4: Sitting on blankets to balance the pelvis.

If sitting with legs extended is uncomfortable, the support of the blankets shown in Figure 9.2.4 will allow you to relax properly, which is more beneficial when it comes to repatterning.

There is no *goal position*. You are not trying to achieve any specific level of flexibility and it's not about *touching your toes*. You are simply tapping into the business of your body's movement to help remap the pattern of your body's tension.

At the end of each pose, you will take three long, deep breaths. Imagine that you can inhale to the area where you feel most tension (even if that means breathing into your toes!). With the subsequent exhalation, imagine you can breathe the tension out for deeper relaxation.

You should move very slowly out of each position as your connective tissue is slow to recoil. There is a counter pose following each yin position. This provides a brief reset before moving to the next asana.

Yin Yoga Forward Folds Instructions

You will need one or two bolsters (or pillows), two blankets, two blocks, an eye pillow, and a yoga mat. This practice will take thirty minutes, including setup, and transitions between poses. You can download the sequence sheet for this yin yoga sequence (Figure 9.2.5) from empoweryourflower.com and place it at the front of your mat when practicing.

You can read the instructions and steps beforehand and follow the poses on the printed copy of Figure 9.2.5 when you are practicing. This will help you to learn the sequence and eventually you will be able to practice it without looking at the sheet.

Yin Yoga Forward Folds Sequence

Total Time: 30 minutes

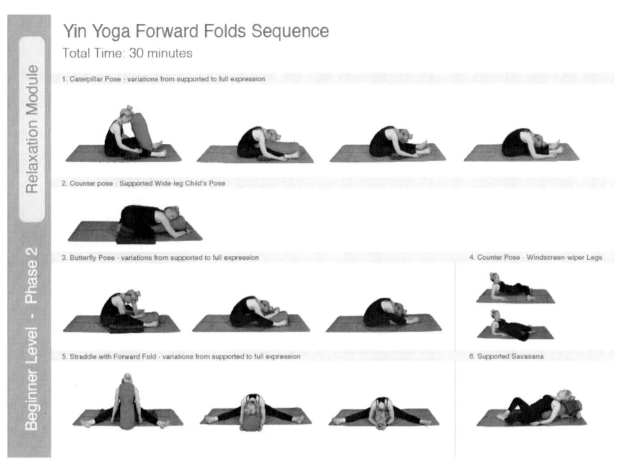

1. Caterpillar Pose · variations from supported to full expression

2. Counter pose · Supported Wide-leg Child's Pose

3. Butterfly Pose · variations from supported to full expression

4. Counter Pose · Windscreen-wiper Legs

5. Straddle with Forward Fold · variations from supported to full expression

6. Supported Savasana

Figure 9.2.5: Phase 2—Relaxation module—Yin yoga forward folds.

Steps to Perform the Yin Yoga Forward Folds Sequence

1 Caterpillar Pose

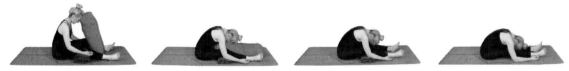

Figure 9.2.5.1: Relaxation module—Yin yoga forward folds—Caterpillar pose.

Caterpillar pose is a yin forward fold, which allows you to round your back as you relax forward. You should feel a stretch through the entire back side of your body, and, in particular, your hamstrings. There are multiple variations demonstrated in Figure 9.2.5.1, using props to support the relaxation. To assume the pose:

1. Sit with your legs hip-distance apart and stretched out in front of you. Allow your legs to be relaxed in this position.

2. Allow yourself to relax forward, letting your head hang, and allowing the weight of your upper body to surrender forward.

3. Props can be used to make this easier. Images display the completely supported version through to the full unsupported expression of the pose (no props).

4. Relax in your version of this position for five minutes. You will feel your tissues release as time passes.

5. Very slowly, mindfully bring energy into your hands, and slowly press your hands to bring yourself back to a seated position.

2 Counter Pose— Supported Wide-Leg Child's Pose

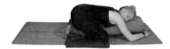

Figure 9.2.5.2: Relaxation module—Yin yoga forward folds—Counter supported child's pose.

1. Slowly move to the supported wide-leg child's pose, staying in this position for one minute.

3 Butterfly Pose

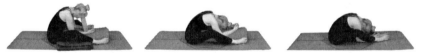

Figure 9.2.5.3: Relaxation module—Yin yoga forward folds—Butterfly pose.

Butterfly pose is a yin forward fold that allows you to feel the stretch on the insides of your legs, particularly the adductor muscles. Props can be used to make this easier, which is demonstrated in Figure 9.2.5.3, showing the completely supported version through to the full unsupported expression of the pose (no props).

To assume the pose:

1. Place a bolster between your legs and slightly bend your knees, rotating at the hip to allow the legs to fall open.

2. Bring your feet to touch the bolster (or to touch each other in the unsupported version).

3. Allow your legs to be relaxed in this position. You should feel the tension on the insides of your legs.

4. Allow yourself to relax forward, letting your head hang and surrendering the weight of your upper body. Allowing the palms to face up will help prevent any pulling into this position.

5. Relax in your version of this position for five minutes. You will feel your tissues release as time passes.

6. After five minutes, very slowly, mindfully bring energy into your hands and slowly press your hands into the floor to come back up.

4 Counter Pose— Windscreen Wiper Legs

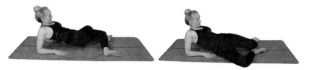

Figure 9.2.5.4: Relaxation module—Yin yoga forward folds—Counter windscreen wipers.

1. Slowly move to the counterpose, windscreen-wiper legs, by resting back on your elbows and windscreen-wiping your legs from side to side, rolling over your glutes. This is my version of a free butt massage.

5 Straddle with Forward Fold

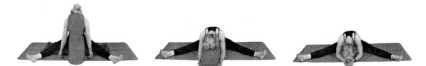

Figure 9.2.5.5: Relaxation module—Yin yoga forward folds—Straddle forward fold.

Straddle pose with a forward fold is a yin asana that will allow you to feel the stretch on the insides and back of your legs but with a different pattern of tension than in the caterpillar and butterfly poses. Figure 9.2.5.5 demonstrates the completely supported version through to the full unsupported expression of the pose (no props).

To assume the pose:

1. Take your version of a straddle, this could be with legs very wide apart or closer together depending on your flexibility. You can use a blanket under your hips and knees if needed.

2. Fold forward when in the straddle position. Again, depending on your flexibility, you can use a bolster to support your forward fold. Ensure you fold forward with a relaxed spine (rounding is OK). Relax your legs in this position. You may feel the tension on the insides or backs of your legs all the way from the ankles. Allowing your palms to face up will prevent any pulling into this position.

3. Relax in your version of this position for five minutes. You will feel your tissues release as time passes.

4. After five minutes, very slowly, mindfully bring energy into your hands, and slowly press your

hands into the floor to come back up to seated. Use your hands under your knees to release your legs from the straddle rather than using the strength of your legs. Shake your legs out before moving to the final position.

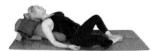

Supported Baddha Konasana

Figure 9.2.5.6: Relaxation module—Yin yoga forward folds—Supported Baddha Konasana.

Note: You will need a blanket, a bolster, two blocks, and eye pillow for this pose and can optionally cover yourself with a blanket.

1. Stack two blocks on your mat and rest the bolster on the blocks.
2. Rest back over the bolster, placing a blanket behind your head and covering your eyes with the eye pillow if that feels comfortable.
3. Relax in this position for five minutes.

Yin is a practice that I like to visualize as wringing out the sponge, where your connective tissues are the sponge and the yin poses create the compression/stretch to release fluids. This movement of fluids can be helpful if you have inflammation. Motion is lotion, and yin yoga is one of my favorite lotions. This completes the relaxation module. You will perform the exercises from this module on the days specified in your weekly schedule.

Phase 2: Mind & Meditation Module

Flex Your Mind to Flex Your Muscles

Having completed Phase 1 of the pelvic floor training, you should be very familiar with performing the contractions on different parts of your pelvic floor. You will need that knowledge for this module. You should also be well practiced in yoga nidra, which is a great way to reduce physical tension and stress. What a wonderful gift to give yourself!

Objective

The objective of the mind/meditation module in Phase 2 is to combine your ability to relax your entire body with your knowledge of how it feels to contract the different parts of your pelvic floor. In Chapter Six, we learned about the research that shows it is possible to improve the tone of a muscle by imagining contracting that muscle. We will utilize this research with this meditation as we will flex our minds to virtually flex our muscles thus improving our potential for rehabilitation. If you are suffering from pelvic pain, you can swap this meditation with the yoga nidra, which is more beneficial for relaxing your pelvic floor.

Success Metric

Success is achieved when you can perform this meditation, imagining strong contractions while keeping your body completely relaxed. This is harder than it sounds and does require practice.

Additional Notes

It is good to perform this meditation in a place where you can be completely comfortable and relaxed while remaining undisturbed. Turn off your phone and eliminate any distractions. This meditation should take less than ten minutes, although you can practice for longer if you choose to.

It can be easier to imagine your contractions if you practice this meditation immediately after performing your actual contractions as your awareness of your pelvic floor will be heightened at that point. You should read through the instructions before you begin and meditate with these instructions in your mind. Alternatively, listen to the guided audio for this meditation on empoweryourflower.com.

Flex Your Mind to Flex Your Muscles' Instructions

For this exercise, you will focus on completely relaxing your body while imagining strong pelvic floor contractions. You will practice this meditation twice per week.

Steps to Perform the Meditation Exercise

1. Get yourself into a comfortable starting position, lying down with your eyes closed.
2. Perform five calming breath cycles before you begin, focusing on relaxing your entire body as you breathe.
3. Bring your awareness to your pelvis and pelvic floor, making sure it is completely relaxed. You can gently press the different parts of your pelvic floor to help heighten your awareness if you struggle to feel it with your mind.
4. Relaxing your hands by your side, begin to imagine performing a full Kegel equal to a score of ten on your strength assessment. This will be a strong contraction with a strong lift. You could imagine that if your finger was in your vagina, this contraction would squeeze your finger strongly.

5. Hold your imagined contraction for five natural breath cycles before imagining complete relaxation of your pelvic floor.

6. Begin your second imagined contraction. Imagine that this contraction is so strong that the opening to your vagina closes while drawing deep within. Allow your body to be completely relaxed as you imagine this strong contraction.

7. Hold your imagined contraction for five natural breath cycles before imagining complete relaxation of your pelvic floor.

8. Repeat eight more times, performing ten imagined contractions in total.

If you suffer specifically from stress incontinence, you could focus on imagining closing the external urethral sphincter rather than the whole pelvic floor.

That completes the mind and meditation module and brings us to the end of the Phase 2 training. You will perform the exercises from this module on the days specified in your weekly schedule.

At the end of each week, if you feel that you may be ready to progress to the next phase of training, you can perform the phase checkpoint review using Figure 9.2.6, which checks your progress against the success metric for each module, and helps you to decide if you should proceed to Phase 3 (beginner level). You can download a blank version of this form from empoweryourflower.com.

Phase 2 Checkpoint Review

Phase Start Date:_____

Checkpoint Date:_____

Pelvic Floor Module

Success

Strength: Success is achieved when you can perform a controlled squeeze of a finger inserted in the vagina giving a score of 4 on the strength scale which is the equivalent to a weak contraction with weak lift. You should be able to maintain this contraction with weak lift for the count of 5, while breathing calmly and having your body relaxed

Yes ☐
No ☐

Relaxation: Success is achieved when you can relax your pelvic floor fully in all the positions specified and no longer feel the symptoms of hypertonicity. Note: Reverse Kegels can help to release pelvic tension, however, you will continue to practice the reverse Kegels module through the entire program and so if you do not achieve success with the pelvic floor relaxation at this phase, this should not prevent you from proceeding to the next phase.

Yes ☐
No ☐

Breathing Module - Breath Strengthening

Success

Success is achieved when you can inhale sufficiently and perform the exercise of filling the balloon without the feeling of exhaustion, all the while maintaining balanced intra-abdominal pressure.

Yes ☐
No ☐

Movement Module - Yoga Basics Sequence

Success

Success is achieved when you can comfortably move through the sequence. It should be easy for you to complete the session without getting out of breath.

Yes ☐
No ☐

Relaxation Module - Yin Yoga Forward Folding Sequence

Success

Success is achieved when you can relax into your own body's pattern of tension, meeting the very edge of your discomfort without moving into pain.

Yes ☐
No ☐

Mind & Meditation Module - Flex your mind to flex your muscles

Success

If you performed the "flex your mind to flex your muscles" meditation, success is achieved when you can perform this meditation imagining strong contractions while keeping your body completely relaxed. This is harder than it sounds and does require practice. If you replaced that meditation with Yoga Nidra, success is achieved when you can completely relax your entire body for the duration of the meditation..

Yes ☐
No ☐

Phase 3 Checkpoint Review

Success

Have you achieved the success objectives and do you feel that you are ready to proceed to the next phase of training?

Yes ☐
No ☐

If no, please continue with the phase 2 training until you are ready to proceed or regress to the phase 1 training if you felt this phase was too difficult.

If yes, proceed to Phase 3 training. Remember, you can regress to the phase 2 training if you find phase 3 to be too difficult. Listen to your body and good luck!

Figure 9.2.6: Phase 2—Checkpoint review form.

Welcome to Phase 3 of the eight-phase training program. This is the second phase of the beginner level of the training, which increases the physical and mental effort versus Phase 2. The following section details the Phase 3 training modules, which are highlighted in Figure 9.3.1.

Eight-Phase Modules	Prep	Beginner			Intermediate		Advanced	
	Phase 1	Phase 2	Phase 3	Phase 4	Phase 5	Phase 6	Phase 7	Phase 8
Pelvic Floor	Kegel Breakdown	Full Kegel	Endurance Kegel	Speed Kegel	Co-Contract	Maximize Strength	Standing Rotations	Functional Training
Breathing	Nasal Breathing	Breath Strengthening	Breath Remapping	Nadi Shodhana	Basic Hypopressive Exercise	Intermediate Hypopressive Sequence	Advanced Hypopressive Sequence	Kapalabhati Breathing
Movement	Yoga Preparation	Yoga Basics	Core Re-tensioning	Rebalancing Yoga	Bandha Strength Yoga	Max Kegel Yoga	Ball Routine	Dynamic Power Yoga
Relaxation	Restorative Yoga	Yin Yoga Forward Folds	Yin Yoga Backward Bending	Yin Yoga Twists & Lateral Movement	Yin Yoga Hip Opening	Yin Yoga Pelvic Floor	Yin Yoga Happy Hips	Yin Yoga All Body
Mind & Meditation	Yoga Nidra	Flex your mind to flex your muscles	ANT therapy	Conquer your fear	Kirtan Kriya	Self Affirmations	Journaling	Blossoming Goddess

Figure 9.3.1: Phase 3—Beginner level.

The exercises and activities for the Phase 3 modules, highlighted in green in Figure 9.3.1, are intended to increase pelvic floor endurance (for strength focus), increase ribcage mobility, and enhance your core strength. This phase progresses the effort to rebalance length-tension relationships throughout the body, which should benefit both those working on pelvic floor strength and relaxation.

Remember, if your goal is pelvic floor relaxation, you will work on the reverse Kegels activity, which is detailed in Phase 1 Pelvic Floor module for all phases of the training. Make sure you listen to your body as the intensity increases in the movement practice, relaxing your pelvic floor on each inhalation, and skipping any poses that make you feel tense in your pelvic floor.

The frequency of practice changes as you progress through the training so, make sure to read through all modules for Phase 3 before you begin, and update your schedule accordingly.

Phase 3
Modules

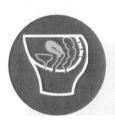

Pelvic Floor

Endurance Kegel

Breathing

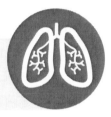

Breath Remapping

Movement

Core Re-tensioning

Relaxation

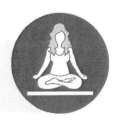

Yin Yoga Backward Bending

Mind & Meditation

ANT Therapy

Phase 3: Pelvic Floor Module

Endurance Kegel

Having completed Phase 2, you should have increased your pelvic floor strength and should be seeing some lift when you perform your pelvic floor exercises. Great work!

Objective

The objective of the pelvic floor module in Phase 3 is to increase endurance by focusing on slow-twitch fibers within the pelvic floor muscles. It is at this stage that you will focus on holding your contraction through multiple breath cycles, instead of contracting on exhalation and relaxing on inhalation. This will improve your pelvic floor endurance.

Success Metric

Success is achieved when you can hold your pelvic floor contraction for ten calming breath cycles (inhaling for four, exhaling for eight). You should be able to maintain the contraction with some lift while breathing with your body relaxed.

Endurance Kegel Exercise Instructions

For this exercise, you will focus on performing and sustaining full pelvic floor contractions. You will continue to practice six days per week while alternating your position each day as per Phase 1 (Figures 9.1.3 a & b):

Day 1:   Hook lying.
Day 2:   Cross leg sitting.
Day 3:   Side-lying (top leg bent).
Day 4:   Side-lying (bottom leg bent).
Day 5:   Kneeling up.
Day 6:   Sitting & standing.

Initially, you may find it difficult to hold your contraction throughout the breath cycles, particularly in upright positions, but this should improve as you continue to practice. It can be helpful to perform five calming breath cycles before you begin the exercise.

Steps to Perform the Endurance Kegel Exercise

1. Get yourself into a comfortable starting position.

2. Begin your first breath cycle, inhaling for a count of four.

3. On your next exhalation, begin to perform your full pelvic floor contraction as you continue to exhale for a count of four. Keep holding the contraction as you inhale for a count of four.

4. Continue for five breath cycles (This is one set). You may lose your contraction or lift before your fifth breath cycle is complete, particularly in upright positions. Do not despair as this will improve with consistent steady practice. Make sure to keep the rest of your body relaxed as you perform the exercise.

5. Repeat the exercise until you have performed five sets in total.

When you first begin with endurance Kegels, it may feel impossible to hold your contraction for five breath cycles, particularly in the standing position. Stick with it, consistent steady practice will make it easier. When you find that holding the contraction for five breath cycles is easy, you can increase it to ten for an extra challenge. This completes the pelvic floor (strength) module.

Phase 3: Breathing Module

Breath Remapping

Having completed Phase 2, you should be nasal breathing with improved diaphragmatic strength. This is a great achievement, give yourself a round of applause!

Objective
The objective with the breathing module in Phase 3 is to begin the process of neurologically remapping your breathing, and helping to ensure you make use of your full lung capacity. We will use some floor exercises that help to increase ribcage mobility for this purpose.

Success Metric
Success is achieved when you can easily perform the exercise while maintaining good core stability.

Additional Notes
This exercise can be difficult if you have a limited ROM in your shoulders, in which case you can use a yoga bolster behind your head to elevate the floor as shown in Figure 9.3.2.

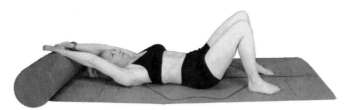

Figure 9.3.2: Using bolster for support if shoulder ROM is limited.

If you are using the bolster as demonstrated in Figure 9.3.2, you should find over time that your shoulder ROM increases. Strive to reduce the size of the bolster until you are eventually reaching your hands onto the floor behind you.

Breath Remapping Exercise Instructions

For this exercise, you will need a yoga mat. A bolster is optional (as shown in Figure 9.3.2) if you have limited shoulder ROM. You will perform the exercise in a hook-lying position and will practice this breathing exercise every second day.

Steps to Perform the Breath Remapping Exercise

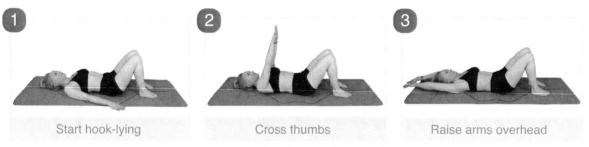

Figure 9.3.3: Breath remapping exercise.

1. Come to a hook-lying position on your mat. Make sure that you are not pressing any part of your body into the mat, just relax.
   a. Close your mouth keeping your lips together with your teeth slightly apart, tongue resting on the roof of your mouth behind your front teeth.
   b. Inhale gently through your nose while relaxing your shoulders and chest. Your breath should be quiet and soft.
   c. Take a few breaths in this position and notice how it feels.
2. Reach your arms out in front of you protracting your shoulder blades (spreading them away from each other) and hooking your thumbs.
3. Depress your ribcage (lowering the bottom of your ribs down, low back will flatten on the mat).
4. Begin to exhale while maintaining the depressed rib cage, and reaching your arms up over your head

toward the floor (or bolster). You should use forced exhalation to empty your lungs completely until you have no air left while continuing to reach out through the fingers.

    a.   With empty lungs, hold your breath out for a count of five.

    b.   **Inhale** through your nose, maintaining a depressed rib cage with your arms still overhead.

    c.   **Exhale** completely until you have emptied your lungs

    d.   **Hold** your breath out for a count of five, gently inhaling when done (this is one set).

    e.   Repeat this inhalation, exhalation, hold pattern for five breath cycles (sets).

    f.   On your final exhalation, bring the arms back down, relaxing them by your sides.

Take 10 soft nasal breaths with your arms relaxed beside your body after the exercise and notice the difference in your breathing after working your diaphragm in the stretched position. Your breathing should feel free and easy. This breathing exercise can help to restore ROM around the shoulders as well as improving the mobility of the rib cage, both beneficial to functional breathing. This exercise also contributes to core stability, which we will focus on in the core re-tensioning sequence in the movement module that follows.

This concludes the breathing module. You will perform the exercises from this module on the days specified in your weekly schedule.

Phase 3: Movement Module

Core Re-tensioning

Having completed Phase 2, your ability to tolerate peripheral load through the limbs should have improved. This should ensure an optimized balance of load when performing basic functional tasks. Go you!

Objective

The objective of the movement module in Phase 3 is to shift focus from the periphery to the management of tension through the center of the body. Your breathing function should have improved somewhat through the breathing exercises in phases 1 and 2, which should ensure you reap the benefits with this module.

Success Metric

Success with this module is achieved when you can properly activate your glutes and core and have increased your ability to tolerate load through these muscle tissues.

Additional Notes

Weak glutes and core can have a negative impact on pelvic floor function. The exercises in this module should help to improve your core stability, which can have a positive impact on your symptoms. Remember that you can raise the floor using yoga blocks (as demonstrated in Figure 9.1.8) if you lack sufficient ROM to complete the full expression of the pose. Listen to your body and practice from where you find it.

Core Re-tensioning Sequence Instructions

You will need a yoga mat and a long resistance band for this exercise routine. The sequence should take thirty minutes. You can download the sequence sheet for this core re-tensioning sequence (Figure 9.3.4) from empoweryourflower.com and place it at the front of your mat when practicing.

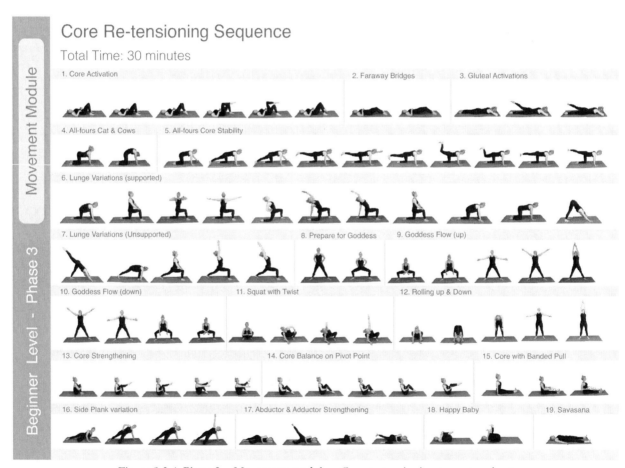

Figure 9.3.4: Phase 3—Movement module—Core re-tensioning sequence sheet

You can read the instructions and steps beforehand and follow the poses on the printed copy of Figure

9.3.4 when you are practicing. This will help you to learn the sequence and eventually you will be able to practice it without looking at the sheet. Repeated practice creates change in the body.

Steps to Perform the Core Re-tensioning Sequence

1 Core Activation

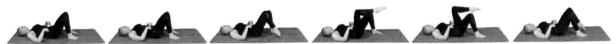

Figure 9.3.4.1: Movement module—Core re-tensioning—Core activation.

1. Lie down in a hook-lying position in preparation for core activation. Using your index fingers, find your ASIS joints at the front of your hips. *Note*: They will be more prominent in the hook-lying position.
2. Step your fingers in and down 1 inch (2.5 cm) from these ASIS joints to find the lower portion of the transversus abdominis (deep ab muscles). You will notice that it is soft.
3. Press your low back into the floor and notice how this spot becomes harder.
4. Point your right toe with just the tip of your toe touching the ground with your knee bent at a 90-degree angle.
5. Maintaining the bent knee, raise the foot from the floor, keeping the low back pressed hard against the floor.
6. Bring the toe to touch the floor again, raising and lowering the foot 5 times.
7. Switch to the left side and repeat the raise and lower of the foot 5 times on that side.

2 Faraway Bridges

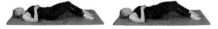

Figure 9.3.4.2: Movement module—Core re-tensioning—Faraway bridges.

1. Reduce the bend in the knees so that the feet are reaching further away, hands resting on the bottom of your ribcage.
2. Press into your midfoot to lift your hips about 1 inch (2.5 cm) from the floor, and hold the hips up for a count of three.
3. Repeat three times.

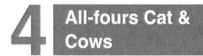

3 Gluteal Activations

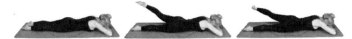

Figure 9.3.4.3: Movement module—Core re-tensioning—Gluteal activations.

1. Turn onto your stomach, using the back of your hands as a pillow.
2. Relax your left leg as you extend your right leg reaching your toes away from you, pressing the right hip into the floor, and lifting the right leg as high as possible while squeezing your right glutes hard for a count of three before lowering.
3. Repeat three times.
4. Flex the right foot and externally rotate at the hip so the inside of the foot faces the floor.
5. Press right hip into the floor raising the right leg as high as possible while squeezing your right glutes hard for a count of three before lowering.
6. Repeat three times.
7. Perform Steps 2 to 6 on the left side.

4 All-fours Cat & Cows

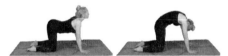

Figure 9.3.4.4: Movement module—Core re-tensioning—All-fours cat & cows.

1. Place your hands under your shoulders and press into the mid-hand to push yourself up to an all-fours position.
2. Begin cat-cow breathing in all-fours position for five breath cycles before returning to neutral.

5 All-fours Core Stability

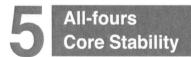

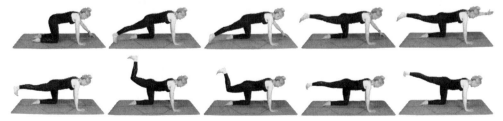

Figure 9.3.4.5: Movement module—Core re-tensioning—All-fours core stability.

Note: Keep the hips level throughout and rest in a child's pose if needed.

1. From neutral all-fours, extend the left fingertips forward touching the floor, maintaining a strong core and keeping shoulders and hips level. Hold for a count of three before returning to neutral.

2. Release the right leg back, keep the toes touching the floor while maintaining a strong core and keeping shoulders and hips level. Hold for a count of 3 before returning to neutral.

3. Release the left hand forward and the right leg back with fingers and toes touching the floor.
   a. If you feel balanced here, release your right leg from the floor, bringing it up in line with your hip.
   b. If you feel balanced here, release your left hand from the floor, extending the arm forward, maintaining a strong core with hips and shoulders aligned. Reach from left fingertips to right toes.
   c. Hold for a count of five then repeat Steps 1 through 3 for the opposite side (right hand, left leg) before returning to a neutral all-fours position.

4. Keeping both hands planted under shoulders, release your right leg from the floor, flexing the foot and bringing the leg up in line with the right hip.
   a. Flex your knee to a 90-degree angle so the sole of your foot faces up toward the ceiling.
   b. Keeping your hips level, reach your foot up toward the ceiling. You should feel a contraction of the right glutes as you do this. Reach as high as possible for a count of three, then lower back down to 90 degrees.
   c. Repeat three times before repeating on the left side.

5. Keeping both hands planted under shoulders, release your right leg from the floor, flexing your right foot and rotating at the hip so the inside of your foot is facing the floor.
   a. While keeping the leg straight, raise the foot as high as possible. You should feel a contraction at the side of your hip while you perform this movement. Reach as high as you can before lowering the leg back in line with the hip.
   b. Repeat three times before repeating on the left side.

6 Lunge Variations (Supported)

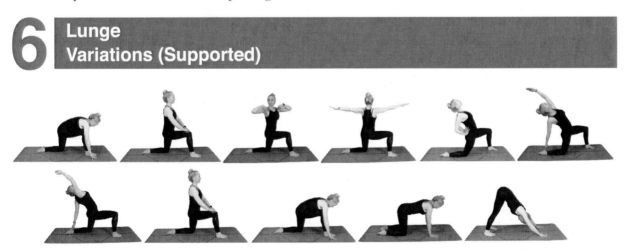

Figure 9.3.4.6: Movement module—Core re-tensioning—Lunge variations (supported).

1. Return to an all-fours position and step your right foot forward between your hands before inhaling as you rise for a low lunge, left knee remains on the floor, resting your hands on your right knee.

2. Bring your hands onto your shoulders and twist to the right side pointing your elbows to the front and back of your mat before extending your arms out, reaching your hands away from each other.

3. Perform three breath cycles here.

4. Return to the center and take the twist to the opposite side, again bringing your hands onto your shoulders, pointing your elbows to the side, and extending your arms.

5. Perform three breath cycles here before returning to the neutral position resting your hands on your knee.

6. Place your hands on your low back and lift your ribcage away from your hips as you shift the hips forward taking a back-bending lunge. Perform three breath cycles here.

7. On your third exhalation, drop your left hand onto your left heel and deepen your backbend as you reach your right hand over your head.

8. Perform three breath cycles here before coming back to a neutral position by lifting your ribcage away from the hips while engaging your core to bring yourself up.

9. Place your hands on the mat and return to all-fours before stepping your left foot forward and repeating Steps 1 to 7 on the right side.

10. Return to your all-fours position, turn out your toes, and press back to downward-facing dog. Find stillness in your downward-facing dog for three breath cycles.

7 Lunge Variations (Unsupported)

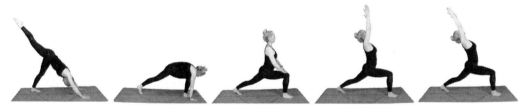

Figure 9.3.4.7: Movement module—Core re-tensioning—Lunge variations (unsupported).

1. On your next inhalation, lift your right leg for the three-legged dog, making sure to keep your hips level.

2. Exhale as you step the right foot forward between your hands.

3. Inhale as you use the strength of your legs, come up to a lunge, keeping the left leg straight, left heel is off the ground. Exhale here.

4. Inhale as you raise your hands over your head, keeping strong legs as you take a small backbend lifting your ribcage away from your hips. *Note:* This backbend should feel easier than those in Phase 2

as your body is becoming stronger and more flexible.

5. Perform three breath cycles here.

6. On your next exhalation, place both hands on the floor on either side of your feet and bring your right leg back for the three-legged dog before exhaling for the downward-facing dog.

7. Repeat Steps 1 to 5 on the left side. *Note*: Do not return to the downward-facing dog when you take the pose on the left instead, **finishing in the lunge position**, bringing your hands back down onto your knee.

8 Prepare for Goddess

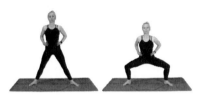

Figure 9.3.4.8: Movement module—Core re-tensioning—Prep for goddess flow.

1. From the lunge position, inhale as you straighten your left leg, placing your hands on your waist and turning your body so you are standing longways on the mat. Turn your toes out to face the corners of the mat.

2. Keeping your hands on your waist, exhale as you bend your knees to come into goddess pose. *Note*: Make sure that your knees do not fall inwards in this position. The middle of your knee should be tracking over your second and third toes. Your spine should remain neutral as much as possible.

9 Goddess Flow

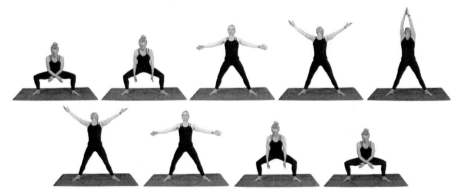

Figure 9.3.4.9: Movement module—Core re-tensioning—Goddess flow.

1. Release your hands in front of your body and inhale as you begin to straighten your legs while you

sweep your hands out to the sides bringing them over your head. *Note*: At the top of the inhalation, you should have your hands together over your head with your legs straight.

2. Exhale as you sweep your hands back down, bending your knees to come back to goddess pose.

3. Flow through Steps 1 and 2 for five full breath cycles, finish by exhaling without bending your knees, and bring your hands back to your waist.

10 Squat with Twist

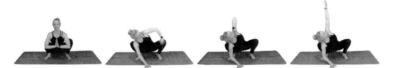

Figure 9.3.4.10: Movement module—Core re-tensioning—Squat with twist.

1. Heel-toe your feet closer together until you are standing a little more than hip-distance apart.

2. Inhale here before exhaling to lower down into a yoga squat. *Note*: If your heels do not reach the ground in a squat, you can elevate them using a rolled-up towel or some yoga blocks. If you struggle to find balance in a squat, you can place a block under your backside to rest on.

3. Press your hands together in front of your heart, keeping your wrists in line with your elbows with the inside of your knees pressing against the outside of your arms. Take three breath cycles here. *Note*: Elongate your spine trying to bring your chest towards your thumbs.

4. Release your right hand to the centre of the mat, placing your left hand on your left knee for a twist. If you feel comfortable in the twist, bring your left hand onto your shoulder, pointing your elbow toward the ceiling. Extend the arm for the full expression of this twist.

5. Exhale as you lower your left hand to the floor coming out of the twist.

6. Repeat Steps 4 and 5 on the other side finishing with both hands resting on the floor.

11 Rolling Up & Down

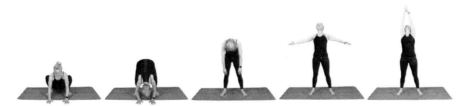

Figure 9.3.4.11: Movement module—Core re-tensioning—Rolling up and down.

1. Inhale as you release your hips from the squat, pressing through the midfoot and sending your hips

up toward the ceiling as you bend forward. *Note*: Allow your head, rib cage, and upper body to hang completely, keeping your knees bent.

2. Keeping softly bent knees, press through your midfoot, and slowly roll up through the spine one vertebrae at a time, sweeping your arms out to the side. The inhalation finishes with your hands together above your head, gaze at your thumbs, weight evenly balanced between the feet.

3. Exhale as you lower back down in the same way, curing the spine forward and letting the weight of the upper body and head release forward. *Note*: Weight shifts back toward the heels as you come back to the squatting position.

4. Repeat Steps 1 to 3 for three breath cycles, flowing up on the inhalation and down on the exhalation. Try to be fluid in your movement and finish back in the squatting position, releasing your backside to the floor in preparation for the core strengthening sequence.

12 | Core Strengthening

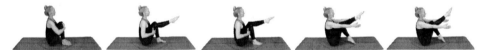

Figure 9.3.4.12: Movement module—Core re-tensioning—Core strengthening.

1. Make sure you are resting on your sitting bones and bring your knees together as you grow taller through the spine, hugging your knees closer, trying to touch knees to nipples. *Note*: In this position, you should engage your core by bringing the bottom of your rib cage closer to your hips, posteriorly tilting your pelvis. This flattens out the curve in your lower back as we did during the core activation at the beginning of this practice.

2. Grip with your hands behind your knees, and without losing the knee to nipple connection, inhale, releasing your right foot from the floor, pointing your toe, and lifting it upwards.

3. Exhale as you release the foot back to the floor before repeating for the left leg (this is one set)

4. Repeat Steps 2 to 3 until you have completed three sets on each leg.

5. **Progression**: If you were able to maintain the strong active core with hands behind knees, try to repeat the sequence again, this time releasing the hands forward as demonstrated in the last two images in Figure 9.3.4.12. Listen to your body as you choose whether to take the progression.

13 Core Balance on Pivot Point

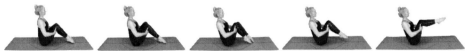

Figure 9.3.4.13: Movement module—Core re-tensioning—Core balance on pivot point.

1. Maintaining a strong core activation, allow your feet to walk forward a little so you have a 90-degree angle at your knees in preparation for *navasana* pose.
2. Keeping your hands behind your knees while maintaining a long spine, point your toes and start to walk the toes backward until you find the "pivot" point (where your toes lift from the floor without effort).
3. When you have found your pivot, allow your feet to lift from the floor, and only if you have good control over your core in this position, bring your lower legs in line with the floor.
4. Hold this position for five breath cycles before bending your knees to bring your feet back onto the floor and then straighten your legs preparing for a dandasana pose.

14 Core with Banded Pull

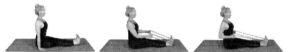

Figure 9.3.4.14: Movement module—Core re-tensioning—Core with banded pull.

1. Place your hands on the floor on either side of your hips, engage your quads and lengthen through the spine and you gaze toward your toes for dandasana pose. Hold this position for three breath cycles.
2. Take your long resistance band and bring it around your feet for the first pulling exercise of the eight-phase training. You will maintain a gentle activation of your core throughout this pulling exercise.
3. Starting with the arms forward, inhale as you draw the elbows back behind you. *Note*: Your chest should stay open, and you should squeeze the muscles in your mid-back as you do this.
4. Exhale as you release the arms forward again. This is one repetition.
5. Perform 10 repetitions.

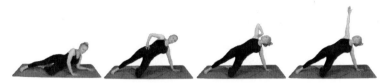

Figure 9.3.4.15: Movement module—Core re-tensioning—Side plank variation.

1. Lie on your left side with the left elbow bent, right hand in front of your body for support, and left knee bent beneath you. Your right leg is straight.
2. Place your left hand under your left shoulder and inhale as you push up into a supported side plank, placing your right hand on your right hip.
   a. If you feel stable here, place your right fingertips onto your right shoulder and point your elbow up toward the ceiling, extending the fingers up toward the ceiling only if you have good balance in this position. *Note*: Keep your gaze on the floor if you struggle with balance.
3. Stay in this position for three breath cycles while maintaining an active core.
4. Repeat Steps 1 to 3 on the opposite side.

16 Abductor & Adductor Strengthening

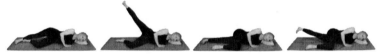

Figure 9.3.4.16: Movement module—Core re-tensioning—Abductor & adductor strengthening.

1. Lie on your left side using your left arm as a pillow, bend your left knee for support. Bend your right elbow and place your right hand in front of you for balance. Your right leg is straight.
2. Inhale as you raise the right leg as high as possible, keeping the leg straight and the foot flexed.
3. Exhale lowering the leg, repeating this raising and lowering for five breath cycles.
4. Straighten your left leg and bend your right knee to 90 degrees placing it in front of you for support.
5. Inhale as you raise the left leg as high as possible, keeping the leg straight and the foot flexed.
6. Exhale as you lower the leg, repeating this raising and lowering for five breath cycles.
7. Repeat Steps 1–5 on the opposite side.

17 | Happy Baby

Figure 9.3.4.17: Movement module—Core re-tensioning—Happy baby.

1. Lie on your back, hugging your knees into your chest. Taking a breath or two here.
2. Release your knees and grab your feet for a happy husband pose, kicking into your hands as you pull into your feet. Try to keep your sacrum on the mat as you do this.

18 | Savasana

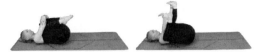

Figure 9.3.4.18: Movement module—Core re-tensioning—Savasana.

1. Release your feet and take your final savasana (resting position) for five minutes.

You may have looked at this practice and assumed it would be easy as it is performed mostly on the floor, but this is deceptive. If your core has been sleeping for a long time, this practice will wake it up, encouraging your abdominal employees (muscles) to get back to working in the business of your body's movement. This completes the movement module. You will perform the exercises from this module on the days specified in your weekly schedule.

Phase 3: Relaxation Module

Yin Yoga Backward Bending

Having completed Phase 2, you should be familiar with the practice of yin and should be beginning to see the benefits of repatterning the lines of tension through your body, such a nice gift to yourself!

Objective

The objective of the relaxation module in Phase 3 is to continue the process of repatterning the lines of tension shifting the focus from forward folds to backward bends.

Success Metric

As with Phase 2, success with yin yoga is achieved when you can relax in the various positions. We tend to find it easier to relax in the forward fold positions versus the backward bending, so give yourself time and be consistent with your practice.

Additional Notes

As backward-bending poses tend to be less comfortable than the forward folding poses, make sure to be kind to yourself and practice the variation of the pose that feels right for you. The backward-bending positions create some compression and decompression of the spine. Remember it's OK to feel some tension/discomfort but not pain.

Yin Yoga Backward Bending Exercise Instructions

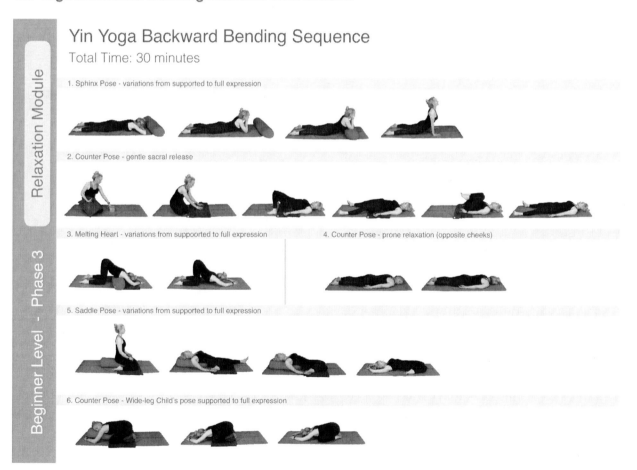

Figure 9.3.5: Phase 3—Relaxation module—Yin yoga backward-bending sequence sheet.

You will need one or two bolsters (or pillows), two blankets, two blocks, an eye pillow, and a yoga mat. This practice will take twenty minutes including setup and transitions between poses. You can download the sequence sheet for this yin yoga back-bending sequence (Figure 9.3.5) from empoweryourflower.com and place it at the front of your mat when practicing.

You can read the instructions and steps beforehand and follow the poses on the printed copy of Figure 9.3.5 when you are practicing. This will help you to learn the sequence and eventually you will be able to practice it without looking at the sheet.

Steps to Perform Yin Yoga Backward-Bending Sequence

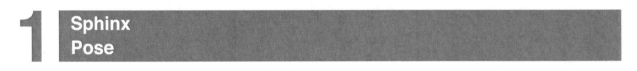

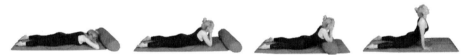

Figure 9.3.5.1: Relaxation module—Backward bending—Sphinx pose.

Sphinx pose is a yin backbend that focuses on spinal extension. It provides some compression on the back side of the spine while decompressing on the front side. There are multiple options demonstrated using props to support the relaxation. *Note*: You begin in the easiest version of this position, only progressing if you meet the requirements for the next level. To assume the pose:

1. Place the bolster in front of your body and bring your feet slightly wider than hip-distance apart. Lift your rib cage up and forward, and then rest it onto the mat while resting your forehead on your hands. If you feel tension in your low back in this position, this is your backbend, otherwise, move to Step 2.

2. Come up onto your elbows, making a platform for your chin using your hands. Relax here. If you feel tension in your low back in this position, this is your backbend, otherwise, move to Step 3.

3. Bring your elbows up onto the bolster and relax here. *Note*: if at any point you feel like you have moved beyond your edge, regress to the previous version.

4. Remain in your backbend for five minutes, making sure to relax your glutes, let your belly hang, relax your shoulders, and try to rest with as minimal effort as possible. *Note*: If you had progressed to Step 3 and had not met your edge during the first four minutes of the relaxation, you can come to the full expression *but* only for the last minute. For the full expression, press into your hands, straightening your arms and allowing a deeper backbend while relaxing your body.

5. Very slowly, mindfully come out of the position, bending at the knees and pushing back to the

close-leg child's pose for a few moments before moving to the counter position.

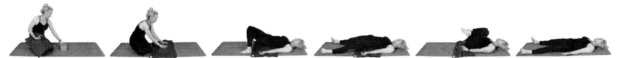

Figure 9.3.5.2: Relaxation module—Backward bending—Counter sacral release.

This counterpose provides a gentle release of the sacrum following your sphinx pose. You will need a block and a blanket for this position. To set up, place a yoga block biggest-side-down on your mat and place a folded blanket over it making sure to smooth out any creases. To come into the position:

1. Place your sacrum on the block with your shoulder blades and head relaxed on the floor. Keep your knees bent to start. *Note*: If you feel any tension in your low back at this stage, you will keep your knees bent for the full duration of the counterpose. If the tension moves you beyond your edge, remove the block and lie flat on the floor with legs extended for a savasana pose as your counterpose, otherwise, you can extend your legs with your sacrum resting on the block for the full version of this counterpose.

2. Stay in your version of the counterpose for one minute.

3. To come out of the position, move slowly, bend your knees, and hug them toward your chest. Push the block and blanket away from beneath you.

4. Relax in savasana for one minute before moving to the next pose. *Note*: If your version of this release was savasana, place a bolster under your legs here.

3 **Melting**
Heart

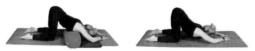

Figure 9.3.5.3: Relaxation module—Backward bending—Melting heart.

Melting heart pose is a backbend that focuses more on the thoracic spine (back of your ribcage). This can help with rib cage flexibility for breathing. You may need a bolster and blanket for this pose. To assume this position:

1. Come to an all-fours position, keeping the hips directly above the knees and allow your chest to lower onto the bolster while your head rests on the blanket and your arms rest on the mat. If this

feels easy, you can remove the props and allow your chest to relax down to the mat. If it is more comfortable, you can rest your chin on the floor instead of your forehead.

2. Allow your belly to hang, relax your shoulders and try to surrender any effort while you remain in the pose for three minutes.

3. Move very slowly out of the position by gently bringing the arms back and pushing back to a brief child's pose before moving props away and coming to lie on your stomach.

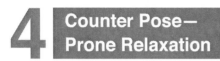
Counter Pose— Prone Relaxation

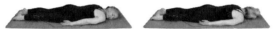

Figure 9.3.5.4: Relaxation module—Backward bending—Counter prone relaxation.

1. Counter by lying flat on your tummy, feet hip-distance, arms alongside your body with your palms facing up.

2. You should place your right cheek on the mat for 1 minute before lifting your head and switching to the left side for one minute. *Note*: It is normal to find one side less comfortable than the other, but please do both sides for balance.

Saddle Pose

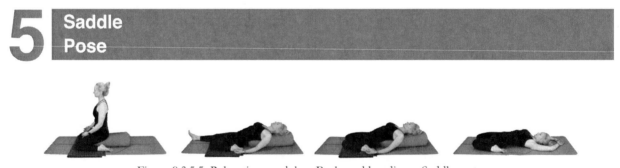

Figure 9.3.5.5: Relaxation module—Backward bending—Saddle pose.

Half saddle pose focuses on internal hip rotation and offers a gentle backbend if you rest backward during the pose. There are multiple progressions, depending on your flexibility. You will need to place a folded blanket on your mat and have a bolster to hand if needed. Saddle pose requires that you can sit your backside on the floor with your feet on either side of your hips, soles of the feet facing the ceiling. If you are unable to do that, you can sit on the bolster with feet on either side as shown in the first image of Figure 9.3.5.5. Otherwise, to assume the position:

1. Sit with your backside on the blanket with the bolster behind your back, both legs extended in front of you.

2. Bend your right knee, sealing the knee, and then internally rotate at the hip, placing the top of your

right foot on the floor beside your right hip. If you have met your edge here, this is your pose, otherwise, progress to Step 3.

3. Place your hands on the floor alongside your hips and bend your elbows to lower your back onto the bolster. Allow the arms to relax, palms facing up. If you do not meet any tension in the quads or low back in this position, you can try a full saddle pose with the bolster. To do this, you will sit on your backside with both feet alongside your hips. Lower down onto the bolster. If you do not meet your edge in supported full saddle, you can try the full expression where you lie back on the floor without support from a bolster. You can raise your arms overhead if this is your version.

4. You should perform either half-saddle for two-and-a-half minutes on each side, or the full version for five minutes.

5. Release from the pose very slowly and mindfully in the same way you came into the pose.

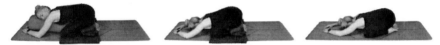

5   Counter Pose—Wide-Leg Child's Pose

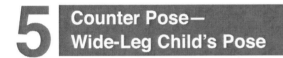

Figure 9.3.5.6: Relaxation module—Backward bending—Counter wide-leg child's pose.

1. Counter the saddle pose with a close-legged child's pose, which is also your final rest so you should stay in this position for five minutes.

Backward-bending poses are also heart-opening poses. An emotional release can be triggered when you allow yourself to relax into the tension that exists in these poses. It is not unusual for at least one person to have an emotional release in each yin yoga class. This can come in the form of tears and sadness, or even joy and laughter. Just know that such releases of emotion are part of the process and nothing to be worried about. This completes the relaxation module. You will perform the exercises from this module on the days specified in your weekly schedule.

Phase 3: Mind & Meditation Module

ANT Therapy

Having completed Phase 2, you should be finding it easy to relax when you feel tension anywhere in your body and you should be able to visualize potential future strength. You should reward yourself by doing something that makes you feel pampered!

Objective

The objective of the Mind & Meditation module in Phase 3 is to begin the process of questioning your negative thoughts, turning them around so you can choose to think more positively. This is an empowering process and should help to improve the quality of your life.

Success Metric

Success is achieved when you are feeling happier because you are automatically boarding positive thought trains instead of continuing to travel through old patterns of negative thinking.

Additional Notes

If you are tormented by negative thought patterns (like my example of the kitchen drawer), you could greatly benefit from doing ANT therapy, which is based on Byron Katy's *The Work*. You can use this system to help change your mind with regards to your views on the female flower, your pelvic health, or any other patterns that drag you down.

Negative thought trains can relate to everything and anything—I want sweets, I need a drink, I'm not pretty, people don't like me, I'm stupid. You will know which trains are relevant to you.

By questioning the thoughts that exist in your mind, you begin to lay the foundations for changing your mind. The process of doing the work may let you see how illogical some of these thought trains really are (like my kitchen drawer example).

When you change your mind, you can let go of many things. I believe that this letting go contributes to the "let go" that is required to have great orgasms. If you want to bring your sex life to the next level, get off those thought trains. Remember that life is not so serious, you should empower yourself to have fun and enjoy it.

ANT Therapy

For this exercise, you will need a notepad and pen. *The Work* is available free of charge on Byron Katy's website: https://thework.com/ where you can download the "Judge thy neighbor" worksheet, which will be used to address any issues that are causing you to follow negative trains of thought.

You should print out the worksheets from Byron Katy's website. Alternatively, you can subscribe to mybrainfitlife.com and perform the ANT therapy exercise there. This exercise should be performed twice per week, although you can perform it more often if you suffer from constant negative thinking.

Steps to Perform This Exercise:

1. Sit down at your table with your notepad and pen to hand.
2. Perform five relaxing breath cycles before you begin.
3. Write a paragraph or two on any negative thoughts that are impacting your QoL.
4. Use this paragraph as input for the "Judge thy neighbor" worksheet, which you printed from the Byron Katy website.
5. Do "the work" in relation to each negative statement that you have written, which involves asking the following questions:
   a. Is this thought true?
   b. Can you be sure that it is true?
   c. How does this thought make you feel?
   d. How would you feel if you did not have that thought?

You will then be asked to turn your thought around a few different ways. For example, if you thought was "He has ruined my life" you can turn that around to "He has not ruined my life" or even "I have ruined his life." These turnarounds give you an opportunity to look at the thought from a different perspective.

After you do the work, consciously decide how you would like to think and feel instead of your current negative thoughts and feelings and make an agreement with yourself to change your mind. The next time that thought appears in your mind, consciously question it and choose to turn it around, thus beginning the process of laying new tracks on which positive thought trains can travel.

Once you have done the work on your own thoughts, I would like you to do the exercise on your thoughts regarding the taboo that surrounds PFD. Work through any guilt or shame that exists around your female flower and sexuality. For doing this work, I thank you from the bottom of my heart as this will contribute to breaking the taboo, **together we can and will make a difference!**

That completes the mind module and brings us to the end of the Phase 3 training.
You will perform the exercises from this module on the days specified in your weekly schedule.

At the end of each week, if you feel that you may be ready to progress to the next phase of training, you can perform the phase checkpoint review using Figure 9.3.6, which checks your progress against the success metric for each module and helps you to decide if you should proceed to Phase 4 (beginner level). You can download a blank version of this form from empoweryourflower.com.

Phase 3 Checkpoint Review

Phase Start Date:_____

Checkpoint Date:_____

Pelvic Floor Module

Strength: Success is achieved when you can hold your pelvic floor contraction for 10 calming breath cycles (inhaling for 4, exhaling for 8). You should be able to maintain the contraction with some lift, while breathing with your body relaxed.

Relaxation: Success is achieved when you can relax your pelvic floor fully in all the positions specified and no longer feel the symptoms of hypertonicity. Note: Reverse Kegels can help to release pelvic tension, however, you will continue to practice the reverse Kegels module through the entire program and so if you do not achieve success with the pelvic floor relaxation at this phase, this should not prevent you from proceeding to the next phase.

Success
Yes ☐
No ☐

Yes ☐
No ☐

Breathing Module - Breath Remapping

Success is achieved when you can easily perform the exercise while maintaining good core stability.

Success
Yes ☐
No ☐

Movement Module - Core Re-tensioning Sequence

Success with this module is achieved when you can activate your glutes and core and have increased your ability to tolerate load through these muscle tissues.

Success
Yes ☐
No ☐

Relaxation Module - Yin Yoga Backward Bending Sequence

As with phase 2, success is achieved when you can relax into your own body's pattern of tension, meeting the very edge of your discomfort without moving into pain.

Success
Yes ☐
No ☐

Mind & Meditation Module - ANT Therapy

Success is achieved when you are feeling happier because you are automatically boarding positive thought trains instead of continuing to travel through old patterns of negative thinking. Extra success if you have managed to change your mind regarding the taboo surrounding Pelvic Floor Dysfunction.

Success
Yes ☐
No ☐

Phase 3 Checkpoint Review

Have you achieved the success objectives and do you feel that you are ready to proceed to the next phase of training?

If no, please continue with the phase 3 training until you are ready to proceed or regress to the phase 2 training if this phase felt too difficult.

If yes, proceed to Phase 4 training. Remember, you can regress to the phase 3 training if you find the phase 4 to be too difficult. Listen to your body and good luck!

Success
Yes ☐
No ☐

Figure 9.3.6: Phase 3—Checkpoint review form.

Phase 4
Beginner Level

Welcome to Phase 4 of the eight-phase training. This is the third and final phase at the beginner level of this training, which will challenge you to get your fast-twitch pelvic floor muscles firing. This phase also challenges your ability to balance and works to lengthen with lateral twisting yin poses. The Phase 4 training modules are highlighted in Figure 9.4.1.

Eight-Phase Modules	Prep	Beginner			Intermediate		Advanced	
	Phase 1	Phase 2	Phase 3	Phase 4	Phase 5	Phase 6	Phase 7	Phase 8
Pelvic Floor	Kegel Breakdown	Full Kegel	Endurance Kegel	Speed Kegel	Co-Contract	Maximize Strength	Standing Rotations	Functional Training
Breathing	Nasal Breathing	Breath Strengthening	Breath Remapping	Nadi Shodhana	Basic Hypopressive Exercise	Intermediate Hypopressive Sequence	Advanced Hypopressive Sequence	Kapalabhati Breathing
Movement	Yoga Preparation	Yoga Basics	Core Re-tensioning	Rebalancing Yoga	Bandha Strength Yoga	Max Kegel Yoga	Ball Routine	Dynamic Power Yoga
Relaxation	Restorative Yoga	Yin Yoga Forward Folds	Yin Yoga Backward Bending	Yin Yoga Twists & Lateral Movement	Yin Yoga Hip Opening	Yin Yoga Pelvic Floor	Yin Yoga Happy Hips	Yin Yoga All Body
Mind & Meditation	Yoga Nidra	Flex your mind to flex your muscles	ANT therapy	Conquer your fear	Kirtan Kriya	Self Affirmations	Journaling	Blossoming Goddess

Figure 9.4.1: Phase 4—Beginner level.

The exercises and activities for the Phase 4 modules, highlighted in green in Figure 9.4.1, will encourage you to conquer your fears, preparing you both mentally and physically for the intermediate-level training that will follow.

Remember, if your goal is pelvic floor relaxation, you will work on the reverse Kegels activity for all phases of training. It is detailed in Phase 1 pelvic floor module.

The frequency of practice can change as you progress through the training so make sure to read through all modules for Phase 4 and update your schedule accordingly before you begin training.

Phase 4
Modules

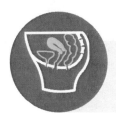

Pelvic Floor

Speed Kegel

Breathing

Nadi Shodhana

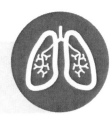

Movement

Rebalancing Yoga

Relaxation

Yin Yoga Twists & Lateral Movement

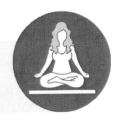

Mind & Meditation

Conquer Your Fear

Phase 4: Pelvic Floor Module

Speed Kegel

Having completed Phase 3, your pelvic floor endurance should have increased allowing you to sustain a full pelvic floor contraction in multiple positions. This is a great achievement; you should be really proud!

Objective

The objective of the pelvic floor (strength) module in Phase 4 is to improve the speed at which you can contract and relax. This helps to train the fast-twitch fibers of your pelvic floor. You will need to ensure that you relax completely in the relaxation phase of these "quick flick" contractions.

Success Metric

Success is achieved when you can perform 10 quick flick contractions with a good contraction and complete relaxation each time. If you suffer from stress incontinence, you should see an improvement in symptoms as you get better at performing these contractions.

Speed Kegel Exercise Instructions

For this exercise, you will focus on performing full pelvic floor contractions followed by full pelvic floor relaxations in quick successions. You will continue to practice six days per week while alternating your position each day as per Phase 1 (Figures 9.1.3 a & b):

Day 1: Hook lying.
Day 2: Cross leg sitting.
Day 3: Side-lying (top leg bent).
Day 4: Side-lying (bottom leg bent).
Day 5: Kneeling up.
Day 6: Sitting & standing.

Initially, you may find it difficult to perform fast contractions, but this should improve as you continue to practice. It is important that you are calm when doing these exercises as there can be a tendency to contract other muscles when you are required to perform fast contractions, for this reason, it can be helpful to perform ten calming breath cycles before you begin the exercise.

Steps to Perform the Speed Kegel Exercise

1. Get yourself into a comfortable starting position.
2. Begin your first breath cycle, inhaling for a count of four.
3. On your next exhalation, fully contract your pelvic floor, and then relax and then contract, and then relax. Continue with rhythmic contact and relax cycles in a pulsing motion until you have performed a full ten contractions (this is one set). Maintain a calm steady breath throughout, making sure to keep the rest of your body relaxed as you perform the exercise.
4. Repeat four times so you will have performed five sets in total.

I cannot emphasize enough the importance of the relaxation phase of these exercises. Try to relax as much, if not more, than your contraction. You can look back at Figure 2.3 to see how the sarcomere looks fully contracted and at rest. We would ideally reach full contraction and return to resting length during each cycle of these quick contractions. Practice makes perfect, stick with it.

That concludes the pelvic floor module. You will perform the exercises from this module on the days specified in your weekly schedule.

 # Phase 4: Breathing Module
Nadi Shodhana

Having completed the breathing module in Phase 3, you should be feeling the benefits of the improvements in your breathing patterns. A deep joyful breath is your reward!

Objective

The objective of the breathing module is to try to balance breathing between your nostrils. For this purpose, we will practice a breathing technique known in yoga as *nadi shodhana* (alternate nostril breathing). This breathing technique will help to balance breathing between your nostrils while teaching you to extend the exhalation. This technique will take advantage of any increase in lung capacity that you have achieved from the earlier modules.

Success Metric

Success is achieved when you can easily perform the exercise without instruction with a comfortable sixteen count exhalation.

Additional Notes

Nadi shodhana in yoga is touted to have many benefits, including clearing toxins, balancing hormones, and creating balance between the left and right brain. I was unable to find any scientific studies to back up these claims. From my perspective, the true benefit is that you are practicing breathing and training in the use of your full lung capacity while communicating safety to your nervous system. You may notice that one nostril "works" better than the other when you begin this practice, but you should find that it balances out with consistent steady practice.

Nadi Shodhana Exercise Instructions

For this exercise, you will need a yoga mat with a small towel to sit on or a meditation chair. You will perform the exercise in a comfortable seated position. This is typically cross-legged, although you have the option to choose a different seated position if cross-legged is uncomfortable for you. You will practice this breathing exercise every second day and it should take five minutes or so.

Steps to Perform This Breathing Exercise

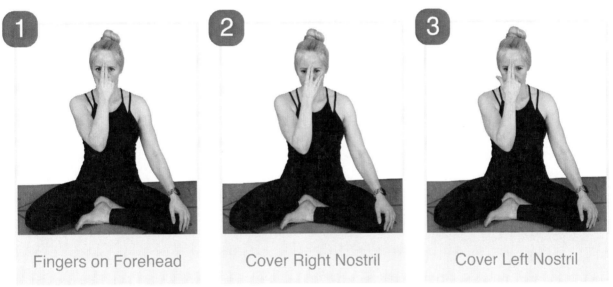

Fingers on Forehead   Cover Right Nostril   Cover Left Nostril

Figure 9.4.2: Nadi shodhana breathing exercise.

1. Come to a comfortable seated position. Make sure that you are not pressing any part of your body into the mat, just relax.
2. Close your mouth keeping your lips together with your teeth slightly apart, tongue resting on the roof of your mouth behind your front teeth.
3. Place your index and middle fingers of your right hand on your forehead and close your right nostril with your thumb.
4. Inhale through the left nostril for the count of four, before holding both nostrils closed for the

count of four (use your ring finger and baby finger to close the left nostril).

5. Release the thumb from the right nostril and exhale for the count of four.

6. Inhale deeply through the right nostril for the count of four before holding both nostrils closed for the count of four.

7. Release the ring and baby finger from the left nostril and exhale for a count of four.

8. Inhale deeply through the left nostril for the count of four before holding both nostrils closed for the count of four.

9. Repeat Steps 5 to 8, extending the count on your exhalation, with each repetition going from four to eight to twelve to sixteen. You should keep the same counting pace, which means you have to slow down your exhalation. *Note*: Make sure that your shoulders remain relaxed throughout this breathing exercise.

10. After the last round, rest your right hand on your lap, and breathe a few relaxing breaths.

Hopefully, you will notice that your ability to extend your exhalation is increasing as you continue to practice. If you are consistent, you will become a master of this breathing technique, which will help to improve your lung capacity. That concludes the breathing module. You will perform the exercises from this module on the days specified in your weekly schedule.

Phase 4: Movement Module

Rebalancing Yoga

Having completed Phase 3, you should be noticing an improvement in your normal functional movement. You should hopefully also see a general improvement in your overall strength and fitness, keep up the fantastic work!

Objective

The objective of the movement module of Phase 4 is to progress the yoga practice through balancing asanas with some additional focus on improving hip strength. This phase takes advantage of your increased ability to load tension through your tissues. The goal of this practice is to optimize length-tension relationships throughout your body.

Success Metric

Success with this module is achieved when you can comfortably flow through the yoga practice without feeling off-balance. It should feel good in your body and you shouldn't feel pain in any of your joints.

Additional Notes

When practicing yoga, resist the temptation to force yourself into positions that your body is not ready for. Listen to the subtle signals that your body sends as you breathe in each pose. Yoga is movement with breath, allowing you to build a connection with your body rather than a pose-focused goal.

I explained in Chapter Two that it is said, "Yoga is not about touching your toes, it's about what you learn on the way down." I forced myself down, which was not good for my body. It is better to view the practice as an opportunity to breathe your way into balance, and to feel your body with the increased awareness that you should be developing through the Mind & Meditation module exercises.

Your yoga practice is yet another opportunity for you to communicate with your nervous system. It allows you to positively contribute to the relationship you have with yourself, so treat your body with the love and compassion it deserves.

Rebalancing Yoga Sequence Instructions

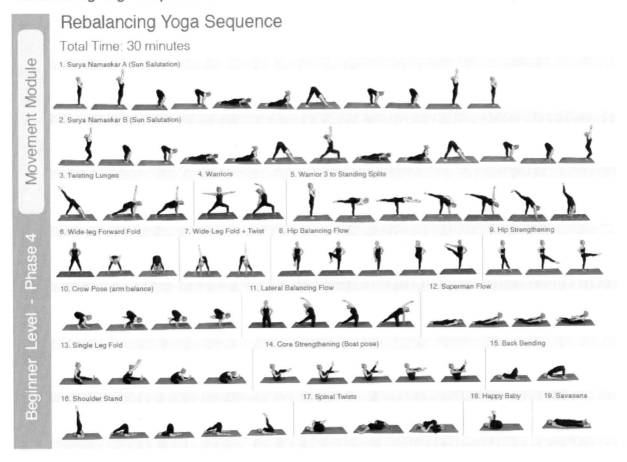

Figure 9.4.3: Phase 4—Movement module—Rebalancing yoga sequence sheet.

You will need a yoga mat, a yoga block, a strap, and optionally an eye pillow and blanket for this practice. The practice should take thirty minutes including final relaxation. The sequence will begin with sun salutations (*surya namaskar*), a staple of a regular yoga practice. Both the A and B versions of sun salutations will be used to warm up the body.

You can download the sequence sheet for this rebalancing yoga sequence (Figure 9.4.3) from empoweryourflower.com and place it at the front of your mat when practicing. You can read the instructions and steps beforehand and follow the poses on the printed copy of Figure 9.4.3 when you are practicing. This will help you to learn the sequence and eventually you will be able to practice it without looking at the sheet. Repeated practice creates change in the body.

Steps to Perform the Rebalancing Yoga Sequence

1 Surya Namaskar A (Sun Salutation)

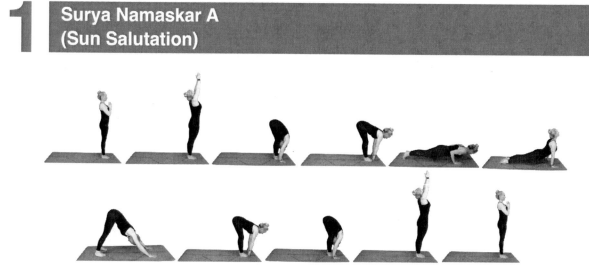

Figure 9.4.3.1: Movement module—Rebalancing yoga—Surya namaskar A.

1. Begin standing in tadasana pose with hands in front of your heart.
2. Inhale and raise the hands over the head gazing toward the thumbs.
3. Exhale folding forward.
4. Inhale to lengthen the spine. *Note*: Come up as high as you need to in order to have a long spine rather than a rounded back. This may require that your hands be on your thighs and not the floor (listen to your body!).
5. Exhale planting your hands on the mat, bending your knees as much as required to keep the heel of your hands on the mat.
6. Inhale as you take a step back with your right leg and then your left leg for plank position.
7. Exhale as you lower down into chaturanga, dropping your knees if you have to.

8. Inhale for an upward-facing dog, making sure to open your chest forward and keep your shoulder blades protracted as you press into your hands.

9. Exhale, rolling over your toes to a downward-facing dog. Perform three breath cycles here.

10. On your next exhalation, look forward between your hands and step the right foot forward followed by the left foot.

11. Inhale to lengthen your spine, coming as high as you need to for a long spine.

12. Exhale, folding forward.

13. Inhale pressing into the midfoot, knees softly bent as you come back up, reaching the arms overhead gazing toward the thumbs.

14. Exhale bringing your hands back to your heart for tadasana.

15. Repeat Steps 1 to 14 twice more for three rounds in total.

2 Surya Namaskar B (Sun Salutation)

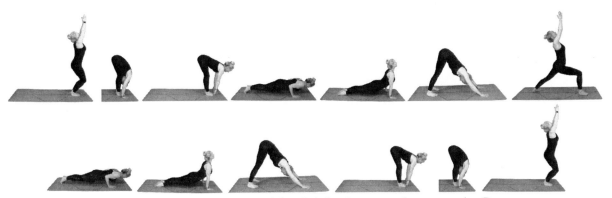

Figure 9.4.3.2: Movement module—Rebalancing yoga—Surya namaskar B.

1. Begin standing in tadasana pose with hands in front of your heart.

2. Inhale and raise the hands over the head gazing toward the thumbs while bending the knees sitting into chair pose (*utkatasana*).

3. Exhale, folding forward.

4. Inhale to lengthen the spine.

5. Exhale planting your hands on the mat, bending your knees as much as required to keep the heel of your hands on the mat. *Note*: when you become stronger, you will exhale directly to chaturanga.

6. Inhale as you take a step back with your right leg and then your left leg for plank position.

7. Exhale as you lower down into chaturanga, dropping your knees if you have to.

8. Inhale for an upward-facing dog, making sure to open your chest forward, and keep your shoulder blades protracted as you press into your hands.

9. Exhale, rolling over your toes to a downward-facing dog.

10. The left foot turns to 45 degrees, and the right foot steps forward between the hands. Inhale, coming up to Warrior 1 and exhale there. Inhale again and on the exhalation, plant your hands and step back to plank position. *Note:* When you become stronger, you will complete your Warrior 1 in a single breath cycle where you inhale up to Warrior 1 and exhale back down to chaturanga.

11. Exhale lowering to chaturanga (dropping your knees if you have to).

12. Inhale for an upward-facing dog.

13. Exhale for a downward-facing dog.

14. Repeat Steps 10 to 13 to perform your Warrior 1 on the left side finishing in downward-facing dog for three breath cycles.

15. On your next exhalation, look forward between your hands and step the right foot forward followed by the left foot.

16. Inhale to lengthen your spine.

17. Exhale, folding forward.

18. Inhale, standing and reaching the arms overhead gazing toward the thumbs.

19. Exhale bringing your hands back to your heart for tadasana.

20. Repeat Steps 1 to 19 for three rounds **finishing on Step 13 (downward-facing dog)**.

3 Twisting Lunges

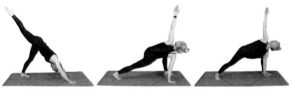

Figure 9.4.3.3: Movement module—Rebalancing yoga—Twisting lunges.

1. From the downward-facing dog, inhale and raise the left leg, stepping it forward between the hands.

2. Allow the back heel to come off the floor as you release the left hand from the floor, placing your fingertips on your shoulder, pointing your elbow up toward the ceiling for a twist. If you feel balanced here, release your fingertips up toward the ceiling. If you don't have the flexibility to twist in this position, you can elevate the floor using a block. Perform three breath cycles in this position.

3. Exhale turning your gaze toward the mat and place your left hand on the floor to the inside of your left foot and lower your right heel.

4. Inhale as you twist to the opposite side, placing your right fingertips on your right shoulder and pointing your elbow up toward the ceiling. If you feel balanced, release your fingertips reaching

your hand toward the ceiling. Perform three breath cycles here.

5. Exhale, dropping your hands, and coming back to your three-legged dog before lowering your leg for downward-facing dog.

6. Repeat Steps 1 to 5 starting with the right leg.

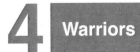

4 Warriors

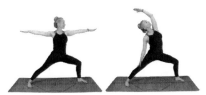

Figure 9.4.3.4: Movement module—Rebalancing yoga—Warriors.

1. From downward-facing dog, step your left foot forward and come up to Warrior 2, dropping your right heel, opening your hips to the long end of the mat, and place your hands on your shoulders pointing your elbows toward the front and back end of your mat.

2. Inhale as you extend your arms, imagining simultaneous expansion from fingertips to fingertips. Your gaze should shift over your left fingers. Exhale here.

3. Inhale and drop your right hand onto your right leg as you reach your left hand up and back taking a small backbend. Make sure to keep a good bend in the left knee keeping it over the ankle. Perform three breath cycles here.

4. On your final exhalation, windmill both hands onto the floor.

5. Inhale raising your left leg for a three-legged dog before lowering the leg to come back to downward-facing dog.

6. Repeat Steps 1–5 on the right. You can then flow through Steps 10 to 15 of surya namaskar A to come to tadasana from downward-facing dog. Take a moment in tadasana to find your breath and feel your balance.

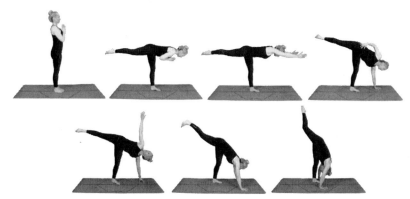

Figure 9.4.3.5: Movement module—Rebalancing yoga—Warrior 3 to standing splits.

1. Inhale as you release your right foot from the floor, flexing at the left hip and keeping one solid line from your shoulders to your right ankle as you allow your body to lower forward; raising your right leg to come to a Warrior 3 pose. *Note*: This is a balance posture. You can stop before your body is parallel with the floor if you feel that you are losing balance.

2. If you feel balanced and comfortable and have reached a parallel position, you can release your hands, stretching them out in front of you. In this outstretched position, you should be reaching through your right toes and your fingertips, this will help you to maintain balance. Perform three breath cycles here.

3. Exhale and lower your hands to the floor preparing for half-moon pose. You can use a block to raise the floor if needed. If using a block, do not shift your gaze toward the ceiling as you could fall off the block. Open your right hip so that the inside of your right foot faces toward the floor. You can place your right hand on your hip and keep your gaze toward the mat where your right hand would be if you were in plank (this helps to maintain balance).

4. If you feel stable, place your right fingertips on your right shoulder and point your elbow toward the ceiling. If you can maintain balance in this position, you can release your right hand and reach it up toward the ceiling as you also turn your gaze to the ceiling.

5. Perform three breath cycles here.

6. Exhale looking back down toward the floor as you release the right hand back to the floor.

7. Walk your hands back toward your feet and extend your right leg up toward the ceiling for a standing split. Remember the goal is to find balance. Reaching a full split is not your goal, so just play with the balance in the pose while listening to your body.

8. Perform three breath cycles in this position.

9. Inhale as you lower your right leg and come back to standing in tadasana.

10. Repeat Steps 1–9 on the left side.

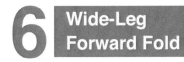
6 | Wide-Leg Forward Fold

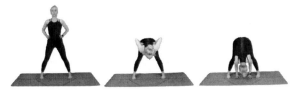

Figure 9.4.3.6: Movement module—Rebalancing yoga—Wide-leg forward fold.

1. Turn to face the long end of your mat, placing your hands on your hips and legs one leg distance apart, toes pointing inwards to prepare for a wide-leg forward fold (*prasarita padottanasana A pose*). Inhale here. This pose stretches the hamstrings as well as requiring some balance. Resist the temptation to open the legs excessively wide.

2. Exhale, folding forward from the waist in a hip hinging motion maintaining a long spine, and open chest. Make sure that you are engaging your quads to allow the hamstrings to stretch (they are an antagonistic pair). Place your hands on the floor (or on blocks if the floor is far away).

3. Once your hands reach the floor and you can balance comfortably, you can bring your fingertips in line with your toes, allow your elbows to bend, and lengthen your spine, encouraging your head to move toward the floor. *Note*: In a more advanced practice, when your head reaches the floor, you can lift into the tripod headstand from this position.

4. Perform three breath cycles in this position before placing your hands back on your waist and inhaling to come up.

7 | Wide-Leg Fold + Twist

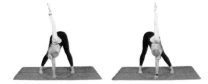

Figure 9.4.3.7: Movement module—Rebalancing yoga—Wide-leg forward fold with twist.

1. Inhale with your hands on your waist and exhale to fold forward once again, placing your hands on the floor.

2. Place your right hand on the floor right beneath your face, keep your gaze on the hand, placing

your left hand on your left hip.

3. If you feel comfortable and balanced here, inhale to twist your spine, placing your left fingertips on your left shoulder and pointing them up toward the ceiling.

4. If your elbow is pointing directly upwards and you feel balanced, you can release your left fingertips from your shoulder and reach your hand directly above.

5. Perform three breath cycles in your version of this pose.

6. Exhale lowering your gaze and your left hand to the floor.

7. Repeat Steps 2 to 6 on the opposite side

8. Place both hands on your waist and inhale to come up, bringing your feet back together for tadasana.

8 Hip Balancing Flow

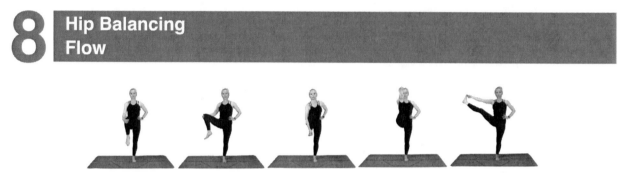

Figure 9.4.3.8: Movement module—Rebalancing yoga—Hip balancing flow.

For the hip balancing flow, we will perform the extended-hand-to-big-toe pose (*utthita hasta padangusthasana*). There are two options for this pose, the first is a gentler version where you hold the knee and the second is the full expression where you hold the big toe with the index and middle fingers. For both poses, you must keep your hips level and resist the temptation to lean backward as shown in Figure 9.4.3.8.a.

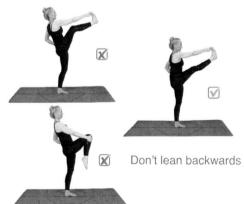

Don't lean backwards

Figure 9.4.3.8.a: Proper torso position for utthita hasta padangusthasana.

Figure 9.4.3.8.a shows the correct alignment marked with the green tick, where the shoulders remain balanced over the hips.

1. From tadasana, shift your weight over the left leg and release the right leg from the floor, bending

at the knee and flexing your hip to 90 degrees. Reach around the outside of your right leg to grab your big toe and extend the leg straight while maintaining your balance (or just grab around your knee if you lack the flexibility/balance).

2. Perform three breath cycles here.

3. Externally rotate your hip, allowing your leg to come to the right while maintaining your balance.

4. Perform three breath cycles here.

5. Inhale, bringing your leg back to the front before releasing the foot/knee and coming back to tadasana.

6. Repeat Steps 1 to 5 for the left leg.

9 Hip Strengthening

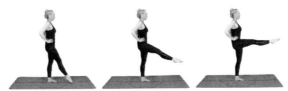

Figure 9.4.3.9: Movement module—Rebalancing yoga—Hip strengthening.

1. From tadasana, shift your weight over your left foot with the hips staying level, while straightening your right leg and pointing your toes.

2. Inhale as you use the strength of your quads to lift your leg as high as possible while maintaining a straight spine and keeping your shoulders stacked over your hips (don't lean back). You can use a block to raise the floor if you find it hard to lift the leg high. Work toward achieving sufficient strength to lift your leg until it is parallel with the floor. *Note*: Although the focus of this pose is hip strengthening, it is important that you maintain balance while you practice.

3. Hold for three breath cycles before exhaling to lower your leg back to the floor.

4. Repeat Steps 1–3 on the left side.

10 Crow Pose (Arm Balance)

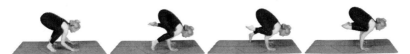

Figure 9.4.3.10: Movement module—Rebalancing yoga—Crow pose (arm balance).

1. Bring your feet a little wider than hip distance apart and exhale as you squat down, allowing the insides of your knees to press against the backs of your arms.

2. Perform three breath cycles here preparing for crow pose (*bakasana*), which is an arm balance. You will maintain the connection between the inside of your knees and the outside of your arms in crow pose.

3. Place your hands shoulder-distance apart in front of you, bending your elbows and shifting your gaze forward. Your gaze should land the same distance in front of your hands as the width you have between your hands. This creates a virtual tripod that will be the base of support for balance in this position. If you gaze between your hands instead of looking forward, your base of support will shift causing you to roll over, so make sure you are gazing forward creating your virtual tripod.

4. While maintaining the connection between the insides of your knees and the outsides of your arms, shift your weight forward and raise your hips up while keeping your toes on the ground. Your arms, bent at the elbows, provide a platform onto which your legs will rest.

5. Keeping your tripod gaze, inhale as you release your right foot from the floor, pointing your toes and feeling for balance through your arms.

6. Exhale, lowering the foot down.

7. Inhale as you lift the left foot up, point your toes and exhale, lower the foot down.

8. Repeat steps 5 to 7 a few times and if you feel sufficiently balanced, try to release both feet and touch your toes together.

9. Progress only if you find the balance to do so and perform three breath cycles in the full position before returning to your squat.

11 Lateral Balancing Flow

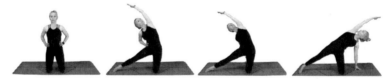

Figure 9.4.3.11: Movement module—Rebalancing yoga—Lateral balancing flow.

1. Come to kneel on the center of your mat with your knees hip-distance apart, hands on your hips.

2. Release your left leg out to the left side, pointing your toes and extending the right arm overhead toward the left. Try to shift your hips to the right as you do this, creating a stretch through the right side of your body.

3. Perform three breath cycles in this position.

4. If you felt balanced, exhale and release your left hand into your right heel while ensuring you continue to lift the rib cage away from the hips on each inhalation throughout this posture.

5. Perform three breath cycles here before inhaling to release your left hand from your right heel,

coming up with your body.

6. Exhale, dropping your right hand to the floor and reaching your left hand overhead, taking a stretch all the way from your left toes to your left fingertips.

7. Perform three breath cycles here before inhaling to come back to kneeling with hands on hips.

8. Repeat Steps 1–7 on the opposite side.

12 Superman Flow

Figure 9.4.3.12: Movement module—Rebalancing yoga—Superman flow.

1. Lie face down on your mat, arms stretched alongside your body, palms facing up toward the ceiling preparing for *shalabhasana* (locust/superman pose).

2. Inhale as you release your chest from the floor, using the strength of your back to lift you as you reach your hands backward while shifting your gaze forward.

3. Perform three breath cycles here before exhaling to lower back down taking a breath cycle of rest.

4. Inhale as you release your chest and legs from the floor, using the strength of your back to lift you as you reach your hands backward, keeping your legs zipped together.

5. Perform three breath cycles here before lowering down for another resting breath cycle.

6. Inhale as you release your chest from the floor, using the strength of your back to lift you as you reach your hands backward, this time allowing your legs to come apart.

7. Perform three breath cycles here before lowering back down.

8. Press your hands under your shoulders and push yourself up, lowering your hips backward for the child's pose. Kneel up and swing your legs around in front of you, preparing for *janu sirsasana* pose (single leg forward fold).

13 Single Leg Fold

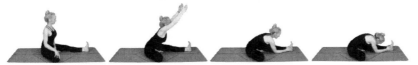

Figure 9.4.3.13: Movement module—Rebalancing yoga—Single leg forward fold.

1. Bend your right knee in, sealing the knee closed and externally rotating from the hip to release your right knee to the floor.

2. Inhale, reaching your hands up overhead, and exhale, folding forward while maintaining a long spine. Your gaze should be toward your toes, hands reaching for the foot. *Note*: The goal here is to stretch the hamstring on the left leg; resist the temptation to round your back. Only round your back once your tummy rests on your thigh with your left leg straight, at which point, you can drop your chin to your shin.

3. Perform three breath cycles here before inhaling back up.

4. Repeat Steps 1–3 on the left side.

14 Core Strengthening (Boat Pose)

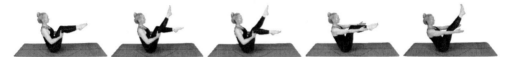

Figure 9.4.3.14: Movement module—Rebalancing yoga—Core strengthening (boat pose).

1. Prepare for *navasana* (boat pose) placing the hands behind the knees, pointing the toes, and walking the toes toward you to find your pivot point before releasing your toes and bringing the lower legs parallel with the floor.

2. Inhale, pointing the right toe to the ceiling, straightening the right leg, exhale to lower it.

3. Inhale, pointing the left toe to the ceiling, straightening the left leg, exhale to lower it.

4. Repeat Steps 2 and 3 twice more.

5. Release your hands from behind your knees and stretch your fingertips forward. Make sure that your legs are zipped together all the way from your ankles to your hips. *Note*: In the full expression of the pose, both legs are straight. When this practice becomes easy, try the full expression.

6. Perform three breath cycles here.

15 Back Bending

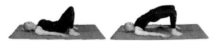

Figure 9.4.3.15: Movement module—Rebalancing yoga—Backward bending.

1. Lie down and bring your heels under your hips. Your middle fingertip should be able to touch your heels in this position. Feet are hip-distance apart (heels in line with sitting bones).

2. Inhale, pressing into your feet as you raise your hips upwards for *setu bandha sarvangasana* (shoulder supported bridge pose).

3. Hold the pose for three breath cycles, with each inhalation bringing the ribcage closer to the chin, each exhalation holding the rib cage there. Your hips should be fully extended here by using the strength of your glutes to lift them.

4. Exhale lowering the hips back down and taking a resting breath here.

5. Repeat Steps 2–4 twice more before hugging your knees to your chest.

16 Shoulder Stand

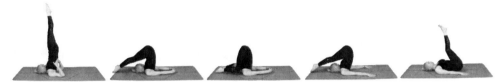

Figure 9.4.3.16: Movement module—Rebalancing yoga—Shoulder stand.

1. Prepare for a shoulder stand in the usual way, coming first to your feet touching the floor behind you (*halasana pose*).

2. Hold shoulder stand for ten breath cycles.

3. Exhale, lowering to halasana, release your hands, and interlock your fingers, press straight arms into the floor, and inhale here.

4. Exhale, bending your knees, and squeezing your ears with your knees.

5. Perform three breath cycles here before releasing the hands, press the palms into the ground, straighten the legs, and slowly roll the spine down, finishing lying flat on your mat.

17 Spinal Twists

Figure 9.4.3.17: Movement module—Rebalancing yoga—Spinal twists.

1. Hug your knees toward your chest and shift your hips slightly to the right before dropping the knees to the left for a spinal twist for three breath cycles.

2. Inhale back to the center and repeat the twist on the right side.

18 Happy Baby

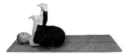

Figure 9.4.3.18: Movement module—Rebalancing yoga—Happy baby.

1. Reach around your feet pulling the knees toward the underarms while keeping the sacrum on the floor. Take five breaths here.

19 Savasana

Figure 9.4.3.19: Movement module—Rebalancing yoga—Savasana.

1. Come to your savasana for final rest. You should rest for five minutes.

Balance takes practice, and this beginner-level routine requires a lot of practice to achieve balance in the various poses. If you are unsteady, the arm balancing pose (Figure 9.4.3.10) may prove to be quite a challenge. You can work with your healthcare provider to decide if any poses should be skipped. Mastering this practice will prepare you for the intermediate and advanced practices later in this program.

Make sure to work where you find your body rather than trying to push yourself into more advanced versions of these balances before you are ready. When the practice becomes easier, you can stay in poses for five breath cycles instead of three. Maintain consistency and you will achieve your goals.

That completes the movement module. You will perform the exercises from this module on the days specified in your weekly schedule.

Phase 4: Relaxation Module

Yin Yoga Twists & Lateral Movement

Having completed Phase 3, you should have learned to relax in your yin yoga poses. Learning to relax into tension *"on your mat,"* can help you to find your calm center during difficult and stressful situations *"off your mat."* Good on you!

Objective

The objective of the relaxation module in Phase 4 is to bring the spine into lateral and twisting movements to enhance the rebalancing of length-tension relationships.

Success Metric

As with Phase 3, success with yin yoga is achieved when you can relax into the positions. Moving into the side body might reveal some unnoticed tensions and imbalances between the left and right sides of your body. This yin practice may offer you the added benefit of improving bilateral movements and twists in your yoga practice.

Additional Notes

As with the other yin practices, you should ensure you avoid moving into pain. You can download the sequence sheet for this yin yoga twists and lateral movement sequence (Figure 9.4.4) from empoweryourflower.com and place it at the front of your mat when practicing.

You can read the instructions and steps beforehand and follow the poses on the printed copy of Figure 9.4.4 when you are practicing. This will help you to learn the sequence and eventually you will be able to practice it without looking at the sheet.

Yin Yoga Twists & Lateral Movement Sequence

Total Time: 30 minutes

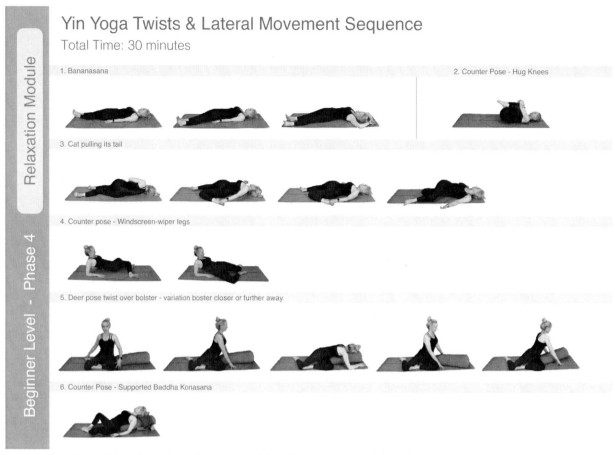

1. Bananasana
2. Counter Pose - Hug Knees
3. Cat pulling its tail
4. Counter pose - Windscreen-wiper legs
5. Deer pose twist over bolster - variation boster closer or further away
6. Counter Pose - Supported Baddha Konasana

Figure 9.4.4: Phase 4—Relaxation module—Yin yoga twists & lateral movement sequence sheet.

Yin Yoga Twists & Lateral Movement Instructions

You will need one or two bolsters (or pillows), two blankets, two blocks, an eye pillow, and a yoga mat. This practice will take twenty minutes including setup, transitions, and final rest.

Steps to Perform the Yin Yoga Twists & Lateral Movement Sequence

1 Bananasana Pose

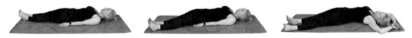

Figure 9.4.4 .1: Relaxation module—Yin yoga twists & lateral—Bananasana.

Bananasana pose focuses on lateral flexion of the spine. It offers a stretch along the entire side of your body. If you have issues with your shoulders, it might be more comfortable to keep your arms resting on your lower rib cage or on the floor beside you. To assume the pose:

1. Lay your body on the left side of your mat.

2. Step your feet to the right corner of your mat.

3. Lift your upper body and rib cage and lower them to the right side of your mat, stretching your arms overhead.

4. Rest in this position for two-and-a-half minutes.

5. Repeat on the right side.

2 Counter Pose— Hug Knees

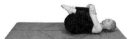

Figure 9.4.4.2: Relaxation module—Yin yoga twists & lateral—Counter hug knees.

1. Lie on your back and hug your knees into your chest for 1 minute, rocking a little from side to side.

3 Cat Pulling its tail

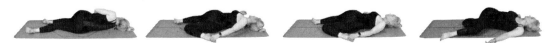

Figure 9.4.4.3: Relaxation module—Yin yoga twists & lateral—Cat pulling its tail.

Cat pulling its tail pose offers a spinal twist, while encouraging a release of tissues in the quads and hip flexors. To assume the pose:

1. Lie on your right side with your left knee bent resting on the floor in front of you and your right arm stretched out in front of you.

2. Bend your right leg, reaching around to grab your right foot with your left hand.

3. Try to allow your spine to twist allowing the left shoulder to rest on the mat while maintaining the position of your hips. You can place a blanket under your left shoulder for support if needed.

4. Relax in this position for two-and-a-half minutes before repeating the pose on the opposite side.

Counter Pose—
Windscreen Wiper Legs

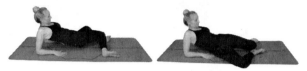

Figure 9.4.4 .4: Relaxation module—Yin yoga twists & lateral—Counter windscreen wiper legs.

1. Slowly move to the counterpose: windscreen wiper legs, by resting back on your elbows and rotating your legs from side to side in a windscreen wiper motion, rolling over your glutes.

5
Twisted
Deer Pose

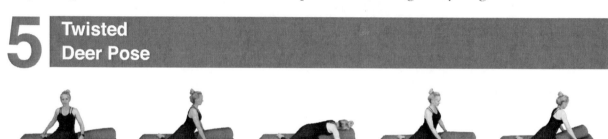

Figure 9.4.4.5: Relaxation module—Yin yoga twists & lateral—Twisted deer pose.

The *twisted deer pose* is a deep twisting pose using the support of a bolster. Your tummy will rest on the bolster during this position. If you cannot lay your tummy on the bolster, decrease the angle between the bolster and your front leg for a shallower twist.

Likewise, if you feel that this is very easy and would like a deeper twist, you can increase the angle between your front leg and the bolster for a deeper twist. The deeper and gentler bolster angles are shown in the two images on the right of Figure 9.4.4.5.

To assume the pose:

1. Place your bolster on the top of your mat and sit with the side of your left hip against the bolster.
2. Take deer pose with your legs by bending both knees with the left hip externally rotated, foot resting on the right thigh and the right leg internally rotated, foot resting beside you. Approximately 45-degree angle in both legs.
3. Turn to face the bolster, inhaling to lift your rib cage away from your hips and exhaling to lower your tummy onto the bolster.
4. Rest your arms on the floor, facing your head away from your knees for a deeper twist or toward your knees for a gentler twist.
5. Stay in this position for two-and-a-half minutes
6. Repeat the pose on the opposite side.

6 Counter Pose— Supported Baddha Konasana

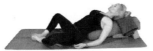

Figure 9.4.4.6: Relaxation module—Yin yoga twists & lateral—Counter baddha konasana.

1. Counter the twisted deer pose and take the final rest in a supported *baddha konasana* position. You can use an eye pillow and place supports under your knees if desired.

Twisting poses can feel quite challenging but are beneficial. As your body becomes accustomed to this yin practice, you should find that your moving yoga practice becomes easier. You should find more flexibility with lateral flexion and twists. This can help dramatically with rebalancing the distribution of tension in your body which should improve balance in your pelvic floor muscles.

That completes the relaxation module. You will perform the exercises from this module on the days specified in your weekly schedule.

Phase 4: Mind & Meditation Module

Conquer Your Fear

Having completed Phase 3, you should have started the process of changing your negative thought patterns, choosing positive thoughts instead. This is such a major achievement that will help you immensely as you move forward with your empowerment. You should be extremely proud!

Objective

The objective of the Mind & Meditation module in Phase 4 is to help you to conquer your fears. Many of the symptoms of PFD are coupled with fears; for example, the fear of embarrassment if someone notices your urine leakage or the fear of penetration if you suffer from vaginismus. This meditation will build on your ability to relax completely while reinforcing your positive thought patterns from the ANT therapy.

Success Metric

Success is achieved when you conquer the fears that prevent you from living your best life.

Additional Notes

This mediation requires that you first do ANT therapy on your fear, so you can begin the mediation knowing how you would like to feel in place of your current feelings of fear. You should read through the meditation beforehand and then go through the steps in your mind while you meditate. Additionally, you can listen to the audio-guided meditation on empoweryourflower.com.

Fear is not always mental. Excessively tense pelvic floor muscles can be painful, which can induce fear of movement or of touching or being touched. Some people like to touch their pain, while others are afraid to do so. If physical pain is your issue, you should still do "the work" on your fear of the physical pain and decide how you would like to physically feel in place of that pain. You can use this meditation to help you overcome your fear of pain.

As you go about your days, when you meet your fear, you should use the calming breath cycles to trigger your "rest and digest" system while relaxing the areas where your fear is physically manifesting. Try to remember the positive feelings that you would like to replace those feelings of fear.

Conquer Your Fear Meditation Instructions

This meditation is typically performed lying down; however, you may choose to do this meditation seated (useful if you have a tendency to fall asleep when lying down). Before you begin the meditation, you should do "the work" on your fear and note down how you would like to feel in place of your current fear.

Steps to Perform This Exercise

1. Get yourself into a comfortable starting position making sure to relax your body completely.
2. Close your mouth keeping your lips together with your teeth slightly apart, tongue resting on the roof of your mouth behind your front teeth.
3. Perform five relaxing breath cycles before you begin.
4. From this relaxed space, allow yourself to feel your fear.
5. Feel the part of your body where that fear manifests; is it a sensation in your gut, around your heart, or some other part of your body? Notice how it physically feels.
6. Inhale for a count of four, extending your exhalation for a count of eight while you send calming relaxation to the part of your body where you physically feel the fear. This will help to calm your nervous system, helping to communicate safety.
7. I want you to imagine a place where you feel safe. Allow yourself to go there to that safe place in your mind.

8. Imagine the scenery in your safe place. See that place in great detail and allow yourself to feel safe and relaxed in that place.

9. In that safe place in your mind, allow yourself to experience the new feelings that you have chosen to manifest in place of your fear. Feel the part of your body where these new positive feelings manifest. Maybe the new feelings make you feel warm around your heart. Maybe the feeling is a reduction in physical pain.

10. Imagine the best possible feeling in place of your fear and try to physically feel these new positive feelings. Notice how this new feeling manifests in your body.

11. Perform five calming breath cycles as you soak up these new positive feelings. You can remain as long as you like in this safe place soaking up the positive feelings.

12. Now, slowly leave that safe place, taking those positive feelings with you. Feel the warmth in your body and notice the beat of your heart.

13. Branch your awareness outwards from your heart reaching all the way to your fingers and toes and begin to gently introduce movement.

14. Make small circles with your wrists and ankles before reaching your hands up over your head taking a long deep stretch.

15. Hug your knees into your chest and roll to your right side, maintaining closed eyes and an internal focus.

16. Gently come to a comfortable seated position by pressing your left hand into the floor to bring yourself up.

17. Take a few moments here before you begin to move and bring those positive feelings with you as you go about your day.

18. In the next situation where you feel your fear, go back to that safe place in your mind, perform five calming breath cycles and try to feel those positive feelings in place of your fear.

This meditative practice should help you to sense the manifestation of fear in your tissues and will encourage the release of that visceral fear response in favor of another more positive feeling.

That completes the Mind & Meditation module and brings us to the end of the Phase 4 training. You will perform the exercises from this module on the days specified in your weekly schedule.

At the end of each week, if you feel that you may be ready to progress to the next phase of training, you can perform the phase checkpoint review using Figure 9.4.5, which checks your progress against the success metric for each exercise and helps you to decide if you should proceed to Phase 5 (intermediate level).

You can download a blank version of this form from empoweryourflower.com. As this is also the end of the beginner difficulty level, you will be prompted in the phase checkpoint review to retake your initial assessments to verify your progress toward your beginner level goal.

Phase 4 Checkpoint Review

Phase Start Date:_____

Checkpoint Date:_____

Pelvic Floor Module	Success

Strength: Success is achieved when you can perform 10 quick flick contractions with a good contraction and complete relaxation each time. If you suffer from stress incontinence, you should see an improvement in symptoms as you get better at performing these contractions.

Yes ☐
No ☐

Relaxation: Success is achieved when you can relax your pelvic floor fully in all the positions specified and no longer feel the symptoms of hypertonicity. Note: Reverse Kegels can help to release pelvic tension, however, you will continue to practice the reverse Kegels module through the entire program and so if you do not achieve success with the pelvic floor relaxation at this phase, this should not prevent you from proceeding to the next phase.

Yes ☐
No ☐

Breathing Module - Nadi Shodhana	Success

Success is achieved when you can easily perform the exercise without instruction with a comfortable 16 count exhalation.

Yes ☐
No ☐

Movement Module - Rebalancing Yoga	Success

Success with this module is achieved when you can comfortably flow through the yoga practice without feeling off balance. It should feel good in your body and you shouldn't feel pain in any of your joints.

Yes ☐
No ☐

Relaxation Module - Yin Yoga Twists & Lateral Movement	Success

Success is achieved when you can relax into your own body's pattern of tension, meeting the very edge of your discomfort without moving into pain. In this phase particular focus was given to lateral and twisting movements.

Yes ☐
No ☐

Mind & Meditation Module - Conquer your Fear Meditation	Success

Success is achieved when can let go of your fears, allowing you to go forward with living your best life.

Yes ☐
No ☐

Phase 4 Checkpoint Review	Success

Have you achieved the success objectives and do you feel that you are ready to proceed to the next phase of training?

Yes ☐
No ☐

If no, please continue with the phase 4 training until you are ready to proceed, or regress to the phase 3 training if this phase felt too difficult.

If yes, this is also the end of the Beginner difficulty level. You should retake your assessments to measure your progress after against your earlier results.

Progress Milestone Review - Beginner Level	Success

Have you already achieved your beginner level goal?

If no, you have the option to repeat phase 4 of the beginner level training.

Yes ☐

If yes, proceed to the intermediate level starting with Phase 5. Good Luck!

No ☐

Figure 9.4.5: Phase 4—Checkpoint review form.

Phase 5
Intermediate Level

Welcome to Phase 5 of the eight-phase training program. This is the first phase at the Intermediate Level. There are two phases at this level, Phase 5 and 6, which you should master before proceeding to the Advanced level of training. The following section details Phase 5 training modules, which are highlighted in Figure 9.5.1.

Eight-Phase Modules	Prep	Beginner			Intermediate		Advanced	
	Phase 1	Phase 2	Phase 3	Phase 4	Phase 5	Phase 6	Phase 7	Phase 8
Pelvic Floor	Kegel Breakdown	Full Kegel	Endurance Kegel	Speed Kegel	Co-Contract	Maximize Strength	Standing Rotations	Functional Training
Breathing	Nasal Breathing	Breath Strengthening	Breath Remapping	Nadi Shodhana	Basic Hypopressive Exercise	Intermediate Hypopressive Sequence	Advanced Hypopressive Sequence	Kapalabhati Breathing
Movement	Yoga Preparation	Yoga Basics	Core Re-tensioning	Rebalancing Yoga	Bandha Strength Yoga	Max Kegel Yoga	Ball Routine	Dynamic Power Yoga
Relaxation	Restorative Yoga	Yin Yoga Forward Folds	Yin Yoga Backward Bending	Yin Yoga Twists & Lateral Movement	Yin Yoga Hip Opening	Yin Yoga Pelvic Floor	Yin Yoga Happy Hips	Yin Yoga All Body
Mind & Meditation	Yoga Nidra	Flex your mind to flex your muscles	ANT therapy	Conquer your fear	Kirtan Kriya	Self Affirmations	Journaling	Blossoming Goddess

Figure 9.5.1: Phase 5—Intermediate level.

The exercises and activities for the Phase 5 modules, highlighted in orange in Figure 9.5.1, begin the process of moving away from isolated pelvic floor exercises and instead, working to get your pelvic floor muscles co-contracting with your abdominal muscles. Breathing will focus on learning a basic hypopressive exercise, and we will work to improve the length-tension relationship across the hips with our yin practice.

Remember, if your goal is pelvic floor relaxation, you will work on the reverse Kegels activity for all phases of training. It is detailed in Phase 1 pelvic floor module.

The frequency of practice can change as you progress through the training so make sure to read through all modules for Phase 5 and update your schedule accordingly prior to beginning.

Phase 5
Modules

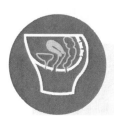

Pelvic Floor

Co-Contractions

Breathing

Basic Hypopressive Exercise

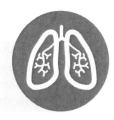

Movement

Bandha Strength Yoga

Relaxation

Yin Yoga Hip Opening

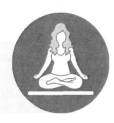

Mind & Meditation

Kirtan Kriya

Phase 5: Pelvic Floor Module

Co-Contractions

Having completed Phase 4, your ability to perform "quick flick" contractions in multiple positions marks a major milestone in your pelvic floor training. This is a fantastic achievement, you should celebrate!

Objective

The objective of the pelvic floor module in Phase 5 is to move away from isolation exercises and begin to focus more on functional pelvic floor exercises where we train an increased balance of tension by co-contracting other muscle groups. This involves progressively increasing the load you will place on the pelvic floor and the rest of your body.

Success Metric

Success is achieved when you can achieve a steady co-contraction of your deep core (transverse abdominals) and pelvic floor during active functional movements. This will require balanced intra-abdominal pressures, which should be achievable due to having completed the earlier phases of training.

This training is essentially neurologically remapping the pathways of tension within your body and should result in the eventual automatic co-contractions without your conscious control, which will go a long way to alleviating your symptoms and reinstating thoughtless, fearless movement patterns.

Additional Notes

It is at this point that I would like you to understand how to define your effort level. For this purpose, I have created the rate of perceived effort scale (RPE Scale), which is shown in Figure 9.5.2. Each level of the scale provides a description of that level from one, which is a very gentle contraction, to ten, which is maximal effort. Very strong and maximal effort contractions will activate co-contractions.

The purpose of the RPE scale is to define varying effort levels, which you will need to exert for the exercises that follow in the intermediate and advanced modules. The control that you have achieved from training your endurance and your strength will be used to achieve the desired effort level. You may be wondering how this is different from the strength assessment scale that you used when assessing your pelvic floor.

10	Maximum Effort - This is the maximum achievable contraction.
9	Very strong - Almost maximum strength and cannot be held for long.
7 - 8	Strong - At this level, periphery muscles (eg: core) will co-activate.
5 - 6	Moderately strong - This involves effort that can be held for a few breaths.
4	Moderate - You can breathe but cannot hold this level for extended periods.
2 - 3	Gentle - Easy with little effort and feels like it can be held for hours.
1	Very gentle - almost no effort. Can be held constantly regardless of the task.

Figure 9.5.2: Pelvic floor RPE scale.

To give you a visualization of the difference between your strength and your RPE, we will use the example of a bicep curl. Two people, side by side, perform a bicep curl with the heaviest dumbbell they can lift. One is lifting a 6 lbs (~3 kg) dumbbell while the other is lifting a 35 lbs (~15 kg) dumbbell. They are both working at an RPE of 10, however, they are not equally strong hence the big difference in the amount of weight they are lifting.

By setting a target for a specific rate of effort, we can ensure that both people are being sufficiently challenged to achieve hypertrophy (an increase in muscle mass) thus building additional strength.

By increasing your effort levels, you can work outside the boundaries of your existing strength. The training in this intermediate module should be challenging and is designed to further increase the strength and coordination of your pelvic floor.

Co-contractions Instructions

The co-contractions for this pelvic floor training are part of a short exercise sequence during which you will add abdominal contraction (*uddiyana bandha*) to your pelvic floor contraction (*mula bandha*). These contractions will have an RPE of 4 so you could view them more as "activations" as they are gentle contractions. You will perform an exercise sequence in two static positions, sitting and standing. You will also perform an active functional variation where you walk while maintaining the co-contraction. The movement module at this phase of training will also use these activations.

Steps to Perform the Co-contractions Exercise

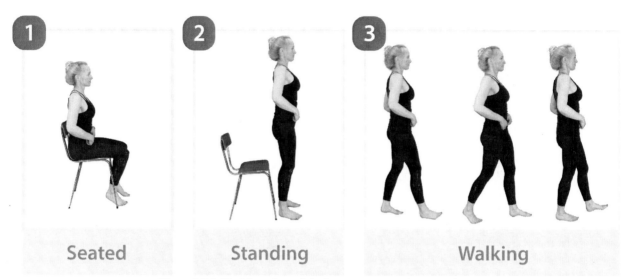

Figure 9.5.3: Positions for pelvic floor co-contraction exercises.

1. Come to your starting position (seated, standing, or standing in prep for walking).
2. Find the bony protrusions at the front of your hips, also known as ASIS.
3. Step your fingers in and down 2.5 cm (1 inch) from the ASIS.
4. Press gently, your core muscles should feel soft and relaxed.
5. On your next exhalation, gently engage your deep abdominals by pulling your belly button toward your spine. You will feel your abs getting firm under your fingertips. This should be a gentle contraction (RPE-4). Resist the urge to create a stronger contraction as that will activate your superficial abdominal muscles (obliques) instead of your deep abdominals (transverse abdominals).
6. Relax your abdominals as you inhale
7. On your next exhalation, initiate a pelvic floor contraction (RPE-4) while at the same time gently co-contracting your abdominals (RPE-4). Make sure to keep the rest of your body relaxed as you perform the exercise.
8. Take 10 calming breaths while holding the co-contraction in either a seated or standing position. For the walking (functional active exercise), you will walk around the room for one minute while maintaining the co-contraction. You should notice a higher level of resting tone in your abdominals when you are standing/walking.

With practice, you will enhance your body's ability to instigate co-contractions. Consistent steady practice will help your nervous system relearn this pattern, eventually making it a reflexive pattern, which will result in bottom-up coordination of movement where you no longer need to actively think about creating these co-contractions. This should have a dramatic impact on your functional movement, which ultimately should result in better management or alleviation of symptoms and an improved QoL. You will practice these co-contractions six days per week as with the earlier phases of pelvic floor training.

That concludes the pelvic floor module.

Phase 5: Breathing Module
Basic Hypopressive Exercise

Having completed Phase 4, your ability to fully utilize your lung capacity should have increased. Your diaphragm is strong, and your breathing pattern is optimized. This is quite an achievement; you should tell your friends and family how well you are doing!

Objective
The objective of the breathing module in Phase 5 is to utilize the hypopressive breathing technique to tap into the relationship between the pelvic floor and the diaphragm. In yoga, this is known as *uddiyana kriya* (Kriyas are cleansing rituals).

Success Metric
Success is achieved when you can perform a stomach vacuum.

Additional Notes
In Chapter Three, we performed an exercise that allowed you to feel the apnea from a stomach vacuum. You can revisit that activity if you struggle with this exercise. A strong stomach vacuum will draw the stomach inwards and upwards, and will also pull in around the collar bone and around the low back as the abdominal chamber is pulled toward the space where your lungs sit. You should also feel your pelvic floor lifting with this motion.

Basic Hypopressive Instructions
For this exercise, you will perform a basic hypopressive while standing bent over. You will practice this breathing exercise every second day. Your pelvic floor should remain relaxed throughout.

Steps to Perform the Basic Hypopressive Exercise

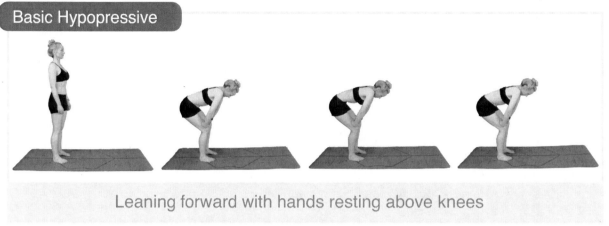

Basic Hypopressive

Leaning forward with hands resting above knees

Figure 9.5.4: Basic hypopressive exercise.

1. Stand with feet hip-distance apart, bending your knees slightly and resting your hands on your knees with your elbows pointing out to the sides.

2. Close your mouth keeping your lips together with your teeth slightly apart, tongue resting on the roof of your mouth behind your front teeth.

3. Perform three rounds of full breaths using the power of your diaphragm while keeping your shoulders relaxed.

4. Take a deep inhalation for a count of four and then exhale all the air out of your lungs.

5. Once you have emptied your lungs, hold the air out from the back of your throat, making sure that you are not holding a pocket of air in your mouth or your throat.

6. With your breath held, relax your tummy and expand your ribs out to the side in the same motion you feel when you are inhaling. This should cause your stomach to form a vacuum. Hold the exhalation for a count of four. *Note*: Do not pull or suck the stomach in manually. The stomach muscles remain relaxed throughout with the vacuum coming from the expansion of the ribcage which is similar to making a breathing motion with empty lungs.

7. Relax your rib cage, allowing your belly to hang before you begin your next inhalation. This will prevent a choking feeling that you can get if you try to breathe into your vacuum.

8. Repeat for five breath cycles.

Once you establish a regular uddiyana kriya practice, you enhance the flexibility of your diaphragm and pelvic floor. This is helpful both for conditions of hyper- and hypo- tonicity of the pelvic floor. Consistent practice will prepare you for the hypopressive sequences in the upcoming phases of training. That concludes the breathing module. You will perform the exercises from this module on the days specified in your weekly schedule.

Phase 5: Movement Module

Bandha Strength Yoga

Having completed Phase 4, you should be feeling more balanced and fit, keep up the momentum, you can do it!

Objective

The objective of the movement module in Phase 5 is to increase the intensity of the yoga practice with a specific focus on bandha activation (both mula bandha—pelvic floor activation, and uddiyana bandha—transversus abdominis activation).

Success Metric

Success with this module is achieved when you can maintain the co-contraction of your bandhas throughout your strong yoga practice. This will have a dramatic impact on your functional pelvic floor control.

Additional Notes

As we increase the intensity of our yoga practice, it becomes even more important to listen to your body. If you are working to overcome a symptomatic POP or stress incontinence, it is crucial that you pay attention to what shows up for you and adapt your practice accordingly. Do not hesitate to skip a pose if it triggers any symptoms.

The same holds true for those with NR-PFD or hypertonicity disorders, where the pelvic floor modules focus on relaxation and has therefore been replaced with the reverse Kegels module. If you have been practicing only reverse Kegels, you do not need to focus on bandha activation throughout this practice, but instead, focus on relaxing your pelvic floor on each inhalation, maintaining relaxaiton on exhalation.

Bandha Strength Yoga

You will need a yoga mat, two yoga blocks, a resistance band, a broomstick, and optionally an eye pillow and blanket. The practice should take twenty-five minutes including setup and final relaxation. You can download the sequence sheet for this bandha strength yoga sequence (Figure 9.5.5) from empoweryourflower.com and place it at the front of your mat when practicing.

Bandha Strength Yoga Sequence

Total Time: 25 minutes

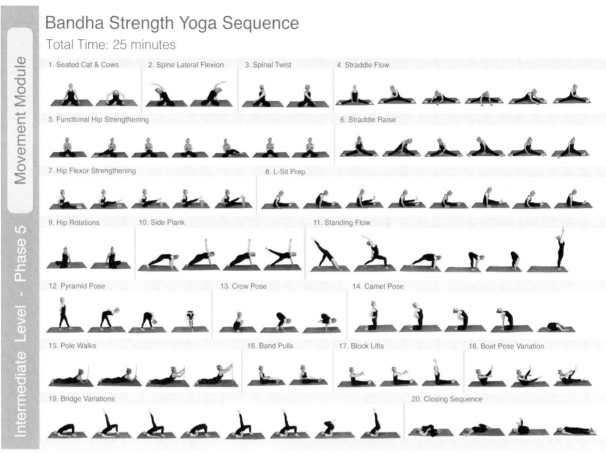

1. Seated Cat & Cows
2. Spine Lateral Flexion
3. Spinal Twist
4. Straddle Flow
5. Functional Hip Strengthening
6. Straddle Raise
7. Hip Flexor Strengthening
8. L-Sit Prep
9. Hip Rotations
10. Side Plank
11. Standing Flow
12. Pyramid Pose
13. Crow Pose
14. Camel Pose
15. Pole Walks
16. Band Pulls
17. Block Lifts
18. Boat Pose Variation
19. Bridge Variations
20. Closing Sequence

Figure 9.5.5: Phase 5—Movement module—Bandha strength sequence sheet.

You can read the instructions and steps beforehand and follow the poses on the printed copy of Figure 9.5.5 when you are practicing. This will help you to learn the sequence and eventually you will be able to practice it without looking at the sheet. Repeated practice creates change in the body.

Steps to Perform the Bandha Strength Yoga Routine

1 Seated Cat & Cows

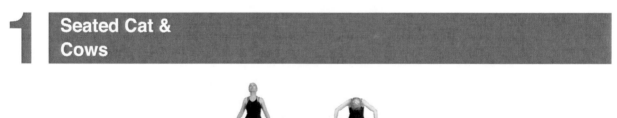

Figure 9.5.5.1: Phase 5—Movement module—Bandha strength yoga—Seated cat & cows.

1. Start in a comfortable cross-legged position, activating your pelvic floor with a contraction RPE-4 while co-contracting your lower abdominals with a similar level of contraction. This co-contraction is the engagement of your bandhas, the same co-contraction you are practicing in the pelvic floor

training on in this phase of training. Maintain your bandhas for the entire practice. *Note*: If you are practicing the reverse Kegels module, avoid co-contraction, focusing instead on pelvic floor relaxation on each inhalation and maintaing relaxation on each exhalation.

2. Initiate cat and cow breaths to warm the spine for five breath cycles.

2 Spine Lateral Flexion

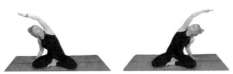

Figure 9.5.5.2: Phase 5—Movement module—Bandha strength yoga—Spine lateral flexion.

1. Place your left hand beside you as you inhale, and your right hand over your head for a lateral stretch for three breath cycles.

2. Place your right hand beside you as you inhale, and your left hand over your head for a lateral stretch.

3. Stay in the position for three breath cycles.

3 Spinal Twist

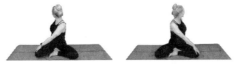

Figure 9.5.5.3: Phase 5—Movement module—Bandha strength yoga—Spinal twist.

1. Bring your left hand onto your right knee, and your right hand behind your back, lengthening your spine as you inhale, twisting as you exhale.

2. Hold the position for three breath cycles before repeating on the opposite side.

4 Straddle Flow

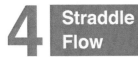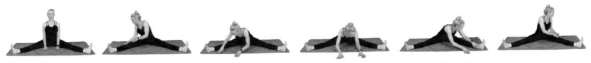

Figure 9.5.5.4: Phase 5—Movement module—Bandha strength yoga—Straddle flow.

1. Release your legs, coming to a straddle position as you inhale.

2. Exhale, beginning to make hip circles starting by moving your body over to the left side and rotating around to the right. You can start with small hip circles and exaggerate the movement as your hips warm up, closing your eyes and really feeling into your hip sockets. Continue for a count of five.

3. Change the direction making the same circles beginning with moving to the right and then rotating around to the left. Continue for a count of five.

5 Functional Hip Strengthening

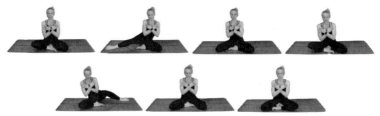

Figure 9.5.5.5: Phase 5—Movement module—Bandha strength yoga—Functional hip strength.

1. Return to a cross-legged position placing your left leg in front of the right, crossing your hands over your upper chest.

2. Release your left leg and swing the leg around, placing your foot down beside your hip and lowering your hip and then allowing your knee to rest on the floor.

3. Inhale, lifting your left knee, then your hip and lastly your foot, swinging the leg back around to the front, and exhaling placing it back in the cross-legged position. This is one set

4. Repeat Steps 1–3 four more times on the left side completing five sets.

5. Swap the cross on your legs so your right foot is in front of your left.

6. Repeat Steps 1–4 five times on the right side completing five sets.

6 Straddle Raise

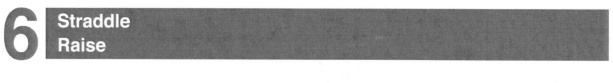

Figure 9.5.5.6: Phase 5—Movement module—Bandha strength yoga—Straddle raise.

1. Returning to the straddle position, you will begin the practice of *hasta upavistha konasana* (straddle lift-up pose). To prepare, place blocks on either side of your left leg.

2. Press into the hands, lifting your backside from the floor, shifting your hips backward but keeping

your heels on the mat.

3. Hold for three breath cycles.

4. Repeat Steps 2 and 3 on the right side. This completes a full set.

5. Perform three sets in total before trying to lift feet and hips with the support of blocks.

6. If you felt strong, you can try to lift without the blocks as shown final image of Figure 9.5.5.6.

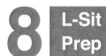

Hip Flexor Strengthening

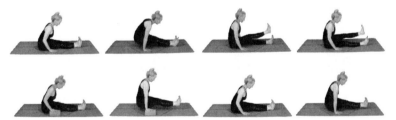

Figure 9.5.5.7: Phase 5—Movement module—Bandha strength yoga—Hip flexor strengthening.

1. Sit with your right leg outstretched and your left leg externally rotated with a block beside your right foot preparing for hip flexor strengthening. (Option to keep left leg straight if that feels better).

2. Keeping your hands on your hips and resisting the urge to lean backward, use the strength in your quads to lift your right foot over the block. *Note*: As your strength increases, you can increase the height of the block as demonstrated in Figure 9.5.5.7. This practice should also improve your standing balance.

3. Lift the foot back to the right of the block. Repeat the lift over and back five times.

4. Repeat Steps 1–3 on the left leg.

L-Sit Prep

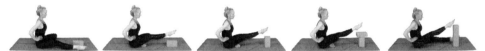

Figure 9.5.5.8: Phase 5—Movement module—Bandha strength yoga—L-sit prep.

1. Sit with both legs outstretched, placing your hands on the mat halfway between your hips and your knees in preparation for an L-sit practice.

2. Inhale as you engage your quads, pulling your knees up toward your hips, keeping your feet flexed. At the same time, push into your hands to straighten your arms, lifting your backside off the mat, sending your hips backward. Your feet might drag backward a little as you shift your hips backward.

This would be a good indication that you have the strength to try the full expression of this pose.

3. Repeat three times.

4. Keep your hands in position beside your legs, allow your hips to remain on the floor but lift your right leg and then your left leg.

5. Repeat five times for each leg.

6. If you felt strong with Steps 1 to 5, you can try the full expression using blocks. For this progression, place blocks beneath your hands, engage your quads, keep your feet flexed and press into your hands lifting the hips and legs fully from the floor.

7. Hold for three breath cycles.

8. If you can lift fully with the blocks, you can try the full expression without blocks. A strong contraction between your core and pelvic floor will help you to lift higher in this pose. Progressions should only be tried if you have the strength available to lift while maintaining your bandhas.

9. Hold for three breath cycles.

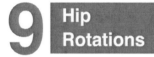

9 Hip Rotations

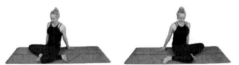

Figure 9.5.5.9: Phase 5—Movement module—Bandha strength yoga—Hip rotations.

1. Place your hands behind your back and bend your knees placing your feet a little wider than hip-distance apart on the mat.

2. Windscreen-wiper your legs from side to side by rotating through the hips.

3. Repeat for a count of ten.

10 Side Plank

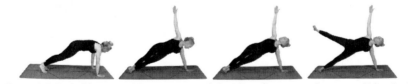

Figure 9.5.5.10: Phase 5—Movement module—Bandha strength yoga—Side plank.

1. Come to the plank position; place your left hand in the center of your mat, turn your body so you are resting on the outside of your left foot. Lift your hips, and extend your right hand upwards for side plank. Keep your gaze to the floor if you find it difficult to balance.

2. If you feel comfortable here, you can increase the difficulty further by extending your right leg up toward the ceiling as shown. This should be playful; if you lose your balance, try again.

3. Hold your version of the side plank for three breath cycles.

4. Come back to plank and take your version of this side plank on the opposite side for three breath cycles.

5. Return to plank position before pushing your hips back to come to a downward-facing dog.

11 Standing Flow

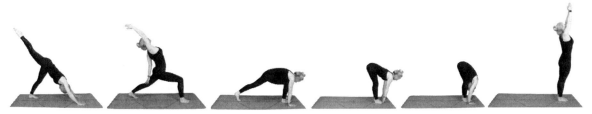

Figure 9.5.5.11: Phase 5—Movement module—Bandha strength yoga—Standing flow.

1. From downward-facing dog, inhale while lifting the right leg, keeping the hips level before exhaling to step the right foot forward.

2. Inhale pressing up into a lunge, lowering your left hand onto your left leg and reaching your right hand overhead taking a small backbend.

3. Perform three breath cycles here.

4. On your last exhalation, windmill the hands back down to the floor, inhaling to step the right leg back up for the three-legged downward-facing dog.

5. Exhale, lowering your leg for the downward-facing dog.

6. Repeat Steps 1 to 5 on the left side finishing in downward-facing dog

7. From the downward-facing dog, inhale as you step the right foot forward, followed by the left.

8. Inhale to lengthen your spine,

9. Exhale to fold forward, straightening your legs.

10. Inhale, with a soft bend in the knees, push through the midfoot to come up, extending the arms overhead, and gazing to the thumbs.

11. Exhale hands to heart center for tadasana pose.

12 Pyramid Pose

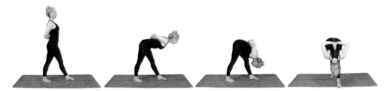

Figure 9.5.5.12: Phase 5—Movement module—Bandha strength yoga—Pyramid pose.

1. Take a small step backward with your right leg and grab opposite elbows behind your back.
2. Inhale to lengthen your spine and open your chest.
3. Exhale to fold over your straight legs, pivoting from the hips and trying to keep both hips level.
4. If your tummy rests on your thighs, allow your chin to reach down toward your shin. *Note*: if shoulder flexibility allows, you can perform a *reverse namaskar pose* (prayer hands) behind your back instead of grabbing opposite elbows (shown in the right image of Figure 9.5.5.12).
5. Hold for three breath cycles.
6. Press into your feet, using the power of your legs to bring your body back up as you inhale.
7. Step forward to tadasana.
8. Repeat Steps 1 to 7 stepping back with the left leg.

13 Crow Pose

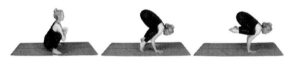

Figure 9.5.5.13: Phase 5—Movement module—Bandha strength yoga—Crow pose.

1. Standing in the center of your mat, lower down into a yoga squat in preparation for crow pose.
2. Place your hands shoulder-distance apart in front of you, shifting your gaze to make the virtual tripod. Make sure to keep your gaze forward to prevent you from rolling over.
3. Place your knees into your underarms and inhale as you lean your weight forward, releasing your feet from the floor and bring your toes to touch each other. *Note*: If you did not reach the full expression of the crow pose during your Phase 4 practice, you should continue to practice your current version here or remain in squat if arm balancing is not part of your practice.
4. Perform five breath cycles here, straightening your arms as much as you can.
5. Exhale, bringing your feet back to the mat.

14 | Camel Pose

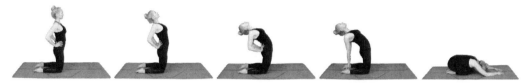

Figure 9.5.5.14: Phase 5—Movement module—Bandha strength yoga—Camel pose.

1. Kneel on the center of your mat, placing your hands into your lower back, fingertips pointing upwards.
2. Inhale, lifting your ribcage away from your hips and shifting your hips forward coming to a backbend. Don't overextend your neck, try to stay long in your neck, bringing the backbend into the low and mid-back.
3. If your backbend is sufficient that you can see the wall behind you, release the right hand from your hip to your right heel, followed by the left hand, placing it on the left heel.
4. Perform three breath cycles in your version of this backbend, lifting the rib cage away from the hips on inhalation and bending a little deeper each exhalation.
5. On your last inhalation, use the strength of your quads to lift your body back up.
6. Exhale coming down to a close-legged child's pose.

15 | Pole Walks

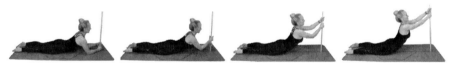

Figure 9.5.5.15: Phase 5—Movement module—Bandha strength yoga—Pole walks.

1. Lie on your stomach while holding a broomstick in front of you on the mat and preparing for a second backbend.
2. Inhale as you begin to walk your hands up the pole, keeping your hips on the mat as you do so. Walk your hands as high as you comfortably can and then hold for three breath cycles.
3. Walk your hands back down the pole and rest for a full breath cycle.
4. Repeat Steps 1 to 3 once more.

16 | Band Pulls

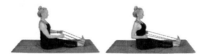

Figure 9.5.5.16: Phase 5—Movement module—Bandha strength yoga—Band pulls.

1. Bring yourself to a seated position on your mat with your legs extended, placing a long resistance band around your feet.
2. Starting with the arms forward, inhale as you draw the elbows back behind you. Your chest should stay open and you should compress the mid-part of your back as you do this. As you get stronger, increase the resistance by swapping for a stiffer band.
3. Repeat ten times.

17 | Block Lifts

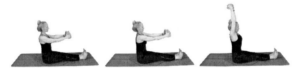

Figure 9.5.5.17: Phase 5—Movement module—Bandha strength yoga—Block lifts.

1. Stay seated with the legs extended, feet flexed, gripping a yoga block holding it straight out in front of you, inhaling here.
2. Exhale as you reach the block away from you, spreading your scapula.
3. Inhale as you reach the block up over your head, keeping your scapula protracted and elbows straight.
4. Exhale lowering the block back in front of you as you maintain scapular protraction and straight elbows.
5. Repeat four more times.

18 | Boat Pose Variation

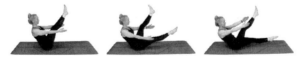

Figure 9.5.5.18: Phase 5—Movement module—Bandha strength yoga—Boat pose variation.

1. Prepare for *navasana* (boat pose), bringing your hands behind your knees, pointing your toes, and walking your feet back to find your pivot point.

2. Release your hands, straightening your legs, and pointing your toes , holding this position for three breath cycles.

3. From navasana, begin to alternate lowering and raising the right leg and left leg, continuing five times on each leg before coming down to lie on your back.

19 Bridge Variations

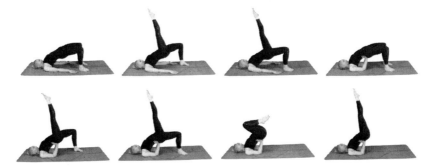

Figure 9.5.5.19: Phase 5—Movement module—Bandha strength yoga—Bridge variations.

1. Prepare for a shoulder-supported bridge, bringing your feet in line with your hips, touching your middle fingers off your heels.

2. Inhale, pressing into your feet, lifting your hips high, exhale here.

3. Inhale as you extend your right leg and point your toes, exhale, lower your right leg, and plant your foot so it is back in its starting position.

4. Repeat this lifting and lowering on the left side. This is one set. You should perform three sets.

5. Lower your hips down and take three breath cycles, resting with feet mat-width and knees together, before once again placing your feet in line with your hips in prep for the second round.

6. Inhale, pressing into your feet, lifting your hips high.

7. Bend your elbows and place your hands in your low back, fingertips pointing toward your face. This creates a platform with your hands that you can use to balance your hips on. *Note*: If you struggled with lifting your legs in the previous backbend, you should continue to practice that version. Progress only when your body is comfortable with the earlier version.

8. Inhale as you release your right leg from the floor, pointing your toe toward the ceiling. Then, exhale, lowering your right leg.

9. Repeat this motion for the left leg. This is one set. You should perform three sets.

10. If you can feel good support from your hands when lifting one leg, you can try releasing both feet, bending your knees, and then extending both legs together, pointing your toes toward the ceiling.

11. Stay in this bridge for three breath cycles.

12. Lower one leg at a time to come back to your supported bridge before lowering your hips back to the mat.

20 | Closing Sequence

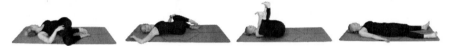

Figure 9.5.5.20: Phase 5—Movement module—Bandha strength yoga—Closing sequence.

1. Hug your knees into your chest, rocking a little from side to side.

2. Release your knees, shift your hips a little to the right and drop your knees to the left for a spinal twist.

3. Take the twist on the opposite side.

4. Come to happy husband pose for three breath cycles.

5. Take your final rest (savasana) for five minutes.

Even though a lot of the positions are floor-based, holding your bandhas through this strong practice is quite challenging. If you struggle to hold your bandhas with this strong practice, you can practice holding your bandhas with a sequence from an earlier phase until your strength increases.

You also have the option to swap out more difficult versions of poses with their regressions (for example, side plank, which you practiced as a supported version in the core re-tensioning sequence from the movement module of Phase 3). Consistent steady practice will produce results so keep working. That concludes this movement module. You will perform the exercises from this module on the days specified in your weekly schedule.

Phase 5: Relaxation Module

Yin Yoga Hip Opening

Having completed Phase 4, you should be noticing an improvement in your ability to shift weight laterally. Your ability to twist should also have improved, this is a great achievement!

Objective

The objective of the relaxation module in Phase 5 is to focus on improving length-tension relationships around your hips. We will do this by relaxing into a range of yin hip opening poses.

Success Metric

As with Phase 4, success with yin yoga is achieved when you can relax into the positions. The hips are often the location of excess tension and one of the key locations where we store "issues in our tissues." Pay attention when you are in stressful situations and notice if you hold any tension in your hips. This practice will give you a chance to release some of that tension.

Additional Notes

As with the other yin practices, you should ensure you avoid moving into pain.

Yin Yoga Hip Openers

You will need one or two bolsters (or pillows), two blankets, two blocks, an eye pillow, and a yoga mat. This practice will take twenty minutes, including setup and transitions between poses. You can download the sequence sheet for this yin yoga twists and lateral movement sequence (Figure 9.5.6) from empoweryourflower.com, and place it at the front of your mat when practicing.

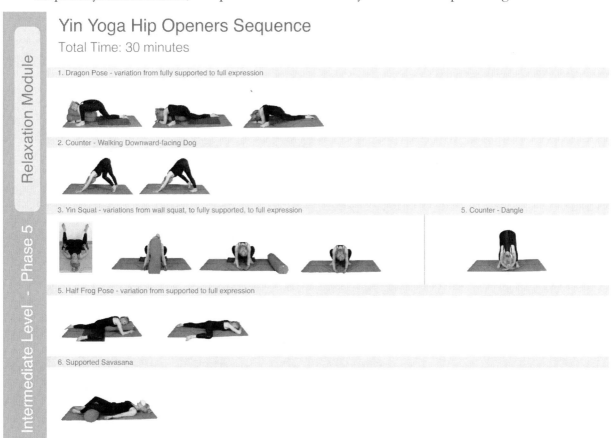

Figure 9.5.6: Phase 5—Relaxation module—Yin yoga hip openers sequence sheet.

You can read the instructions and steps beforehand and follow the poses on the printed copy of Figure 9.5.6 when you are practicing. This will help you to learn the sequence and eventually you will be able to practice it without looking at the sheet.

Steps to Perform the Yin Yoga Hip Openers Sequence

1 Dragon Pose

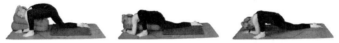

Figure 9.5.6.1: Phase 5—Relaxation module—Yin yoga hip openers—Dragon pose.

Dragon pose is a deep hip and groin opener. It also stretches the hip flexors and quads on the back leg. There are multiple supported versions of this pose shown from the most supported to the full expression. To assume the pose:

1. Start in an all-fours position, stepping your left foot forward. *Note*: you can place a blanket under your back knee if needed.

2. Allow yourself to relax forward, surrendering the weight of your hips toward the floor as you rest on your elbows, allowing your head to hang. You can rest on one or two bolsters if you lack the openness in your hips for the full expression.

3. Relax in your version of this pose for two-and-a-half minutes. You will feel your tissues release as time passes.

4. Very slowly, mindfully bring energy into your hands and slowly press your hands to bring yourself back releasing your left foot back to all-fours.

5. Repeat steps 1–4 for the right leg.

2 Counter Pose— Walking Downward-Facing Dog

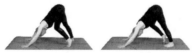

Figure 9.5.6.2: Phase 5—Relaxation module—Yin yoga hip openers—Counter pose walking dog.

1. From all-fours, press up into a gentle yin, walking downward-facing dog for one minute. *Note*: You can move your hips around in this yin dog, taking whatever movement your body is craving after that deep hip stretch.

Yin Squat

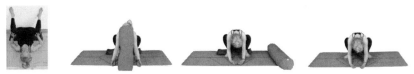

Figure 9.5.6.3: Phase 5—Relaxation module—Yin yoga hip openers—Yin squat.

A *yin squat* is a supported squat where you surrender yourself to gravity in the squatting position. You will fold forward in this squat to allow a deeper relaxation into the hips. There are multiple supported versions of this pose shown from the most supported, which is a wall squat, to the full expression, which is a squat with no props.

If your physiotherapist or healthcare provider has advised you against upright squatting positions, you should check with them if you can practice the wall squat, which would allow you to work your hip flexion without loading weight into the hips. To assume the pose:

1. Come into a squatting position (or in your wall squat position if indicated) using whatever props you need to.
2. Once in position, allow your upper body to relax forward, allowing the palms to face upward to resist the temptation to grip the floor.
3. Adjust the placement of your hands until you find a position that allows you to remain effortlessly balanced in your squat, then relax completely.
4. Stay relaxed in your squat for five minutes.
5. Very slowly, mindfully bring energy into your hands and slowly press your hands bringing them closer to your body, fingertips touching the mat.

4 Counter Pose— Dangle

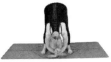

Figure 9.5.6.4: Phase 5—Relaxation module—Yin yoga hip openers—Counter pose dangle.

1. Press into your feet to bring your hips up so you are standing, knees bent, upper body resting on your thighs and your hands relaxed on the floor for the counterpose, which is a yin dangle.
2. Sway a little from side to side here if you feel you need movement.
3. After one minute, lower your hips back down to the mat to prepare for the next pose.

5 | Half Frog Pose

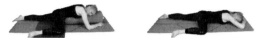

Figure 9.5.6.5: Phase 5—Relaxation module—Yin yoga hip openers—Half frog pose.

The *half frog pose* is a yin pose which offers a deep external rotation of the hip. Opening one hip at a time allows for a deeper relaxation versus the full frog pose in which both hips are open at the same time. To assume the pose:

1. Lie on your stomach, opening your right leg out to the right side bringing the knee in line with the hip, and keeping the ankle in line with the knee. This creates a 90-degree angle at the knee. You have the option to rest your body on a bolster, reducing the degree of external rotation, and placing a blanket under your knee for padding.
2. Relax into the pose for two-and-a-half minutes.
3. Very slowly, mindfully bring energy into your right hand, pressing into your hand to roll your body onto the left side. From there, you can gently come to the child's pose for a few moments before repeating Steps 1 and 2 on the left side.

6 | Supported Savasana

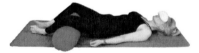

Figure 9.5.6.6: Phase 5—Relaxation module—Yin yoga hip openers—Supported savasana.

1. Come to a supported savasana to counter the half-frog pose. This is the final relaxation, which you should enjoy for five minutes.

It can take time to create an opening in the hips, particularly if you have spent many years in sedentary seated positions. Give yourself the grace of time as you undertake this yin practice and continue to listen to your body, making sure not to pass your edge.

This concludes the Relaxation module. You will perform the exercises from this module on the days specified in your weekly schedule.

Phase 5: Mind & Meditation Module

Kirtan Kriya

Having completed Phase 4, you should have conquered some of your fears and should be moving toward a higher QoL, that is absolutely amazing!

Objective

The objective of the Mind & Meditation module in Phase 5 is to exercise your brain with the yogic meditation known as Kirtan Kriya (kriya being a cleansing ritual).

Success Metric

Success is achieved when you have established a regular practice of this meditation, which you should feel comfortable with adopting as part of your normal life.

Additional Notes

The Kirtan Kriya is a meditation that involves a combination of mantra (chanting), mudra (repetitive finger movements), and stillness (seated with eyes closed). The mantra that is repeated is, "Saa, Taa, Naa, Maa," which is said to mean birth, life, death, rebirth. It is used as a treatment for Alzheimer's and is believed to reduce stress while increasing activity in the parts of the brain linked to memory.

As you repeat the mantra, you are touching a finger and thumb together (mudra) while repeating the relevant sound (mantra). This combination of mudra and mantra is believed to enhance the neurological benefits of this meditation.

The meditation takes twelve minutes to complete. You will need a meditation timer to alert you when to move to the next step. You will set the timer as follows:

First alert: 0 minutes (begin to repeat the mantra aloud)

2nd alert: 2 minutes (begin to whisper the mantra)

3rd alert: 4 minutes (begin to think the mantra)

4th alert: 8 minutes (begin to whisper the mantra)

5th alert: 10 minutes (repeat the mantra aloud)

Last alert: 12 minutes (meditation end)

Alternatively, you can listen to a guided audio of the meditation on <u>empoweryourflower.com</u>.

Kirtan Kriya Meditation

This meditation is typically performed in a seated position as shown in Figure 9.5.7 but you can choose a different position if this is uncomfortable for you.

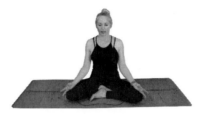

Figure 9.5.7: Seated Kirtan Kriya meditation—mudra + mantra.

You can see that I am speaking the mantra while making the mudra in Figure 9.5.7. In the suggested schedule, you will perform this meditation twice per week. However, it can be of great benefit to practice this meditation every day if you feel so inclined. The table below shows the mantra and mudra. You can sing the mantra or speak it by repeating "Saa, taa, naa, maa" while touching the relevant finger to the thumb as shown in Figure 9.5.8.

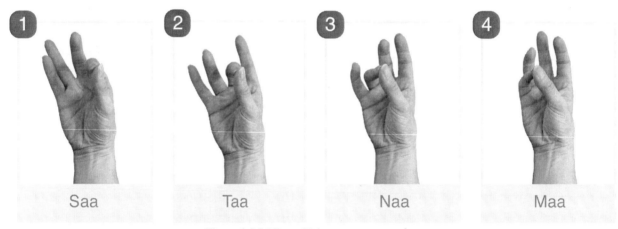

Figure 9.5.8 Kirtan Kriya mantra + mudra.

You continue to perform the mudra shown in Figure 9.5.8 even when you are at the "thinking" stage of the meditation.

Steps to Perform the Kirtan Kriya Meditation

1. Find a comfortable seated position with your spine elongated, with your body relaxed.
2. Perform five calming breath cycles before you begin the meditation.
3. Start your meditation timer and allow your gaze to lower to the floor.
4. When you hear the first alert, say or sing the mantra while at the same time performing the mudra on both hands, continuing for two minutes until you hear the second timer alert.
5. Whisper the mantra as you perform the mudra for the next two minutes until you hear the third alert.

6. Think the mantra while performing the mudra for four minutes until you hear the forth alert. *Note*: It can be hard to concentrate on thinking the mantra when your head is full of thoughts. Try to use the mudra to keep your mind focused on repeating the mantra in your head.

7. Whisper the mantra as you perform the mudra until you hear the fifth alert.

8. Say or sing the mantra while performing the mudra until you hear the sixth and final alert.

9. Inhale deeply as you raise your hands above your head.

10. Exhale as you lower your hands to your heart, holding them in prayer position with your thumbs resting over your heart for a moment as you relax. Notice if you can feel your heartbeat as you relax.

11. Perform five calming breath cycles before slowly blinking your eyes open to end the meditation, being sure to get up slowly as your legs may be sleeping.

This meditation is a nice addition to your day and should help to bring some peace and equanimity. That completes the mind/meditation module. You will practice the meditation according to your weekly schedule

At the end of each week, if you feel that you may be ready to progress to the next phase of training, you can perform the phase checkpoint review using Figure 9.5.9, which checks your progress against the success metric for each exercise and helps you to decide if you should proceed to Phase 6 (intermediate level). You can download a blank version of this form from empoweryourflower.com.

Phase 5 Checkpoint Review

Phase Start Date:_____

Checkpoint Date:_____

Pelvic Floor Module

Success

Strength: Success is achieved when you can achieve a steady co-contraction of your deep core (transverse abdominals) and pelvic floor during active functional movements. This will require balanced intra-abdominal pressures which should be achievable due to having completed the earlier phases of training.

Yes ☐
No ☐

Relaxation: Success is achieved when you can relax your pelvic floor fully in all the positions specified and no longer feel the symptoms of hypertonicity. Note: Reverse Kegels can help to release pelvic tension, however, you will continue to practice the reverse Kegels module through the entire program and so if you do not achieve success with the pelvic floor relaxation at this phase, this should not prevent you from proceeding to the next phase.

Yes ☐
No ☐

Breathing Module - Basic Hypopressive

Success

Success is achieved when you can perform a stomach vacuum.

Yes ☐
No ☐

Movement Module - Bandha Strength Yoga

Success

Success with this module is achieved when you can maintain the co-contraction of your bandhas throughout your strong yoga practice. This will have a dramatic impact on your functional pelvic floor control.

Yes ☐
No ☐

Relaxation Module - Yin Yoga Hip Openers

Success

As with phase 4, success with Yin yoga is achieved when you can relax into the hip opening positions which are often the location of excess tension and one of the key locations where we store "issues in our tissues".

Yes ☐
No ☐

Mind & Meditation Module - Kirtan Kriya Meditation

Success

Success is achieved when you have established a regular practice of this meditation, which you should feel comfortable with adopting as part of your normal life.

Yes ☐
No ☐

Phase 5 Checkpoint Review

Success

Have you achieved the success objectives and do you feel that you are ready to proceed to the next phase of training?

Yes ☐
No ☐

If no, please continue with the phase 5 training until you are ready to proceed or regress to phase 4 if this phase felt too difficult.

If yes, please proceed to Phase 6 which is the final phase at the intermediate level. You are more than half way, keep up the great work!

Figure 9.5.9: Phase 5—Checkpoint review form.

Phase 6
Intermediate Level

Welcome to Phase 6 of the eight-phase training program. This is the final of the two phases at the intermediate level. The modules for Phase 6 are highlighted in Figure 9.6.1.

Eight-Phase Modules	Prep	Beginner			Intermediate		Advanced	
	Phase 1	Phase 2	Phase 3	Phase 4	Phase 5	Phase 6	Phase 7	Phase 8
Pelvic Floor	Kegel Breakdown	Full Kegel	Endurance Kegel	Speed Kegel	Co-Contract	Maximize Strength	Standing Rotations	Functional Training
Breathing	Nasal Breathing	Breath Strengthening	Breath Remapping	Nadi Shodhana	Basic Hypopressive Exercise	Intermediate Hypopressive Sequence	Advanced Hypopressive Sequence	Kapalabhati Breathing
Movement	Yoga Preparation	Yoga Basics	Core Re-tensioning	Rebalancing Yoga	Bandha Strength Yoga	Max Kegel Yoga	Ball Routine	Dynamic Power Yoga
Relaxation	Restorative Yoga	Yin Yoga Forward Folds	Yin Yoga Backward Bending	Yin Yoga Twists & Lateral Movement	Yin Yoga Hip Opening	Yin Yoga Pelvic Floor	Yin Yoga Happy Hips	Yin Yoga All Body
Mind & Meditation	Yoga Nidra	Flex your mind to flex your muscles	ANT therapy	Conquer your fear	Kirtan Kriya	Self Affirmations	Journaling	Blossoming Goddess

Figure 9.6.1: Phase 6—Intermediate

The exercises and activities for the Phase 6 modules, highlighted in orange in Figure 9.6.1, are intended to maximize your pelvic floor strength in many positions. If you have been working on pelvic floor relaxation using the reverse Kegels from Phase 1, you will focus on relaxing on inhalation rather than maximum strength contractions. The relaxation at this phase offers a deep pelvic floor relaxation.

The frequency of practice can change as you progress through the training so make sure to read through all modules for Phase 6 and update your schedule accordingly before you begin

Phase 6
Modules

Pelvic Floor

Maximize Strength

Breathing

Intermediate Hypopressive Sequence

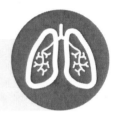

Movement

Max Kegel Yoga

Relaxation

Yin Yoga Pelvic Floor

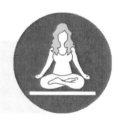

Mind & Meditation

Self Affirmations

Phase 6: Pelvic Floor Module

Maximize Strength

Having completed Phase 5, you should have mastered the ability to co-contract your deep abdominals and pelvic floor. This may seem quite basic, but it adds an additional layer of functional control that should help you to balance intra-abdominal pressures. Give yourself a gold star!

Objective

The objective of the pelvic floor module in Phase 6 is to move you beyond the basic pelvic floor contractions and co-contractions to maximum strength contractions. This should help you to build substantial pelvic floor strength.

You will practice every second day while alternating your position as follows:

Day 1: Hook lying.

Day 2: Sitting.

Day 3: Standing.

The rest days in between practice will give your pelvic floor time to recover as these sessions use maximum effort.

Success Metric

Success is achieved when you can perform a controlled squeeze of a finger inserted in the vagina giving a score of eight on the strength scale, which is equivalent to a good contraction with a strong lift. You should be able to sustain a strong contraction for a count of ten with the co-contractions happening naturally.

Additional Notes

When you perform the maximum strength contractions in this module, you could imagine that your pelvic floor is like your fist. If you were holding a little marble in your fist, you could easily hold it all day (RPE-4). Now if you were to squeeze that marble as hard as possible, you would not be able to sustain that contraction for long. When squeezing your fist as tightly as possible, your forearm muscles will also co-contract, and potentially your biceps too.

In the same way, when you contract your pelvic floor, squeezing as strongly as possible, you will feel your core, your glutes, and the muscles that support your hips will be holding increased tension. The center of your contraction remains within your pelvic floor, while the extra tension is triggered to distribute the load to other relevant muscles (employees) in a balanced way, rather than from you deliberately contracting these other muscles. This load distribution is an important function in the business of your body's movement.

Steps to Perform This Exercise

1. Perform five calming breath cycles before you begin.
2. Get yourself into a comfortable starting position.
3. Begin inhaling for a count of four
4. On your next exhalation, initiate a pelvic floor contraction with an RPE-4 and maintain that contraction (like gently holding the marble in your fist).
   a. Inhale here.
   b. Exhale and perform a maximum strength contraction with an RPE-10
   c. Inhale releasing the contraction back to an RPE-4.
   d. Exhale performing another maximum strength contraction with RPE-10.
   e. Inhale releasing the contraction to an RPE-4.
   f. Figure 9.6.2 shows a graphic representation of this pattern. As you can see from this, the RPE-4 contraction remains in place until the end of the set.

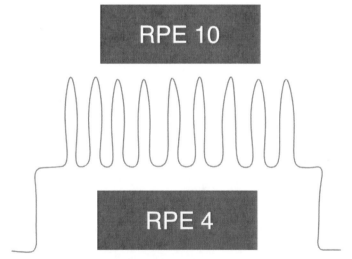

Figure 9.6.2—Maximum Strength Contraction—RPE 4 to RPE 10.

5. Continue the cycle until you have performed a full ten contract/release cycles moving from RPE-4 to RPE-10. Try to maintain a calm steady breath throughout. This is one set. You should perform five sets.

As well as producing hypertrophy, maximum strength contractions may help to relax hypertonic pelvic floor muscles[78]. If you are suffering from an NR-PFD or pelvic pain condition, you should check with your pelvic floor physio or healthcare provider if maximum strength contractions could be helpful for you.

That concludes the pelvic floor module. You will perform the exercises from this module on the days specified in your weekly schedule.

Phase 6: Breathing Module

Intermediate Hypopressive Sequence

Having completed Phase 5, you have successfully learned to perform a hypopressive stomach vacuum. This puts you in the same league as Arnold Schwarzenegger who was the master of the stomach vacuum on the bodybuilding stage, go you!

Objective

The objective of the breathing module is to begin to add movement to your hypopressive practice. This will help you work on the relationship between your diaphragm and pelvic floor so you can train on your balance of directional tension. This practice should also increase your core stability.

Success Metric

Success is achieved when you can comfortably perform the hypopressive routine achieving a stomach vacuum in all positions.

Additional Notes

It is common to feel a stronger apnea (vacuum) in positions where you are bent over or on all-fours. By adding movement to this practice, you have the opportunity to feel the relationship between your diaphragm and pelvic floor through different lines of tension as you move.

Intermediate Hypopressive

You will need a yoga mat to perform this intermediate hypopressive routine. You will practice this short sequence every second day and it should take no more than fifteen minutes to complete.

You can download the sequence sheet for this intermediate hypopressive sequence (Figure 9.3.6) from empoweryourflower.com and place it at the front of your mat when practicing.

Intermediate Hypopressive Sequence

Total Time: 15 minutes

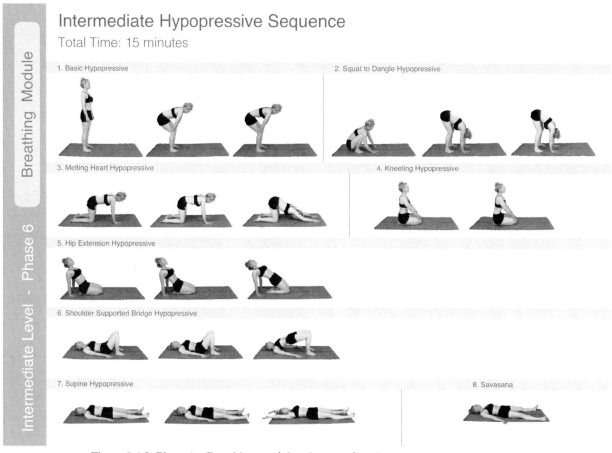

1. Basic Hypopressive

2. Squat to Dangle Hypopressive

3. Melting Heart Hypopressive

4. Kneeling Hypopressive

5. Hip Extension Hypopressive

6. Shoulder Supported Bridge Hypopressive

7. Supine Hypopressive

8. Savasana

Figure 9.6.3: Phase 6—Breathing module—Intermediate hypopressive sequence sheet.

You can read the instructions and steps beforehand and follow the poses on the printed copy of Figure 9.6.3 when you are practicing. This will help you to learn the sequence and eventually you will be able to practice it without looking at the sheet.

Steps to Perform This Intermediate Hypopressive Sequence

1 Basic Hypopressive

Figure 9.6.3.1: Intermediate hypopressive—Basic Hypopressive.

1. Stand, feet hip-distance apart, bend your knees slightly, and rest your hands on your knees with your elbows out to the side.

2. Close your mouth keeping your lips together with your teeth slightly apart, tongue resting on the roof of your mouth behind your front teeth.

3. Perform three rounds of full breaths using the power of your diaphragm while keeping your shoulders relaxed.

4. Inhale deeply for a count of four and then exhale all the air out of your lungs holding your breath out. Expand your rib cage as though breathing into your empty lungs to achieve your apnea.

5. Relax your rib cage allowing your belly to hang before you begin your next inhalation

6. Repeat the hypopressive in this position twice more.

2 Squat to Dangle

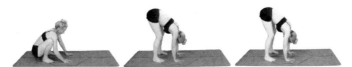

Figure 9.6.3.2: Intermediate hypopressive—Squat to dangle.

1. On your next inhalation, bring your hands to the floor and lower into a squat position.

2. In your squat, keeping your hands gently resting on the floor in front of you, begin to take a deep exhalation, finishing the exhalation when your hips are raised, hands planted on the floor.

3. With the hips in the air, allow your abs to relax and hold your breath out to perform your vacuum, expanding the rib cage as though breathing into your empty lungs.

4. Relax your ribcage and let your belly hang before you begin your next inhalation while lowering the hips to come back to your squat.

5. Repeat this squat to dangle hypopressive twice more.

3 Melting Heart

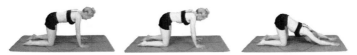

Figure 9.6.3.3: Intermediate hypopressive—Melting heart.

1. Come down to all-fours and take a full breath cycle before inhaling in preparation for apnea.

2. Exhale all the air out and hold the breath out to take your vacuum, expanding your ribcage as though you could breathe into your empty lungs.

3. Hold the apnea as you reach the hands forward for the melting heart pose, keeping your hips stacked above your knees.

4. Allow your ribcage to relax and your belly to hang as you inhale back to neutral all-fours.

5. Repeat the melting heart hypopressive twice more taking a resting breath cycle in between.

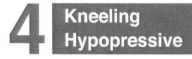 ## Kneeling Hypopressive

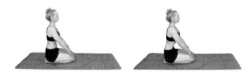

Figure 9.6.3.4: Intermediate hypopressive—Kneeling Hypopressive.

1. Come to a kneeling position and take a calming breath cycle before inhaling in preparation for taking your apnea.

2. Exhale and take your apnea holding for a count of four.

3. Before inhaling, allow your ribcage and stomach to relax.

4. Repeat twice more to complete three hypopressives in the kneeling position.

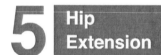 ## Hip Extension

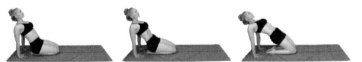

Figure 9.6.3.5: Intermediate hypopressive—Hip extension.

1. From the kneeling position, place your hands on the floor behind your back, making sure to stack shoulders over elbows, over wrists. Take a calming breath cycle here before inhaling in preparation for your apnea.

2. Exhale to empty your lungs and create your apnea. Once you have achieved a vacuum, press into your hands as you squeeze your glutes to lift your hips up, opening through the chest as you do this.

3. Hold the apnea in this elevated position for a count of four.

4. Allow your ribcage and stomach to relax before inhaling as you lower back down.

5. Repeat twice more to complete three hypopressives with hip extension.

6 Shoulder Supported Bridge

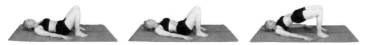

Figure 9.6.3.6: Intermediate hypopressive—shoulder supported bridge.

1. Lie on your back planting your ankles under your knees, arms alongside your body. Inhale here.
2. Exhale and create your apnea. Once you have achieved a vacuum, press into your feet as you lift your hips up. Try to lift the rib cage closer to the chin when you do this.
3. Hold the apnea in this elevated position for a count of four.
4. Allow your ribcage and stomach to relax before inhaling and lowering back down.
5. Repeat twice, hugging your knees to your chest after the final round.

7 Supine Hypopressive

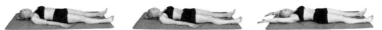

Figure 9.6.3.7: Intermediate hypopressive—Supine hypopressive.

1. Lie on your back in a savasana position with your arms alongside your body. Inhale here.
2. Exhale and create your apnea. Once you have achieved a vacuum, raise your arms up over your head reaching for the floor as you activate the legs, pointing your toes. You should have a small space under your low back and your shoulders should remain on the mat.
3. Hold the apnea in this position for a count of four.
4. Allow your ribcage and stomach to relax before inhaling and lowering your hands.
5. Repeat twice.

8 Savasana

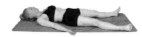

Figure 9.6.3.8: Intermediate hypopressive—Savasana.

1. Perform a final savasana for a few minutes, allowing your body to relax completely with quiet breathing.

Hypopressives are a great way to get some movement into your diaphragm and pelvic floor. By following a routine, you can establish a positive habit that can help to reduce your symptoms, particularly for those suffering from POP. Remember, it takes 40 days to break a habit, 90 days to gain a new habit, in 120 days you are the habit, and at 1000 days, you are the master of it.

That concludes the breathing module. You will perform the exercises from this module on the days specified in your weekly schedule.

Phase 6: Movement Module

Max Kegel Yoga

Having completed Phase 5, you should have good control of your bandhas, having learned how to practice with both mula bandha and uddiyana bandha engaged. This shifts you into a new league in the pelvic floor control category, go you!

Objective

The objective of the movement module in Phase 6 is to increase the pelvic floor strength (or relaxation) during the yoga practice. We will incorporate some bands into the practice and will perform max-strength Kegels in some challenging positions. If you are focused on pelvic floor relaxation, I want you to practice maximum relaxation in place of contraction.

Success Metric

Success with this module is achieved when you can perform max-strength Kegels in yoga poses without compromising the balance of tension throughout your limbs.

Additional Notes

You should already have a good feeling for the capabilities of your current body. Make sure to progress to more difficult asanas only when your body gives you the go-ahead. If you are struggling with a pose, regress to a more basic version to hold the pose while performing a max-strength Kegel. You can skip inversions if you feel you don't have the strength or balance.

I personally found my inversion practice provided some relief from prolapse sensations, and inevitably challenged my balance of abdominopelvic tension in a new way. Be persistent and you will reap the benefits of this practice.

Remember, if you are working on the reverse Kegels activity in place of pelvic floor strength training, you will perform this sequence without performing max strength Kegels. Instead, focus on maximum pelvic floor relaxation on each inhalation. You should pay close attention to your body and skip any poses that trigger your symptoms. By training your body for movement with relaxation in the pelvic floor, you enhance your potential for living an active life without excess pelvic floor hypertonicity.

Max Kegel Yoga

You will need a yoga mat, small and large bands, some blocks, and optionally an eye pillow and blanket. The practice should take thirty minutes including setup and final relaxation. You can download the sequence sheet for this max Kegel yoga sequence (Figure 9.6.4) from empoweryourflower.com and place it at the front of your mat when practicing.

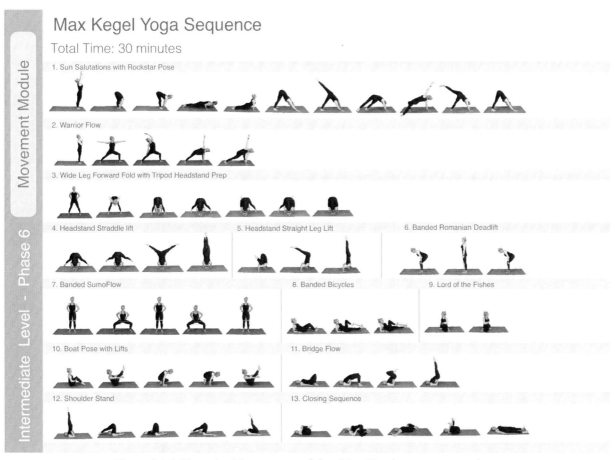

Figure 9.6.4: Phase 6—Movement module—Max Kegel yoga sequence sheet.

You can read the instructions and steps beforehand and follow the poses on the printed copy of Figure 9.6.4 when you are practicing. This will help you to learn the sequence and eventually you will be able to practice it without looking at the sheet. Repeated practice creates change in the body.

Steps to Perform the Max Kegel Yoga Sequence

1 Sun Salutations with Rockstar Pose

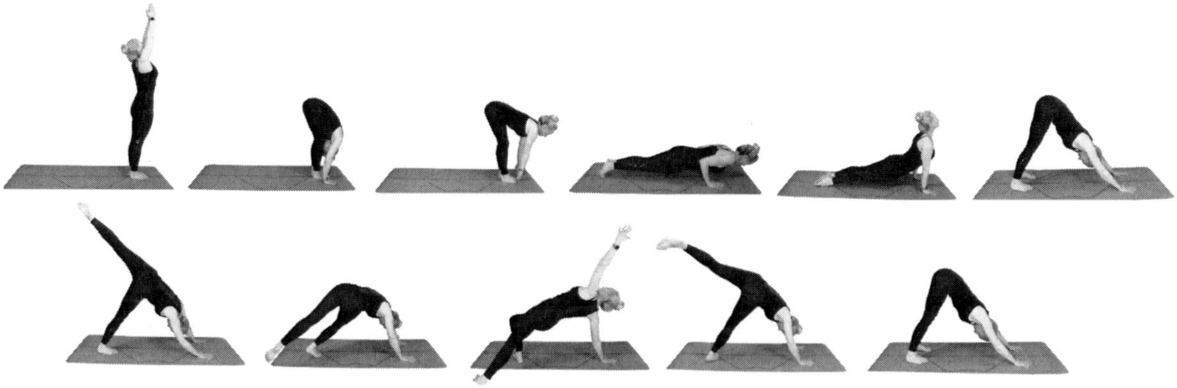

Figure 9.6.4.1: Phase 6—Max Kegel yoga—Sun salutation with rock star pose.

1. Stand in tadasana pose with hands in front of your heart, engaging your bandhas with an RPE-4 pelvic floor contraction.
2. Flow through a sun salutation coming to a downward-facing dog for three breath cycles.
3. Inhale your left leg high, preparing to come to rock star pose.
4. Open your left hip, bringing your foot all the way behind you to place it on the floor, then release your left hand from the mat and opening your heart up toward the ceiling. *Note*: If you have shoulder issues, skip rockstar and perform your max strength Kegels in three-legged dog.
5. Perform two breath cycles in rock star pose while performing your max strength Kegel during each exhalation.
6. Inhale as you bring your left hand back to the mat and release your left foot.
7. Exhale, taking a max strength Kegel as you bring the leg back up for a three-legged dog before lowering your left leg for the downward-facing dog.
8. Take a couple of breaths in downward-facing dog.
9. On your next exhalation, look forward between your hands, stepping or jumping forward (landing softly).
10. Inhale to lengthen your spine.
11. Exhale, folding forward.
12. Inhale, pressing into the midfoot, knees softly bent as you come back up, reach the arms overhead, and gaze toward the thumbs.
13. Exhale, bringing your hands back to your heart for tadasana.
14. Repeat steps 2 to 12, taking the rock star pose on the right side.

2 Warrior Flow

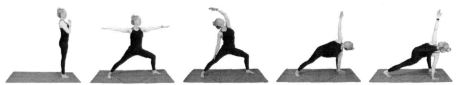

Figure 9.6.4.2: Phase 6—Max Kegel yoga—Warrior flow.

1. Inhale, taking a big step back with your right leg coming to Warrior 2.
2. Perform three breath cycles here, performing a max strength Kegel on each exhalation.
3. Inhale, releasing your right hand onto your right leg, and reaching your left hand overhead for reverse warrior.
4. Perform three breath cycles here, performing a max strength Kegel on each exhalation.
5. Release your left hand down to the floor outside your left foot while reaching your right arm overhead toward the ceiling.
6. Perform three breath cycles here, performing a max strength Kegel on each exhalation.
7. Place your right hand on the mat, releasing your right heel from the floor going for a twist while reaching your left arm straight up overhead. *Note*: Use blocks to raise the floor if needed.
8. Perform three breath cycles here, performing a max strength Kegel on each exhalation.
9. Drop your left hand and come back up to your warrior 2 before stepping forward to tadasana.
10. Repeat Steps 1–9 on the opposite side.

3 Wide-Leg Fold to Tripod Prep

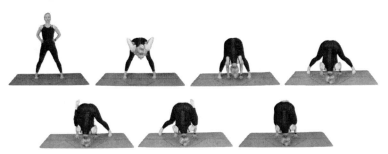

Figure 9.6.4.3: Phase 6—Max Kegel yoga—Wide-leg fold to tripod prep.

1. Turn to face the long end of your mat with legs apart and hands on hips.
2. Inhale to lengthen your spine and exhale to fold over, placing your hands on the floor in line with your toes, for a wide leg forward fold as a tripod headstand preparation.

3. Exhale, folding forward from the waist. If your hamstring flexibility prevents your head from reaching the mat, you can widen your stance slightly, but not so much as to overstretch your adductors.

4. Take a few breaths in forward fold before inhaling to come back up.

5. Repeat steps 2 and 3 to come back into the forward fold. This is an inversion practice that you should skip if advised by your healthcare provider. If you are not practicing headstand, you will perform three rounds of forward fold. Otherwise, move to step 6.

6. Place your head on the floor, bending your elbows and placing your hands as far away from your head as there is space between your hands. *Note*: For the headstand, the very top of your head rests on the floor. If you place your forehead on the floor, this can cause injury. If you place the back of your head, this can also cause injury. The correct spot is directly in the center of your head above your ears. **Your tripod needs to be an equilateral triangle in order to provide sufficient support. If you place your hands too close to your head, your base of support will be too small. Your elbows should be bent and should be parallel with your shoulders.**

7. Inhale, releasing your right foot from the floor, bending your knee, and resting it on the back of your right elbow. Exhale, lowering the leg back down. Inhale, releasing your left leg from the floor, bending your knee, and resting it on the back of your left elbow. If you feel balanced, you can try the tripod headstand prep position by releasing your right leg resting the knee on your elbow, and bringing your toes to touch. This pose is shown both from a front view in figure 9.6.4.3.

8. Perform three breath cycles in this position before coming back up.

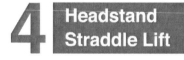
Headstand Straddle Lift

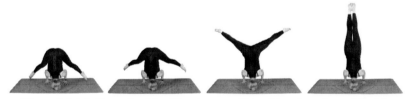

Figure 9.6.4.4: Phase 6—Max Kegel yoga—Tripod headstand straddle lift.

1. If you felt comfortable balancing in the tripod headstand prep position, you can try lifting both legs from the straddle position, bringing your legs together as you raise them up. *Note:* Never jump into a headstand or use momentum. The strength you are building in your core and pelvic floor, combined with the balance and flexibility you are gaining through the eight-phase training will bring you into an effortless and controlled headstand when your body is ready.

2. Stay in the tripod headstand for five breath cycles.

3. Lower down the same way you came in and come back to tadasana.

5 Headstand Straight Leg Lift

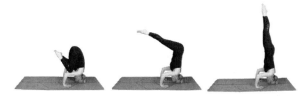

Figure 9.6.4.5: Phase 6—Max Kegel yoga—Tripod headstand straight leg lift.

1. If you felt comfortable lifting to the tripod headstand from the straddle position, you can try lifting with straight legs, either from the floor or from balancing your knees on your elbows.
2. Stay in the tripod headstand for five breath cycles.
3. Lower the legs straight down to the floor and take childs pose before coming back to tadasana.

6 Banded Romanian Deadlift

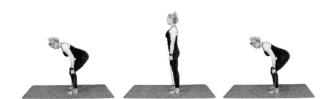

Figure 9.6.4.6: Phase 6—Max Kegel yoga—Banded Romanian deadlift.

You will need a long resistance band for this exercise, which is similar to a Romanian deadlift. For this exercise, we will brace the core and pelvic floor, holding the brace while coming up and back down. This is an important addition to your practice if you plan on lifting weights at any point.

1. Starting with the band under your feet, have your knees bent, and hips shifted back while having a long neutral spine.
2. Brace your core and pelvic floor and perform one rep of this exericse. To do this:
   a. Exhale, initiating a max strength Kegel while also engaging your core (close the space between your ribcage and your hips but without taking the curve out of your low back).
   b. Inhale and hold your breath. You should feel that you are using the tension in your pelvic floor and core to hold and support the increased intra-abdominal pressure that comes from holding your breath. You should be familiar with this control of intra-abdominal pressure as you have learned to deploy it in the breath strengthening exercise in Phase 2 (when blowing the balloon). You can imagine that your abdominopelvic cavity becomes a solid canister with the muscular tension solidifying and balancing the tension supporting this space. This creates good low back

support should you try to lift a heavy weight.

    c. With the breath held, press through the mid-foot while contracting your glutes to press your hips forward to bring you to standing, maintaining the balance of pressure in the abdominopelvic cavity keeping the breath held.

    d. When you are fully standing (breath still held), squeeze your glutes as hard as possible before sending your hips back to lower yourself back down, keeping a neutral spine and lowering back down and exhaling at the bottom of that movement relaxing core and pelvic floor.

3. Perform the next repetition by bracing once more at the end of your exhalation.

4. Repeat until you have performed ten repetiations. *Note*: there is no resting breath between repetitions. Bands don't require breath holding but this teaches bracing for lifting heavy weights.

7 | Banded Sumo Flow

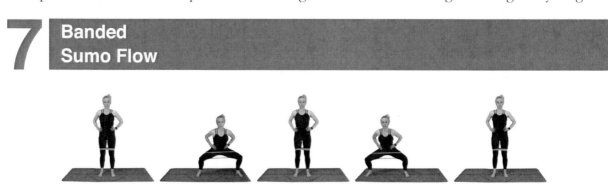

Figure 9.6.4.7: Phase 6—Max Kegel yoga—Banded sumo flow.

You will need a short resistance band for this exercise, which works your abductors. Step into the resistance band, bringing it to rest just above your knees, feet hip-distance apart, and hands on your waist. *Note*: You do not need to perform max strength Kegels in this flow, just keep bandhas engaged.

1. Take a big step to the left as you exhale to a wide squat.

2. Inhale and step the left foot back to its starting position beneath your hip.

3. Take a big step to the right as you exhale to a wide squat.

4. Inhale, stepping the right foot back to its original starting position.

5. Repeat Steps 1–4 four more times.

8 | Banded Bicycles

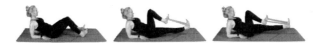

Figure 9.6.4.8: Phase 6—Max Kegel yoga—Banded bicycles.

1. Bring yourself to laying on the mat, placing the small band around your feet, flexing your feet, and

resting back on your elbows keeping your knees bent.

2. Begin to bicycle the legs by bringing the right knee up toward the chest with the left leg extended, before extending the right leg forward and bringing the left knee toward your chest.

3. Repeat this bicycling motion ten times for each leg with bandhas engaged.

9   Lord of the Fishes Pose

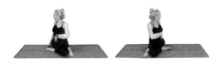

Figure 9.6.4.9: Phase 6—Max Kegel yoga—Lord of the fishes pose.

1. Bend your left leg, placing your heel on the floor alongside your right hip as you cross the right leg over the left, placing your foot standing on the floor beside your left knee.

2. Inhale, bringing your right hand behind you, crossing your left arm over your leg, and taking a twisting pose. Make sure to keep both sitting bones planted as you take this twist, inhaling to lengthen, lifting the rib cage away from the hips, exhale to twist, gazing behind you.

3. Hold the twist for three breath cycles.

4. Repeat Steps 1–3 on the opposite side.

10   Boat Pose with Lifts

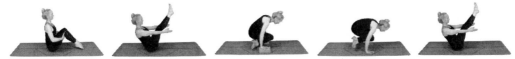

Figure 9.6.4.10: Phase 6—Max Kegel yoga—Boat pose with lifts.

1. Preparing for *navasana* (boat pose), place your hands behind your knees, point your toes and walk your toes back toward you until you find your pivot point.

2. Straighten your legs and release your hands stretching them forward while maintaining your bandhas.

3. Hold boat pose for three breath cycles.

4. Inhale for a lift up (*lolasana pose*), bending your knees, crossing your feet in front of you, placing your hands on the floor (or on blocks) alongside your hips, and lifting yourself up. Try to touch your knees to your nipples as you do this. It can take a long time to build the strength needed, consistent practice will be required.

5. Exhale, placing your hips back on the floor, returning to boat pose. This is one set

6. Repeat Steps 2 to 5 twice more for three sets in total.

11 Bridge Flow

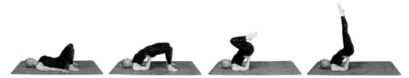

Figure 9.6.4.11: Phase 6—Max Kegel yoga—Bridge flow.

1. Prepare for the shoulder-supported bridge, bringing your feet in line with your hips, touching your middle finger off your heel. Perform one shoulder support bridge before progressing to step 2.

2. Inhale, pressing into your feet, lifting your hips high, and then exhale.

3. Bend your elbows and place your hands in your low back, fingertips pointing toward your face.

4. Inhale, releasing your right foot, bend your knee and then the left foot, bring both knees above your hip, and exhale.

5. Inhale, extending both legs together, pointing your toes toward the ceiling.

6. Hold for three breath cycles.

7. Lower one leg at a time to come back to your supported bridge before lowering your hips back to the mat.

12 Shoulder Stand

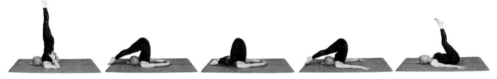

Figure 9.6.4.12: Phase 6—Max Kegel yoga—Shoulder stand.

1. Hug your knees toward your chest, performing a relaxing breath cycle as you rock a little from side to side.

2. Lie flat, preparing for a shoulder stand, coming first to halasana pose.

3. Hold shoulder stand for ten breath cycles.

4. Exhale, lowering to halasana, interlocking the fingers, and pressing straight arms into the floor, take an inhalation here.

5. Exhale, bend your knees, and squeeze your ears with your knees.

6. Perform three breath cycles here before releasing the hands, pressing the palms into the ground, straightening the legs, and slowly rolling the spine down, finishing lying flat on your mat.

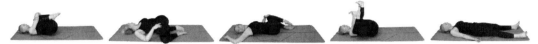

13 Closing Sequence

Figure 9.6.4.13: Phase 6—Max Kegel yoga—Closing sequence.

1. Hug your knees in toward your chest, then shift your hips a little to the left, dropping your knees to the right side for a spinal twist.
2. Perform three breath cycles in this twisting position before taking the twist on the opposite side.
3. Come to happy husband pose for three breath cycles.
4. Take your final rest (savasana) for five minutes.

Prior phases offered inversions in the form of downward-facing dog variations and shoulder stand. This practice, as well as adding resistance and bracing with a deadlift style pull, introduces the first full inversion with the tripod headstand. Make sure to start slowly if you are choosing to practice headstands.

That completes the movement module. You will perform the exercises from this module on the days specified in your weekly schedule.

Phase 6: Relaxation Module

Yin Yoga Pelvic Floor

Having completed Phase 5, you should be feeling more openness and less tension, both physically and mentally. If you have been suffering from pelvic pain, you should, hopefully, also be seeing a drop in pain levels. What a lovely gift to yourself!

Objective
The purpose of the relaxation module in Phase 6 is to reach through the hips to increase the relaxation of the pelvic floor. All previous relaxation modules also offer some pelvic floor relaxation, but from my perspective, the poses in this sequence provide the most direct release. Having worked to release

tension in the earlier modules, your body should now be ready for this practice and it should help to optimize pelvic floor length-tension.

Success Metric

As with Phase 5, success with yin yoga is achieved when you can relax into the positions. When we reach the pelvic floor through the hips, there can sometimes be an emotional release. This is a deep letting go and I always feel great following this type of release. It may come as a flood of tears or even a burst of laughter. It is not certain that you will have an emotional release but it is good to be aware so you don't get a shock should it happen to you.

Additional Notes

As with the other yin practices, you should ensure you avoid moving to a place of pain. Listen to your body and practice with compassion. You can download the sequence sheet for this yin yoga pelvic floor sequence (Figure 9.6.5) from empoweryourflower.com and place it at the front of your mat when practicing.

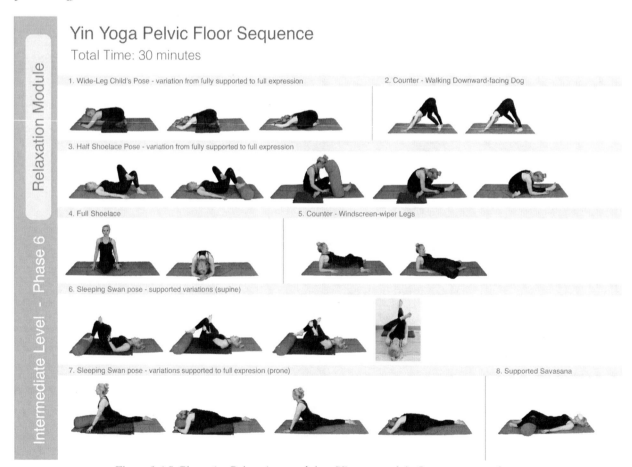

Figure 9.6.5: Phase 6—Relaxation module—Yin yoga pelvic floor sequence sheet.

You can read the instructions and steps beforehand and follow the poses on the printed copy of Figure 9.6.5 when you are practicing. This will help you to learn the sequence and eventually you will be able to practice it without looking at the sheet.

Yin Yoga Pelvic Floor Sequence Instructions

You will need one or two bolsters (or pillows), two blankets, two blocks, an eye pillow, and a yoga mat. This practice will take thirty minutes, including setup and transitions between poses.

Steps to perform the yin yoga pelvic floor sequence

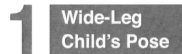 **Wide-Leg Child's Pose**

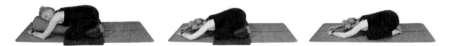

Figure 9.6.5.1: Phase 6—Yin yoga pelvic floor—Wide-leg child's pose.

The *wide-leg child's pose* is a gentle hip opener, which prepares your body for the subsequent asanas. There are multiple supported versions of this pose shown from the most supported to the full expression. To assume the pose:

1. Start kneeling with your legs together, then maintaining the toes touching, bring your knees almost mat width apart. You can place a blanket under your knees and between your bum and heels if needed. A blanket under the knees is also good, particularly if you have knee issues.
2. Relax forward, resting your forehead on the floor. You can rest on a bolster if needed.
3. Relax in your version of this pose for five minutes, allowing your hips to open as time passes.
4. Very slowly, mindfully bring energy into your hands and slowly press your hands to bring yourself up, coming to the all-fours position.

2 Counter— Walking Downward-Facing Dog

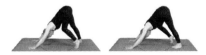

Figure 9.6.5.2: Phase 6—Yin yoga pelvic floor—Counter walking dog.

1. From all-fours, press up into a gentle yin, walking dog for one minute. You can move your hips around in this yin dog, taking whatever movement your body is craving after.

3 | Half Shoelace

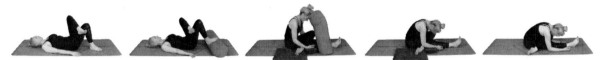

Figure 9.6.5.3: Phase 6—Yin yoga pelvic floor—Half shoelace.

Half shoelace pose is a deep yin hip opener. There are multiple supported versions of this pose, either a lying prone or seated shoelace. You should choose a version to practice based on your flexibility.

1. **Supine**: From the hook-lying position, externally rotate the left hip so the space above your left ankle rests on your right thigh. You should feel the tension across your left buttock and on the back of your left thigh. If you don't feel any tension, try elevating your right foot on a bolster.

2. **Seated**: Start sitting with both legs extended, bending the left knee and sealing the knee before rotating at the hip and placing the left foot alongside the right hip. You can place a blanket under the right knee if hamstring flexibility creates too much tension. Release the upper body into a forward fold. You can rest your head on a bolster if folding over creates too much tension.

3. Remain in your version for three minutes then repeat on the opposite side.

4 | Full Shoelace

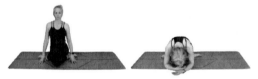

Figure 9.6.5.4: Phase 6—Yin yoga pelvic floor—Full shoelace.

If you find half-shoelace easy, you can opt to perform a full shoelace pose. To perform the full shoelace:

1. Externally rotate at the right hip, placing the right foot alongside the left hip.

2. Externally rotate at the left hip, bringing the left leg over the right, placing the left foot on the floor alongside the right hip. The left knee should be resting above the right knee.

3. Release your body forward allowing your arms to relax onto the floor in front of you, palms facing up toward the ceiling.

4. Relax in your version of this pose for three minutes.

5. Very slowly, mindfully bring energy into your hands and slowly press your hands to bring yourself back up.

6. Repeat your version of the pose on the opposite side.

5 Counter— Windscreen Wiper Legs

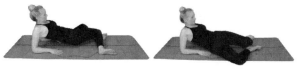

Figure 9.6.5.5: Phase 6—Yin yoga pelvic floor—Counter windscreen wiper legs.

1. Counter the shoelace with windscreen wiper legs, allowing the knees to drop over from right to left for one minute

6 Sleeping Swan Pose Supported Supine

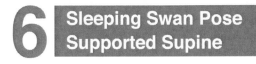

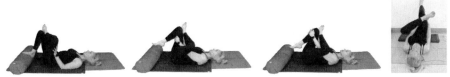

Figure 9.6.5.6: Phase 6—Yin yoga pelvic floor—Sleeping swan supported supine.

The *sleeping swan pose* is the yin version of a pigeon pose. There are multiple supported versions with the gentlest lying on your back (*supine*) and the full expression laying on your front. If you have limited hip flexibility, you should practice supine. To assume the pose:

1. Start in a hook-lying position with your feet on a bolster.
2. Externally rotate at the left hip, placing the space above your ankle on the right thigh above your knee. You should feel the stretch in your buttocks and back of your left thigh.
3. Deepen the stretch by grabbing behind the right thigh.
4. Deepen more by grabbing in front of the right knee. Deepen further by elevating your right foot from the bolster and onto a wall. You will relax in your version for three minutes on each side.

7 Sleeping Swan Pose Prone

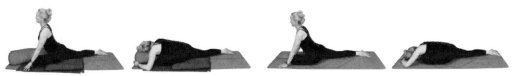

Figure 9.6.5.7: Phase 6—Yin yoga pelvic floor—Sleeping swan prone.

If you have reasonable flexibility in your hips, you should perform the prone version either using bolster/blankets for support or in the full expression without props. To assume the position:

1. Come to an all-fours position with a bolster lain in front of your body and a folded blanket close to hand.
2. Inhale, bringing the left knee forward, rotating at the hip, and allowing the left foot to rest in front of the right hip. Use a blanket under your left hip if needed.
3. Allow your body to rest forward, surrendering either onto a bolster or the floor.
4. Relax in your version of this pose for three minutes on each side, making sure to keep shoulders and hips very relaxed throughout.
5. Very slowly, press into your hands, coming out of the pose in the same way as you came in.

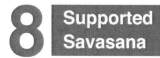

Supported Savasana

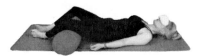

Figure 9.6.5.8: Phase 6—Yin yoga pelvic floor—Supported savasana.

1. Come to a supported savasana as your final rest for five minutes.

These poses utilize the ring of support surrounding the pelvic floor (which we viewed in Figure 2.14) by tapping into the piriformis and obturator internus muscles. This triggers a lengthening and release of the pelvic floor muscles. This practice can be helpful if you are suffering from pelvic pain or conditions that are triggered by hypertonicity.

That concludes the relaxation module. You will perform the exercises from this module on the days specified in your weekly schedule.

Phase 6: Mind & Meditation Module

Self Affirmations

Having completed the Phase 5 mind & meditation module, you should be noticing an improvement in your memory and further reductions in your stress levels, this is phenomenal!

Objective

The objective of the Mind & Meditation module in Phase 6 is to provide an opportunity for you to work on the relationship you have with yourself through self-affirmations. This is an exercise where you validate and affirm the positive aspects of your personality. It involves seeing the good in yourself and reminding yourself of your positive attributes.

Success Metric

Success is achieved when you see an increase in your self-esteem, which is a crucial step on your journey of empowerment.

Additional Notes

Self-affirmations were popularized in the 1980s by a psychologist named Claude Steele as a method to increase self-esteem. It is an exercise where you identify and confirm your positive attributes to yourself. Most people have done some form of affirmation therapy during their lifetime. This is an important tool for people who are overly critical of themselves.

In order to truly empower yourself, you must nurture the relationship you have with yourself and self-affirmations are a very useful tool for this purpose. Examples of self-affirmations are:

I am kind

I am beautiful

I am considerate

I am lovable

I am brave

Self-affirmations

For this exercise, you will need a notepad, a pen, and a mirror. The exercise should be performed twice per week, although you can perform it more often if you find it beneficial.

Steps to Perform This Exercise

1. Find a quiet space where you can sit to write.
2. Perform five calming breath cycles before you begin.
3. Think about the positive aspects of your personality and write ten affirming statements that begin with "I am."
4. Read these statements to yourself while looking in the mirror finishing with, "I love you XXXX" where XXXX is your name.
5. Repeat the process of reading the statements to yourself ten times. As you speak the words, feel

the warmth of their meaning in your heart and believe fully in the words that you speak. You can record your words to listen to at times when your self-esteem feels low.

6. To finish, thank yourself and carry those affirmations in your heart for the day, taking the opportunity to listen to recordings of your affirmations if you feel the need.

If you struggle to believe the lovely affirmations that you have written/recorded, you should think about examples of why they are true and remind yourself of those when you practice. This practice of self-affirmation can help to enhance the positive thought trains that you have created through your ANT therapy.

That completes the Mind & Meditation module. You will perform the self-affirmation exercise from this module on the days specified in your weekly schedule.

At the end of each week, if you feel that you may be ready to progress to the next phase of training, you can perform the phase checkpoint review using Figure 9.6.6, which checks your progress against the success metric for each exercise and helps you to decide if you should proceed to Phase 7 (Advanced level).

You can download a blank version of this form from empoweryourflower.com. As this is also the end of the intermediate difficulty level, you will be prompted in the phase checkpoint review to retake your initial assessments to verify your progress toward your intermediate level goal.

Phase 6 Checkpoint Review

Phase Start Date:_____

Checkpoint Date:_____

Pelvic Floor Module

Success

Strength: Success is achieved when you have the ability to perform a controlled squeeze of a finger inserted in the vagina giving a score of 8 on the strength scale which is equivalent of a good contraction with a strong lift. You should be able to sustain a strong contraction for the count of 10 with the co-contractions happening naturally.

Yes ☐

No ☐

Relaxation: Success is achieved when you can relax your pelvic floor fully in all the positions specified and no longer feel the symptoms of hypertonicity. Note: Reverse Kegels can help to release pelvic tension, however, you will continue to practice the reverse Kegels module through the entire program and so if you do not achieve success with the pelvic floor relaxation at this phase, this should not prevent you from proceeding to the next phase.

Yes ☐

No ☐

Breathing Module - Intermediate Hypopressives

Success

Success is achieved when you can comfortably perform the hypopressive routine achieving a stomach vacuum in all positions.

Yes ☐

No ☐

Movement Module - Max Kegel Yoga

Success

Success with this module is achieved when you can perform max strength Kegels in yoga poses without compromising the balance of tension throughout your limbs.

Yes ☐

No ☐

Relaxation Module - Yin Yoga Pelvic Floor

Success

As with phase 5, success with Yin yoga is achieved when you can relax into the positions. When we reach the pelvic floor through the hips, there can sometimes be an emotional release. This is a deep letting go and I always feel great following this type of release. You should be feeling that your pelvic floor is less tense.

Yes ☐

No ☐

Mind & Meditation Module - Self Affirmations

Success

Success is achieved when you see an increase in your self-esteem which is a crucial step on your journey of empowerment.

Yes ☐

No ☐

Phase 6 Checkpoint Review

Success

Have you achieved the success objectives and do you feel that you are ready to proceed to the next phase of training?

Yes ☐

No ☐

If no, please continue with the phase 6 training until you are ready to proceed, or regress to the phase 5 training if this felt too difficult.

If yes, this is also the end of the advanced difficulty level. You should retake your assessments to measure your progress against your earlier results.

Progress Milestone Review - Intermediate Level

Success

Have you already achieved your Intermediate level goal?

If no, you have the option to repeat the phase 6 of the intermediate level training.

Yes ☐

No ☐

If yes, proceed to the advanced level starting with Phase 7. Good Luck!

Figure 9.6.6: Phase 6—Checkpoint review form.

Phase 7
Advanced Level

Welcome to Phase 7 of the eight-phase training program. You have now progressed to the Advanced Level, which has two phases, 7 and 8. The following section details Phase 7 training modules, which are highlighted in Figure 9.7.1.

Eight-Phase Modules	Prep	Beginner			Intermediate		Advanced	
	Phase 1	Phase 2	Phase 3	Phase 4	Phase 5	Phase 6	Phase 7	Phase 8
Pelvic Floor	Kegel Breakdown	Full Kegel	Endurance Kegel	Speed Kegel	Co-Contract	Maximize Strength	**Standing Rotations**	Functional Training
Breathing	Nasal Breathing	Breath Strengthening	Breath Remapping	Nadi Shodhana	Basic Hypopressive Exercise	Intermediate Hypopressive Sequence	**Advanced Hypopressive Sequence**	Kapalabhati Breathing
Movement	Yoga Preparation	Yoga Basics	Core Re-tensioning	Rebalancing Yoga	Bandha Strength Yoga	Max Kegel Yoga	**Ball Routine**	Dynamic Power Yoga
Relaxation	Restorative Yoga	Yin Yoga Forward Folds	Yin Yoga Backward Bending	Yin Yoga Twists & Lateral Movement	Yin Yoga Hip Opening	Yin Yoga Pelvic Floor	**Yin Yoga Happy Hips**	Yin Yoga All Body
Mind & Meditation	Yoga Nidra	Flex your mind to flex your muscles	ANT Therapy	Conquer your fear	Kirtan Kriya	Self Affirmations	**Journaling**	Blossoming Goddess

Figure 9.7.1: Phase 7—Advanced level.

The exercises and activities for the Phase 7 modules, highlighted in red in Figure 9.7.1, are designed to increase the intensity of your practice to enable you to have pelvic floor control in all planes of movement. The intermediate phase should have prepared your body for this physically demanding phase that will challenge your pelvic floor.

Remember, if your goal is pelvic floor relaxation, you will work on the reverse Kegels activity for all phases of training. It is detailed in Phase 1 pelvic floor module.

The frequency of practice can change as you progress through the training so make sure to read through all modules for Phase 7 and update your schedule accordingly before you begin with the exercises.

Phase 7
Modules

Pelvic Floor

Standing Rotations

Breathing
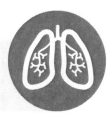

Advanced Hypopressive Sequence

Movement

Ball Routine

Relaxation
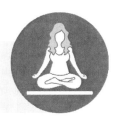

Yin Yoga Happy Hips

Mind & Meditation

Journaling

Phase 7: Pelvic Floor Module

Standing Rotations

Having completed Phase 6, you should have achieved excellent pelvic floor strength. This is a major achievement for anyone suffering from PFD. I suggest you play your favorite music and dance around the room in celebration!

Objective

In Phase 7, you will add directional strength to your pelvic floor by incorporating twists into your performance of maximum strength Kegels. You will continue to practice every second day while alternating your position as shown in Figure 9.7.2.

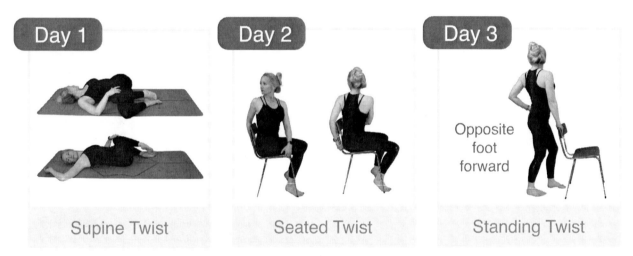

Figure 9.7.2: Phase 7—Pelvic floor exercise positions.

Day 1: *Supine Twist*—Lying down, knees bent with legs rotated to right for one round and then to the left for the second round as shown in Figure 9.7.2.

Day 2: *Seated Twist*—Sitting with torso rotated to right for the first round and then the left for the second round.

Day 3: *Standing Twist*—Standing with feet hip-distance apart, your left foot should be slightly forward with your right foot toes in line with your left foot heel. Rotate your torso to the right. You will do a second round where you take the same pose on the opposite side.

The rest days in between practice days will give your pelvic floor time to recover as these sessions use maximum effort.

Success Metric

Success is achieved when you can manage a controlled squeeze of a finger inserted in the vagina with a score of eight when rotating the body to either side. You should be able to sustain this strong contraction for a count of ten with the co-contractions happening naturally.

Additional Notes

Twisting may reveal a directional weakness in what is otherwise a strong pelvic floor. You shouldn't worry, as consistent steady practice will help you to improve directional strength.

If you have been practicing the reverse Kegel exercises detailed in Phase 1, you should replace the positions for that exercise with the positions listed above. Learning to relax your pelvic floor in twisted positions should help to ensure your pelvic floor can maintain its optimized length-tension relationship regardless of your position. You can continue practice relaxation six days per week.

Steps to Perform the Pelvic Floor Exercises

1. Get yourself into a comfortable starting position.
2. Begin inhaling for a count of 4.
3. On your next exhalation, initiate a pelvic floor contraction with an RPE-4 and maintain that contraction (like gently holding the marble in your fist).
   a. Inhale here.
   b. Exhale and perform a maximum strength contraction with an RPE-10.
   c. Inhale releasing the contraction back to an RPE-4.
   d. Exhale performing another maximum strength contraction with RPE-10.
   e. Inhale releasing the contraction to an RPE-4 .
4. Continue the cycle until you have performed a full ten contract/release cycles moving from RPE-4 to RPE-10 .

This practice can seem difficult in comparison to performing the Kegels in the earlier phases. Maintain consistency and you should find they become easy before long.

This concludes the pelvic floor module and is the last pelvic floor training module that requires static contractions. In the next and final module of the pelvic floor training, you will perform dynamic Kegels as part of other exercises. You should already be feeling empowered, and the advanced level training should solidify that feeling. You will perform the exercises from this module on the days specified in your weekly schedule.

Phase 7: Breathing Module

Advanced Hypopressive Sequence

Having completed Phase 6, you are now well-practiced at hypopressive vacuums in many positions. This puts you ahead of Arnold Schwarzenegger in the stomach vacuum masters league. Sorry, Arnie!

Objective

In Phase 7 of the breathing module, you will incorporate unilateral movements and pelvic floor contractions into your hypopressive practice. This will stimulate some new lines of tension to enhance your core stability.

Success Metric

Success is achieved when you can achieve a good stomach vacuum with a strong pelvic floor contraction during a unilateral movement.

Additional Notes

Unilateral movements will create an unequal balance of tension between the left and right sides of the pelvic floor. This presents an increased challenge when training muscles involved in core stability, including the diaphragm, pelvic floor, abdominals, psoas, and muscles of your back, thus improving your ability to handle physical stressors in a balanced way which can reduce symptoms such as urine leakage.

We will add maximum strength Kegels during the apnea in this sequence. You may notice that your apnea is not as deep due to the co-contraction of the abs when you peform a maximum strength contraction. Don't worry, you will still make progress.

If you have been working with the reverse Kegels module, focus instead on relaxing your pelvic floor.

You can download the sequence sheet for this advanced hypopressive sequence (Figure 9.7.3) from empoweryourflower.com and place it at the front of your mat when practicing. You can read the instructions and steps beforehand and follow the poses on the printed copy of Figure 9.7.3 when you are practicing. This will help you to learn the sequence and eventually you will be able to practice it without looking at the sheet.

Advanced Hypopressive Sequence

Total Time: 15 minutes

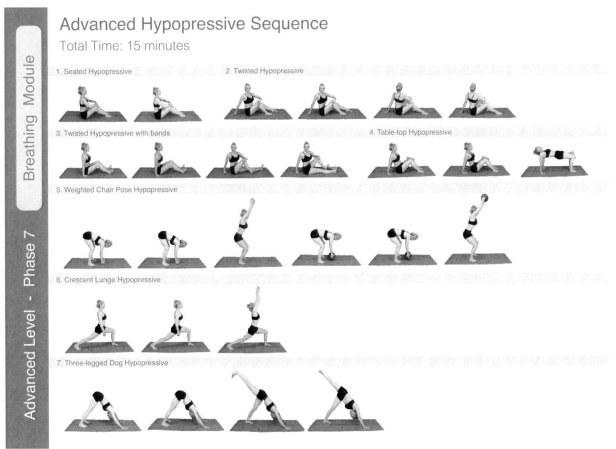

1. Seated Hypopressive

2. Twisted Hypopressive

3. Twisted Hypopressive with bands

4. Table-top Hypopressive

5. Weighted Chair Pose Hypopressive

6. Crescent Lunge Hypopressive

7. Three-legged Dog Hypopressive

Figure 9.7.3: Phase 7—Breathing module—Advanced hypopressive sequence sheet.

Advanced Hypopressives

You will need a yoga mat, a block, and a short resistance band to perform this advanced hypopressive routine. You also have the option to add a weighted medicine ball. You will practice this short sequence every second day, and it should take no more than fifteen minutes to complete.

Steps to Perform the Advanced Hypopressive Sequence

1 Seated Hypopressive

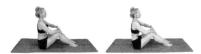

Figure 9.7.3.1: Phase 7—Advanced hypopressives—seated hypopressive.

1. Sit tall with your spine elongated, knees bent, feet hip-distance apart, hands resting on knees, and elbows pointing out to the sides.

2. Close your mouth keeping your lips together with your teeth slightly apart, tongue resting on the roof of your mouth behind your front teeth.

3. Perform three rounds of full breaths using the power of your diaphragm while keeping your shoulders relaxed.

4. Initiate a max strength Kegel as you exhale all the air out of your lungs, then hold your breath out. Expand your rib cage as though breathing into your empty lungs.

5. Relax your rib cage, let your belly hang, and release your Kegel before beggining your next inhalation.

6. Repeat the hypopressive in this position twice more.

2 Twisted Hypopressive

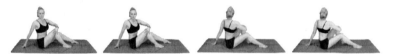

Figure 9.7.3.2: Phase 7—Advanced hypopressives—Twisted hypopressive.

1. Reach your left foot forward a little, your right foot back a little, twisting your body to the right side, placing your right hand behind your back and your left hand on your right knee.

2. Take a full breath cycle before initiating a max strength Kegel as you exhale all the air out and hold the breath out to take your vacuum, expanding your ribcage as though you could breathe into your empty lungs. Hold both your max strength kegel and your apnea.

3. Allow your ribcage to relax, your belly to hang, and release your Kegel before your next inhalation.

4. Turn back to the center and repeat a hypopressive on the opposite side. This is one set.

5. Repeat steps 1 to 4 twice more to perform three sets total.

3 Twisted Hypopressive with Bands

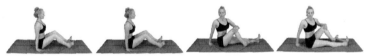

Figure 9.7.3.3: Phase 7—Advanced hypopressives—Twisted hypopressive with bands.

1. Place a small resistance band around your feet, flexing them while your heels remain on the mat. Sit tall with your hands on the floor beside your hips taking three full breath cycles.

2. Initiate a max strength Kegel as you exhale all the air out and hold the breath out to take your vacuum, expanding your ribcage as though you could breathe into your empty lungs.

3. With your apnea held, step the right foot back, the left foot forward and twist, placing your left

hand on your right knee for support.

4. Maintain the apnea and step the left foot back and the right foot forward, supporting the left knee with your left hand.

5. Bring both legs back to the start position, facing your body forward, and relase your apnea, relaxing your tummy, releasing your Kegel, and allowing an inhalation. Reset by taking a full breath cycle.

6. Repeat Steps 2 to 5 while twisting to the opposite side for one full set and perform three sets total.

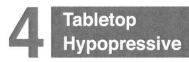

Tabletop Hypopressive

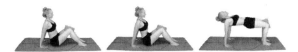

Figure 9.7.3.4: Phase 7—Advanced hypopressives—Tabletop.

1. Place a block between your knees, feet hip-distance apart, knees bent and hands slightly behind you with fingertips facing forward, preparing for a tabletop position. Take three breath cycles here.

2. Initiate a max strength Kegel as you exhale all the air out and hold the breath out to take your vacuum, expanding your ribcage as though you could breathe into your empty lungs.

3. With your apnea held, press into your midfoot as you lift your hips up to be in line with your knees and shoulders maintaining the apnea for a count of four.

4. Lower your hips to the floor, relax your tummy, release your Kegel, and inhale. This is one set.

5. Take three breath cycles and repeat steps 2 to 4 for a second round of this exercise.

Weighted Chair Pose

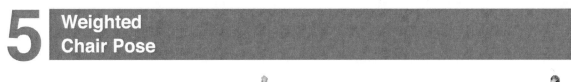

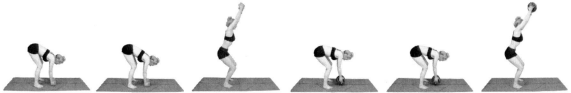

Figure 9.7.3.5: Phase 7—Advanced hypopressives—Weighted chair pose.

1. Stand with feet hip-distance apart, knees bent, flexed at the hip holding a block with straight arms.

2. Take three breath cycles and initiate a max strength Kegel as you exhale all the air out and hold the breath out to take your vacuum.

3. With your apnea held, press into your midfoot come to chair pose (*utkatasana*), holding the block overhead while maintaining the apnea for a count of four.

4. Lower back down to the starting position before relaxing your tummy, releasing your Kegel, and

allowing an inhalation. This is one set. Perform three sets total. *Note*: If you find this easy with the block, you can replace the block with a weighted medicine ball as demonstrated.

6 Crescent Lunge

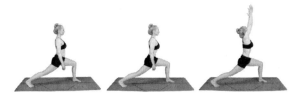

Figure 9.7.3.6: Phase 7—Advanced hypopressives—Crescent lunge.

1. Come to a lunge position with the left leg forward and the right heel off the floor, arms resting by your side. Take three breath cycles here.
2. Initiate a max strength Kegel as you exhale all the air out and hold the breath out to take your apnea, expanding your ribcage as though you could breathe into your empty lungs.
3. With your apnea held, reach your hands up overhead coming to *anjaneyasana* (crescent lunge), shifting your gaze to your thumbs while maintaining the apnea.
4. Lower your hands before relaxing your tummy, releasing your Kegel, and allowing an inhalation.
5. Step forward and repeat steps 1 to 4 on the opposite side.

7 Three-Legged Dog

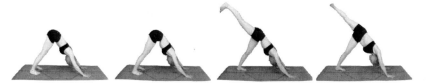

Figure 9.7.3.7: Phase 7—Advanced hypopressives—Three-legged dog.

1. Come to a downward-facing dog. Take a few breath cycles here.
2. Initiate a max strength Kegel as you exhale all the air out and hold the breath out to create your vacuum; expand your ribcage as though you could breathe into your empty lungs.
3. With your apnea held, extend your right leg with foot flexed, while keeping your hips parallel.
4. Maintaining the apnea, open your right hip.
5. Still holding the apnea, bring the hip back to level again.
6. Lower your leg back to the mat, relax your tummy, release your Kegel, and allow an inhalation.
7. Repeat the hypopressive on the opposite side to complete one set.
8. Perform two sets total to finish your hypopressive routine. Savasana is optional.

This concludes the breathing module. You will perform the exercises from this module on the days specified in your weekly schedule. This advanced hypopressive routine may feel challenging at first. The combination of the max strength Kegels (if that is part of your practice) and the apnea, adds increased demand on your tissues. Practice makes perfect so stick with it and you will reap the rewards.

Phase 7: Movement Module

Ball Routine

Having completed Phase 6, your pelvic floor should be feeling really strong. Are you pleased with your progress? You should be!

Objective

The objective of the movement module in Phase 7 is to challenge the pelvic floor and core by adding an element of instability by using a stability ball. This compliments the pelvic floor training for this phase, where the emphasis is on contracting in unilateral twisted positions.

In addition to this ball routine, you can also take a normal yoga class, aerobics, Zumba, or some other fitness class that is interesting for you. Regardless of what you choose to add from a training perspective, you must use a *pelvic floor first* approach and ensure that you are not pushing your body beyond your limitations. Remember that you always have the option of practicing sessions from earlier modules or regressing your training if you feel your body needs that on any given day. Listen to your body and let it be your guide.

Success Metric

Success with this module is achieved when you feel comfortable working through this sequence while maintaining balanced intra-abdominal pressure.

Additional Notes

When we add the ball, we add instability. This requires heightened awareness when you practice as you can injure yourself if you come off the ball due to a lack of balance. Be careful and continue to listen to your body, being mindful of your limits.

You will need a yoga mat and a stability ball. Your feet should be able to rest flat on the floor while you sit on the ball as shown in Figure 9.7.4.

Figure 9.7.4 shows how you should be able to sit on a ball with your feet resting flat on the floor. You should ensure that the ball has sufficient firmness to support you.

Ball Routine Instructions

If you have never practiced on a stability ball before, you can use a wall for support as you learn to balance. You will need a wall for some of the positions so make sure to set up beside one. The practice should take fifteen minutes including setup and final relaxation.

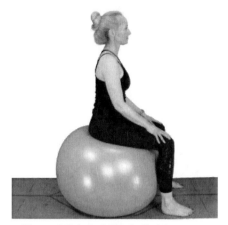

Figure 9.7.4: Stability ball sizing.

You can download the ball routine sequence sheet (Figure 9.7.5) from <u>empoweryourflower.com</u> and place it at the front of your mat when practicing.

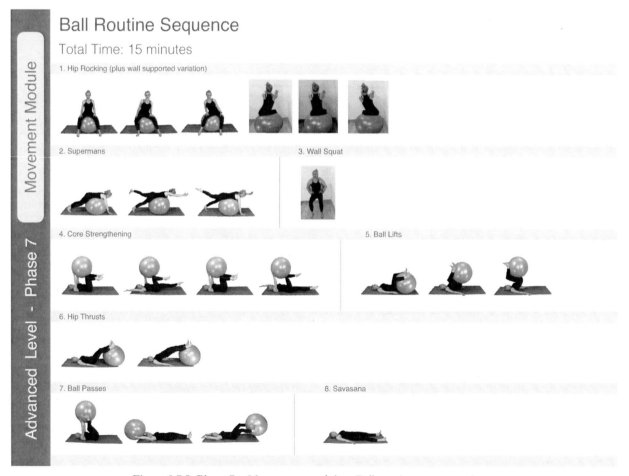

Figure 9.7.5: Phase 7—Movement module—Ball routine sequence sheet.

You can read the instructions and steps beforehand and follow the poses on the printed copy of Figure

9.7.5 when you are practicing. This will help you to learn the sequence and eventually you will be able to practice it without looking at the sheet. Repeated practice creates change in the body.

Steps to Perform the Ball Routine

1 Hip Rocking

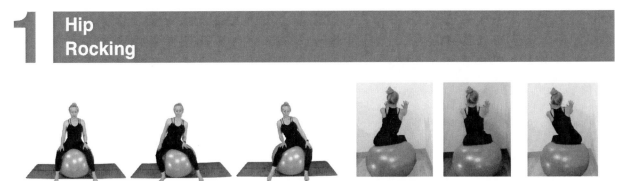

Figure 9.7.5.1: Phase 7—Movement module—Ball routine—Hip rocking.

1. Begin by sitting on the ball in the middle of your mat with your hands resting on your knees. *Note*: You have the option of resting your hands on a wall as you perform this movement (as shown in Figure 9.7.5.1). This can be a useful support if you have never practiced on a stability ball before. Eventually, you should be able to do this without the support of a wall.

2. Shift your hips from left to right on the ball for one minute, maintaining your balance as you do so. The movement is coming mostly from your hips with your chest and shoulders staying reasonably level throughout. Think of this as a practice of moving into the tissues on the sides of your hips. You can make circles and exagerate the movement as you practice. Enjoy it!

2 Supermans

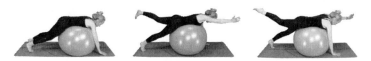

Figure 9.7.5.2: Phase 7—Movement module—Ball routine—Supermans.

1. Rest your stomach on your ball in a supported plank position with both your hands and feet touching the ground. If your hands and feet can't reach the floor in this position, you should use a smaller ball or let a little air out (but not so much that it loses integrity)

2. Inhale as you release your right hand and your left leg from the floor, balancing through the core to stabilize.

3. Perform three breath cycles in this position before returning the supported plank.

4. Repeat steps 2 and 3 on the opposite side for one set. Perform two sets total.

3 | Wall Squat

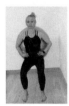

Figure 9.7.5.3: Phase 7—Movement module—Ball routine—Wall squat.

1. Come to the wall, standing, place the ball behind your back, and rest against the ball.
2. Move your feet out in front of you to a sufficient distance so that your ankles will be stacked above your knees when sitting into an imaginary chair.
3. Exhale as you squat down into your imaginary chair with your knees bent to 90 degrees, thighs parallel with the mat. Stay in this wall squat for five breath cycles.
4. Repeat the wall squat once more.

4 | Core Strengthening

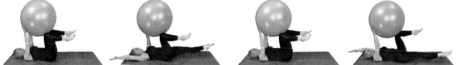

Figure 9.7.5.4: Phase 7—Movement module—Ball routine—Core strengthening.

1. Come to a hook-lying position, hold the ball between your hands and your knees; inhale using your legs to lift the ball so your shins are now parallel with the floor and the ball is held in place between your hands and knees.
2. Engage your core here, pressing the low back into the floor strongly. You will maintain that strong core engagement throughout this exercise.
3. Exhale, lowering your right arm straight on the floor behind you while you reach your left leg out pointing your toe sending energy from fingertips to toes. If you feel your low back lifting at any point, this indicates that your core is not strong enough to maintain stability. Only lower the arm/leg to a point where you can maintain a strong core. It will improve with practice.
4. Inhale, returning to the neutral position while keeping your low back pressed into the floor with a strong pelvic floor.
5. Exhale taking the position on the opposite side. This completes one set.
6. Repeat Steps 3 to 5 until you have performed ten sets in total.

5 | Ball Lifts

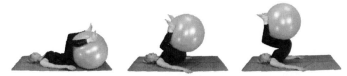

Figure 9.7.5.5: Phase 7—Movement module—Ball routine—Ball lifts.

1. Place the ball beneath your legs with your knees bent, and grip the ball with your legs; exhale here, preparing to do ball raises.
2. Inhale as you curl your spine up off the mat, raising the ball and keeping your hands outstretched with palms pressing into the floor. This should be a slow controlled movement, using a strong contraction of the core muscles to create the lift.
3. Exhale as you roll your spine back down again but keeping the ball off the floor. Your shoulders should remain in contact with the ground throughout. This is one set.
4. Repeat Steps 2 and 3 until you have performed ten sets in total.

6 | Hip Thrusts

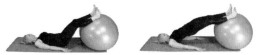

Figure 9.7.5.6: Phase 7—Movement module—Ball routine—Hip thrusts.

1. Roll the ball away from you slightly so just your calves and heels are resting on it. Your legs are hip-distance apart. Your arms should still be by your side, palms pressing into the floor.
2. Inhale as you press into your heels, extending your hips into the air to bring them in line with the rest of your body. Your bodyweight should balance evenly between your shoulders/arms and your heels, with your glutes powering the movement.
3. Hold this extended position for five breath cycles before lowering down. This is one set.
4. Roll the ball towards your backside, hugging your knees into your chest for a rest between sets.
5. Perform three sets total.
6. Take a short happy baby following your third set to release your low back.

7 Ball Passes

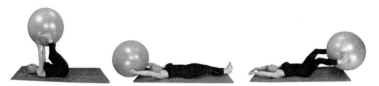

Figure 9.7.5.7: Phase 7—Movement module—Ball routine—Ball passes.

1. Lie flat on your back, with your legs and arms extending, holding the ball between your feet.
2. Press your low back into the floor to engage your core (you will maintain this activation throughout this exercise).
3. Lower the ball to the floor with the hands, keeping your arms straight while at the same time, lowering your legs until they are close to the floor. You should stop when the ball is almost on the floor.
4. Bring the ball back up while at the same time, bringing your legs up to meet the ball.
5. Grip the ball with your feet and lower it toward the floor as you reach your arms overhead. *Note*: You should keep your low back firmly connected with the floor throughout. If you find your low back is lifting, this is an indication that your core is not yet strong enough to support this movement. Practice taking the ball as low as possible without losing the connection between your low back and the floor. Over time this will improve.
6. Bring the ball back up reaching to grab it with your hands. This completes one set.
7. Repeat Steps 3 to 6 until you have performed ten sets in total.
8. Rest your feet on the ball and catch your breath before moving into your final rest.

8 Savasana

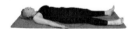

Figure 9.7.5.8: Phase 7—Movement module—Ball routine—Savasana.

1. Release the ball and take your final rest (savasana) for five minutes.

This ball practice should solidify your core stabilization, which will help immensely when you undertake the final module in the advanced level of this training. That completes the movement module. You will perform the exercises from this module on the days specified in your weekly schedule.

Phase 7: Relaxation Module

Yin Yoga Happy Hips

Having completed Phase 6, you should be reaping the rewards of a regular yin practice. You should be very proud of your dedication and determination.

Objective

The objective of the relaxation module is to continue the process of rebalancing the tissues around the hips. This should contribute to a deeper relaxation of your pelvic floor. Listen to your body as it tells you which poses it craves.

Success Metric

As with Phase 6, success with yin yoga is achieved when you can relax into the positions. Your body may be sufficiently open that you no longer find an edge in these poses. If so, just enjoy the deep relaxation as your reward for consistent practice.

Additional Notes

As with the other yin practices, listen to your body and respond with grace and love.

Yin Yoga Happy Hips

You will need one or two bolsters (or pillows), two blankets, two blocks, an eye pillow, and a yoga mat. You will also need a wall with sufficient space for your legs to straddle. This practice will take thirty minutes, including setup and transitions between poses.

You can download the sequence sheet for this yin yoga happy hips sequence (Figure 9.7.6) from empoweryourflower.com, and place it at the front of your mat when practicing.

You can read the instructions and steps beforehand, and follow the poses on the printed copy of Figure 9.7.6 when you are practicing. This will help you to learn the sequence and eventually you will be able to practice it without looking at the sheet.

Yin Yoga Happy Hips Sequence

Total Time: 30 minutes

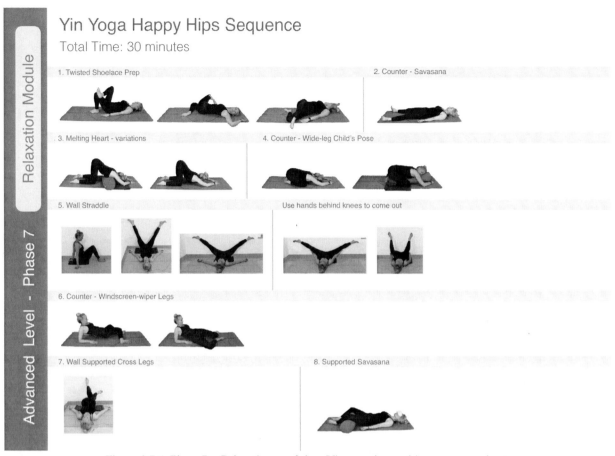

Figure 9.7.6: Phase 7—Relaxation module—Yin yoga happy hips sequence sheet.

Steps to Perform the Yin Yoga Happy Hips Sequence

1 Twisted Shoelace Prep

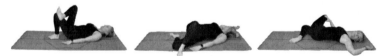

Figure 9.7.6.1: Phase 7—Happy hips—Twisted shoelace prep.

Twisted shoelace prep is a twisted version of one of the gentler versions of the supported shoelace pose. To assume the pose:

1. Lie on your back, releasing your right leg, rotate at the hip, and place the space just above your right ankle onto your left thigh above your knee.

2. While maintaining the connection between your right ankle and left leg, lower your right foot so it rests on the floor with your left leg resting sideways on the floor. Your shoulders should remain level on the floor throughout this twist. You can use a bolster or block to raise the floor under your

legs if you find they cannot reach the floor without losing the connection between your shoulders and the mat. You can also use your hand for support as shown in the right image of Figure 9.7.6.1.

3. Stay in this position for three minutes.
4. Repeat the pose on the opposite side.

2 Counter Pose— Savasana

Figure 9.7.6.2: Phase 7—Happy hips—Counter pose—Savasana.

1. Counter with a one-minute wide-leg savasana.

3 Melting Heart

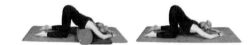

Figure 9.7.6.3: Phase 7—Happy hips—Melting heart.

You have already learned *melting heart pose* in the relaxation module of Phase 3 where the focus was on backward-bending. You can choose to do either the supported version or full expression of the pose but shift your focus from the backbend to releasing tension around your hips.

1. Start from an all-fours position, keeping the hips directly above the knees and allow your chest to lower down. Use a bolster under your chest if you feel this more in your chest than your hips.
2. Allow your belly to hang, relax your shoulders and try to surrender any effort in this position. Stay in the pose for five minutes.
3. Move very slowly out of the position coming back to a wide child's pose

4 Counter Pose— Wide-Leg Child's Pose

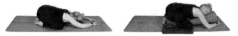

Figure 9.7.6.4: Phase 7—Happy hips—Counter pose—Wide-leg child's pose.

1. Remain in wide-legged child's pose for one minute.

5 Wall Straddle

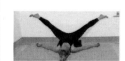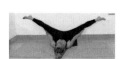

Figure 9.7.6.5: Phase 7—Happy hips—Wall straddle.

Wall straddle is a yin pose that allows you to focus on releasing the adductors without unnecessary tension in the hamstrings. To assume the pose:

1. Come to the wall and place a folded blanket right against it. Sit with your right hip touching the wall and rotate, swinging your legs up against the wall as you lay your upper body down, shuffling closer to the wall if needed. Allow your backside and legs to be tight against the wall.

2. Relax into the widest straddle available to your body, remaining in this position for five minutes.

3. Use your hands behind your knees to support your legs when slowly and mindfully releasing from the pose, bending your knees and hugging them toward your chest.

6 Counter Pose— Windscreen Wiper Legs

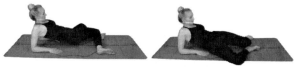

Figure 9.7.6.6: Phase 7—Happy hips—Counter pose—Windscreen wiper legs.

1. Counter with windscreen wiper legs for one minute.

7 Wall-Supported Cross Legs

Figure 9.7.6.7: Phase 7—Happy hips—Wall-supported cross legs.

The *wall-supported cross legs* is a yin pose that allows you to compress some of the tissues surrounding the hips without the weight of your body bearing down. To assume this position:

1. Come close to the wall as you did for the wall straddle, then cross the left leg over the right as you

would if you were sitting in a chair.

2. Bend the right knee as much as is comfortable, allowing the right foot to remain resting against the wall. You can place a blanket between your stomach and your left knee for extra support if needed.

3. Release your hands on either side of your body, palms facing up, and relax into this position for three minutes.

4. Repeat the position on the opposite side.

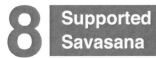
Supported Savasana

Figure 9.7.6.8: Phase 7—Happy hips—Supported savasana.

1. Finish in a supported savasana as your final rest where you let go completely.

At this stage in the program, you should be finding that your hip mobility and stability have improved. These hip-opening poses may still present some tension, but it is also possible that you are finding more relaxation. Enjoy whatever is showing up in your yin practice and, as always, stay away from pain.

This completes the relaxation module. You will perform the exercises from this module on the days specified in your weekly schedule.

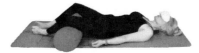

Phase 7: Mind & Meditation Module

Journaling

Having completed the Phase 6 mind & meditation module, you should be feeling more confident in yourself. That's a great result.

Objective

The objective of the mind & meditation module in Phase 7 is to build on the earlier written exercises (ANT therapy and self-affirmations). Journaling presents an opportunity to verbalize problems and concerns that may be affecting your mood. By writing your thoughts and feelings, you can see things from a new perspective. This practice can be helpful when managing stress and anxiety.

Success Metric

Success is achieved when you find yourself feeling that you have more control over your thoughts and moods and that you are learning to accept all parts of yourself.

Additional Notes

When writing a journal, you should write your truth. If you are worried about writing what you honestly think for fear someone may read your deepest thoughts, you can burn or shred what you have written at the end of the exercise.

It is especially important that you can be really honest with yourself as journaling is more effective if you don't have to hold back. You may find that journaling helps you to open a small valve in your brain to let out some steam, releasing the pressure and allowing stress levels to drop.

We each have the potential to feel a great many emotions. Work on practicing acceptance and changing negative patterns where you can.

Journaling

For this exercise, you will need a notepad and pen. The exercise should be performed twice per week, although you can perform it more often if desired.

Steps to Perform This Journaling Exercise

1. Find a quiet space where you can sit to write.
2. Perform five calming breath cycles before you begin.
3. Begin to freely write how you truly feel. If nothing comes to mind, ask yourself a question, such as "What am I afraid of?" or "What would I like to do with my life?" and watch as you write the answer. If you are still struggling, write your story, or the story of a specific event in your life.
4. Write for as long as you feel you need to.
    a. If what you have written is negative, you can do "the work" on your statements.
    b. If what you have written is very self-critical, you should do the self-affirmations exercise when you have finished.
5. When you are finished writing, you can choose whether to read what you have written.
6. Put your journal away once you have finished, or you can burn/shred your writing if you are more comfortable with that.

Journaling can be very rewarding if you use it as a type of brain dump, especially if you are under a lot of stress. For me, journaling often brings me solutions to problems I have been tossing around in my head. I hope that it is helpful for you.

That completes the mind & meditation module of phase 7. You will practice this journaling exercise on the days specified in your weekly schedule.

At the end of each week, if you feel that you may be ready to progress to the next phase of training, you can perform the phase checkpoint review using Figure 9.7.7, which checks your progress against the success metric for each exercise and helps you to decide if you should proceed to Phase 8 (advanced level), which is the final phase of the eight-phase training. You can download a blank version of this form from empoweryourflower.com.

Phase 7 Checkpoint Review

Phase Start Date:_____

Checkpoint Date:_____

Pelvic Floor Module	Success

Strength: Success is achieved when you can achieve a controlled squeeze of a finger inserted in the vagina with a score of 8 when rotating the body to either side. You should be able to sustain this strong contraction for the count of 10 with the co-contractions happening naturally.

Yes ☐
No ☐

Relaxation: Success is achieved when you can relax your pelvic floor fully in all the positions specified and no longer feel the symptoms of hypertonicity. Note: Reverse Kegels can help to release pelvic tension, however, you will continue to practice the reverse Kegels module through the entire program and so if you do not achieve success with the pelvic floor relaxation at this phase, this should not prevent you from proceeding to the next phase.

Yes ☐
No ☐

Breathing Module - Advanced Hypopressive	Success

Success is achieved when you can achieve a good stomach vacuum with a strong pelvic floor contraction during a unilateral movement (with maximum strength Kegel if you are working on pelvic floor strength).

Yes ☐
No ☐

Movement Module - Ball Routine	Success

Success with this module is achieved when you feel comfortable working through this sequence while maintaining balanced intra-abdominal pressure.

Yes ☐
No ☐

Relaxation Module - Yin Yoga Happy Hips	Success

As with phase 6, success with Yin yoga is achieved when you can relax into the positions. Your body may be sufficiently open that you no-longer find an edge in these poses. If so, just enjoy the deep relaxation as your reward for consistent practice.

Yes ☐
No ☐

Mind & Meditation Module - Journaling	Success

Success is achieved when you find yourself feeling that you have more control over your thoughts and moods and that you are learning to accept all parts of yourself.

Yes ☐
No ☐

Phase 7 Checkpoint Review	Success

Have you achieved the success objectives and do you feel that you are ready to proceed to the next phase of training?

Yes ☐
No ☐

If no, please continue with the Phase 7 training until you are ready to proceed, or regress to the Phase 6 training if you felt that you are not ready for Phase 7.

If yes, please proceed to Phase 8 which is the final phase of the Eight-phase training. Your empowerment is within reach!!!

Figure 9.7.7.: Phase 7—Checkpoint review form.

Phase 8
Advanced Level

Welcome to Phase 8 of the eight-phase training, you have reached the final phase in this training program! At this stage, you should be seeing the benefits of your journey to empowerment. The following section details the Phase 8 training modules that are highlighted in Figure 9.8.1.

Eight-Phase Modules	Prep	Beginner			Intermediate		Advanced	
	Phase 1	Phase 2	Phase 3	Phase 4	Phase 5	Phase 6	Phase 7	Phase 8
Pelvic Floor	Kegel Breakdown	Full Kegel	Endurance Kegel	Speed Kegel	Co-Contract	Maximize Strength	Standing Rotations	**Functional Training**
Breathing	Nasal Breathing	Breath Strengthening	Breath Remapping	Nadi Shodhana	Basic Hypopressive Exercise	Intermediate Hypopressive Sequence	Advanced Hypopressive Sequence	**Kapalabhati Breathing**
Movement	Yoga Preparation	Yoga Basics	Core Re-tensioning	Rebalancing Yoga	Bandha Strength Yoga	Max Kegel Yoga	Ball Routine	**Dynamic Power Yoga**
Relaxation	Restorative Yoga	Yin Yoga Forward Folds	Yin Yoga Backward Bending	Yin Yoga Twists & Lateral Movement	Yin Yoga Hip Opening	Yin Yoga Pelvic Floor	Yin Yoga Happy Hips	**Yin Yoga All Body**
Mind & Meditation	Yoga Nidra	Flex your mind to flex your muscles	ANT therapy	Conquer your fear	Kirtan Kriya	Self Affirmations	Journaling	**Blossoming Goddess**

Figure 9.1.1: Phase 1 training—Preparation level.

The exercises and activities for the Phase 8 modules, highlighted in red in Figure 9.8.1 are physically more demanding. At this phase of training, you are challenging your strength, balance, and coordination with dynamic and sometimes explosive movements, such as jumping. This phase of training is the final preparation for returning to a life of thoughtless, fearless movement where reflexes are managing the balance of tension and you can just get on with living your best life.

Phase 8
Modules

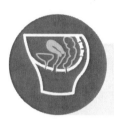
Pelvic Floor

Functional Training

Breathing
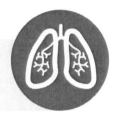

Kapalabhati Breathing

Movement

Dynamic Power Yoga

Relaxation
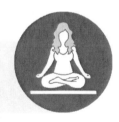

Yin Yoga All-Body

Mind & Meditation

Blossoming Goddess

Phase 8: Pelvic Floor Module

Functional Training

Having completed Phase 7, you are now at the final stage of your training. You deserve a medal, very well done on making it this far!

Objective

The objective of the pelvic floor training at Phase 8 is to practice pelvic floor contractions during dynamic functional movements including pulling, jumping, and lifting. These pelvic floor exercises are functional as they involve a physical movement or activity rather than a static position.

At this stage of the training, you should practice the functional Kegel activities three days per week choosing a different activity each day of practice. For example:

Day 1: Pulling.
Day 2: Jumping.
Day 3: Lifting.

Rather than repetitions of Kegel exercises, you will engage your bandhas during functional activities.

Success Metric

Success is achieved when you can perform these dynamic activities thoughtlessly and fearlessly without needing to use conscious effort to engage your bandhas. Pelvic floor control at this level should become automatic.

Additional Notes

With functional training, we will feel the patterns of tension throughout the body when we move. This training should promote good coordination of tensegrity through your body.

This is the module that takes the strength you have created and helps you to apply it intelligently to the different movements that form the pattern of your life. These may range from lifting heavy things, to jumping, running, reaching up for something, or pulling yourself up. We will train the pelvic floor to optimize the management of all stresses that come its way.

It is important that you continue to listen to the signals from your pelvic floor at this stage. If you decide to squat 100 kg at the gym and it makes you leak, you need to drop weight and work with good pelvic floor activation (your bandhas) until you have the strength to maintain urethral closure pressure during a 100 kg squat.

Your goals do not have to be so extreme. Maybe you just want to be able to run around kicking a ball with your kids without fear of leaking. This is also something you can achieve through this training.

You are free to do these exercises at a gym or to incorporate them in a fitness class. It is less important where you practice, but rather that you stress the tissues in these various directions.

Functional Exercise— Pull

For the pull exercises, you will need a pull-up bar or other stable bar that you can pull against. You will also need strong resistance bands as you will not be pulling your entire weight. Regular pull-ups are used to train your upper back; however, our focus is to train your pelvic floor to manage increased pressures during the pulling motion.

If the only pull training you have done to this point is the one or two banded pull exercises in the earlier phases, you should not start directly with pull-ups (unless you are already pull-up strong). Start instead from a bar that you can squat under. Bend your knees and take very little weight in your hands. Most of your weight can be in your legs but you still get to perform the pulling motion. You will need your pull-up bar and bands for this exercise.

Steps to Perform the Pull Exercises

1 Pull-Up Bar and Band

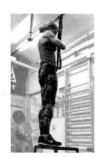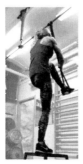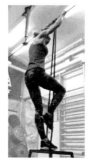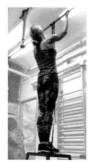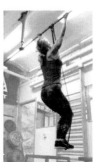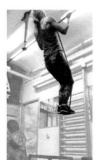

Figure 9.8.2.1: Functional exercise pull using pull-up bar and band.

1. Make sure your pull-up bar is stable and wrap your bands around the bar. You can loop two together if needed.
2. Initiate a pelvic floor contraction with an RPE-4.
3. Stretch the band down and step into it with one foot. You can then hold the bar with both hands and step your second foot in the band.
4. On your next exhalation, initiate a strong pelvic floor contraction (RPE-10) as you pull yourself up. You may need to bend your knees if you can reach the platform with your feet as shown in Figure 9.8.2.1 but bear in mind that bent knees will equal less resistance from your bands.
5. Inhale as you lower back down, softening the pelvic floor contraction to an RPE- 4.
6. Repeat ten times.

2 Cable Machine Pull

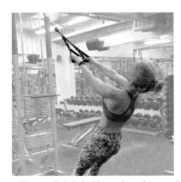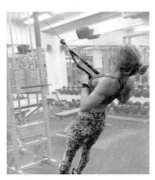

Figure 9.8.2.2: Functional exercise pull using a cable machine.

1. Alternatively use a cable machine, TRX bands, or a weighted pull-up machine that is close to your body weight. You can gradually work to full pull-ups. Technique is the same as for exercise 1.
2. Changing the angle of the pull, with the cable machine, as demonstrated in Figure 9.8.2.2, produces a different line of tension, which is also useful for this functional pelvic floor training. If you are a gym-goer, approach each pulling exercise from the perspective of your *pelvic floor first* and you will greatly enhance your pelvic floor strength.

Training your body to have a strong pelvic floor with a variety of pulling motions will help you to manage pulling actions in your everyday life, without urine leakage, or excessive downward pressure that can irritate POP.

Functional Exercise— Lift
For the lifting exercises, you will need some weights. These can be actual weights, such as kettlebells or

dumbbells, or full water bottles. If you choose to use bottles of water, make sure you weigh them and don't lift heavier than you can comfortably manage. You can swap the exercises detailed below for a structured gym session or fitness class that uses weights.

Steps to Perform Lifting Exercises

3 Light & Heavy Squat

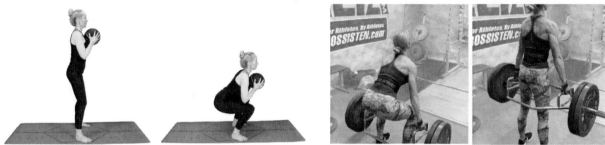

Figure 9.8.2.3: Functional exercise lift—Light & heavy squat.

1. Stand with feet a little wider than hip-distance apart, soft knees, and a long spine. Hold your weight close to your chest (like a goblet squat). You will use the brace technique detailed below (which you have already practiced in Figure 9.6.4.6.). *Note*: Bracing is important, particularly if you lift heavier weights. A waist belt (shown in the heavy version of Figure 9.8.2.3) can help with bracing as it allows you to feel the abdominopelvic canister when lifting heavy.
2. Initiate a max strength Kegel while also engaging your core.
3. Inhale and hold your breath in against the strong canister of your core and pelvic floor.
4. Squat down while maintaining the brace, weight shifting to the heels.
5. Press through the midfoot to come up again, exhaling as you release the brace once you are standing.
6. Repeat ten times. *Note*: The heavy squat shown would brace at the bottom, not from standing.

4 Revolving Split Squat

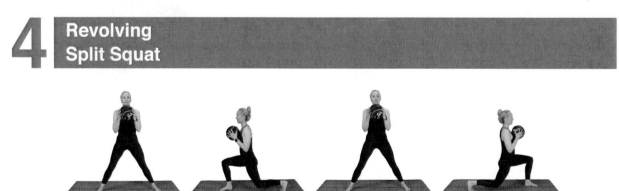

Figure 9.8.2.4: Functional exercise lift—Revolving split squat.

1. Stand sideways on your mat in a straddle position while holding your weight close to your chest as before, inhale.

2. Exhale as you pivot on your heels, turning to face the left side, and coming into a lunge while performing a max strength Kegel (RPE-10).

3. Inhale coming back up, releasing the Kegel and returning to the neutral position.

4. Exhale as you pivot on your heels turning to face the right side and coming into a lunge while performing a max strength Kegel (RPE-10).

5. Inhale coming back up, releasing the Kegel and returning to the neutral position. This completes one set.

6. Perform Steps 1 to 5 until you have performed ten sets in total.

5 Pelvic Floor First Biceps & Triceps

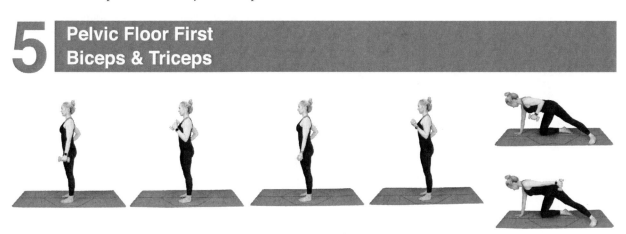

Figure 9.8.2.5: Functional exercise lift—Revolving split squat.

Although the pelvic floor is not directly connected to the arms, training biceps and triceps with a pelvic floor focus, trains the pelvic floor to manage intra-abdominal pressure during these movements..

1. Stand tall, holding your dumbbell in your right hand and placing your left hand on your waist. You will perform two different types of biceps curls, as shown in Figure 9.8.2.5, which involves rotating the forearm to change the angle of the dumbbell. Start with the hammer curl (short side of dumbbell faces forward). Engage your bandhas before you begin, creating an RPE-4 activation.

2. Inhale, keeping your elbow close to your body, and use the strength of your bicep to lift the dumbbell as you increase your pelvic floor contraction to RPE-10.

3. Exhale while lowering the dumbbell and releasing the pelvic floor back to the RPE-4 activation.

4. Perform ten hammer curls on each arm before rotating your forearm so the long side of the dumbbell faces forward in prep for standard bicep curls.

5. Perform 10 standard bicep curls on each arm using steps 2 and 3 for your pelvic floor.

6. Come to the all-fours position on your mat and extend your left foot behind you for support.

7. Pick up your dumbbell, bringing your elbow up so it is in line with your shoulder, parallel with the

mat as you activate an RPE-4 on your pelvic floor.

8. Inhale as you extend your elbow, raising the dumbbell behind you, bringing your arm parallel with the floor while at the same time activating an RPE-10 contraction of the pelvic floor.

9. Lower the dumbbell back to the starting position, making sure the elbow remains fixed in position, as you release back to RPE-4 on your pelvic floor.

10. Perform ten of these triceps extensions before repeating on the opposite side.

6 Light & Heavy Pullovers

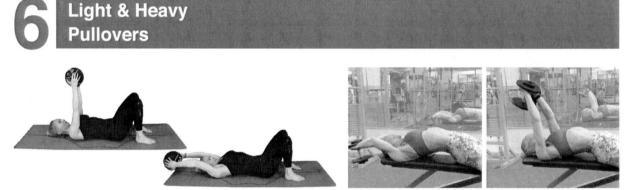

Figure 9.8.2.6: Functional exercise lift—Light & heavy pullovers.

Pullovers must be one of my favorite pelvic floor exercises of all time! That is right, I consider this back/shoulder strengthening exercise to be an amazing option for building integrated strength in the pelvic floor. We will practice a very regressed version of a dumbbell pullover using a medicine ball for this weighted exercise. When you perform this exercise with heavier weights at the gym, you should do so on a weight bench as demonstrated in Figure 9.8.2.6. Your feet should remain on the floor. Use the same pelvic floor contractions as explained in this exercise.

1. Start in a hook-lying position on your mat and raise your medicine ball or dumbbell straight out in front of your chest. Inhale as you activate your core and pelvic floor to RPE-4 without flattening your low back.

2. Exhale as you lower the weight behind you with straight arms as you perform an RPE-10 contraction. Allow the ball to touch the floor.

3. Inhale raising the ball back up as you release the RPE-10 back to RPE-4.

4. Repeat until you have performed this exercise ten times.

This is just a small sample of many potential lifting exercises that you can utilize to improve pelvic floor strength and control. This practice should translate to an improvement in the management of intra-abdominal pressure when you lift things.

When I began my bodybuilding journey, my first trainer told me that I should expect some leakage when lifting, which is the wrong advice to give to anyone with a pelvic floor, so I quickly changed trainers. I focused on my *pelvic floor first* in all lifting exercises, using the techniques explained in this module, and made it to my stage debut without a single leakage episode even though I pulled, pushed, and lifted a lot of weight. Make sure to practice *pelvic floor first* regardless of the type of exercise you are performing.

Functional Exercise— Jump

For the jump exercises, you will need your yoga mat. If you have access to a trampoline, you could use it as a progression when you have completed the program; however, before you start jumping on a trampoline, you should be aware that a study[79] into in female trampolinists found that 72.7% of participants experience urine leakage. There was a significant association between the volume of practice and the severity of continence.

Trampolines do have a place in pelvic floor training, and can be useful for training to return to running, which we will discuss more in Chapter Ten, but they should not be used excessively (unless you actually are a trampolinist).

Jumping substantially stresses the pelvic floor. Up to Phase 7, we have been training to maximize strength and coordination. In this final training, the addition of jumping introduces fast dynamic blasts of movement, which can prepare the body for that sudden potential burst of intra-abdominal activity that would traditionally have triggered stress incontinence. By training for these sudden bursts, we teach the nervous system to program reflexes for bottom-up control allowing us to return the things we love to do.

The exercises below can be swapped for an aerobics class, Zumba, some dancing, or even skipping. Any sport that adds dynamic bursts of energy. Just remember that your focus should remain *pelvic floor first* and activity second. For this exercise, you will be jumping from one end of your mat to the other.

Steps to Perform the Jump Exercises

These dynamic jumping movements may already be easy for you, having completed the first seven phases of the training. That's wonderful if they are. If not, practice consistently and you should see results.

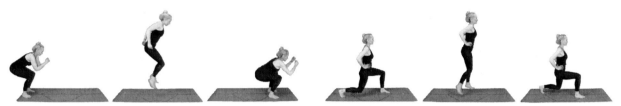

Figure 9.8.2.7: Functional exercise lift— Mat jumps (left) & split-squat jumps (right).

1. Stand at the back end of your mat and inhale, initiating a pelvic floor contraction (RPE-4).

2. Squat down, bringing your weight toward your heels, shift your arms forward, elbows bent.

3. Exhale as you press through your midfoot to jump as high as you can while swinging your arms behind you and creating a strong pelvic floor contraction (RPE-10) when you are in the air. Think of this mid-air pelvic floor contraction as pre-tensioning for landing.

4. As you land, allow your knees to bend and your hips to flex coming back to a squat to help absorb the ground reaction forces, while at the same time releasing your pelvic floor contraction back to RPE-4.

5. Turn to face the other end of your mat and repeat. You should perform ten jumps in total.

6. Take a split squat in the middle of your mat with your hands on your hips. Initiate a pelvic floor activation RPE-4 as you exhale.

7. Inhale as you jump up, contracting RPE-10 mid-air and landing in a split squat with the opposite leg forward while releasing your pelvic floor back to RPE-4. Perform ten jumps total.

It is important to initiate the max strength Kegel while "in the air" with these jumps as though you are pre-tensioning in preparation for landing. I found this strategy to be the most beneficial when training to overcome stress incontinence when jumping and in preparation to return to running.

That concludes the pelvic floor module. You will practice the exercises as defined in your weekly schedule.

Phase 8: Breathing Module

Kapalabhati Breathing

Having completed Phase 7, you should be noticing increased tone around your abdominals and maybe even a tighter waist, which is one of the benefits of regular hypopressive exercises, fantastic work!

Objective

The objective of the breathing module in Phase 8 is to further enhance lung capacity and elasticity. The kapalabhati yogic breathing technique utilizes the lower abdominals (uddiyana bandha) to explosively exhale while inhalation happens passively. This works the lower abdominals, which are typically harder to target with isolated exercises, while also training the diaphragm.

Success Metric

Success is achieved when you can relax your entire body while using your lower abdominals to power the exhale. When you master this breathing technique, you will feel energized following this practice.

Additional Notes

Like *nadi shodhana*, there are many perceived benefits touted in yoga for this breathing technique, which is a *kriya* (cleansing ritual). The scientific research into kapalabhati shows a clear benefit for those suffering from metabolic syndrome, with one study[80] suggesting that those benefits could also help women suffering from PCOS due to the similarities between the two syndromes.

We have waited until this late stage of the training to introduce this breathing technique as it is important that you have good pelvic floor strength before beginning this practice. It is also helpful to have reasonable lung capacity and flexibility of the diaphragm and rib cage before you begin this practice. The breathing exercises in the earlier phases should have achieved this.

Kapalabhati Breathing

For this exercise, you will need a yoga mat with a small towel, which you can place under your knees as you will perform the exercise in a kneeling position. You will practice this breathing exercise every second day and it is best practiced on an empty stomach, so I suggest you practice first thing in the morning before breakfast (if your schedule permits).

This is a practice that uses a forced expiration, which then triggers a powerful and automatic inspiration. You do not intentionally inhale but, rather, you allow your body to inhale for you. Imagine that your lungs are billows, and you are using your abdominals to force the air quickly out of the billows, which, in turn, causes them to refill.

This practice can leave you feeling a little breathless when you first try. Make sure to stop if you start to feel breathless or dizzy, and perform some calming breath cycles before trying again.

The practice includes a strong pelvic floor contraction. If you have been practicing reverse Kegels throughout all the phases due to pelvic floor hypertonicity, do not contract your pelvic floor as you perform this breathing technique.

Steps to Perform This Exercise

1. Find a comfortable kneeling position on your yoga mat placing a small towel under your knees for cushioning if required. Rest your hands on your lap.
2. Perform three relaxed breath cycles and then inhale deeply.
3. Exhale explosively through the nose by pulling your lower abdominals upwards and inwards toward your spine while at the same time performing a strong pelvic floor contraction.
4. Relax your abs and pelvic floor completely. Inhalation will happen automatically.
5. Immediately and explosively pull your lower abdominals in toward your belly button again while performing a strong pelvic floor contraction for a forceful exhalation and then relax your abs and pelvic floor completely.
6. Repeat this motion as though you are pulsing your lower abdominals and pelvic floor rhythmically. This is like the pulse you use for your speed Kegels—Contract, relax, contract, relax. The inhalation happens naturally when you relax. Continue to pulse your explosive exhalations for twenty breath cycles.
7. Finish by performing ten relaxing breath cycles where you inhale for four and exhale for eight with a relaxed pelvic floor.

This breathing exercise helps to increase core and pelvic floor strength, adding nicely to the layers of strength you have been building throughout the eight-phase program. That concludes the breathing module. You will practice the kapalabhati exercises on the days specified in your schedule.

Phase 8: Movement Module

Dynamic Power Yoga

Having completed Phase 7, you should be feeling empowered and may have already restarted some of the activities your PFD was preventing, I'm so proud of you!

Objective

The objective of the movement module is to increase the intensity of the yoga practice, adding strong core work, pistol squats, and the little ball of balance, which is a precursor to a full headstand.

This type of strong yoga helped me immensely with my own journey of empowerment. The challenging little ball of balance is shown in Figure 9.8.3.

The little ball of balance is harder than the tripod headstand from Phase 6. Inversions are fantastic if you are suffering from pelvic pain or POP, but you should always practice with guidance from your healthcare provider, and skip poses that are not recommended for your specific condition.

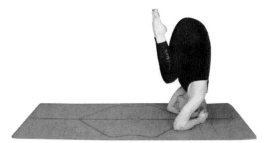

Figure 9.8.3: The little ball of balance.

Having completed the first seven phases of this program, your strength and flexibility should be sufficient to undertake this level of practice. Remember to listen to your body as always, you are your own best teacher after all.

Success Metric

Success with this module is achieved when you feel empowered to do the things that your pelvic floor dysfunction was previously preventing.

Additional Notes

Only practice inversions if approved to do so by your healthcare provider. Stay present as you practice, listening to your breath and practicing with inner equanimity.

Dynamic Power Yoga

You will need a yoga mat, some socks, and a surface that is slippery when you have socks on (such as a wooden floor). If you have limited floor space, you can roll up your mat so you have just a small portion of mat onto which you can place your hands (to prevent your hands from slipping). An eye pillow and blanket are optional for savasana at the end of practice.

The practice should take thirty minutes, including setup and final relaxation. You can download the sequence sheet for this dynamic power yoga sequence (Figure 9.8.4) from empoweryourflower.com and place it at the front of your mat when practicing.

You can read the instructions and steps beforehand and follow the poses on the printed copy of Figure 9.8.4 when you are practicing. This will help you to learn the sequence and eventually you will be able to practice it without looking at the sheet.

Dynamic Power Yoga Sequence

Total Time: 30 minutes

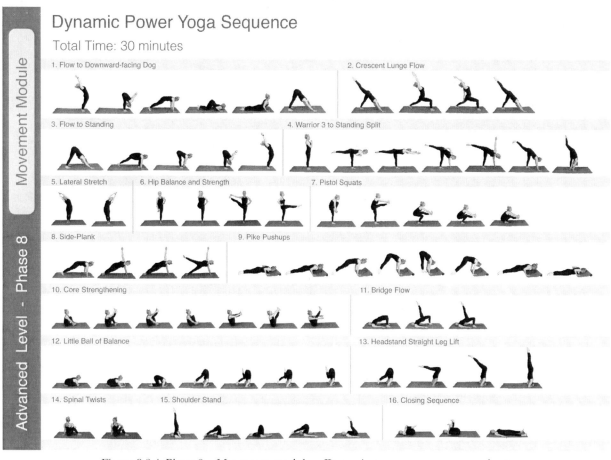

Figure 9.8.4: Phase 8—Movement module—Dynamic power yoga sequence sheet.

Steps to Perform the Dynamic Power Yoga Sequence

1 Flow to Downward-Facing Dog

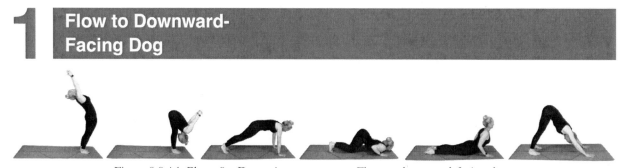

Figure 9.8.4.1: Phase 8—Dynamic power yoga—Flow to downward-facing dog.

1. Come to tadasana at the front of your mat with hands in prayer in front of your heart.

2. Inhale, raising the arms above your head and sending your hips forward, taking a small backbend.

3. Exhale, bending your knees as you fold forward, interlocking your hands, straightening your arms and legs as you finish your exhalation.

4. Inhale, lengthening your spine as you gaze forward.

5. Exhale, planting your hands and stepping back right leg, left leg coming to plank and in the same exhalation lowering your knees, chest, and chin to the floor.

6. Inhale for cobra pose, elbows tight to the body, using your back muscles to lift your chest.

7. Exhale coming to the downward-facing dog.

8. Perform three breath cycles in your downward-facing dog.

2 Crescent Lunge Flow

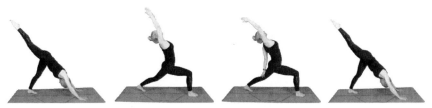

Figure 9.8.4.2: Phase 8—Dynamic power yoga—Crescent lunge flow.

1. Inhale, raising the right leg for the three-legged dog.

2. Stepping the right leg forward on the exhalation.

3. Inhale coming up to a lunge, reach your hands up and back as you take a backbend.

4. Perform three breath cycles here, inhaling to lift the rib cage away from hips, exhaling to reach a little further back.

5. On your third exhalation, drop your left hand onto your left leg, allowing you to go a little deeper into your backbend as you continue for three more breath cycles.

6. Exhale, windmill your hands back down to the mat, and inhale back to the three-legged dog.

7. Repeat Steps 1 to 6 on the opposite side finishing in a downward-facing dog.

3 Flow to Standing

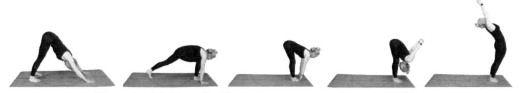

Figure 9.8.4.3: Phase 8—Dynamic power yoga—Flow to standing.

1. From downward-facing dog, exhale looking forward, stepping or floating forward landing softly.

2. Inhale as you lengthen your spine gazing forward.

3. Exhale, bending your knees, interlocking your hands behind your back, and straightening your knees and your arms as you bow forward finishing your exhalation.

4. Inhale, releasing your hands, bending your knees, and pushing through the midfoot to come back up, reaching the arms overhead for a backbend as you shift your hips forward.

5. Exhale, bringing your hands back in front of your heart, finding your tadasana.

4 | Warrior 3 to Standing Split

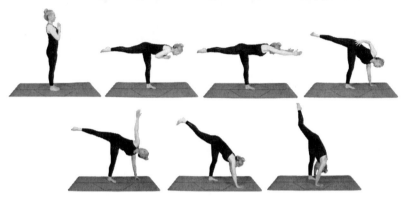

Figure 9.8.4.4: Phase 8—Dynamic power yoga—Warrior 3 to standing split.

1. Come to tadasana at the center of your mat, hands in prayer position in front of your heart.

2. Inhale, as you shift your weight onto your left leg, and exhale as you pivot in the left hip joint, allowing your body to come forward as you send your right leg backward so, it is now parallel with the back of your mat.

3. Release your hands, and extend your arms forward. Your body should be parallel with the floor, and hips level.

4. Perform three breath cycles here.

5. Exhale as you release your fingertips to the floor in preparation for a half-moon pose.

6. Inhale, opening your right hip so that the inside of your flexed right foot is parallel with the floor, extending your right hand up toward the ceiling and gazing toward your thumb.

7. Perform three breath cycles here.

8. Exhale, lowering your right hand back to the floor, walking your hands toward your feet as you reach your right leg up above your left leg for a standing split.

9. Perform three breath cycles here.

10. Exhale, pivoting in the left hip joint as you lower your right leg, simultaneously raising your upper body, and coming back to a tadasana pose.

11. Repeat Steps 2 to 10 on the left side.

5 | Lateral Stretch

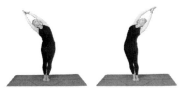

Figure 9.8.4.5: Phase 8—Dynamic dower yoga—Lateral stretch.

1. From tadasana, inhale with your arms above your head, press your palms together, and close the space around your ears with your upper arms as you lift your rib cage away from your hips.
2. Exhale shifting your hips toward the left, bringing your hands over toward the right side.
3. Perform three breath cycles here, returning to the center on your fourth inhalation.
4. Repeat Steps 2 and 3 on the opposite side.

6 | Hip Balance and Strength

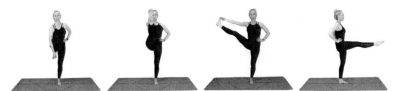

Figure 9.8.4.6: Phase 8—Dynamic power yoga—Hip balance and strength.

1. Exhale as you lower your hands, placing them on your waist.
2. Shift your weight over the right foot, releasing the left foot from the floor as you reach around the outside of your left leg to grab your big toe with peace-sign fingers.
3. Inhale, extending the right leg straight in front of you while maintaining level hips, keeping your shoulders above your hips.
4. Perform three breath cycles here.
5. Exhale as you open your left hip, bringing your left leg out to the side.
6. Perform three breath cycles here gazing towards the right if you feel balanced.
7. Inhale, closing your left hip to bring your left leg back to the front, releasing your grip without dropping your leg to the floor, pointing through the toes, and keeping your leg parallel with the floor.
8. Perform three breath cycles here before exhaling to lower the leg to the floor.
9. Repeat Steps 2 to 8 on the opposite side.

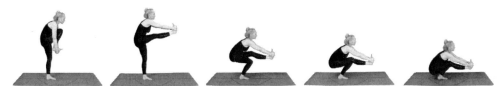

7 Pistol Squats

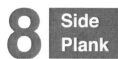

Figure 9.8.4.7: Phase 8—Dynamic power yoga—Pistol squats.

1. Inhale, bend your right knee, and reach your hands around the sole of your right foot, interlocking your fingers. Your weight should be shifted over your left foot for balance. Straighten your right leg, preparing for a pistol squat. Your bandhas, which should be automatically engaged by this phase of the training, will support you in this movement.

2. Exhale, bending your left knee and lowering yourself down toward the floor.

3. Inhale pressing through the midfoot to come back up again. This completes one set. *Note*: If your strength and balance are insufficient to power you for the raising phase of this pistol squat, allow yourself to come to the floor, release your foot and stand up.

4. Repeat the pistol squat until you have performed three sets on each side.

8 Side Plank

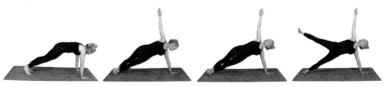

Figure 9.8.4.8: Phase 8—Dynamic power yoga—Side plank.

1. Come to plank position in preparation for side plank.

2. Inhale as you bring your left hand to the center of the mat, turning your feet so you are resting on the outside of your left foot as you find your side plank. Turn your gaze toward the fingertips of your right hand when you feel balanced.

3. Perform three breath cycles here.

4. Inhale to raise your right leg as high as you can while maintaining your balance.

5. Take three breath cycles here, coming back to your side plank if you fall out.

6. Exhale, lowering your right leg and bringing your gaze back toward the mat before lowering the right hand back to plank position.

7. Repeat Steps 2 to 6 on the opposite side.

9 | Pike Pushups

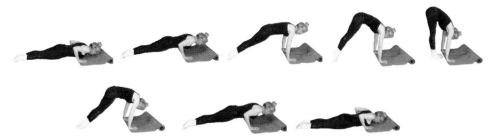

Figure 9.8.4.9: Phase 8—Dynamic power yoga—Pike push-ups.

1. Roll your mat as shown in Figure 9.8.4.9, and put your socks on your feet.
2. Lie on the floor with your hands under your shoulders. Ensure your bandhas are engaged.
3. Inhale as you press through the mid-hand to lift yourself into plank, keeping your toes pointed, toenail side down.
4. Rather than stopping in plank, keep pressing and lifting your hips higher, sliding your feet forward. This requires a strong activation where you try to bring the bottom of your rib cage closer to your hips. Your shoulders will shift forward beyond your wrists as you do this, so ensure that you keep the heel of your hand pressed into the floor for stability.
5. Bring your feet as close to your hands as you can, turning out your toes and stepping forward with your feet when you can draw them no closer.
6. Inhale here.
7. Come to your tippy toes and exhale as you slide back down the same way you came in, finishing back at the starting position.
8. Repeat for five breath cycles in total, taking child's pose to rest if needed.
9. Unroll your mat and remove your socks when finished.
10. Dry the sweat off the floor!

10 | Core Strengthening

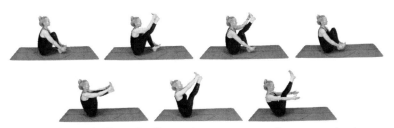

Figure 9.8.4.10: Phase 8—Dynamic power yoga—Core strengthening.

1. Sit on your mat, engage your core, and bring your knees toward your nipples, hold the sole of each flexed foot with your hand as your heels rest on the floor.

2. Inhale, release the right foot from the floor, and straighten your leg.

3. Exhale and lower the heel back to the floor.

4. Inhale, release the left foot from the floor, and straighten your leg.

5. Exhale, and lower the heel back to the floor. This is one full set

6. Repeat Steps 2 to 5 four more times so you have completed five sets in total.

7. Inhale, release both heels from the floor, and allow yourself to rest on your pivot point before extending your legs while still holding the soles of your flexed feet.

8. Gaze toward your toes, and perform three breath cycles here while maintaining a strong core.

9. Exhale, release your feet, and extend your arms forward for a high boat pose (navasana), trying to maintain the position of your body and legs.

10. Perform three breath cycles here before slowly lowering your legs and upper body to the floor while maintaining a strong core.

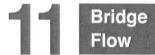 **Bridge Flow**

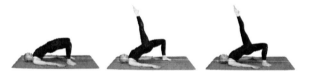

Figure 9.8.4.11: Phase 8—Dynamic power yoga—Bridge flow.

1. Prepare for the shoulder-supported bridge (*setu bandha sarvangasana*), bring your feet in line with your hips, and touch your middle finger to your heel.

2. Inhale, press into your feet, lift your hips high, and exhale.

3. Inhale, extend your right leg, and point your toes.

4. Exhale, lower your right leg, and plant your foot.

5. Inhale, extend your left leg, and point your toes.

6. Exhale, lower your left leg, and plant your foot.

7. Repeat this lifting and lowering of legs until you have raised each leg three times.

8. Lower down and take one rested breath cycle.

12 Little Ball of Balance

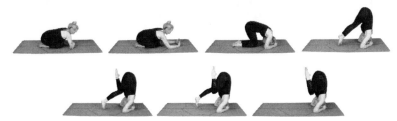

Figure 9.8.4.12: Phase 8—Dynamic power yoga—Little ball of balance.

1. Come to kneel on your mat in preparation for the little ball of balance (headstand prep).

2. Lean forward, and bring your elbows to the floor in front of you. Reach your hands around opposite elbows. This ensures that your elbows are placed in line with your shoulders. Keep your elbows planted exactly where they are. There is a tendency for beginners to allow the elbows to come wider when bringing the head to the floor. Pay attention to your elbow position keeping them in line with your shoulders.

3. Release your hands and interlock your fingers, leaving your hands open and your thumbs free.

4. Rest the top of your head on the floor, but without dumping all your weight on it. Press through the forearms as you spread your scapula to engage the shoulder girdle. Weight in the headstand is distributed through the forearms, upper arms, and across the shoulder girdle, not dumped into the head and neck. It should be possible to slip a piece of paper under your head when you are in this position due to the light touch of the head on the ground.

5. Turn your toes out and walk forward on your toes to bring your hips up above your shoulders. Like navasana prep, you will find a pivot point as you walk the toes forward, where the toes will lift naturally from the floor without effort. Stop just short of this pivot point.

6. Keeping your left toes on the floor, release the right foot, keeping the toes pointed as you bring your knee to touch your nipple. Lower the right toes to the floor.

7. Keeping your right toes on the floor, release the left foot, keeping the toes pointed as you bring your knee to touch your nipple. Lower the left foot to the floor.

8. Repeat Steps 6 to 7 four more times as you sense the effortlessness of balance when the knee is tight to the nipple.

9. Once you feel the balance, you can bring your right knee to your nipple, holding it there while releasing your left knee to your nipple to find the little ball of balance. The little ball of balance requires no momentum and should feel quite effortless.

10. Perform three breath cycles in your little ball of balance, before lowering one leg at a time and

coming down to a child's pose when done. Only progress to the headstand with a straight leg lift when you are comfortable in your little ball of balance.

13. Headstand Straight Leg Lift

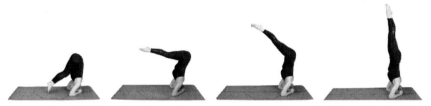

Figure 9.8.4.13: Phase 8—Dynamic power yoga—Headstand with straight leg lift.

Once you have found comfort in the little ball of balance, you can try for a full headstand. **This requires no momentum—you do not need to leap or jump into the headstand position**. Your bandhas will support the lifting of your legs.

1. Set up for your headstand in the same way as for the little ball of balance by walking your toes forward until you find your pivot point where your toes lift effortlessly from the floor.
2. From your pivot point, engage your legs by pointing your toes. Imagine that your legs have been zipped together using an imaginary zip from the ankles to the groin.
3. Allow your hips to move backward a little beyond your shoulders as your straight legs begin to lift, this allows the legs to lift with minimal effort. You can bring your legs halfway up (known as half balance) before lowering them back down. If you feel comfortable in half balance, you can attempt a full headstand using Step 4 below. Otherwise, skip to Step 5.
4. From the half balance position first, allow your legs to continue lifting, bringing your hips back over your shoulders, finishing in a straight line with toes engaged pointing toward the ceiling, legs zipped.
5. Stay in your version of the headstand for ten breath cycles.
6. Lower from the headstand in the same way you came in, with control coming down through half balance.
7. Take a child's pose after every headstand as coming up quickly from this position can cause dizziness.

14. Spinal Twists

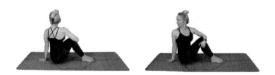

Figure 9.8.4.14: Phase 8—Dynamic power yoga—Spinal twists.

1. Come to a seated position, knees bent to 90 degrees and feet flat on the floor in front of you, preparing for a spinal twist.

2. Inhale to lengthen the spine, twist to the right side, bring the left hand around the knees, and place the right hand behind your back.

3. Perform three breath cycles here, as you inhale to lengthen the spine, and exhale to twist.

4. Return to facing forward and repeat Steps 2 to 3 on the opposite side.

15 Shoulder Stand

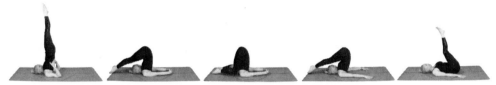

Figure 9.8.4.15: Phase 8—Dynamic power yoga—Shoulder stand.

1. Lie flat, preparing for a shoulder stand, and come first into a halasana pose.

2. Hold shoulder stand for ten breath cycles.

3. Exhale, lowering to halasana, interlocking the fingers, and pressing straight arms into the floor, take an inhalation here.

4. Exhale, bending your knees, and squeezing your ears with your knees.

5. Perform three breath cycles here before releasing the hands, press the palms into the ground, straighten the legs and lower them.

6. Slowly roll the spine down before finishing by lying flat on your mat.

16 Closing Sequence

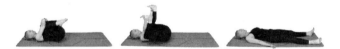

Figure 9.8.4.16: Phase 8—Dynamic power yoga—Closing sequence.

1. Hug your knees in toward your chest, and rock a little from side to side.

2. Come to happy husband pose for three breath cycles.

3. Take your final rest (savasana).

Having worked through the previous seven phases of the training, your body should be ready for this advanced practice. You can replace this practice with a studio yoga class or some other instructor-led practice of your choice. Remember to focus on managing intra-abdominal pressure using your bandhas.

Giving yourself the gift of yoga is the equivalent of gifting yourself agility. As time passes by, you gracefully flow toward the later years of your life with a strong and flexible body. Your goals can shift from short-term improvements to long-term maintenance. You have truly empowered yourself to live your best life.

That completes the movement module. You will practice this dynamic yoga sequence on the days specified in your schedule.

Phase 8: Relaxation Module

Yin Yoga All-Body

Having completed Phase 7, you should feel very empowered with your yin practice. A full yin toolkit is a great gift to yourself!

Objective
The objective of the relaxation module is to maintain the length-tension relationships you have created through the course of this training. We will revisit some great yin poses from earlier modules to get an all-body-focused yin session. These are my favorites. If you have favorites, you can swap the asanas in this workout with your preferred yin poses.

Success Metric
As with Phase 7, success with yin yoga is achieved when you can relax into the positions. At this point, you should have a well-established yin practice and should be seeing the benefits with reduced pelvic floor hypertonicity and enhanced flexibility in all planes of movement.

Additional Notes
Remember to continue being kind to yourself as you practice. Use the practice to release any remaining excess tension as you work toward your final goal.

Yin Yoga All-Body
You will need one or two bolsters (or pillows), two blankets, two blocks, an eye pillow, and a yoga mat. This practice will take thirty-five minutes including setup and transitions between poses. You can download

the sequence sheet for this all-body yin yoga sequence (Figure 9.8.5) from <u>empoweryourflower.com</u> and place it at the front of your mat when practicing.

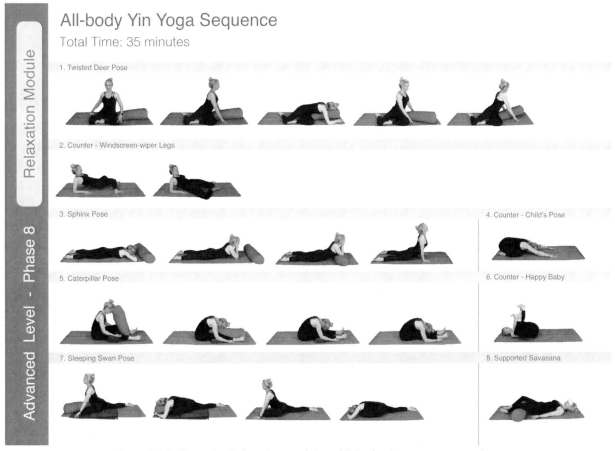

Figure 9.8.5: Phase 8—Relaxation module—All-body yin yoga sequence sheet.

You can read the instructions and steps beforehand and follow the poses on the printed copy of Figure 9.8.5 when you are practicing. This will help you to learn the sequence and eventually you will be able to practice it without looking at the sheet.

1 Twisted Deer Pose

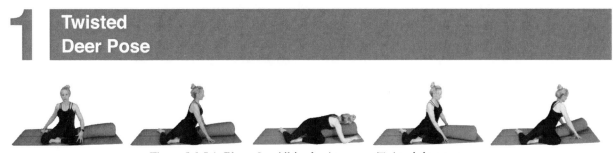

Figure 9.8.5.1: Phase 8—All-body yin yoga—Twisted deer pose.

The *twisted deer pose* is a deep twisting pose using the support of a bolster. You will need a bolster for this position. If you cannot lay your tummy down on the bolster, decrease the angle between the bolster and your left leg for a shallower twist. Likewise, if you feel that this is very easy and would like a deeper twist, you can increase the angle between your left leg and the bolster for a deeper twist. The deeper and gentler bolster angles are shown in the two images on the right in Figure 9.8.5.1. To assume the pose:

1. Place your bolster on the top of your mat and sit with the side of your left hip against the bolster.
2. Take deer pose with your legs by bending both knees with the left hip externally rotated, foot resting on the right thigh and the right leg internally rotated, foot resting beside you. Approximately 45-degree angle in both legs.
3. Turn to face the bolster, inhaling to lift your rib cage away from your hips and exhaling to lower your body onto the bolster.
4. Rest your arms on the floor, facing your head away from your knees for a deeper twist or toward your knees for a gentler twist.
5. Stay in this position for two-and-a-half minutes before repeating on the opposite side.

2 Counter Pose— Windscreen Wiper Legs

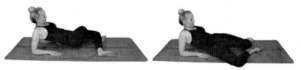

Figure 9.8.5.2: Phase 8—All-body yin yoga—Counter windscreen wiper legs.

1. Slowly move to the counterpose: do windscreen-wiper legs by resting back on your elbows and windscreen wiping your legs from side to side, and rolling on your glutes.

3 Sphinx Pose

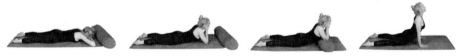

Figure 9.8.5.3: Phase 8—All-body yin yoga—Sphinx pose.

Sphinx pose is a yin backbend that focuses on spinal extension. It provides some compression on the back side of the spine while decompressing on the front side. There are multiple options demonstrated, using props to support the relaxation. *Note*: You begin in the easiest version of this position, only progressing if you meet the requirements for the next level. To assume the pose:

1. Place the bolster in front of your body and bring your feet slightly wider than hip-distance apart

424

before lifting your rib cage up and forward, and then resting it on the floor and placing your forehead on your hands. If you feel tension in your low back in this position, this is your backbend, otherwise, move to Step 2.

2. Come up onto your elbows, making a platform for your chin, using your hands. Relax here. If you feel tension in your low back in this position, this is your backbend, otherwise, move to Step 3.

3. Bring your elbows up onto the bolster and relax here. *Note*: if at any point you feel like you have moved beyond your edge, regress to the previous version.

4. Remain in your backbend for five minutes, making sure to relax your glutes; let your belly hang, relax your shoulders, and try to rest with as minimal effort as possible. *Note*: If you progressed to step 3 and had not met your edge during the first four minutes of the relaxation, you can come to the full expression *BUT* only for the last minute. For the full expression, press into your hands, straightening your arms and allowing a deeper backbend while relaxing your body.

5. Very slowly, mindfully come out of the position, bending at the knees

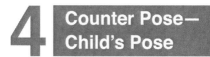

Counter Pose— Child's Pose

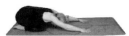

Figure 9.8.5.4: Phase 8—All-body yin yoga—Counter child's pose.

1. Push back to the close-leg child's pose for a minute before moving to the next position.

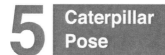

Caterpillar Pose

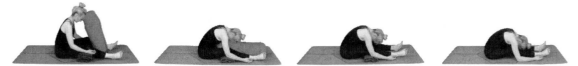

Figure 9.8.5.5: Phase 8—All-body yin yoga—Caterpillar pose.

Caterpillar pose is a yin forward fold that allows you to round your back as you relax forward. You should feel a stretch through the entire back side of your body and, in particular, your hamstrings. There are multiple variations demonstrated in Figure 9.8.5.5, using props to support the relaxation. To assume the pose:

1. Sit with your legs hip-distance apart and stretched out in front of you. Allow your legs to be relaxed in this position.

2. Allow yourself to relax forward, letting your head hang and allowing the weight of your upper

body to surrender forward.

3. Props can be used to make this easier. Images display the completely supported version through to the full unsupported expression of the pose (no props).

4. Relax in your version of this position for five minutes. You will feel your tissues release as time passes.

5. Very slowly, mindfully bring energy into your hands and slowly press your hands to bring yourself back to a seated position.

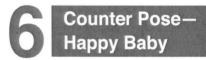

6 Counter Pose—Happy Baby

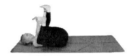

Figure 9.8.5.6: Phase 8—All-body yin yoga—Counter happy baby.

1. Come to a happy husband pose for one minute, and gently rock from side to side to counter this position.

7 Sleeping Swan

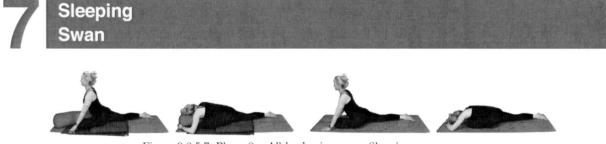

Figure 9.8.5.7: Phase 8—All-body yin yoga—Sleeping swan pose.

The *sleeping swan pose* is the yin version of a pigeon pose. You have the option to practice the supine version if that is part of your practice. Listen to your body when choosing your version. To assume the prone verison of this pose:

1. Come to an all-fours position with a bolster lain in front of your body and a folded blanket close to hand.

2. Inhale, bringing the left knee forward, rotating at the hip, and allowing the left foot to rest in front of the right hip. Use a blanket under your left hip if needed.

3. Allow your body to rest forward, surrendering either onto a bolster or the floor.

4. Relax in your version of this pose for three minutes on each side, making sure to keep shoulders and hips very relaxed throughout.

5. Very slowly, press into your hands, coming out of the pose in the same way as you came in.

8 | Supported Savasana

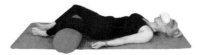

Figure 9.8.5.8: Phase 8—All-body yin yoga—Support savasana.

1. Come to a supported savasana as your final rest for five minutes.

If you had started out suffering from pelvic pain, this yin practice should have helped immensely to reduce hypertonicity and reduce pain levels. You will always have a full toolkit of yin poses at your disposal should your symptoms return.

That completes the relaxation module. You will practice this all-body yin sequence on the days specified in your schedule.

Phase 8: Mind & Meditation Module

Blossoming Goddess

Having completed Phase 7 of the mind/meditation module, you have reached the eighth Mind & Meditation module where you reach the pinnacle of your empowerment, you have done amazingly well to reach this stage in the process, well done!

Objective

The objective of the mind & meditation module in Phase 8 is to give you an opportunity to meditate on all you have achieved. You will perform the final meditation, which is aptly named blossoming goddess. The meditation is designed to allow you to feel the depth of what you have achieved and to raise your feminine energy in anticipation of a wonderful life ahead.

Success Metric

Success is achieved when you feel you are truly empowered to live your best possible life.

Additional Notes

This meditation is your chance to feel blessed in the abundance of your feminine energy. This is the pinnacle of the empowerment of your flower and the blossoming of a lifelong wonderful relationship with yourself. From this point forward, ensure that you always give yourself the love and compassion that you deserve. As your empowerment blossoms, share your wonderful energy with those lucky enough to be graced by your presence.

Blossoming Goddess Meditation

For this meditation, you will lie in a savasana position. You can use an eye pillow and blanket if you prefer. You will practice this meditation twice per week. You can listen to the audio version of this meditation on empoweryourflower.com. Read through the instructions before you begin and either step through the meditation in your mind or listen to the meditation audio as you mediate.

Steps to Perform This Exercise

1. Get yourself into a comfortable savasana position with your eyes closed.
2. Perform five calming breath cycles before you begin, focusing on relaxing your entire body as you do so.
3. Bring your awareness to your heart, feeling the gentle pulse as it beats.
4. As you feel the gentle beat of your heart, visualize a golden staircase in front of you. Walk toward the staircase feeling light under your feet as you gracefully move toward it.
5. Resting your hand on the stair-rail, begin to walk up the stairs feeling the smooth golden rail and noticing its warmth. At the top of the stairs, see an expansive room, beautifully decorated.
6. Feel the soft carpet under your feet.
7. Notice the mirror with a golden frame in the corner of the room and walk toward it, feeling the warmth of its golden glow.
8. As you reach the mirror, speak your self-affirmations while looking into your own eyes. While speaking those kind words feel the warmth around your heart. Imagine that the golden warmth is flowing around your body with each beat.
9. Visualize flowers beginning to blossom at your feet. As those flowers blossom and begin to grow taller, watch in your golden mirror as you begin to emanate a golden glow.
10. Watch in amazement as flowers blossom all around you as you glow in golden warmth, your inner beauty shining outwards
11. Feel your pulse moving from the base of your spine to the very top of your head as the golden energy begins to flow upwards toward your crown, each beat of your heart causing golden light to blossom from your crown into the sky above you.
12. Feel the joy in your heart as your inner feminine beauty blossoms out into the world. You are a goddess. You are amazing. You are love itself. Feel it in every cell, as the sparkling fluctuations of

potential become your reality and you fulfill your empowerment.

13. Take five calming breaths as you gaze lovingly at the blossoming goddess in the mirror. Feel her feminine power. Own it, it is yours.

14. Turn back toward the golden staircase, you are the golden goddess.

15. Gracefully descend the staircase, coming back to the beat of your heart and the feeling of the golden energy that is flowing through you. Feel the energy moving out to your fingers and your toes. Feel it flowing up to your crown. Feel your power.

16. Bring your awareness to your pelvis, feeling into the depths of your vagina. Imagine calling all your power to this area, as though harnessing it in the very root of your being.

17. Visualize your golden goddess energy coming together, bringing power to your flower. Feel the warmth of your flower as it absorbs your golden energy. Embrace your divine feminine energy and carry it with you into your future.

18. Come back to your breath, inhaling deeply and exhaling slowly.

19. Bring energy to your fingers and your toes, as you gently move them.

20. Make small circles with your wrists and your ankles.

21. Reach your hands up overhead, reach your feet out in front of your body and have a nice, long, deep stretch.

22. Hug your knees into your chest and roll to your right side, taking a moment in the fetal position, holding your divine feminine energy deep inside.

23. Press gently into the ground with your left hand to bring you to a comfortable seated position, maintaining closed eyes and an internal focus.

24. Slowly blink open your eyes bringing your hands over your heart, feeling it beating in your chest.

25. Smile to yourself and affirm your love in words.

And with that, you have come to the end of module eight. You will practice this meditation on the days specified in your weekly schedule.

At the end of each week, if you feel that you may be ready to progress to living your life filled with thoughtless, fearless movement, you can perform the phase checkpoint review using Figure 9.8.6, which checks your progress against the success metric for each exercise and helps you to decide if you should finish the training and get back to enjoying life. You can download a blank version of this form from empoweryourflower.com.

Phase 8 Checkpoint Review

Phase Start Date:_____

Checkpoint Date:_____

Pelvic Floor Module	Success

Strength: Success is achieved when you can perform these dynamic activities thoughtlessly and fearlessly without needing to use conscious effort to engage your bandhas. Pelvic floor control at this level should become automatic.

Yes ☐
No ☐

Relaxation: Success is achieved when you can relax your pelvic floor fully in all the positions specified and no longer feel the symptoms of hypertonicity.

Yes ☐
No ☐

Breathing Module - Kapalabhati Breathing	Success

Success is achieved when you can relax your entire body using only your lower abdominals to power the breath. When you master this breathing technique, you will feel energized following this practice.

Yes ☐
No ☐

Movement Module - Dynamic Power Yoga	Success

Success with this module is achieved when you feel empowered to do the things that your pelvic floor was previously preventing.

Yes ☐
No ☐

Relaxation Module - Yin Yoga All Body	Success

As with phase 8, success with Yin yoga is achieved when you can relax into the positions. At this point, you should have a well-established yin practice and should be seeing the benefits with reduced pelvic floor hypertonicity and enhanced flexibility in all planes of movement.

Yes ☐
No ☐

Mind & Meditation Module - Blossoming Goddess	Success

Success is achieved when you feel you are truly empowered to live your best possible life.

Yes ☐
No ☐

Phase 8 Checkpoint Review	Success

Have you achieved the success objectives and do you feel that you are ready to proceed to finish the training and get on with your life?

Yes ☐
No ☐

If no, please continue at the with the Phase 8 training until you are ready to proceed, or regress to the Phase 7 training if you feel that you are not ready for Phase 8.

If yes, proceed with the Progress Milestone review where you repeat the initial assessments checking your progress against the advanced level goal that you had set for the program.

Progress Milestone Review - Advanced Level	Success

Have you already achieved your advanced level goal?

If no, you have the option to repeat the phase 8 of the advanced level training.

Yes ☐
No ☐

If yes, well done, you have empowered your flower and can get on with your life!

Figure 9.8.6: Phase 8—Checkpoint review form.

What to Do Once You Have Completed the Eight-Phase Training

If you have worked through all eight phases while utilizing the symptom management and life strategies that are detailed in Chapter Ten, you should have fully empowered your flower. I would like to congratulate you on getting to this stage.

I would also like to encourage you to think about what comes next. Your empowerment does not have to end here. Having set goals to get back to doing what your symptoms had been preventing, you can now move forward by setting new goals. You can strive to reach new heights, achieving even more than you considered possible. I did exactly that.

When I was completely symptom-free, I embarked on a bodybuilding journey. I worked tirelessly with an amazing coach, John Meadows (also known as Mountain Dog), and built a strong physique that brought me to the bodybuilding stage in December 2019. I lifted way more than a kettle of water (the advice I was given when leaving the hospital in 2015).

John was an amazing and inspirational coach, who unfortunately passed away a few weeks before the publication of this book. He helped me to believe that I could do more than I had allowed myself to believe possible, and for that I am forever grateful.

Strive to do more, be the best version of yourself. I would say the sky's the limit, but there are footsteps on the moon, so *reach for the stars!*

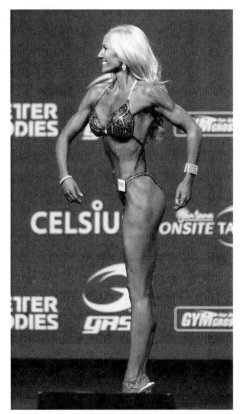

Figure 9.8.7: Body Building December 2019.

Part three

Symptom management,
tools and strategies for empowerment

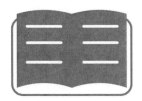

Overview of Part Three

Having read through the eight-phase training, you will have seen that a multi-modal approach is being taken to tackle PFD from many different angles:

1. **Directly**: By performing pelvic floor strength or relaxation exercises.
2. **Through Breathing**: Tapping into the diaphragmatic relationship.
3. **Through Movement**: Working to rebalance strength and flexibility in the entire body.
4. **Through Relaxation**: Working to rebalance length-tension in the entire body.
5. **Through Mind & Meditation**: Working on the mental and emotional aspects of PFD.

This approach improves your chances of empowering your flower, however, there are many symptoms relating to PFD, and it can also be very helpful to approach your symptoms directly. The objective of Part Three book is to explore *what* you can do to manage symptoms, *what* treatments are available, *when* and *why* you should use tools and strategies, and *who* can help you on your journey.

Chapter Ten: Strategies for living with PFD

Chapter Ten utilizes the assessments you performed in Chapter Eight to guide you in selecting symptom management and life strategies that can complement your eight-phase training. These include symptom-specific strategies, posture adaptation exercises, life pattern adaptation strategies, massage techniques, and self-care strategies. This comprehensive list of strategies can help you decide *what* you can do to conservatively manage your PFD. Even if you choose not to undertake the eight-phase training, this chapter can help you to manage your PFD.

Chapter Eleven: Pelvic Floor Dysfunction Treatments

Chapter Eleven begins with the shocking history behind the use of mesh devices to treat POP and stress urinary incontinence (SUI). This is a must-read, especially if you are considering surgery. This chapter details the various conditions that fall under the umbrella term PFD, and explains *what* non-invasive and invasive treatments are available, including surgeries with and without mesh devices.

Chapter Twelve: Devices and Tools

Chapter Twelve details the devices and tools that are on the market to help deal with the symptoms of PFD and shares my opinions on these devices, explaining *when* and *why* you would use them.

Chapter Thirteen: Medical Professionals and Therapists

Chapter Thirteen is a short chapter that shares details of the different healthcare specialists *who* can help you on your journey of empowerment. You should always seek medical advice before beginning any training program or implementing any changes to manage your symptoms.

Chapter Ten:
Symptom Management and Life Strategies

In this chapter, we will detail strategies and exercises that can help to manage your symptoms and maintain the changes to your patterns that you are working to achieve. The various conditions that fall under the umbrella of PFD are explained in detail in Chapter Eleven, which also explains the non-surgical and surgical treatment options for PFD conditions.

You should read Part Three fully before implementing any changes, and always consult with your healthcare provider before selecting and adopting any of the outlined strategies and exercises. Remember also that you should never self-diagnose. Your healthcare provider can perform a full assessment and give the relevant diagnosis. You may be following this program as a preventative measure rather than to address symptoms. If that is the case, there are some valuable little nuggets in this chapter that may help to ensure that you remain symptom-free throughout the course of your life so do read on.

There are five sections in this chapter, which will use the assessments from Chapter Eight to help you choose which strategies may be helpful for you. The purpose of the strategies and activities is to support you on your journey of empowerment by offering methods to manage your condition. These sections and associated assessments are:

1. **Symptom-management strategies**: using the symptom assessment.
2. **Posture adaptations**: using the posture assessment.
3. **Massage**: using the flexibility assessment.
4. **Self-care and diet**: using the life pattern and mind assessments.

Symptom-Management strategies

We will now utilize the symptom assessment that you completed in Chapter Eight to help choose which symptom-management strategies may be helpful for you. These strategies should help you to manage and improve your symptoms to support you on your empowerment journey. This section covers strategies for the following categories:

Symptom Management
Strategies

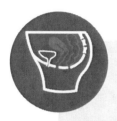

1. Urinary Symptoms

a. Overactive bladder/urgency (OAB)
b. Stress incontinence (SUI)
c. Mixed incontinence (MUI)
d. Urinary retention (UR)

2. Fecal Symptoms

a. Flatulence/skid-marks
b. Fecal incontinence (FI)
c. Chronic constipation (CC)

3. POP Symptoms

a. Heaviness, dragging and "golf-ball" sensations
b. Incomplete defecation

4. Pelvic Pain Symptoms

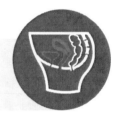

a. Chronic pelvic pain syndrome (CPPS)
b. Bladder pain syndrome (BPS)
c. Vaginismus, dyspareunia (painful sex), and vulvodynia

Symptom Management Strategies for Urinary Symptoms

In this section, we will review the symptom-management strategies for urinary symptoms, which are outlined in Table 10.1 below.

	OAB Overactive Bladder	SUI Stress Incontinence	MUI Mixed Incontinence	UR Urinary retention
Strategy 1	Tap into your superpower	Leak Management	Use OAB & SUI strategies	Timed Voiding
Strategy 2	Retrain your bladder	Learning "the knack"		Pelvic Floor Relaxation Practices
Strategy 3		Remembering continence		Uretharal Splinting
Strategy 4		Post void "free" Kegels		Hokey Cokey double void HCDV
Strategy 5		Sit to stand pressure management		Self-catheterization
Strategy 6		Return to running		

Table 10.1: Symptom-management strategies for urinary symptoms.

Table 10.1 shows the urinary symptom in the top row with the strategies for that symptom listed beneath.

Before even considering urinary symptoms, I want to tell you not to strain when you pee. You shouldn't pee by pushing the pee out. Your bladder (detrusor muscle) pushes the pee out for you. The only thing you should have to do is to relax your pelvic floor. To relax your pelvic floor, you must sit down (don't hover over the toilet seat). With that out of the way, let's explore strategies to deal with urinary symptoms.

Urinary symptoms including overactive bladder and incontinence are quite common among women. When it comes to incontinence, one in every four women will experience some form of urinary leakage during her adult lifetime. Incontinence is an embarrassing condition and can leave you feeling isolated. If you leak when walking, you might be reluctant to leave your house.

I remember planning my trips around available toilets. This is so detrimental to QoL and can have a big impact on socialization due to fear that someone may smell the leaking urine. Many women reduce their fluid intake when they experience incontinence, which can cause dehydration. Many also decrease their movement, which can accelerate the rate at which muscles atrophy. With this atrophy, the symptoms of incontinence can worsen. This can contribute to the onset of frailty at an earlier age than would otherwise be expected. Remember, motion is lotion… you need to move.

It is imperative that you don't reduce your fluid intake or your movement levels if you find yourself leaking urine. It is also important not to urinate when your body is not telling you that it is time. Often, when experiencing slight leakage, we begin to urinate before going out and when arriving somewhere, "*just in case*". This JIC peeing reprograms the bladder and can contribute to overactive bladder symptoms resulting in mixed incontinence. Don't worry, if you adopt some of the strategies outlined in the following pages, you can make the very best of your situation, whatever that may be.

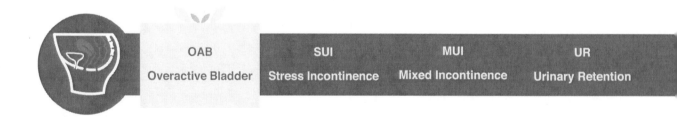

OAB	SUI	MUI	UR
Overactive Bladder	Stress Incontinence	Mixed Incontinence	Urinary Retention

If you have listed OAB with or without incontinence on the symptom assessment sheet, the pelvic floor, relaxation, and mind/meditation modules of the eight-phase program should be helping with your symptoms. This section offers some strategies that can help to manage and relieve the symptoms you are experiencing, making PFD easier to live with.

Sometimes the things you drink can irritate your bladder and create sensations of urgency. If you feel urgency but have not been diagnosed with OAB, you should consider removing caffeinated beverages, acidic beverages, and other potential irritants from your diet to see if that alleviates the issue.

Oftentimes, we stop listening to the subtle language of our bodies—those "sensations" that tell us we are hungry, thirsty, tired, need to pee, need to poop, etc. We work to fit around a busy schedule rather than listening to the rhythms of our biology. Before deciding to change patterns, it is important to know our current pattern.

With OAB, the bladder signals that it is time to urinate when there is only a small amount of urine in the bladder. OAB is typically diagnosed when your doctor/urologist has confirmed that there are no infections present and tissue pathology is negative (meaning tissues are normal).

Remember in Part One of this book, we learned that the nervous system does not automatically default back to a functional movement pattern after you've had an injury or infection. Well, the same can be true for urination.

When a urine infection is present, your nervous system will typically make you urinate more frequently. When the infection is gone, urination doesn't necessarily return to the normal reflexive pattern and this can result in the symptoms of OAB.

JIC peeing can also trigger the symptoms of OAB. As well as triggering urgency sensations, OAB can also be accompanied by bladder spasms and general discomfort within the pelvis. We will utilize the following two strategies to address OAB symptoms:

OAB Strategy 1: "Tap into your superpower"—a strategy to delay urination & reduce bladder spasms.
OAB Strategy 2: Retrain your bladder—a strategy to retrain bladder function ensuring it can fill before emptying.

With both strategies, you will tap into the body's urinary guarding reflex, which we learned about in Chapter Five. I believe the guarding reflex is one of your body's superpowers that helps to relax your bladder, delaying urination until an appropriate time while also reducing bladder spasms.

When you were potty trained, you were taught to sense your bladder signaling that it was full. You were trained to delay urination by "holding on" until you could get to the toilet. You may not have realized at the time that "holding on" involved a contraction of the front portion of your pelvic floor (more specifically the external urethral sphincter). This contraction sends a signal back to your brain to tell your nervous system to relax your bladder. This is the guarding reflex. The following exercise details how to tap into your superpower:

OAB Strategy 1

Tap into your superpower

You should perform this exercise when you feel the sensation of urgency or bladder irritation/spasm at an inappropriate time. This can be when you are out and about and have a sudden urgency sensation or it can be when you are undertaking bladder retraining and are trying to delay urination. We will detail bladder training in the subsequent exercise. The steps to perform this strategy (your superpower):

1. STOP in your tracks when you first feel the urgency sensation. If you are walking STOP. Whatever you are doing, immediately STOP and bring your awareness to your bladder.
2. If possible, sit down, otherwise, stay standing.
3. Relax as much as possible allowing your stomach to be soft and resisting the urge to tighten up your body. If you sit down, assume a pose I like to call "supta gummy-bear" where you relax your legs a little wider than hip-distance apart, rest your back on the chair and let every part of your body relax.
4. Contract the front part of your pelvic floor gently for a count of three.
5. Relax completely after that contraction and then contract again for a count of three.
6. Repeat these contractions a few times until the sensation of urgency or bladder spasm have subsided.

It is important to stay relaxed when you undertake this exercise. It is an exercise in communicating with your nervous system. You want your nervous system to have the bandwidth to listen to this communication, so you need to stay calm and relaxed.

This strategy will help you to delay urination when you are not close to a bathroom. If you are out running or in the middle of a gym class and experience urgency where you don't have the opportunity to go to a bathroom, just use this strategy to delay the need until you have reached a suitable time/ location.

Of course, if your bladder is full and it's time to go, you should find a bathroom and empty your bladder rather than trying to delay. Excessive holding can negatively reprogram your bladder causing it to overstretch, which can dampen the signals from your bladder's stretch receptors, which can lead to symptoms of UR. We are striving for an optimal balance with urinary function so ensure that you empty your bladder every two to four hours (unless you are sleeping).

OAB Strategy 2

Retrain your bladder

It is advisable to seek the advice and guidance of your healthcare provider should you require bladder retraining. The information provided in this book should by no means be considered a substitute for the advice and guidance of qualified healthcare professionals. You can agree with your healthcare provider if the bladder retraining detailed in this section could be helpful for you.

From the perspective of urinary function, it is important that you understand your bladder patterns before you make any changes. This will involve keeping a bladder diary for a few days. A bladder diary is a record of the volume and frequency of fluids that we drink and urinate.

Maybe you are wondering what a "normal" bladder volume is. I've read so many conflicting studies and undertaken training in different countries where I have received conflicting information on what "normal" is for both volume and frequency.

One study, whose purpose was to determine normal ranges for voiding in asymptomatic women concluded that "It is probably inappropriate to apply a single set of normative values to all women"[81]. Another study states that "Normal functional bladder capacity in adults ranges from approximately 300 to 400 ml"[82] while also stating that "the International Continence Society defines urinary frequency as the perception by the patient that he/she voids too often."

Bladder volume depends on the size of the bladder, which depends on the size of the person. Bladder frequency depends on the amount that a person drinks, and the type of drinks/foods/drugs that the person consumes. Level of activity, age, and race can also impact bladder frequency. With my own bladder, I have seen volumes as low as 50ml and as high as 900ml (I was fit to explode by the time I got to the bathroom with that one!).

For one person, emptying 200 to 300 ml on each void could be a normal functional amount, and for another, it could indicate that the person is emptying before the bladder is full. Urologists can perform urodynamics tests using cystometry to assess bladder pressures, filling and voiding rates, etc. I would not rush out to have this type of testing done unless your doctor recommends it as it involves catheterization (inserting small tubes into the bladder through the urethra), which can be a little uncomfortable and sometimes makes symptoms worse. Instead of trying to fit your bladder into some *normal* box, you should ask yourself if your volume and/or frequency are negatively impacting the quality of your life.

It is suggested that normal voiding frequency is 6 to 8 times per day and once during the night (or twice per night after the age of 65). If you sleep 8 hours per night, then you are awake for 16 hours per day so you would expect to urinate every two hours or thereabouts.

If you urinate more than eight times per day, **that does not mean you have a dysfunctional bladder**, but if your frequency of urination impacts your QoL, and if you are experiencing symptoms of bladder spasms or incontinence then it is important to address these issues. You can try the exercise to "tap into your superpower" and that may be sufficient to resolve bladder spasms and urgency sensations. If those sensations persist then create a bladder diary over three days. The following instructions will help you do this.

Instructions for Creating a Bladder Diary

To create a bladder diary, you can download an editable bladder diary from empoweryourflower.com or just use a notebook and pen and record the volumes you drink and pee (or leak) over three days. Don't use delay tactics (like the "tap into your superpower" exercise) when creating your bladder diary as you want to see your baseline before changing anything.

Volumes of liquid can be measured with a measuring cup. You should count all liquids (water, coffee, tea, milk, soft drinks, alcohol, juice, smoothie, soup, etc.). Volumes of urine can be measured with a small measuring jug. Just make sure that you don't use it for anything else... gravy anyone?

An alternative way to measure, and one that you can do anywhere without having to carry a measuring jug is to count your Mississip*pees*! When the flow starts, your count starts, 1 Mississip*pee*, 2 Mississip*pee*, 3 Mississip*pee*, etc. A full bladder would land somewhere around 20 Mississip*pees* (which is approximately twenty seconds). You can record the number of Mississippees instead of the ml if you opt for this method.

Reviewing Your Bladder Diary

Once you have three days' worth of data, you will get to see your pattern. Patterns are a little like habits (remember it takes forty days to break a habit and ninety days to create a new habit). It is normal to output less than your input so don't panic if you notice that you have drunk 2 liters and only urinated 1.5 liters (or vice versa). It is more important to review your frequency and average volumes for drinking and urination. Use the following steps to review your data and to create a schedule for bladder retraining:

Step 1: *Review your fluid intake*—calculate the frequency (e.g., every two hours), average volume (e.g., 200 ml), and total volume (e.g., 1.6 liters) of fluids that you consumed.

a. If you found that you were drinking less than 1.5 liters of fluids in one day, you should consider drinking more as the suggested for females is around 2.2 liters[83]. Do bear in mind that you get approximately 0.5 liter from food.

b. If you found that you were going long stretches without a drink, you should consider timing your fluids, so you are drinking every two to three hours.

c. If you were drinking a lot of coffee or other caffeinated drinks and are experiencing bladder spasms or irritation, you should consider cutting these stimulants out during your bladder retraining.

Step 2: *Review your urine output*—calculate the frequency (e.g., 6 times in the day) and the average time between voids (e.g., three hours), average volume (e.g., 300ml), and the total volume (e.g., 1800ml).

a. If you find that you are urinating less than 200ml with high frequency (more than ten times per day), it can be good to proceed with the bladder training exercise, but only if you feel that this pattern is impacting your QoL.

b. If you were measuring Mississip*pees* and you were urinating for 10 Mississi*pees* with high frequency (more than ten times per day) it can be good to proceed with the bladder retraining exercise.

The Following Steps Are Required to Perform Bladder Retraining

Step 1: *Create a schedule for fluid intake* ensuring that you are drinking similar amounts (e.g.: 200 ml) at regular intervals throughout your day. Try to stick to that schedule during bladder retraining. You should also try to notice your thirst signals and have a drink if you feel thirsty. I suggest drinking after you go to the bathroom as drinking can trigger the need to go for some people and so it presents you with an opportunity to practice overcoming that unnecessary signal to void.

Step 2: *Remove stimulants like caffeine and alcohol* from your regularly consumed beverages and monitor for changes to your symptoms of urgency. You should avoid these beverages for at least a week to see if there is a positive impact.

Step 3: *Create a schedule for voiding.* To do this, you should take your average time between voids and add fifteen minutes to that. For example, if you were voiding every 45 minutes, you would set a schedule to void every hour. You can continue to add 15-minute increments each week as you continue with bladder retraining, stopping when you feel you have reached a function level (usually around 2 to 3 hours between voids).

Step 4: *Use the "tap into your superpower" strategy* to helping to delay the time between voids by contracting the front part of your pelvic floor to send a signal to your nervous system asking it to relax the bladder. This should be done to delay urination according to your voiding schedule during your bladder retraining.

Step 5: *Plan activities that require movement immediately post void* (e.g., for the hour after your void) and plan seated activities closer to void time (e.g., for the hour before your next void). This is a practice that can help during your early bladder retraining as it can help the bladder to stay relaxed while it fills.

If you had been experiencing leakage along with your OAB/urgency, it might be that your pelvic floor is not quite strong enough to hold while your bladder is filling. You can support your bladder as it works to reach capacity by sitting down when you start to feel the first sensations and staying seated while your bladder fills. When you sit, you reduce the tension in your pelvis and around your bladder. You should sit until you feel a strong urge to go, or until you have reached your voiding time.

I used this technique when retraining my bladder after mesh removal. It allowed my reflexes to return to a normal pattern when my pelvic floor muscles were still not quite strong enough to prevent leakage from walking. You can use this time to read a good book or work at your computer. When it comes time to go to the bathroom, use the "tap into your superpower" exercise to activate the guarding reflex before standing. You can perform a full Kegel, which you can maintain as you stand up. Stop and utilize your superpower if needed as you make your way to the bathroom to empty that full bladder.

Step 6: *Try distraction techniques.* Particularly if you feel the urgency immediately after voiding. Distraction techniques involve a focus on something that requires mental focus, such as a puzzle (e.g., Sudoku), a Rubix cube, knitting, painting, or some other craft that requires both attention and motor control (using your hands).

These steps should help you to retrain your bladder, finding a more suitable pattern for urination. Continue with bladder training over six to eight weeks until you have successfully reduced symptoms/frequency and increased bladder volumes.

You may need to reduce your level of physical activity while undertaking bladder training. For example, if you are working through the eight-phase training while retraining your bladder, you could work at the preparation or beginner level rather than the more advanced levels, particularly if strong exercise is triggering your bladder symptoms.

If you have incontinence as well as an overactive bladder (mixed incontinence), prioritize your bladder retraining before tackling your leaking. It's easier to address leakage episodes when the bladder has a happy pattern. I made great progress over a six-week period back in 2015. The bladder retraining resolved the OAB/urgency aspect of my mixed incontinence, which meant that my focus thereafter was on the stress incontinence aspect.

Remember that retraining your bladder is a process that enhances your ability to communicate with your nervous system. Throughout your journey of empowerment, I encourage you to listen to the subtle language that the nervous system uses to communicate through bodily sensations. You should also learn as much as you can about your patterns.

That concludes the strategies for OAB. We will now address strategies for stress incontinence (SUI).

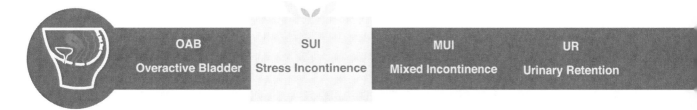

| OAB | SUI | MUI | UR |
| Overactive Bladder | Stress Incontinence | Mixed Incontinence | Urinary Retention |

Stress incontinence is leakage as a result of an imbalance in intra-abdominal pressures. When the downward intra-abdominal pressure is greater than the urethral closure pressure, leakage can occur. If you have listed stress incontinence on the symptom assessment sheet, the pelvic floor, breathing and movement modules of the eight-phase program should be helping you to retrain the balance and management of intra-abdominal pressure.

This section offers some additional strategies that can help to manage and relieve the symptoms you are experiencing. We will utilize the following strategies to address the symptoms of stress incontinence:

SUI Strategy 1: *Leak management* is a strategy to ensure protection is available to soak up or mask embarrassing leaks.

SUI Strategy 2: *Learning "The knack"* is a strategy to pre-tension the pelvic floor before coughing, sneezing, laughing, or other high-pressure activities.

SUI Strategy 3: *"Remembering continence"* is a strategy that attempts to find the continence mechanism that existed prior to the onset of stress incontinence. We will use a balloon analogy for this exercise.

SUI Strategy 4: *Post void "free" Kegels* is a strategy to enhance pelvic floor strength while reducing after pee dribble.

SUI Strategy 5: *Sit to stand pressure management* is a strategy to help maintain continence when moving from sitting to standing and vice versa.

SUI Strategy 6: *Return to running* is a strategy to assist those who experience mild to moderate incontinence when running.

These strategies can be viewed as tools for your incontinence toolkit. Some you may need to use daily, others you may not need but you may still find comfort in knowing that they are there.

Remember that we are all slowly aging, a process of degradation. New symptoms may appear as you age, or when you reach menopause. Having the tools available to manage and improve incontinence symptoms can help to ensure that your QoL remains high even in your later years.

SUI Strategy 1

Leak Management

Pelvic floor training is very effective in reducing and eliminating leakage; however, it takes time. As you work to strengthen your pelvic floor, optimize your breathing, and manage your intra-abdominal pressure, you should also make sure to protect against leakages.

There are many products on the market to help manage leakages. These will allow you to live a somewhat normal life while you work on your rehabilitation. The following products will help to avoid the embarrassment of a wet patch on your clothing while also giving you the confidence to remain active with your movement. The protective products are summarized below but you can find out more about them in Chapter Twelve where we review devices and tools.

Protective Products

Panty-liners, incontinence pads, and disposable underwear: Panty liners, incontinence pads, and disposable underwear are designed to soak up leakage to prevent wet patches in your pants/trousers. With panty-liners being the lightest, suitable for leakages of just a few drops. Incontinence pads (not period pads) are designed for moderate leakage and disposable pants for heavy leakage. These pads often mask smells too.

Incontinence underwear: This underwear is designed to soak up mild leakage. They are used without panty-liners or pads and generally soak up light leakage.

EVB sports pants: These are specially engineered compression pants that can be used to help prevent mild stress incontinence. Originally designed for running, they can also be worn as underwear. They do not provide soakage for leaking but can help to balance intra-abdominal pressure, which can help to prevent leakage. They also provide support for prolapse.

Urethral blockers: These are small sticky pads that cover the urethral opening. Urine can still enter the urethra (pee pipe) but the sticky pad covers the hole from which the urine exits that pipe. Make sure not to become dependent on this type of product as it is better to train your pelvic floor to prevent leakage than to just block the exit!

Disposable incontinence pessaries: These are like tampons that you can use any time of the month. They place some bulk for structural support under the urethra from within the vagina, which can help if your internal urethral sphincter or front vaginal wall are contributing to your incontinence. Pessaries are more commonly used with POP, but can also be helpful if you suffer from incontinence. Disposable pessaries are sold on Amazon or in pharmacies and usually can be purchased in a starter pack that has a few different sizes that you can try. You may need to wet them before use.

Bed pads: These can help with nighttime leakage. They look like a small blanket that you can place underneath your pelvis while you sleep. They can catch leakage and prevent staining of sheets.

Hand warmers: Hand warmers may sound like a strange protection suggestion for stress incontinence, however, if your stress incontinence is triggered by the feeling of cold when you step outside, you can use hand warmers to limit the impact of the cold. Hand warmers are small sachets with a small capsule that you snap to activate the heating mechanism. You can place the sachet in your trouser pocket so it is close to your bladder. This can help to prevent the urgency that triggers leakage due to cold temperatures. Hand warmers typically hold heat for up to eight hours.

You should use whatever products you need to help keep you as fresh and dry as possible. This can give you the confidence to keep moving while remaining social (an absolute requirement for good mental health). The end goal would be to live without these products. We don't want to become dependent on them but should not feel even slightly guilty about using them when needed.

You should also be aware of your menstrual cycle and the varying levels of vaginal secretions that you experience throughout the month (which we visualized in Figure 8.14). For anyone who has already overcome incontinence, you may have experienced how the fertile time of the month, when vaginal discharge is slippery and wet, can cause post-traumatic stress disorder (PTSD) type symptoms and flashbacks to those dreaded days when you were still leaking. If you know your cycle, you can mentally prepare ahead of time, and add a liner if the PTSD is too much to bear.

SUI Strategy 2

Learning "The Knack"

"The knack" is a strategic practice that prepares your pelvic floor to deal with sudden pressure increases. It is a full Kegel exercise performed at the maximum strength you can achieve. It is a technique that pre-tensions the pelvic floor prior to a sneeze, cough, or laugh.

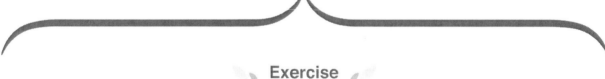

Exercise
to practice "the knack"

You will practice this exercise in two positions—seated and standing. Try to relax the rest of your body as you do this. The actual exercises are the same whether you are seated or standing but it will feel different due to the extra tension in your muscles when you stand. You will need a tissue for this exercise as you will blow your nose to mimic increased downward pressure.

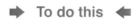

➡ To do this ⬅

1.   Starting seated, relax your body, paying particular attention to your core and glutes to ensure they are relaxed.

2.   Inhale deeply and bring the tissue to your nose.

3.   Perform a maximum strength contraction of your pelvic floor as you blow your nose into the tissue. You will feel that your core also contracts when you are blowing as is normal when sneezing, coughing, or laughing.

4.   Repeat three times seated and then stand up and repeat three times standing.

Practicing this action helps to train the pelvic floor to react should a sudden sneeze or cough manifest. Through practice, this pre-tensioning action should become a bottom-up reflexive action rather than a top-down instruction.

My hand in Figure 10.1 indicates the action of the pelvic floor contraction, which pre-tenses before sneezing, coughing, or laughing.

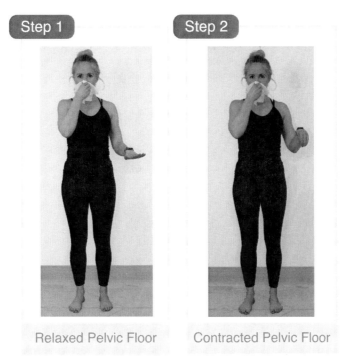

Figure 10.1: Performing "the knack" exercise.

The image on the left in Figure 10.1 shows a relaxed pelvic floor as I prepare to blow my nose. The image on the right in Figure 10.1 shows the maximum strength contraction just before I blow my nose. A properly functioning pelvic floor will create enough closure pressure around the urethra and anus to prevent leakage of urine and fecal matter when there is a sudden pressure change.

SUI Strategy 3

"Remembering Continence"

Many of the suggested strategies in this book have been the subject of scientific study. This strategy could be viewed as an exception. This strategy was, for me, born of necessity. In trying to understand why I couldn't just hold my pee after having my mesh removed, I tried many different techniques and went down one rabbit hole after another looking for answers.

I tried to remember how continence felt for my body but I could not remember ever performing a big strong contraction of my pelvic floor prior to first hearing about Kegels, and yet I had been continent for most of my life. This got me thinking about why I couldn't remember these strong contractions that kept my sphincter closed. That's when I realized, I had been looking at my incontinence the wrong way.

You will recall in Part One, we looked at all the different muscles of the pelvic floor. One of the key muscles involved in continence is the external urethral sphincter. A small circular muscle that is quite unsubstantial compared with the other muscles within the pelvic floor.

I know that "holding" involves the external urethral sphincter holding the urethra closed, but this is a small muscle so why was I expecting to remember a big contraction?

That is when I came up with the balloon analogy. If you fill a balloon full of air, you increase the pressure within that balloon. So much so that if you let go of the balloon, it will fly around the room as air flows out, normalizing the pressure within the balloon to match the pressure outside of the balloon. The bladder (detrusor muscle) is like a balloon. It is filled with urine rather than air, but the principle is the same.

Now, imagine filling a balloon full of air and trying to hold it closed with a clenched fist. It would be much more difficult than closing it with the pinch of your fingers, right? Well, the same is true for the urethra. The external urethral sphincter muscle doesn't require a huge amount of energy to close the urethral opening. It is simply pinching the balloon closed. This is a subtle contraction, not a massive, big strong contraction. The visualization of pinching the balloon closed helped me to remember that subtle sensation that I had previously used to hold my pee and that, for me, changed everything.

➡ To do this ⬅

1. Sit comfortably in a chair with your eyes closed, hands resting on your legs.
2. Bring your mind back to a time when you were continent and try to remember the subtle sensation of holding.
3. Focus your awareness on the area beneath your bladder and try to feel just that area with your mind.
4. With the memory of continence, imagine that your urethra (pee pipe) is a balloon and pinch the balloon closed.
5. Relax your pelvic floor and repeat the exercise 5 times.

Once you have done this exercise a few times, you can begin to use it when you go to the bathroom. Feel yourself "pinch the balloon closed" for a moment before you relax your pelvic floor to urinate. This is a great way to feel control as you consciously decide to release the urine. Once you have finished urinating, you can consiously "pinch the balloon closed" once more, signifying the return to holding.

Once you are familiar with this sensation, you can remember continence in situations where you may normally leak. Interrupt your incontinence episodes with this memory. This can be viewed as a method to steer your nervous system back to the functional reflexive action of holding, helping to reduce the symptoms of your stress incontinence.

Also, a bonus tip for those of you that are still fully continent. Pay attention to how continence feels in your body so you can remember that sensation should you ever need it!

SUI Strategy 4

Post Void "Free Kegels"

Urination is sometimes followed by a secondary/double void also known as "after pee dribble," a few drops that come when you have already finished your void. This after pee dribble can happen before or after you stand up. This strategy helps to reduce and eliminate double voids or "after pee dribble." I call them "free Kegels" because they are not part of a regimented exercise program but instead are free to use as you choose (like a little bonus).

Exercise
to utilize "free Kegels"

➡ To do this ⬅

1. Before wiping following urination, contract the front portion of your pelvic floor for a count of two (this is element three of a full Kegel—"hold your pee").
2. Relax your pelvic floor for a count of two.
3. Repeat ten times.

This exercise should be performed when you have finished urinating before you wipe yourself. Adding these "free Kegels" helps build in additional consistency with your pelvic floor training. Consistency really is the key to success with any training program. I also believe that the best pelvic floor exercises are the ones you do, so do some regular pelvic floor exercises and you will see results.

SUI Strategy 5

Sit to Stand Pressure Management

One of the first things an infant learns when becoming mobile is how to stand up and sit down. If you have ever watched an infant when they begin to become mobile, you will notice that they tend to wobble a bit when getting up and they subsequently "flop" back down. No control or stability. As we grow, we learn how to get up and sit down with control and stability due to the development of strength in the legs and glutes.

Do you ever think about how you make these movements now? As we age, the tendency to "flop" down becomes more prevalent. The tendency to pull ourselves up also increases. A wee touch of laziness can accumulate over time resulting in weakness in the muscles that should power these movements, making it feel like a chore to stand up. This can contribute to pelvic floor instability.

I encourage you to pay attention to how you stand up and sit down. Notice if you are using the big strong muscles in your legs and backside, or if you have begun to flop down instead. Being aware of how you make these movements gives you the opportunity to ensure you are using your legs and glutes.

If you leak when getting in and out of the car or when you transition from sitting to standing (or vise versa), this exercise can help to reduce these leakage episodes. Like "*the knack*", this exercise will pre-tension the pelvic floor before making the movement; However, the difference with this practice is that you will hold the contraction throughout your movement (e.g. from sitting to standing).

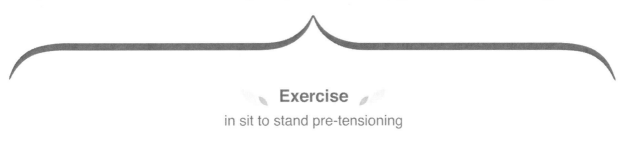

Exercise
in sit to stand pre-tensioning

➡ To do this ⬅

1. Start in a seated position. You should engage your pelvic floor and core before standing by performing a moderate contraction of your pelvic floor (RPE-5 on the pelvic floor RPE scale). This is the level of contraction that you can sustain for a few minutes.

2. With this contraction held, shift your upper body forward to shift your weight toward your feet then press through your midfoot using the strength of your legs to bring you to a standing position.

3. Throughout this movement from seated to standing, maintain the RPE-5 contraction of

your pelvic floor.

4.   Relax your pelvic floor and take a breath in standing.

5.   Recontract your pelvic floor (RPE-5) holding the contraction and use the strength of
      your legs to help you lower, bending at the knees and sitting gently back into the chair.

Similar to the knack, this practice begins as a top-down control of pelvic floor muscles when moving from sitting to standing and vice versa. Eventually, this pre-tensioning of the pelvic floor will become an automated bottom-up reflexive action, which will help to support you moving thoughtlessly and fearlessly without leakage.

SUI Strategy 6

Return to Running

Stress incontinence is quite common in athletes with one study showing 41% of female athletes suffer from the condition[84]. If I had not taken up running, I am unsure if I would have discovered my PFD, at least not in my twenties and possibly not even in my thirties or forties.

Alas, it was running that revealed my pelvic floor weakness and so you may think that strategies to return to running would have been top of my list for the training for this book. To be perfectly honest, I think that returning to running following incontinence should be the subject of its own book.

I have spoken to many women around the world who don't want to stop running while they rehabilitate their pelvic floor. If running is an important part of your life, incontinence can make it feel that your life is over and old age has prematurely set in.

Even though you may feel this way, **you should stop running**, at least for a month or two while you work on the early phases of training, particularly if your incontinence is moderate or severe. Continuing to run could overload your system and exacerbate an already compromised pelvic floor. You should, instead, work on the eight phases of training to help rebalance the tension through your body before you resume running, and then you should take it slowly.

For the return to running strategies, I would like you to think back to the goal-setting exercise in

Chapter Eight. We chose our end goal and reverse engineered our way back to our current situation. If you wanted to run 10 km without leaking, you should first be able to run 5 km or 1 km without leaking. If you want to be able to run 1km without leaking, you need to be able to walk 1 km without leaking. Getting from walking to running without leaking requires progressions that help you adapt to faster more dynamic movements (like those in Phase Eight at the advanced level).

If stress incontinence when running is your most impactful symptom, I expect you have already set running goals, and in that case, these strategies will give you some extra progressive steps that you can include in your program to help you achieve your leak-free running goals. These strategies are as follows:

1. **Leakage management and pessaries for urethral support**: We have already covered multiple leakage management products (pads, liners, EVB shorts, and tampon-style pessaries) in the previous section. These products can be used to manage small leakages while you run. If you also suffer from POP, I recommend you use a pessary to provide support for your prolapse when you run and try to run on softer surfaces (think running track or grass) as this will reduce the ground reaction forces when running.

2. **Cycle timing for running**: Timing your runs in line with your menstrual cycle is something I don't often see discussed, but it is really important to consider where you are in your menstrual cycle, particularly if you are leaking when running. You may recall that in Figure 8.14 we reviewed the cervical position in relation to the menstrual cycle. This can have an impact on your running, particularly if you also suffer from POP.

    If you leak while running, try to avoid running immediately before, during, or just after your period as your cervix is at its lowest during this time. Once you can run in the "high and dry" stages of your cycle without leakage, and you have learned to control intra-abdominal pressures, you can try to resume running during the low-wet times of the month.

3. **Graded running exercises to compliment your empowerment program**: You should have already completed your assessments and selected the correct phase of training based on the results of your assessments. You may recall that your pelvic floor assessment was the primary driver for selecting the training phase. To complement this program, the following exercises should be added to the relevant phase if your goal is to return to running.

    a. **Preparation level running exercises**: You should add a thirty-minute walk to your training each day. The goal is to have a leak-free walk. *Note*: I have not specified a distance. I would like you to walk at a pace that is comfortable for you to take without leakage.

You should STOP if you feel urgency symptoms or if you feel like you may leak. You can "remember continence" or perform the "tap into your superpower" exercise to relax your bladder until the symptoms subside and then resume walking. Only move to the next phase when you can walk for thirty minutes at a comfortable pace without stopping once and with no leakage.

b. **Beginner-level running exercises**: You can perform these exercises every second day. March on the spot for four minutes at a walking pace then march on the spot for one minute at a running pace. Alternate between four min walking and one min running pace for thirty minutes. You are doing this in your home rather than going outside so there should be less fear of leaking.

It can be nice to do this exercise on a small trampoline as it's softer under the feet. You can buy one with a handrail, which you can hold while you march. Alternatively, you can practice similar drills in a swimming pool. The water is very supportive and provides some extra resistance for your legs.

When the exercise begins to feel easy, subtract one minute from the time at walking pace and add it to the time spent at running pace (e.g., three minutes walking and two minutes running). Continue making these time changes until you can comfortably march at a running pace for four minutes and a walking pace for one minute without any leakage, after which, you can progress to the next phase.

c. **Intermediate level running exercises**: At this level, you can take your first run outside. You should begin with a running motion but at a walking pace. Try to run slow and steady, ten minutes out and ten minutes back (rather than focusing on a specific distance).

If you feel any urgency or feel you may leak, STOP and use some of the earlier strategies to stop leakage and delay urination. You can practice this running exercise three times per week, only moving to the next phase when you are able to run comfortably for twenty minutes continuously without leakage.

d. **Advanced running exercise**s: At the advanced level of training, your pelvic floor should be strong and respond well to dynamic movements. The pelvic floor and movement modules at this level of training are already preparing your pelvic floor for fast and dynamic shifts in intra-abdominal pressure. It is at this level that you can work to move beyond just slow steady short distance runs. You should not be experiencing leakage during these drills. If you do, ease off and work at a lower level.

This level of run training is broken into three parts:

i. **Drills**: You will perform running drills over a 20 m stretch of flat terrain (preferably running track or grass). Perform each drill over 20 m and then walk back to the starting point. As a runner, you should already be familiar with how to perform these drills. The drills are as follows: high knees, butt kicks, power skips, Left side to side skips, and right side to side skips. Following these drills, you can work on some sprinting drills with 60%, 70%, and 80% effort. You should be able to complete these drills without leakage.

ii. **Hills**: You can perform your hill work either on a nice hilly terrain (my preference) or on a treadmill with a suitable gradient (3 or above). Take shorter strides on the uphill portion and longer strides on the downhill portion. Choose a distance that suits your goals.

iii. **Endurance**: At this stage, you can begin to build on your running endurance. If you have a target of 10 km as your top goal, you should increase your distance by 1 km each week until you reach this goal. All runs should be comfortable and leak-free.

When you have reached the advanced stage of the program, you should hopefully achieve your running goals without experiencing leakage. You should also have learned a lot about the patterns at play in your body and should adapt your training to complement your natural rhythms. Always meet your body where you find it. Give it the support needed to rehabilitate and the grace of time to do so.

Additional Note

I have consistently advised that you undertake training and add strategies based on the advice from your healthcare provider. **I would like to add further caution here:** if you have just given birth or are recovering from pelvic surgery, make sure to take medical advice before you recommence running. Postpartum running should typically not be resumed until at least twelve weeks postpartum. With recovery from surgery, it can be even longer. Your doctor will tell you what the right time for your specific body is.

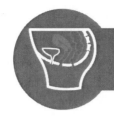

	OAB	SUI	MUI	UR
	Overactive Bladder	Stress Incontinence	Mixed Incontinence	Urinary Retention

Mixed incontinence is a combination of the symptoms of OAB/urgency combined with some elements of stress incontinence. If you are suffering from mixed incontinence (like I was following my mesh-removal surgery), you should focus on the OAB symptoms first before tackling the stress incontinence symptoms. You should use the strategies already outlined for OAB/urgency and stress incontinence to manage your mixed incontinence.

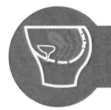

	OAB	SUI	MUI	UR
	Overactive Bladder	Stress Incontinence	Mixed Incontinence	Urinary Retention

With UR, it can be difficult to start the flow or to urinate at all. It can sometimes be caused by the pelvic floor muscles failing to relax sufficiently, however; in women, it is more commonly caused by POP creating a kink in the urethra. As retention can be life-threatening, it is important to seek urgent medical help if you are unable to urinate.

If you are suffering from UR due to a hypertonic pelvic floor, it can help to practice reverse Kegel exercises rather than exercises that contract the pelvic floor. The relaxation and mind/meditation modules can also help in this case. Catheterization (which is the insertion of a pipe through the urethra into the bladder) or medication may also be offered. You can read more about these treatments in Chapter Eleven, section one. The following five strategies can help if you are suffering from UR, your healthcare provider can advise if you should try them:

UR Strategy 1: *Timed voiding*—It can help to void on a schedule if you are suffering from retention. This will help to ensure that you empty sufficient volumes throughout the day, particularly if you are not feeling the urgency to empty. You should empty at least every 3 hours.

UR Strategy 2: *Pelvic Floor Relaxation Practices*—If your retention is due to a hypertonic pelvic floor, make sure that you actually sit on the toilet seat so you can completely relax your pelvic floor, do not hover over the toilet seat. It can help to elevate your feet slightly if you can't fully place your feet on the floor. It can help to have something to lean your upper body on. You can place a chair facing away from the toilet and rest your arms and forehead on it.

Closing your eyes, you can send relaxation through your entire body. It can help to have a tap running so you can listen to the sound of the water running, which sometimes helps to stimulate the bladder to let go. Keep relaxing your vulva as though blossoming your flower as you allow your pelvic floor to relax completely.

UR Strategy 3: *Urethral Splinting*—If your retention is due to a POP, it can help to wear a pessary to help straighten out the kink in the urethra. Urethral splinting, a practice where you use either your fingers or a splinting device to provide some support to the front wall of the vagina can also help.

UR Strategy 4: *Hokey Cokey double void (HCDV)*—Techniques for double voiding are often proposed when the patient suffers from urinary retention. The name HCDV came compliments of one of my clients who coined the term due to having to do the Hokey Cokey in order to fully empty.

These techniques vary from shifting the weight from left sitting bone to right sitting bone when sitting on the toilet, to getting up, and doing a bit of a Hokey Cokey to get things moving before sitting down to go again. Although double voiding can be seen as a dysfunctional voiding pattern, it can be an important tool for those who suffer from retention.

UR Strategy 5: *Self-Catheterization*—Your doctor may offer you a catheter to allow you to empty your bladder manually. This works by inserting a catheter pipe through the urethral opening and up into the bladder in order that it can be emptied. You will be given professional help when learning to use the device and should follow the instructions provided by your healthcare professional and the manufacturer.

UR is less common in women than the other urinary symptoms and tends to require additional treatments so please do see your doctor as soon as possible if you are experiencing UR. That completes the strategies for the management of urinary symptoms. We will now focus on the strategies for fecal symptoms.

Symptom Management Strategies for Fecal Symptoms

In this section, we will review the fecal symptom-management strategies listed in Table 10.2.

	FLATULANCE & Skidmarks	FI Fecal Incontinence	CC Chronic Constipation
Strategy 1	Post defecation "free" Kegels	Leak management	Sena tea
Strategy 2		Post defecation "free" Kegels	Magnesium citrate
Strategy 3		Learning "the knack"	Psyllium husks
Strategy 4		Sit to stand pressure management	Ground flex seed
Strategy 5		Tuning-in to your "superpower"	Probiotics
Strategy 6		Avoiding anal sex	Increase physical activity
Strategy 7			Abdominal massage

Table 10.2: Symptom-Management strategies for fecal symptoms.

Table 10.2 shows the fecal symptom in the top row with the strategies for that symptom listed beneath.

Fecal symptoms tend to be discussed less, in particular, FI, which, although less common than urinary incontinence, affects 20% of women with urinary incontinence. FI is one of the most embarrassing conditions with a huge psychological impact. Sometimes it can be a symptom of another condition, for example, if you have a gastrointestinal infection causing diarrhea, you could experience FI while normally being able to maintain continence. In this section, we will review strategies to help manage and improve fecal symptoms.

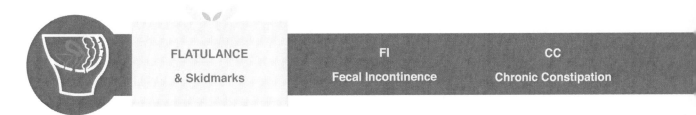

FLATULANCE & Skidmarks	FI Fecal Incontinence	CC Chronic Constipation

Flatulence, skid marks, or a bum that never seems to wipe clean after defecation can all be indications of a weakness of the anal sphincter. Flatulence is considered to be an issue only if you can't hold in a fart in an inopportune moment. Imagine sitting in a job interview, the final round of interviews where you have the HR manager, the CEO, and the Chairman of the board all diligently questioning you about your suitability for the position. If you are unable to hold in a fart in that situation, this is an indication that there could be weakness in the anal sphincter.

While skid marks and a bum that never seems to wipe clean are less obvious and possibly less embarrassing, these are early indications that there may be weakness in your anal sphincter. To help address these symptoms, you can add "free Kegels," following each defecation, before wiping:

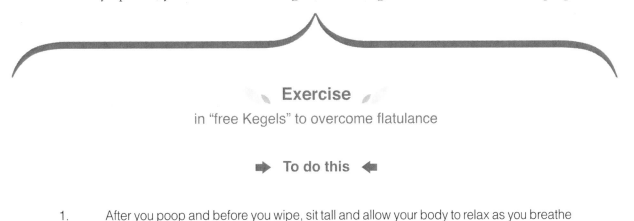

Exercise
in "free Kegels" to overcome flatulance

➡ To do this ⬅

1. After you poop and before you wipe, sit tall and allow your body to relax as you breathe gently.

2.   Contract the anal sphincter for a count of two (this is element four of a full Kegel—"hold your poop").

3.   Relax your pelvic floor for a count of two.

4.   Repeat ten times.

I like to call these "free Kegels" as they are a complement to your pelvic floor training and are "free" rather than being a set part of the phased training. These "free Kegels" will help to strengthen your pelvic floor and should also reduce the amount you need to wipe to get your bum clean after pooping. As your anal sphincter becomes stronger, you should also find it easier to hold your farts.

This tip to do Kegels before wiping was given to me by Beate Carrière, author of *Fitness for the Pelvic Floor*. She is an absolute legend among pelvic floor physiotherapists and I was very privileged to meet her at a conference in Geneva.

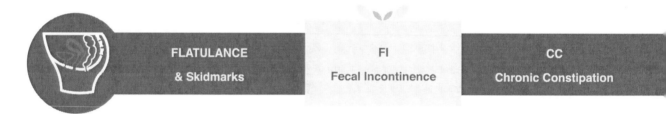

FLATULANCE
& Skidmarks

FI
Fecal Incontinence

CC
Chronic Constipation

Like stress incontinence, FI can be a result of an imbalance in intra-abdominal pressures. If you have listed FI as one of your symptoms on the symptom assessment sheet, the pelvic floor, breathing and movement modules of the eight-phase program can help you to retrain the balance of tension and the management of intra-abdominal pressure, which should contribute to an improvement of symptoms. It is important to seek medical advice if you suffer from FI. Bowel retraining (which is discussed in section two of Chapter Eleven) may be helpful in managing FI but should only be undertaken under the advice and guidance of your healthcare provider.

There are six strategies proposed that can help to manage and improve the symptoms of FI. Some refer to strategies outlined earlier in this chapter. The remaining will be detailed in the upcoming pages. An overview of these strategies is listed below.

FI Strategy 1:   *Leak management*—a strategy to ensure protection is available to delay or mask embarrassing leaks.

FI Strategy 2: *Post defecation "free Kegels"*—For this, you should utilize the "free Kegels" exercise that has been outlined for flatulence. (**See Flatulence Strategy 1**).

FI Strategy 3: *Learning "The knack"*—For this, you should use "*the knack*" strategy that was outlined for stress incontinence. This will teach you to pre-tension the pelvic floor before coughing, sneezing, laughing, or other high-pressure activities. (**See SUI Strategy 2**).

FI Strategy 4: *Sit to stand pressure management*—For this, you should use the sit to stand pressure management strategy that was outlined for stress incontinence. This will help maintain continence when moving from sit to stand and vice versa. (**See SUI Strategy 5**).

FI Strategy 5: *Tuning-in to your "superpower"*—learn to listen and respond to your defecation reflexes.

FI Strategy 6: *Avoiding anal sex*—less of a strategy and more of some general advice.

FI Strategy 1

Leak Management

Managing fecal leakage is unfortunately not as easy as managing urine leakage, however, the following products can help to protect against leakage. These protective products are detailed in Chapter Twelve and are summarized below:

FI pads are available to help with fecal leakage. These are not the same as menstrual pads or incontinence pads. They have a wider section at the back to help prevent embarrassing stains on clothes. They are suitable for mild to moderate leakage.

FI disposable pants are specifically designed to hold fecal matter (again, these are not the same as the incontinence pads). These are similar to pull-ups or nappies and can deal with more severe leakage including more runny poops.

Anal plugs act to block the anal passage until you are in a position to empty your bowel. Similar to a tampon, they can be inserted into the rectum and discretely remain in place. These can be purchased on Amazon or from your local pharmacy and may also be available on prescription.

These products can really make a difference if your FI is preventing you from moving or socializing. It is important to stay active and stay social to maintain good physical and mental health, so use whatever products you need to support you as you work toward your empowerment.

FI Strategy 5

Tuning-In to Your "Superpower"

The process of defecation, like that of urination, involves reflexes that you learn to tune in to as a child. We learned about those reflexes in Chapter Five where we also reviewed the importance of removing the anal kink by elevating the knees above the hips when defecating (please do take heed of that advice). With this strategy, we will aim to enhance our "reflex listening" skills.

Reflexes can be subtle, like a whisper. If we do not listen and respond to the whispers of our nervous system, we are reprogramming those reflexes as our failure to respond by, for example: finding a toilet and emptying the bowels, we are sending a message back to the nervous system that its signals are invalid, which can contribute to dysfunction. With this exercise, we are going to listen and respond to the signals we receive from our reflexes. This technique should help you to make it to the bathroom without leaking:

Exercise

in "tuning in" to help manage FI

➡ To do this ⬅

1. If you refer back to Chapter Five, you will see that the first defecation reflex is the "intrinsic myenteric defecation reflex" or as I like to call it, the "I feel like I need to poop" reflex. This reflex moves the poop toward the exit, which, in turn, relaxes the internal anal sphincter. The first step in this exercise requires that you sense this first reflex, no matter how subtle it feels.

2. If your anal sphincter is relaxed when you get this sensation, defecation can occur. This is why it is so important to sense that first reflex. Immediately upon sensing the reflex, relax your body contract the anal sphincter (this is element four of a full Kegel— "hold your poop"). You should contract with the maximum strength possible for a count of ten. This sends an inhibitory signal to the nervous system. You should feel the urgency reduce when you do this.

3. Relax the contraction of your anal sphincter from the maximum possible down to an RPE of 5 (a contraction that you can hold for a longer time) and make your way immediately to the bathroom to defecate.

This technique becomes more effective the stronger your anal sphincter becomes. It is important to empty when your body sends the signal. If you are defecating frequently, this could indicate some stiffness in the rectum, which could require bowel retraining and visceral mobilization (a massage to help mobilize the rectal tissues to allow for filling). Bowel retraining is beyond the scope of this book so see your healthcare provider if you feel it could be needed in your case.

FI Strategy 6

Avoiding Anal Sex

This strategy may seem contentious, so for clarity: this is not a command, nor a requirement, nor a judgment of your choices. I am simply suggesting that if you are suffering from fecal incontinence, you avoid anal sex for a while, as studies show that anal sex is a risk factor for FI[85].

If you do practice anal sex and suffer from FI, perhaps take a break from anal sex while you work on strengthening your anal sphincter. Then when you do have anal sex again, make sure to use plenty of lubrication, have at least 35 degrees of hip flexion while having anal sex (to remove the kink from the rectum), and perform the pelvic floor exercises from Phase 6 of the pelvic floor module following your intercourse. This should go a long way to helping you to manage and hopefully improve your FI.

That concludes the strategies for fecal symptoms. We will now address strategies for dealing with chronic constipation (CC).

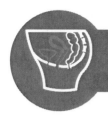

CC is a fecal symptom that can have a detrimental impact on your pelvic floor while also potentially increasing the symptoms of POP. If you suffer from CC, your doctor may have given you medication to help. If you take medication, you should consult your doctor before adding herbal supplements or other dietary supplements. The following strategies can help with CC:

CC Strategy 1: *Senna Tea*—Senna is an herbal tea produced from flowering plants that have laxative properties. Drinking this type of tea can have a stimulating effect that can help to relieve constipation.

CC Strategy 2: *Magnesium Citrate*—A good magnesium citrate supplement can help to promote regular bowel movements. Magnesium citrate pulls water into the intestines, which can help if your poop is dry and hard. You should drink sufficient fluids if you are using this type of supplement.

CC Strategy 3: *Psyllium husks*—Psyllium husks are a dietary fiber supplement that can sometimes help to add bulk to your stools. This supplement soaks up water and so it is important to ensure you are drinking sufficient water. For some people, psyllium husks have a very positive effect on digestion, for others, it can leave stools too bulky making them more difficult to pass. Your healthcare provider can guide you if this is a good option for you.

CC Strategy 4: *Ground flax seeds*—Ground flax seeds can often help to make the poop more slippery while also having a stimulating effect. There have been many studies into the benefits of eating ground flax. Ground flax has similar chemical properties to estrogen and one study showed that it can have a positive impact on menopausal symptoms[86].

However, the European Food Safety Authority (EFSA) issued a report that suggested that ground flax seeds could expose people to toxic levels of cyanide. Ground flax was immediately removed from the market in Sweden and sensational UK headlines suggested potential poisoning from consuming the seeds. Subsequently, the EFSA issued a statement downplaying the impact of flax and pointing out that there have been no reported cases of linseed poisoning[87]. You should speak with your healthcare provider before deciding whether to add ground flax seeds to your diet. *Note*: the unground seeds are not viewed to have the same cyanide issue although they are also believed to have less of an effect on CC.

CC Strategy 5: *Probiotics*—Probiotics are believed to support the healthy bacteria that live in your digestive tract (part of your microbiome). A 2019 study suggested that an imbalance of gut microbiota can contribute to constipation[88]. However, there was no clarity on what type of probiotics could be the basis for treatment, so I believe more research is needed.

CC Strategy 6: *Increase Physical Activity*—Sedentary lifestyles can negatively impact on digestion. One study showed that colon transit time in active females (the time it takes for food to transit through the colon) was significantly faster than in non-active females[89]. Slower digestion can contribute to constipation. By maintaining a good level of physical activity, you are less likely to remain constipated.

By following the eight-phase program of empowerment, you are making a commitment to be consistently more active. You can add a target step count to your day to complement your training. Start by first counting your steps (using a pedometer or smartwatch). When you know your average daily steps, you can incrementally increase your steps by 500 per week, until you are averaging 10,000 steps per day.

CC Strategy 7: *Abdominal massage*—Massage of the large intestine can be a helpful way to stimulate your digestive system. Massage should be performed lying down with knees bent. It can also be nice to use massage oil (I like coconut oil for this purpose). It is good to be close to a bathroom when you perform the massage as it may stimulate the need to poop rather quickly. Figure 10.2 shows the path you should take with the massage.

The green arrow in Figure 10.2 is indicative of the circular motion with the blue arrow showing the direction of the massage. Steps to perform the massage are detailed below:

Steps To Perform Abdominal Massage

1. Starting at the bottom right side of your abdomen just above your hips, make small circular movements progressing those movements up toward your ribcage.

2. When you reach the area just below your ribcage on the right, begin to make small circular movements across your abdomen toward the left.

3. When you reach the left side beneath the rib cage, make small circular movements moving down toward your abdomen on the left just above your hips opposite to where you started.

That covers the strategies for fecal symptoms. You can choose which of these strategies to implement based on your own symptoms.

Next, we will explore strategies for POP. There are some additional strategies for incomplete emptying in the strategies for POP that can also prove useful for those with constipation.

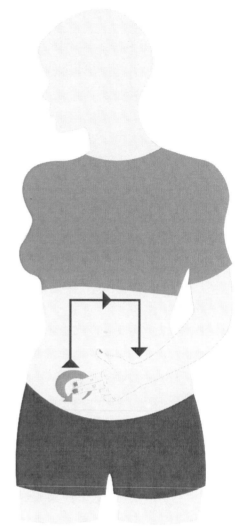

Figure 10.2: How to perform abdominal massage for constipation.

Symptom Management Strategies for Pelvic Organ Prolapse (POP)

In this section, we will review the POP symptom-management strategies shown in Table 10.3.

	HEAVINESS & "golf ball"	FECAL Incomplete defecation
Strategy 1	Intravaginal structural support	Sing while you poop
Strategy 2	Avoid constipation	Don't stay all day
Strategy 3	Avoid excessive coughing	Splint if you need to
Strategy 4	Maintain healthy BMI	Reconsider stimulants
Strategy 5	Manage intra-abdominal pressure	Enema
Strategy 6	Listen to your body	Don't be afraid of straining
Strategy 7	Cycle timing for exercise	

Table 10.3: Symptom-management strategies for POP.

Table 10.3 shows the POP symptom in the top row with the strategies for that symptom listed beneath.

You may have additional urinary or fecal symptoms if you are suffering from symptomatic POP. If so, you can utilise the strategies listed previously in this chapter.

If you have pelvic organ prolapse, it is really important that you visit a pelvic floor PT to have your pelvic floor checked. There could be scaring and fascial adhesions, resulting in an imbalance of tension that exacerbates your symptoms. There are various myofascial release techniques and visceral manipulations that can be performed by aptly trained pelvic floor PTs which can help.

A study[90] in August 2019 on the development of a biotensegrity focused therapy for the treatment of POP found that the release of taut pelvic tissue improved pelvic organ position while improving symptoms. This is just the first study that ties together the tensegrity of pelvic structures with the symptoms of POP.

I believe that this study highlights the importance of understanding the web of connectivity. It shows the benefit of approaching POP from a more therapeutic holistic approach rather than just offering surgery as a first line treatment that introduces even more scarring and taut tissues.

If your POP is producing pain symptoms, you can utlize strategies from the pelvic pain section later in this chapter.

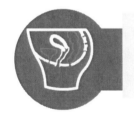

HEAVINESS	FECAL
& "golf ball"	Incomplete defecation

When it comes to dragging, heaviness, the feeling of a golf-ball in the vagina or a sensation like you have a tampon falling out; The pelvic floor, breathing, movement and relaxation modules of the eight-phase program should really help to improve those symptoms. The following strategies can also help to reduce the impact of your symptoms:

Heaviness Strategy 1: *Intravaginal Structural Support*—Pessaries can provide structural support within the vagina that can greatly help to relieve the symptoms of POP. They come in many shapes and sizes and include varieties that are either supportive or space filling (space filling pessaries cannot be used during intercourse). You can read more about pessaries in Chapter Eleven, where we explore the treatment options for POP.

It is best to visit a pelvic floor PT or another pelvic health professional to get fitted for a pessary. Once they are fitted, they are typically left in place and are changed every three to six months. Tampon-style pessaries are useful to try if you have POP, particularly if your POP is low grade. Tampon pessaries can give you a feel for whether you would benefit from a fitted pessary. Wearing a pessary while exercising can also provide extra support, which can be of benefit while you work on the empowerment program.

Heaviness Strategy 2: *Avoid constipation*—I cannot emphasize enough how important it is to avoid constipation if you have POP. A 2005 study by the University of Pennsylvania found that women with POP are at a higher risk for constipation than controls[91]. This increase was partially explained by a lower intake of dietary insoluble fiber by women with prolapse than controls, but it is still an interesting finding as I have personally experienced how bearing down can have a negative impact on prolapse.

Constipation is actually the only thing that makes my POP feel symptomatic. I do not measure the success of my day based on the things I manage to achieve at work or at home. Instead, I measure my success based on my ability to poop. If I manage to poop without straining or constipation, then my day has been a success. You can utilise the CC strategies detailed earlier in this chapter to help you avoid constipation.

Heaviness Strategy 3: *Avoid excessive coughing*—A study into the functional anatomy of the female pelvic floor with stress incontinence found that the intra-abdominal pressure from a sudden hard cough results in increased pressure on the pelvic floor requiring it to stretch by 1 cm. This may not sound like much, but try to lift your pelvic floor by 1 cm—not so easy, right? Each cough is like a little punch. If you keep punching your pelvic floor, you will weaken it. Chronic coughing can worsen the symptoms of POP so it's best to avoid smoking and try to avoid catching colds or getting Covid19 (if you can).

Heaviness Strategy 4: *Maintain a healthy BMI*—Your BMI is calculated by dividing your weight in kilograms by your height in meters squared. A study designed to define "normal" intra-abdominal pressure noted that "Body mass index was positively related to intra-abdominal pressure." This means that a higher BMI will have a higher level of intra-abdominal pressure. Increases in intra-abdominal pressure are believed to impact POP and weight is a risk factor for prolapse with vaginal or uterine prolapse being more common in overweight women[92]. Lots of great reasons to maintain a healthy BMI.

Heaviness Strategy 5: *Manage intra-abdominal pressure*—The management of intra-abdominal pressure will help greatly when suffering from POP symptoms. The eight-phase training program goes a long way toward teaching you to manage pressures and balance tension throughout your body. Supplemental to this, you can utilize "the knack" and "sit to stand pressure management" strategies in the SUI strategy section of this chapter.

Heaviness Strategy 6: *Listen to your body*—Listening to your body is even more important when you have POP. When you suffer from POP, what you can or cannot do is very much dictated by the length-tension relationship at play within your own tissues. For one woman, squatting may cause no issues. For another, it could make her prolapse symptoms more noticeable. The lines of tension in your tissues will not be the same as the lines of tension in the person next to you. By listening to your body, regardless of whether you are exercising, stretching, or just pottering around the house, you gather valuable information on how your body responds to different movements.

You should adapt your exercises and other movements to support your prolapse. There is one yoga pose that triggered my rectocele symptoms and that was *supta kurmasana* also known as sleeping turtle pose, which is shown in Figure 10.3.

As you can see in Figure 10.3, the pose involves bringing the legs over the back

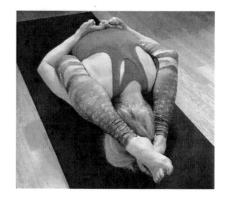

Figure 10.3: Supta kurmasana (sleeping turtle pose).

of the shoulders. Hands are bound behind my back, almost like tying myself up in a knot. The feet should be crossed behind the neck—I clearly did not have the flexibility for this pose. Pushing my body into this position was not good for my prolapse and so I no longer include it in my practice. You will encounter poses or movements that do not suit your body. Do not even hesitate about dropping them from your practice. Remember that you are responsible for your own pelvic health so, listen to your body.

Heaviness Strategy 7: *Cycle timing for exercise*—We have already discussed the menstrual cycle in relation relation to running within the SUI strategy section. This is something that you also need to consider when exercising with prolapse. Figure 8.14 revealed cervical positions in relation to the menstrual cycle. The change in size and position of the womb that is normal during your cycle can have an impact on the level of your symptoms.

If you feel very symptomatic around your period, reduce the level and intensity of your workouts. It can be good to practice Phase 1 restorative yoga (relaxation module). Take the opportunity to sit down when you can and elevate your hips if that helps to relieve your symptoms. As your pelvic floor gets stronger, and you begin to rebalance your body, you should find that your symptoms ease and you may even get through your cycle without feeling symptomatic.

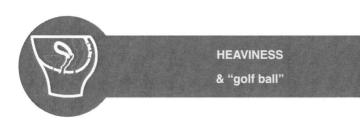

| HEAVINESS & "golf ball" | FECAL Incomplete defecation |

When it comes to the symptoms of incomplete emptying with POP, the strategies are very much centered around managing your defecation experience. These strategies can also be helpful if you suffer from CC.

Fecal Strategy 1: *Sing while you poop*—Singing, humming and other vocal tactics can be used to prevent you from excessively bearing down when you poop. Straining places unnecessary stress on the pelvic floor and can worsen the symptoms of POP.

Singing creates a gentle contraction of the abdominals that helps to maintain balanced intra-abdominal pressure. It also helps to calm the nervous system which provides the conditions needed for peristalsis to function (the contractions of smooth muscle to evacuate poop from your rectum).

Remember you don't have to rush your poop - rushing is stressful. Take your time, and make up a new poop song to help you to relax while you poop. I would rather do a relaxed unforced poop and be late for a meeting than struggle to force a poop out quickly in order to get to the meeting on time... I do measure success in poop after all!

Fecal Strategy 2: *Don't stay all day*—If you get the urge and go to the bathroom but the urge leaves you, don't try to force it out. Walk about for a while, perform abdominal massage, put a hot water bottle on your tummy, drink plenty of water and wait. The urge should return within a day or two.

Fecal Strategy 3: *Splint if you need to*—If you have a rectocele (a POP where the bowel pushes into the vagina), that can prevent you from fully emptying your bowel leaving you with that constant feeling that you have not emptied. In that instance, it is possible to use either your fingers or a "splinting device" to press gently against the back wall of your vagina toward your rectum to help with the evacuation. A spliting device looks a bit like a small shoehorn.

Another splinting method is to make a "V" shape with your fingers. Reaching around behind you, putting the base of the "V" at your tailbone. Place one finger on either side of your anal sphincter and press gently. If you cannot empty fully without splinting, do splint. It's better to splint than to strain hard to get the last of the poop out.

Fecal Strategy 4: *Reconsider stimulants*—Certain stimulants, such as coffee and nicotine can trigger the urge to defecate. I have always been prone to constipation and when I was in my early twenties, I had given up smoking but when I would struggle to poop, I would run to a neighbor's house and take a few drags from her cigarette to stimulate my bowel.

Smoking is an extremely unhealthy bowel stimulant. Did you know your risk of developing PFD increases if you smoke? I would suggest that you do not use cigarettes as a stimulant. In my thirties, I began to drink coffee and it worked like magic. Stimulants can work very well when applied on occasion, however, the stimulating effects diminish as your body adjusts to their presence.

If you drink a lot of coffee, you might find that it eventually fails to stimulate your bowel. It can also irritate your urinary system. If you suffer from cystitis, you need to weigh up the benefit of your morning coffee with the potential bladder irritation. Your need for stimulation will be greatly reduced if you eat a balanced diet, do not snack between meals (to allow for a break between digestion phases), and listen to your reflexes. If you suffer from constipation and get even the slightest wee hint of "I have to poop," go directly to the bathroom.

Fecal Strategy 5: *Enema*—An enema is an injection of fluid into your rectum to help clean out the bowel. There is a lot of disagreement around whether or not they are safe/healthy so the decision to try one should be taken with consultation from your healthcare provider.

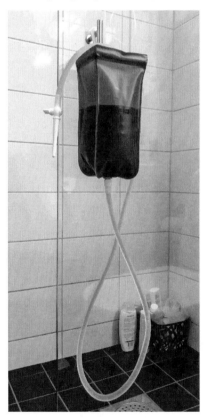

Figure 10.4: A coffee enema.

Enemas range from over-the-counter ready-to-use enemas (can be prescribed by a doctor) to home enema kits. I have one of these kits and have tried the coffee enema (see Figure 10.4), which was rumored to stimulate the liver to release toxins. I subsequently did some research only to find that coffee enemas are not backed by scientific evidence and can have severe adverse events so, I suggest you skip the coffee enema even if you read online that they are great[93].

Fecal Strategy 6:   *Don't be afraid of straining*—After everything I have said about straining, I think it is important to reassure you that you should not be afraid to utilize controlled intra-abdominal pressure to aid defecation. If you do need to strain when pooping, make a gentle *valsalva* (bearing down/straining motion) but not at maximum strength. Try RPE-4 on your "bearing down" scale. Then hold that pressure using your abdominal muscles and begin to sing your poop song. Singing will ensure that you are not excessively straining. If you suffer from prolapse, this method is less likely to make you feel symptomatic than a strong bearing down.

With these symptom-management strategies, you are empowered to manage your prolapse symptoms while you continue to work toward the blossoming of your flower.

That concludes the strategies for POP. We will now focus on the symptoms of pelvic pain, which are the final symptoms listed on our symptom assessment form.

Symptom Management Strategies for Pelvic Pain

In this section, we will review the symptom-management strategies for pelvic pain, which are outlined in Table 10.4, which shows the pelvic pain symptoms on the top with the strategies for that symptom listed beneath.

Pelvic pain is a broad term that encompasses more than just musculoskeletal PFD conditions (which are covered in this book). At the beginning of this book, in the "how to use this book" section, I explained that this book does not cover mensuration, conception, pregnancy, or menopause. At the start of part two, I expanded this list further to include endometriosis, IC, PCOS, and other conditions that can cause PFD symptoms, but are not musculoskeletal in nature.

If you have any of those conditions, or PFD based, you should work with your healthcare provider to decide on your treatment options and follow their guidance regarding any practices, exercises, or activities that you may choose to help you deal with your pain.

Pelvic pain is extremely prevalent and is often accompanied by urinary or fecal symptoms, which we have already explored. The eight-phase program, detailed in Part Two, can help to address some causes of pelvic pain, and we shall explore some additional strategies within this section that may provide further relief from painful symptoms.

	CPPS Chronic pelvic pain syndrome	BPS Bladder pain syndrome	SEXUAL PAIN Vaginismus, dyspareunia, vulvodynia
Strategy 1	Heat or cold	Refer to CPPS and OAB strategies	Avoid vaginal irritants
Strategy 2	TENS		Vaginal dilation
Strategy 3	Reverse Kegels & ball sitting		Doing "the work" on sex
Strategy 4	PNF Stretching		Switching "on" arousal
Strategy 5	Doing "the work" on your pain		Masturbation for self-pleasure
Strategy 6	Massage		Set the scene for sex

Table 10.4: Symptom-management strategies for Pain.

Chronic pelvic pain syndrome (CPPS) also known as CPP is regularly occurring pelvic pain lasting for more than 6 months without a sinister cause (with sinister being infection, disease, or tissue pathology). You should not diagnose yourself with CPPS. It is important to have your pain investigated by a relevant healthcare professional to rule out infection, disease, or other sinister cause. Very often those who receive a diagnosis of CPPS have been through multidisciplinary clinical investigatory tests and tissue pathology assessments with no issues found.

CPPS can dramatically impact physical performance and reduce QoL. A recent World Health Organization (WHO) systematic review of high-quality studies with representative samples found CPPS was prevalent in 2.1%–24% of women[94]. Pain can be debilitating, making you feel old beyond your years.

Remember back to what we learned in Part One of this book when exploring the business of the body's movement. If you become injured, your nervous system will inhibit certain muscles (employees) to protect the area of injury. When the injury has healed and the tissue damage has been repaired, your nervous system will not automatically default back to the original pattern of movement. You must train it actively to return to a functional pattern of movement.

The same can be true for pain. The nervous system initiates pain signals as a protective mechanism to prevent you from using a body part that is under repair. You sense the pain, and you also learn from that pain sensation. If you injure your shoulder, you will likely choose to move it less while it is injured. The challenge arises when the injury has healed. Your nervous system doesn't always know that the injury has resolved, and it may continue to send pain signals following recovery. I believe that increased tension and stiffness from injury contributes to these continuing pain signals.

In order to manage your pain, you first need to have an understanding of the mechanisms of pain. Professor Lorimer Moseley and David Butler do a great job of explaining how pain functions in the *Explain Pain Handbook*[95]. They use a "protectometer" that helps you to identify DIMs (danger in me) and SIMs (safety in me). If you suffer from any pain condition, I advise that you also read their book.

A DIM is something your nervous system interprets as a danger in you. Let's imagine you've had a shoulder injury that has subsequently healed. You go to lift your arm overhead, which you should be able to do as the injury has healed, but your nervous system remembers the danger, so it sends you a pain signal. That is a DIM.

In order to combat the DIM, you need to send a message to your nervous system to communicate that there is safety (a SIM). An example of a SIM is movement. As we learned in Part One, we communicate with the nervous system through movement, thoughts, and touch. Movement provides physiological evidence of safety to your nervous system. Thoughts provide psychological evidence and touch can combine the two.

When rehabilitating that shoulder injury, your physiotherapist will have you perform movement exercises, often moving into your pain, as that communicates a message of safety to your nervous system. They may desensitize the tissues with physical touch, and they will reassure you the whole time, giving you the psychological reassurance that combines to allow your nervous system to let go of the protective tone.

Many of the exercises within the eight-phase program are designed to help communicate safety to your nervous system and they should help to dampen and hopefully eliminate your pain signals.

There are strategies in this section that can be helpful if you have a chronic pelvic pain condition where your healthcare provider has already ruled out any sinister cause. The strategies are summarized below and explained in more detail in the pages that follow:

CPPS Strategy 1: *Heat or cold*—A strategy to apply heat and/or cold to ease pain signals
CPPS Strategy 2: *TENS*—A strategy to use transcutaneous electrical muscle stimulation (TENS).
CPPS Strategy 3: *Reverse Kegels & ball sitting*—A strategy to relax the pelvic floor muscles.
CPPS Strategy 4: *PNF Stretching*—A strategy to inhibit hypertonic muscle contractions.
CPPS Strategy 5: *Doing "the work" on your pain*—A strategy to question your thoughts regarding your pain.
CPPS Strategy 6: *Massage*—A strategy to release excess tension from pelvic floor muscles.

These strategies can be used individually or in combination when you are in pain. You can review them with your healthcare provider before implementing them.

CPPS Strategy 1

Heat or Cold

For some, the use of heat and/or cold can ease the symptoms of pain. For others, heat and/or cold can exacerbate pain. The only way to know if it is helpful for your specific pain is to try it for yourself. Personally, I find that a hot water bottle placed under my low back or on my lower belly can help when I experience pelvic pain. An ice pack (or a hot water bottle that has been in the freezer), for me, does not produce the same pain-relieving effect.

CPPS Strategy 2

TENS

TENS (Transcutaneous electrical nerve stimulation) is a pain therapy that has been around since the 1960s[96] and in portable form since 1974. It is used to treat many different types of pain. In the case of CPPS, TENS is typically used to stimulate nerves that innervate the pelvis and lower limb.

Sometimes TENS can be used to interrupt pain signals to/from the lower limb. In this case, skin electrodes are placed around the tenth thoracic vertebrae. This spinal location is around the same level as your belly button. The idea is that it places a distraction between the brain and your place of pain. One study found this to be an effective treatment having two patients whose pain was completely resolved with many others showing great improvement[97].

As with all PFD treatments, you should only use TENS under the guidance of a healthcare professional, and always follow manufacturer guidelines when using TENS devices. The devices for pelvic floor stimulation are generally not TENS devices and should not be used in place of a TENS device unless indicated by the manufacturer and confirmed by your healthcare provider. You can read more about these devices in Chapter Twelve.

CPPS Strategy 3

Reverse Kegels and Ball Sitting

If you are suffering from pelvic pain, you can perform reverse Kegel exercises in place of the pelvic floor exercises that are detailed in the eight-phase program. You can find instructions on how to do reverse Kegel exercises in the Phase 1 pelvic floor module in Chapter Nine where you will also find information on ball sitting (where you sit on a ball or sock to enhance pelvic floor relaxation prior to performing reverse Kegels).

CPPS Strategy 4

PNF stretching

In Chapter Eight we reviewed the four different types of stretching, one of which was facilitated stretching (also known as PNF). PNF techniques were developed in the 1940s by Dr. Herman Kabat and Physiotherapist Maggie Knott. PNF is a method of stretching that takes advantage of the intricacies of the business of your body's movement by stimulating the department managers (Golgi tendon organs) to inhibit muscle contraction. In yoga, we use the technique to increase flexibility, which is an important aspect of overcoming muscle hypertonicity.

In the relaxation module of the eight-phase program, there are various yin yoga exercises that help to passively release the pelvic floor. The following facilitated stretching exercises offer a more active pelvic floor release. Both techniques can be found on *The Flower Empowered* YouTube channel. If you have knee issues, these exercises may be inaccessible for you. You can check with your healthcare provider if you are unsure.

Figure 10.5 shows the PNF technique for posterior pelvic floor release.

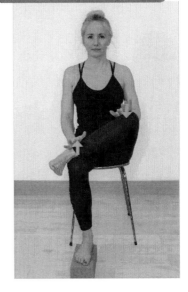

Figure 10.5: Posterior pelvic floor release using PNF stretching.

The image on the left in Figure 10.5 shows the *active stretch* of this PNF technique with the green arrow showing the direction of gentle hand pressure used to actively stretch. The image on the right in Figure 10.5 shows the *counter contraction* of this PNF technique. The green arrow highlights the direction of movement of the contraction, while the blue arrow shows the resistance from the hand. The steps to perform this exercise are detailed below.

Steps to perform posterior pelvic floor release using PNF stretching

1. Sit upright tall in a chair with feet flat on the floor (use a step or yoga blocks if your feet do not comfortably reach the floor).
2. Rotating at the hip, bring your right leg, just above the ankle onto your left leg, just above the knee.
3. Place the palm of your left hand on your right ankle and the palm of your right hand on your right knee.
4. **Active Stretch**: Using your right hand, apply gentle pressure to lower the leg as much as possible into this external hip rotation (as shown in the image on the left in Figure 10.5). Hold for a count of five.
5. **Counter Contraction**: Push your right foot up into your right hand as though you are trying to raise the foot up toward the ceiling, all the while maintaining a neutral spine and resisting the movement of the knee with your hand (as highlighted by the blue arrow in the image on the right of Figure 10.5). Do this for a count of five. *Note*: You can lean your upper body forward slightly to increase the stretch if your leg is lowered to be in line with your hip.
6. Repeat Steps 4 and 5 until you have done each five times, then relax in the position for a count of twenty.
7. Perform the exercise on the opposite side.

You should notice that your ROM increased throughout the exercise, indicating a release in muscular tension, which should help with the release of tone on the posterior (back) of the pelvic floor.

The next technique focuses on releasing the anterior (front) portion of the pelvic floor, which is shown in Figure 10.6. The image at the top in Figure 10.6 shows the active stretch of this PNF technique, with the green arrow showing the direction of gentle pressure to actively stretch.

Unlike the previous exercise, this image does not show the use of the hand to facilitate the active portion, but you can place your hand on your hip, applying gentle pressure to the backside to increase the active stretch. Try to relax the inside of your leg (adductors) while you do this.

The image at the bottom in Figure 10.6 shows the counter contraction of this PNF technique, with the green arrow highlighting the direction of movement of the contraction, and the blue arrow showing the resistance from the hips, which you should keep in position.

The contraction here activates the adductor muscles in the same movement you would use to close your legs.

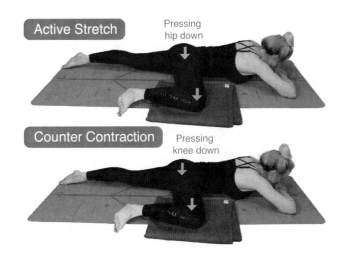

Figure 10.6: Anterior pelvic floor release using PNF stretching.

To perform this technique, you will need a yoga mat and a folded blanket. The blanket is required to create padding under your knee (or knees if you do both legs at the same time).

Steps to Perform Anterior Pelvic Floor Release Using PNF Stretching

1. Lie on your side on your yoga mat with a folded blanket alongside your body.
2. Bend your right knee as you rotate at the hip, resting your knee on the blanket with 90 degrees of hip flexion and 90 degrees of knee flexion. The inside of your foot should be resting on the floor.
3. Turn your body to bring the inside of your leg to rest on the floor.
4. **Active stretch**: Actively send your right hip to the mat as you relax the adductors on the inside of your legs. Your gluteal muscles will drive the contraction in this active stretch.
5. **Counter Contraction**: Making sure your knee is resting on the blanket then press your knee into the blanket as strongly as possible while maintaining the position of your hips. You will notice the adductor muscles have to contract hard for this movement (the equivalent movement to closing your legs). Press for a count of five.
6. Repeat Steps 4 and 5 until you have done each five times, then relax in the position for a count of twenty.
7. Perform Steps 1 to 6 on the opposite side.

You should notice that your ROM increased throughout the exercise, indicating a release in muscular tension. This should help with the release of tone on the anterior (front) of the pelvic floor. These PNF stretches increase flexibility around the hips while helping to trigger inhibitions to various muscles in the hips and pelvic floor. If you find these exercises to be helpful, you can practice them once or twice per week or use them actively to relieve pelvic floor spasms or pain. I sometimes experience painful spasms in the anal sphincter following orgasm and these techniques have been effective in stopping those spasms.

CPPS Strategy 5
Doing "The Work" on Your Pain

In the mind/meditation module of Phase 3, you learned how to do Byron Katie's "the work," on your negative thoughts. If you are suffering from pelvic pain, I would advise that you also do "the work" on your pain. To do this, you should write out everything you think and believe about your pain and follow the steps detailed in the exercise detailed in the Mind/Meditation module of Phase 3.

What you think about your pain can impact how your pain manifests in your body as your thoughts are another mechanism for communicating with your nervous system. As much as possible we want to communicate safety to the nervous system through our thoughts and actions. By doing the work, you can turn negative thoughts around and begin the work of changing your mind.

CPPS Strategy 6
Massage

If you had marked pelvic pain as a symptom on your symptom assessment and your flexibility assessment highlighted tension or pain, you should consider adding vulvar/vaginal massage to your weekly schedule. We will cover two massage techniques in the massage section later in this chapter. Your healthcare provider can help you to decide if either of these techniques could be helpful for you.

That finishes the strategies for dealing with chronic pelvic pain. We will now discuss strategies for BPS.

| CPPS Chronic pelvic pain syndrome | BPS Bladder pain syndrome | SEXUAL PAIN Vaginismus, dyspareunia, vulvodynia |

BPS and bladder spasms sometimes fall under the umbrella of chronic pelvic pain. BPS is a condition where there is no infection, disease, or tissue pathology present. The strategies offered for chronic pelvic pain can sometimes provide benefits if you are suffering from BPS. Additional to these strategies, you can use the "tap into your superpower" strategy from the OAB section as that strategy taps into your guarding reflex to send signals that can trigger bladder relaxation.

That concludes BPS symptom management. We will now review vaginal pain conditions that are commonly associated with painful sex. These include vaginismus, dyspareunia, and vulvodynia.

| CPPS Chronic pelvic pain syndrome | BPS Bladder pain syndrome | SEXUAL PAIN Vaginismus, dyspareunia, vulvodynia |

The final set of symptom strategies relate to sexual pain. Specifically; vaginismus, dyspareunia, and vulvodynia. I have grouped these three conditions together as they can be difficult to differentiate[98,99]. With these conditions, pain isn't necessarily associated with sex, however, all of these conditions can cause painful sex, which will be the focus of this section so the strategies will be marked as "sexual pain" for ease of reference.

Dyspareunia is defined as pelvic or vaginal pain associated with sexual intercourse. Vaginismus is defined as an involuntary contraction of the pelvic floor muscles, which makes sexual intercourse difficult or impossible. With vaginismus, it can also be difficult to insert tampons so the condition is not solely related to sex.

Vulvodynia is another vulvar/vaginal pain condition (without infection, disease, or tissue pathology). It can happen without any specific trigger (such as sex), which differentiates it from vaginismus and dyspareunia, which are triggered by physical touch.

Remember—do not self-diagnose. You should have your pain checked by a healthcare professional.

Another important consideration if you are suffering from one of these conditions is your history in relation to sexual abuse. A study[100] by the University of New Mexico highlighted that a history of sexual abuse was common in women presenting with pelvic floor complaints. Chronic pelvic pain had the strongest association with sexual abuse. I would encourage you to seek therapy to work through the abuse if you have not already done so, or at the very least, do "the work" on your abuse. I have done both (therapy and "the work") and found both to be beneficial.

Once you have been diagnosed, you can use the training in the eight-phase program, along with the strategies for pain management described earlier in this section to help reduce your symptoms. Supplemental to these strategies, you can also utilize the strategies in this section to further manage your symptoms. These strategies are summarized below and detailed in the pages that follow:

Sexual Pain Strategy 1: *Avoid vaginal irritants*—A strategy for happy superficial vulva & vaginal tissues.

Sexual Pain Strategy 2: *Vaginal dilation*—A strategy to train the pelvic floor muscles and tissues to manage penetration.

Sexual Pain Strategy 3: *Do "the work" on sex*—A strategy to change negative thoughts regarding sex and sexuality.

Sexual Pain Strategy 4: *Switching "on" arousal*—A strategy to use clitoral stimulation to turn on the lubrication, relaxation, and lengthening of vaginal tissues.

Sexual Pain Strategy 5: *Masturbation for self-pleasure*—A strategy to learn what turns you on and to encourage you to find pleasure in your genitals.

Sexual Pain Strategy 6: *"Set the scene" for sex*—A strategy to "set the scene" to make your nervous system feel safe for sex.

These strategies can be combined with those from the CPPS strategies if your pain is prolonged or experienced at other times.

Sexual Pain Strategy 1

Avoid Vaginal Irritants

Did you know that the vagina is self-cleaning? Your lovely lady flower is maintained by your vaginal microbiome. One in three women in the United States douche or use other vulvar/vaginal cleaning products even though these products can cause many adverse effects including increased risk of gynecological issues, increased risk of STDs, and increased risk of bacterial infections. One 2010 review[101], which evaluated 181 studies found that "Douching alters the vaginal flora and predisposes women to develop bacterial vaginosis (BV)."

That same review also highlighted that "Douching is associated with adverse pregnancy outcomes including ectopic pregnancy, low birth weight, preterm labor, preterm birth, and chorioamnionitis." Chorioamnionitis is a bacterial infection that can occur before or during labor.

Save yourself all the potential risk by following these tips for good vaginal hygiene:
1. Avoid using baby wipes, scented soap, shampoo, bubble bath, scented lotions, vaginal douching products, or other feminine hygiene products on your vulva/vagina.
2. Avoid soaking in baths with any of the above-listed products in the bathwater.
3. Shower clean using only a small amount of hypoallergenic soap to clean the outer labia majora always cleaning from front to back.
4. Always wipe from front to back after urination or defecation.
5. Ensure your partner has brushed their teeth and washed their hands before sex.
6. Ensure your partner does not rub from back to front during sex as this can bring bacteria from the anus into the vagina and/or the urethra, which can cause BV or urinary tract infections.
7. Always urinate after sex. This will help to flush the urethra should any bacteria have entered.
8. Don't scrub the skin on your vulva.
9. Air dry or gently pat dry with a soft towel.
10. Take an occasional sitz bath: This is just a shallow pool of fresh water with a small amount of salt. It should have a similar salinity to tears. If you mix 4 cups of water (940ml) with 2 teaspoons of salt (12g) that should be sufficient. You can use pre-boiled water (that has cooled sufficiently) and stir the salt in so it dissolves. The small amount of salt can have an antibacterial effect but it's not something you should do every day.

These tips should help to protect your vulva/vaginal health, which is imperative for a functional and healthy sex life.

Sexual Pain Strategy 2

Vaginal Dilation

If you suffer from vaginismus, you may well be familiar with vaginal dilators or "trainers" as they are often referred to. Dr. Amanda Olsen, the founder of Intimate Rose, has developed some nice vaginal dilators in eight different sizes. You can find links to her products from the sexual dysfunction page on theflowerempowered.com.

Dilators are typically sold as devices that "stretch" the vagina; however, we have already learned that we are not necessarily "stretching" tissues but rather communicating safety to the nervous system in order that hypertonicity or overly contracted muscles can relax.

In Part One of this book, in Chapter Five, we learned that the clitoris is the *on* switch for arousal and that vaginal tissue responds to sexual arousal by creating lubrication while relaxing and lengthening. We will explore this further in Sexual Strategy 4. For this exercise, you will learn how to use vaginal dilators without stimulation.

You should set the scene as you have done when taking your pelvic floor assessments in Chapter Eight. Make sure you have some spare pillows for this exercise as well as those that you will place behind your back. Make sure your hands and the dilators have been cleaned with hypoallergenic soap before use. It can also be useful to have lubrication close to hand. I prefer coconut oil. You can lubricate both the dilators and your vagina before you begin. Vaginal dilation can be performed with a partner if you feel comfortable. Lubricate dilators and vaginal opening before you begin.

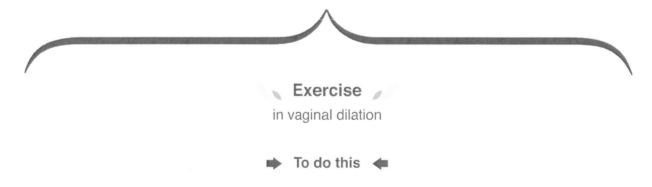

Exercise
in vaginal dilation

➡ To do this ⬅

1. Remove your underwear and lie back on your pillows, starting with your knees bent and your feet under your knees.

2. Relax your legs open. If your legs do not rest comfortably on the bed when you open them, place pillows under your legs for support. This will ensure that your adductor muscles (on the inside of your thighs) can let go of tension. This is important as these muscles have fascial connections to the pelvic floor so they can impact its tension.

3. Close your eyes and perform ten calming breath cycles while thinking calm and safe

thoughts. You can run your fingers along the inside of your thighs as you relax in this position. This will give you an indication if you are relaxed enough to try dilation. If running your fingers on the insides of your legs makes you feel like snapping your legs closed, this could indicate that you are not yet ready to move forward with dilation and should work on feeling safe with your legs spread.

4.   Once you are relaxed, you can begin with the smallest dilator. Bring the tip of the dilator to the opening of your vagina and allow it to gently slide in. If you meet a wall as you insert the dilator, take a few breaths. Make sure your adductor muscles are relaxed and perform some reverse Kegels. This should help the deeper muscles, that are creating the barrier, to relax.

5.   Press the dilator in until the handle is close to the vaginal entrance, then begin to gently slide it out again.

6.   You should slide it in and out ten times. You also have the option of leaving it in but, in my opinion, some movement of the dilator is better as movement communicates more to your nervous system than just leaving it in place.

If you are comfortable with that size, you can try the next size up. If you find the smallest dilator is too big, you can begin with a Q-tip (cotton bud). As with pelvic floor exercises, consistency is key. You should practice dilation six days per week until you can do it without any issue. You don't need to work through every dilator the first time you try, and you are not under time pressure to get to the larger sizes. Remember you are working to communicate safety to your nervous system so try to let go of emotional and physical tension as much as possible.

Sexual Pain Strategy 3

Do "The Work" on Sex

We learned in Chapter Six how to use Byron Katie's "the work" on our thought trains. Performing this exercise on your thoughts around sex can be useful if you suffer from vaginismus, dyspareunia, or vulvodynia. To do this, you should perform the ANT therapy detailed in the Mind/Meditation module of Phase 3. Instead of writing general negative thoughts, I would like you to write your thoughts, fears, and opinions of sex and your sexuality.

You can also complete this exercise with regards to your thoughts about your condition, or even with your thoughts about using tampons or period cups if your condition prevents you from using them.

This is for your eyes only, so be very honest with yourself as you work through those thoughts. This exercise has helped me to drop some of the guilt and shame that was the product of my Catholic upbringing. I hope you find it to be beneficial too.

Sexual Pain Strategy 4
Switch "On" Arousal

You may have heard the term "flick the bean," which is used to denote stimulation of the clitoris (which is very much like a wee bean). Well, in my opinion, you are not flicking the bean when you stimulate the clitoris, you are instead flicking the *on* switch!

We have learned in Part One that the vaginal tissue responds to sexual arousal by lubricating, relaxing, and lengthening. If your partner is male, they may be unaware of the importance of clitoral stimulation. They may well go straight to penetration. That was how the majority of my sexual encounters went until I plucked up the courage to take control sexually.

Vaginismus is a condition in which the pelvic floor muscles contract involuntarily, indicating that the nervous system is protecting rather than becoming aroused and creating the necessary opening. Dyspareunia can be caused by a lack of lubrication, a lack of opening, hypertonicity, or spasms before, during, or after sex.

Flicking the *on* switch could be the difference between success and failure when it comes to sex. Clitoral stimulation is a method you can use to communicate to your nervous system. You are telling your nervous system that you want to become aroused.

It isn't going to magically fix everything if you have been suffering from vaginismus, dyspareunia, or vulvodynia for some time, but it will provide you with a very valuable tool. The strategy here is to always use your *on* switch before you try penetration. Before giving the job of flicking the switch to your partner, you should figure out how your switch works, and that is what we will explore in the next strategy.

Sexual Pain Strategy 5

Masturbation For Self-Pleasure

Hopefully, you already know exactly how to stimulate yourself to orgasm, and hopefully, you are also comfortable with allowing your partner to bring you to clitoral climax. If not, you have work to do!

Orgasms are a treat, and I believe every woman deserves to experience orgasmic delight. The strategy here is to learn how to please yourself, and to learn how to allow someone else to please you.

There are so many techniques that can be used for clitoral stimulation. We have spent so much of this book learning about patterns. When you think of clitoral stimulation, you should also think in terms of patterns. Consistency and repetition are generally key ingredients to good clitoral stimulation. You could opt for a consistent side-to-side stimulation, or maybe a circular motion. Maybe you like the feeling of moving it up and down or perhaps you like the feeling of rhythmically tapping it with your finger. The nervous system tends to like patterns and consistency.

With that said, heightened anticipation when there is no regular pattern can also produce excited arousal. For example, if you use the water spray from your shower to stimulate your clitoris. The water jets are inconsistent. Some will "hit the spot," some will miss. You'll be left guessing and longing for those "hits" that lead to climax.

Of course, you need to ensure that the water pressure isn't strong as that could hurt, and we want to avoid pain. Less water pressure is probably a better option if you want to try that.

If you remember back to the flexibility assessment, you were pressing gently as though you were checking the ripeness of a piece of fruit. You should use a similar level of pressure when you are stimulating the clitoris. Think sensual rub rather than deep tissue massage. It should not take much pressure due to the large number of nerve endings in the area.

You can also use a masturbation session as an opportunity to practice penetration. Clitoral stimulation can produce an aching feeling within the vagina. If you have been suffering from vaginal pain, it can be easy to confuse this ache with a pain signal. Try to imagine instead that it is an ache that can only be resolved by feeling inside your vagina with the dilator (or a penis). Use a size you are comfortable with and try sliding it in and out while you are stimulating your clitoris.

I should also add… if you are having negative thoughts about masturbation, or about that ache to have vaginal penetration, please do "the work" on those thoughts. These are all normal human desires, human nature, managed by your nervous system to ensure the survival of our species. Your vagina will want to have a penis (or a dilator) in there. The corrupt lens of your conditioning can make these sensations and thoughts feel bad, and I am here to tell you that they are not.

When you figure out how to fully pleasure yourself, you can share that wonderful knowledge with someone deserving of it. Teach your partner what it takes to please you and learn what it takes to please your partner. This is very empowering and will greatly improve the quality of your life.

Sexual Pain Strategy 6

"Set The Scene" For Sex

So, this strategy may seem a little silly or out of place after all the masturbation talk, but this is an important step in making your nervous system feel safe. If you have learned how to please yourself, and you want to teach your partner how to please you, doing so in a place where you both feel safe and comfortable is important. This strategy is all about setting the scene for sex.

Setting the scene doesn't just mean lighting a few candles and playing Barry White in the background. You have to think about what makes *you* comfortable. If this is the first time you will be guiding your partner through the proper use of your *on* switch, maybe you want to talk things through first, leaving some time before giving it a try. Every relationship is different. Communicating your intimacy needs with your partner can really strengthen your relationship.

When setting the scene, make a point of leaving judgment and performance pressure outside the door. Use a lighting level that makes you feel safe. If you are turned on by the visuals, maybe you want the full lights on. Otherwise, opt for softer lighting, or even darkness. So long as you are working to overcome your condition, your nervous system should be the one setting the scene.

The goal for your first session shouldn't be penetration. It should be to allow your partner to stimulate you to orgasm. Coming to climax requires that you let go of control. You have to surrender and trust your partner. You can guide your partner's hand and give instructions as needed. You can even show them how it is done by bringing yourself to climax in your partner's presence. Not only are you empowering yourself to let go, but you are also empowering your partner by teaching them how to please you, and that is a beautiful gift in any relationship.

It is important that you also learn how your partner's pleasure works, I am sure they will be happy to teach you. Being open enough to speak and act intimately enables a deepening of trust. The deeper your trust, the safer your nervous system will feel. When you feel ready, you can try again with penetration.

Overcoming pain associated with sex is possible. Don't give up hope. Be really compassionate with yourself as you work through these pain conditions and remember, your empowerment is in your hands.

We are now finished with symptom management and will shift our focus to the life strategies that can contribute to a permanent change in your patterns.

Life Strategies to Support Pelvic Floor Function

In this section, we will review the life strategies listed below:

1. **Posture adaptations**: using the posture assessment.
2. **Massage**: using the flexibility assessment.
3. **Self-care**: using the life pattern and mind assessments.

These life strategies are outlined in Table 10.5 on the next page.

| | POSTURE | MASSAGE | SELF-CARE | | | |
	Adaptations	Techniques	Movement	Diet & Nutrition	Sleep hygiene	Self-Care
Strategy 1	Finding a neutral pelvis	Massage to improve circulation & sensation	Step Goal	Increase NEAT	Sleep Equipment	See a therapist
Strategy 2	Floor sitting	Massage to reduce pain	Stand Goal	Tweak your diet	Wind down before sleep	Pamper yourself
Strategy 3	Kicking off your heels		Stability ball sitting	Avoid stress eating	Sleep Schedule	
Strategy 4	Wall standing		Alternate sitting positions		Spend time in daylight	
Strategy 5	Morning routine for posture				Block out noise	
Strategy 6					Weighted blanket	
Strategy 7					Mouth taping	

Table 10.5: Life Strategies to support your empowerment.

The top row of Table 10.5 shows the areas of focus for our life strategies. These include posture adaptations, massage techniques, and self-care strategies focused on movement, diet & nutrition, sleep hygiene, and other self-care practices. We will begin this section with a review of the posture adaptation strategies.

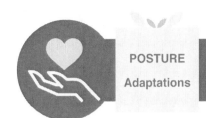
We will now utilize the posture assessment that you completed in Chapter Eight. When you completed the assessment, you were looking for postural imbalances. It is best to visit a structural integrator for a full and proper assessment. If needed, they can help with myofascial massage to adjust the pattern in your tissues in order to help with the rebalancing of your body.

Posture is dynamic, not static. The intention here is not to *force* you into a rigid posture that is considered "*neutral*," but instead to gently support positive adaptations to your posture. Changes from working on the eight-phase training, and any manual therapies you are undertaking for the purpose of improved posture, are more likely to be sustained when you implement the strategies listed in this section.

The pattern of your daily life creates a shape that, over time, is held in place by your connective tissues. You could view this as an evolution from your current shape into a new more functional shape. Evolution takes time therefore the strategies listed in this section should be maintained over a long period.

This posture adaptation section covers the following strategies, which are summarized below and detailed in the pages that follow.

Posture Strategy 1:   *Finding a neutral pelvis*—a strategy that teaches you where your neutral pelvis is. This will act as a guide for its position when moving/sitting.

Posture Strategy 2:   *Floor sitting*—a strategy to encourage more ROM around hips, knees, and ankles.

Posture Strategy 3:   *Kicking off your heels*—a strategy to bring your heels back down to earth, which will help to support your neutral body alignment.

Posture Strategy 4:   *Wall standing*—a strategy for correcting posture at a standing desk.

Posture Strategy 5:   *Morning routine for posture*—a strategy to encourage the use of ROM through your joints upon waking, helping to support more fluid movement during the day.

Remember that your bones, muscles, and connective tissues are as unique as your face. Trying to stack yourself up like your neighbor is not a good strategy. I would like you to get a feel for what normal posture is for your specific body and what postural patterns have been introduced due to suboptimal movement patterns.

Posture Strategy 1

Find a Neutral Pelvis

In Part One of this book, we learned about the ligaments of the uterus, which we viewed in Figure 3.12. These ligaments form part of the connective tissue network that holds our shape. When the pelvis tilts either posteriorly (flat butt) or anteriorly (duck butt), those ligaments will create lines of tension that can potentially pull on the organs.

Tilting the pelvis also changes the relationship between the pelvic floor and the diaphragm. We visualized that relationship in Figure 3.4 when we reviewed the hydraulics of breathing. A disruption in the relationship between the diaphragm and pelvic floor makes it more difficult to balance intra-abdominal pressures.

Now let's imagine that you are sitting slumped in a chair. For the entire time that you are in that slumped position, your pelvis is tucked under in a posterior tilt. This will create a very specific pattern of tension through the ligaments of the uterus. Those ligaments provide a great deal of support deep within your pelvis. Your pelvic position has a direct connection to your spine, with a posterior tilt reducing the lumbar curve (low back) and the anterior tilt increasing it.

The degree of thoracic and lumbar curvature may be associated with the presence and severity of urinary incontinence according to one Japanese study. Another study[101] concluded that postural changes may be seen more often in women with PFD and suggested that conservative treatment for PFD could include postural corrections.

There are many schools of thought when it comes to finding a neutral pelvis. Figure 4.9 demonstrates one possible method for identifying a neutral pelvis where the pubis symphysis aligns with the ASIS joints. Figure 10.7 shows the different pelvic tilts.

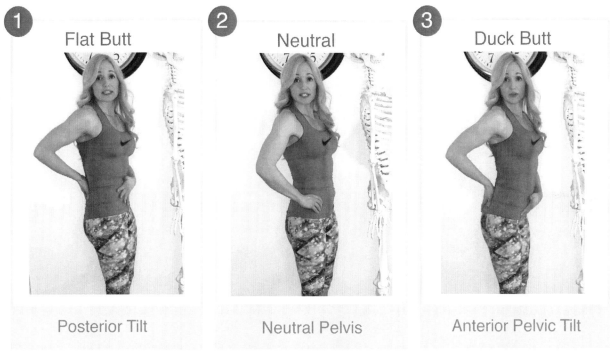

1 Flat Butt	2 Neutral	3 Duck Butt
Posterior Tilt	Neutral Pelvis	Anterior Pelvic Tilt

Figure 10.7: The different pelvic tilts.

The first image in Figure 10.7 shows the posterior pelvic tilt, which has flattened the curve of the low back. The second image shows the neutral pelvis, while the third image shows the anterior pelvic tilt, which exaggerates the curvature of the low back. The following exercise helps you to find your pelvic tilt by feeling an extreme posterior and anterior tilt before coming to a relaxed neutral position.

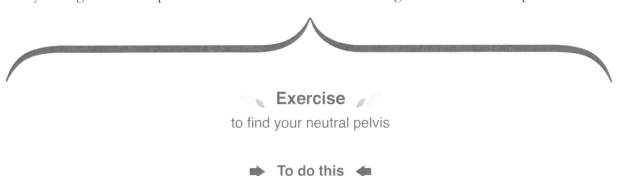

Exercise

to find your neutral pelvis

➡ **To do this** ⬅

1. Stand up, look side-on at a mirror, and identify your ASIS joints. They are the two bony protrusions from the front top side of your hips. I have my finger on these ASIS joints in image 2 of Figure 10.7.

2. Place your left hand on your pubic symphysis, which is where the two hip bones meet just above your mons pubis at the front of your body. I have my left hand on my pubis symphysis in both image 1 and image 3 in Figure 10.7.

3. Place your right hand on your sacrum, which is the fusion of bones below the lumbar spine where the two hip bones meet at the back of your body. I have my right hand on my sacrum in both image 1 and image 3 in Figure 10.7.

4. Tuck your pelvis under so that your pubic symphysis is more forward than your ASIS joints. Notice that this tilt gives the appearance of a flat butt and removes the lumbar curve from your low back.

5. Untuck your pelvis, and stick your sitting bones out behind you so your ASIS joints are more forward than your pubic symphysis. Notice that this gives the appearance of a duck butt and a more accentuated lumbar curve.

6. Bring your pelvis to a central point between these two extremes so your ASIS joints are somewhat in line with your pubic symphysis as shown in image 2 of Figure 10.7. This is a neutral pelvis.

Does the *neutral pelvis* from that exercise feel natural for you? Take a look at your posture assessment. Does your pelvis look neutral in that assessment? It is good to learn what a neutral pelvis feels like, particularly if it was not neutral in your postural assessment. As I have stated previously, body reading is not simple, and, if you feel your pelvis is out of alignment, you should see a structural integrator.

The benefit of learning how to find a neutral pelvis is that you can adjust to a neutral position if you are sitting or standing. For sitting, this would ensure that you are sitting squarely on your sitting bones with a tall spine. For standing, you can tilt your pelvis forward, tilt it backward and then find balance in the middle while extending your spine (imagine a string on the top of your head pulling you upwards). This lengthening of the spine when standing will help you to hold your version of neutral.

Posture Strategy 2

Floor Sitting

When you review your life pattern assessment, if you found that you were sitting in chairs for a large part of your day, I would like you to consider implementing this strategy to help improve your posture.

We learned in Chapter Eight that your connective tissue is the net that holds your shape. We also learned how the pattern of your daily life impacts this shape. You may recall reading that, "If you move every muscle and joint in every direction every day of your life, you are more likely to maintain your agility." This strategy takes this one step further by encouraging you to rest your joints in various positions rather than continually sitting in a single position.

By implementing this change, adding variation to your sitting positions, you will encourage an improvement or restoration of ROM around your hips and spine. This helps to sustain changes in the balance of tension throughout your body that may be coming to fruition if you are working through the eight-phase program.

Sitting on the floor may sound a little childish but you should try it. If you have been sitting on chairs for years, you will most likely find that your body is no longer flexible enough to find a comfortable position on the floor.

Personally, I had not realized that I had lost ROM in my hips and spine until I went to my first yoga class and had to sit on the floor. I discovered that my hips had become extremely inflexible, as had my hamstrings. I am sure my years of running and triathlon combined with sitting in chairs with my tucked pelvis contributed to this loss of ROM. I definitely wasn't using my full ROM on a daily basis and this left me feeling stiff and old.

The strategy is to spend at least thirty minutes each day sitting on the floor. If you watch TV, then that is the most opportune time to practice floor sitting. I suggest you alternate your floor sitting position rather than sitting in a single stiff position. Figure 10.8 shows multiple possible sitting positions that you can cycle through during your thirty minutes on the floor.

You can see in Figure 10.8 that I am sitting in front of my sofa. By sitting in front of your sofa, you provide yourself with a backrest. You can use cushions to help support you so that you can relax into these sitting positions.

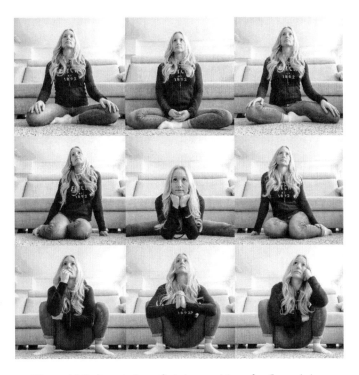

Figure 10.8: A variation of sitting positions for floor sitting.

When I began my practice of floor sitting, I was far from balanced. If you look at Figure 10.8, you will see that I look fairly balanced between left and right. That is due to an accumulation over the past four or five years. My body has rebalanced and the pattern in my tissues has become more functional. You may recall the study where sexologists were able to discern a woman's orgasmic history by observing her gait (walking pattern), which was explained in Chapter Five. This exercise helps to improve hip flexibility, which in turn can improve your gait and, if the results of that study have any bearing, it may also have a positive effect on your orgasms!

You may notice that not all these positions involve actually sitting your bum onto the floor. The positions include:

1. *A passive squat*: This is a great way to get some movement into the connective tissue around your hips.

2. *Resting on one hip*: By bringing both legs to one side or the other, you get a chance to relax asymmetrically into your tissues. This typically highlights a "tighter side." It is very likely that you may be completely comfortable resting to one side and completely uncomfortable resting to the other. I suggest that you spend a little extra time on the uncomfortable side.

3. *Straddle your legs*: Sitting in a straddle position provides an opportunity to stretch the tissues around your low back, hamstrings, and inner thighs. You can also stretch your legs straight out in front of you. In these positions, make sure you sit on your sitting bones rather than slouching. You can put a little towel under your knees if your hamstrings feel very tight.

I like to "opposite myself", meaning that I simply take the opposite position to the one that makes me feel most comfortable. This is similar to what we do when we practice yin yoga relaxing into our own tension/discomfort. When I bend both legs to the right and sit on my left hip, I feel really comfortable. I could sit there all day. When I try the same position on the opposite side, it feels awkward and uncomfortable. I choose to do the opposite of what feels really comfortable as I am trying to passively rebalance my tissues.

If you have dysfunctional patterns in your tissues, moving toward your own discomfort can be equated to moving in the direction of function. You are giving constricted muscles and connective tissues a chance to passively stretch and open. Tiny tissue adaptations will accumulate over time resulting in sustained changes to your posture.

Posture Strategy 3

Kick Off Your Heels

I believe that wearing heels all day every day for 20+ years contributed to my forward-leaning posture. I am not telling you not to wear heels, I am telling you to wear them as seldom as possible. The following tips should allow you to continue to wear your heels without further compounding negative postural patterns.

1. When walking any distance, wear flat shoes. You can bring your heels in your handbag.
2. When wearing heels, try to sit rather than stand.
3. When you take your heels off, massage your feet to get the blood flowing. Curl your toes under and gently press the top of your foot onto the floor to stretch the front of the foot and ankle.
4. Practice picking up a cotton wool ball with your foot (as though it were a hand).
5. Stretch and massage your calves after removing your heels.
6. Roll a tennis ball under each foot for a minute or so before bed.
7. Walk barefoot as often as possible.
8. Walk barefoot on different surfaces such as grass or on sand when the opportunity arises.

Heels really are lovely to look at and they can make you feel sexy while also making the legs look longer, making you feel taller, making the butt look a little perkier. All well and good, but unfortunately not good for your posture. Save them for special occasions and give your pelvic floor the chance to rebalance without them.

Posture Strategy 4

Morning Routine for Posture

The next strategy in our posture adaptation section offers a morning routine that can help to encourage the evolution of your tissues by giving you an opportunity to move your joints when you awaken. You can download the sequence sheet for this morning routine for posture (Figure 10.9) from empoweryourflower.com and keep it by the bed to remind you to practice.

This is a gentle practice, as shown in Figure 10.9, which communicates to your nervous system that you need to have your full ROM available to you. This practice begins in the bed and ends with you standing tall and ready to face the day and should help you to maintain your ROM and agility.

Morning Routine for Posture

Total Time: 5 minutes

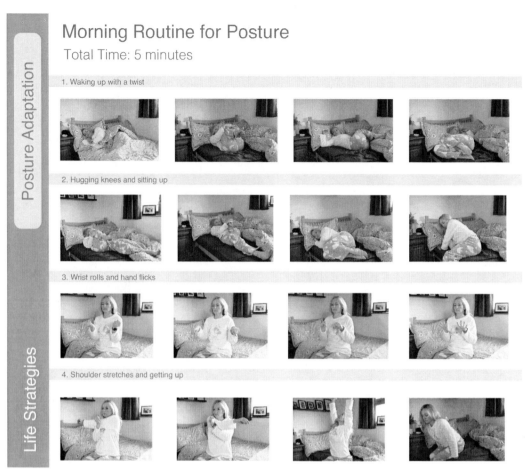

1. Waking up with a twist

2. Hugging knees and sitting up

3. Wrist rolls and hand flicks

4. Shoulder stretches and getting up

Figure 10.9: Morning routine for posture.

Try to rise early enough to perform this routine while leaving sufficient time to get ready before leaving for work. Rising early should also help to minimize the stress levels caused by rushing.

Steps to Perform the Morning Routine for Posture

1 Waking Up With a Twist

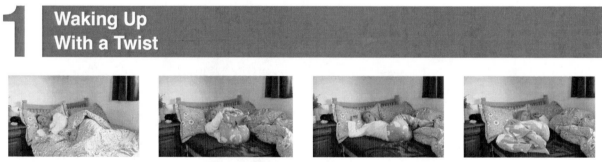

Figure 10.9.1: Waking up with a twist.

1. Ensure that you wake up early enough to go through this routine without rushing or feeling stressed.
2. Hug your knees into your chest, and take a few breaths in this position.

3. Twist your knees to the right side while keeping your shoulders level and gazing gently in the opposite direction.

4. After a few breaths, take the twist to the left.

2 | Hugging Knees and Sitting Up

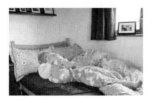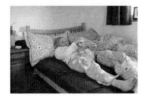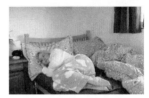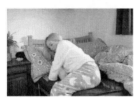

Figure 10.9.2: Hugging knees and sitting up.

1. Extending the right leg, hug the left knee into the chest. Your right leg should stay relaxed on the bed while you make this movement.

2. After a few breaths, take the position on the opposite side.

3. Pull both knees into your chest and turn to face the outside of the bed in preparation for sitting up.

4. Push the upper hand into the bed to gently come to a seated position.

3 | Wrist Rolls and Hand Flicks

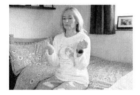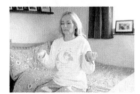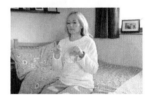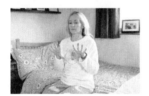

Figure 10.9.3: Wrist rolls and hand flicks.

1. Stretch your hands up over your head, take in a really good stretch with your upper body

2. Make small circles with your wrists first rotating them away from each other and then rotating them toward each other.

3. Close your fists and then flick them open as though you are flicking water on someone.

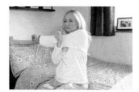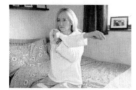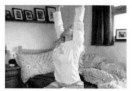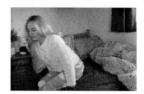

Figure 10.9.4: Shoulder stretches and getting up.

1. Stretch your right arm across your body, gently stretching your shoulder. You can take a few breaths in this position.
2. Take the position on the opposite side.
3. Raise your arms over your head for an enjoyable stretch.
4. Gently bring yourself to a standing position and get on with your day.

Once you are standing and ready to start your day, remember that you are working toward more optimal pelvic floor health and that involves making many small and consistent changes that will accumulate into a fundamental shift away from dysfunction and toward function.

Morning is a great time to implement changes for multiple reasons, my favorite being that you have begun to make improvements before the busy day has started. Rising early ensures that you have time to work out, shower, and eat without stressing about making it to the office on time. Plan accordingly.

Posture Strategy 5

Wall Standing

The final strategy in our posture adaptation section is an exercise to help you to correct your standing posture if you work at a standing desk. When standing, most people have a center of gravity that is not balanced centrally over their base of support (feet). For most of my life, when standing, I would hang all of my weight in one hip, allowing tissues on one side to elongate, while the tissues on the other side had to shorten to support my body. This isn't very good for posture and will result in imbalanced strength and flexibility, which, over time, can accumulate into a dysfunctional posture pattern.

This wall-standing exercise helps to create a little balance before you stand for any length of time. In the office, I do this when I get off my ball to stand at my desk. It ensures I have set a reasonable posture before I settle in to work while standing. It helps you to feel a neutral standing position, which, over time, can teach you to sense when you are off-balance.

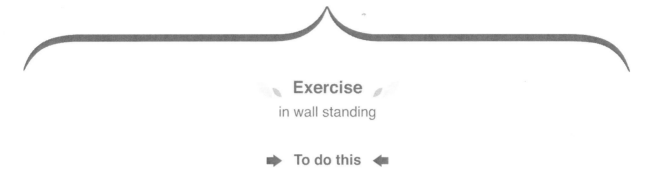

Exercise
in wall standing

➡ To do this ⬅

1. Go to a wall and line your heels with the back of the wall. Notice if your weight is forward. If so, lean backward until your back touches the wall.
2. Check the alignment of your pelvis finding a neutral position where you can elongate your spine.
3. Put one of your hands into the space behind your low back and feel upwards until you come to the bottom of your rib cage. Your ribs here should be touching the wall. If they are not, drop the front your ribcage down a little until the back of your ribcage touches the wall. You should still have that space behind your low back.
4. Relax both arms down by your side. Try to relax the front of your shoulders and gently press your shoulder blades against the wall.
5. Maintain your position against the wall for a minute or so.
6. Step away from the wall, try to maintain that posture as you walk to your desk.
   Note: You shouldn't be rigid. This should be a relaxed position. It gets easier the more you practice it.

This exercise builds postural awareness more than anything else. The eight-phase training program includes many exercises that help to increase strength and flexibility, which should make it easier to perform this exercise as time passes.

This concludes the strategies to help with posture adaptation. We will now review the flexibility assessment and some massage strategies to help with pain relief and reducing tension.

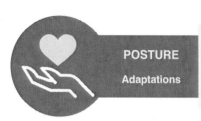
Massage can be an effective tool when suffering from pelvic floor hypertonicity or pain. For this section, we will focus specifically on vulvar/vaginal massage techniques. We will use the pelvic floor flexibility assessment. There are two different massages that you can try depending on your scores. They are summarized below and detailed in the pages that follow.

Massage Strategy 1:   *To improve circulation & sensation*—This is a general massage technique that can be nice to do regardless of your scores.

Massage Strategy 2:   *To reduce pain*—This is a trigger point massage that can be used if you scored four or five for any part of your pelvic floor flexibility assessment.

If you have recently had surgery or are postpartum, you should check with your healthcare provider to see if self-massage should be avoided. You also have the option of going to a pelvic floor PT. They can give your pelvic floor a full assessment as well as releasing any tight or painful areas.

Massage Strategy 1

To Improve Circulation & Sensation

Increasing blood flow and improving sensation can have a very positive impact when you are working to build pelvic floor strength. It can also help if you feel that you have reduced sensation during sex. Like all the exercises in this book, you are using massage as a way to communicate with your nervous system. This massage requests nutrients and encourages repair.

You should set up for this massage in the same way you did for the assessments in Chapter Eight. I like to use coconut oil for lubrication, but you are free to use whichever lubrication you prefer. Massage is all about balance. It should feel nice, not painful.

This is not a deep tissue massage but rather a gentle massage using the same pressure as you would check if fruit is ripe. Happy endings are always allowed when you finish your massage... orgasm is, after all, a great workout for your pelvic floor muscles!

You can refer to Figure 1.3 if you are unsure of the locations of the different parts of the female vulva. For this massage, you will use the vulva clock, shown in Figure 10.10, as a guide to the area that you are massaging.

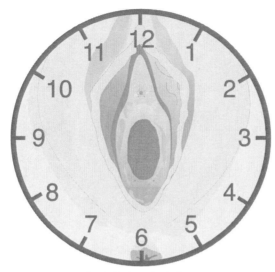

Figure 10.10: Vulva clock for massage.

Figure 10.10 shows the clitoris at 12 o'clock and the anus at 6 o'clock. The massage technique is detailed below.

Massage Technique to Improve Blood Circulation and Sensation

1. Begin by gently massaging the labia majora (outer lips) with a feather-like touch. Gently stroking and noticing the sensation. Keep the touch very gentle, like the brush of a feather. Try to relax and get used to the sensation of a very gentle touch. You can then move the gentle touch onto the labia minora (inner lips). *Note*: If you suffer from chronic pelvic pain, this very gentle touch may feel painful or excessive. In this circumstance, you can utilize the pain strategies listed earlier in this chapter and consult with your healthcare provider to explore other treatment options.

2. Slowly increase your touch with a gentle rubbing motion, eyes closed paying attention to how it feels. You should not be applying a lot of pressure; you are simply feeling the external portion of your vulva.

3. Massage the perineum by placing your thumb just inside your vagina facing toward 6 o'clock on the vulva clock (Figure 10.10) with your index and middle finger outside on your perineum. Make sure that you are relaxed in your pelvic floor muscles when you are doing this.

4. Gently rub the outer part of your perineum with your fingers. Be very gentle with this area,

particularly if you have undergone surgery. Scarred skin can be quite light and susceptible to tearing.

5. Gently rub the inside of the perineum with your thumb, feeling the tissues between your thumb and fingers.

6. Work your way around the vaginal clock from 5 o'clock to 1 o'clock on the vulva clock, massaging the inside of your vagina gently with your thumb. You may want to switch to massaging with your fingers if it is uncomfortable to massage with your thumb. *Note*: If you find a sore spot, stop and press gently to see if that helps. You are looking for a release, not an increase in pain, so listen to your vagina as you go.

7. Once you reach 1 o'clock on the vulva clock, stop and bring your fingers around to 7 o'clock, massaging until you reach 11 o'clock on the vulva clock. *Note*: The space between 11 o'clock and 1 o'clock on your vulva clock should be avoided if you suffer from IC as massage here may cause your cystitis to flare up. If you have no issues with cystitis, you can very gently feel this part of your vagina but do be extremely gentle.

If you find this massage technique to be beneficial, you should add it to your weekly schedule. Once per week is more than enough, unless your healthcare provider has suggested you undertake self-massage more frequently.

 ## Massage Strategy 2

To Reduce Pain

Massage for reduced pain involves feeling inside for "sore spots" and pressing the sore spot to send a signal to your department managers to inhibit muscle contraction. You will need to follow the same setup for this massage technique as for the previous technique. Here you should also use some lubrication. It can be useful to use a massage wand for this type of massage. These can be purchased from Amazon. The technique, detailed below, is similar to trigger point release.

Massage Technique to Reduce Pain

1. Feel around the vulva clock with your thumb, starting at 6 o'clock and working your way around the clock looking for tight/sore spots. *Note*: these spots may have changed since performing your initial assessment as the body is constantly adapting.

2. Press the sore spot gently with the same pressure you would use to check the ripeness of fruit. You are not massaging around but rather holding the gentle pressure on the spot for thirty to ninety seconds (no more than that).

3. Release the pressure and continue to move around the vulva clock looking for additional tight/ sore spots.

This type of pain-relieving massage can be used daily if you have pain. If you choose to use a "wand" for massage, do so only with the guidance of your healthcare provider and follow the manufacturer's instructions. You should ensure that your pressure is gentle. A wand can be a useful alternative to your fingers/thumb as it can be difficult to get the right angle with your thumb for pressing/releasing the tight spot. Wands can also be used to release tight spots in the anus.

You should also note that a pelvic wand is just a tool. Jilly Bond, a UK physiotherapist is a wand advocate, however, she makes it clear that "it's not about the wand." You can check out her website: jillybond.com. More details on wands are provided in the "Devices and tools" chapter in Part Three.

This completes the massage techniques. In the next and final section of this chapter, we will explore strategies to optimize self-care.

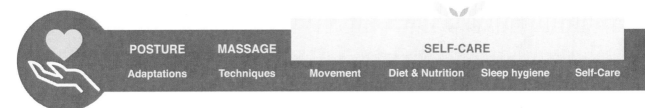

For this section, you will need to review your life pattern and mind assessments. You learned in Part One of this book how inextricably linked everything is. It is not possible to change one aspect of your life without impacting others. You can use your life pattern and mind assessments to help you choose which strategies and exercises from this section could help you to achieve your goals. The strategies are summarized below and detailed in the pages that follow.

1. **Movement**: Strategies to balance daily movement and activity.
2. **Diet & Nutrition**: Strategies to help you with digestive health and weight management.
3. **Sleep**: Strategies to help you with sleep hygiene/quality.
4. **Self-care**: Self-care strategies to help you reduce stress and create balance.

These strategies can be used while you work on the eight-phase training or can be used in isolation. We will begin by exploring movement

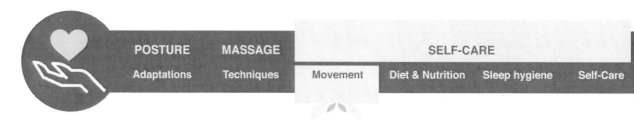

When you completed your life pattern assessment, you created a snapshot of a normal working day in your life. We will begin this movement strategies section by stepping through this snapshot beginning with exploring the breakdown of your daily activity.

You have summarized how much time you typically spend sitting, standing, walking, running, lying down, or performing other activities. Did you find that you were sitting more than nine hours on a normal day? If so, I would highly recommend that you consider implementing some of the movement strategies detailed in this section.

Recent studies have raised the question "Is sitting the new smoking?[102]." In the modern age, people are sitting more than ever before. Lifestyle studies[103] indicate that excessive sitting is bad for your health. A sedentary life pattern could be negatively affecting your posture and your general health.

A 2010 study[104] concluded that affluence in the western world has contributed to a rise in sedentary lifestyles. Many adults spend more than 70% of their waking hours sitting (that's you if you sit for nine or more hours of your normal twenty-four-hour day). The study observed an increase in cardiometabolic disease and all-cause mortality in parallel with this lifestyle change. What does that mean? Too much sitting is bad for you.

Excessive sitting is also bad for your pelvic floor. When you sit, your glutes, pelvic floor, and core all relax. Your hip flexors need to do very little. If you are sitting for the majority of your wakeful hours, these muscles are all underutilized and can easily atrophy. Sitting also impacts the psoas, which crosses the pelvis connecting to the femur.

Think back to Figure 3.11 where we viewed the pattern of connective tissue in sedentary versus active lifestyles. Your movement organizes your connective tissue fibers. Sedentary lifestyles result in disorganized connective tissue fibers, which impacts the connective tissue's ability to evenly distribute load throughout the body when you move. Your connective tissue can develop adhesions, similar to scar tissue, if you are not moving sufficiently. There is a simple solution if you are sitting too much—
Move more!

Strategies to Help You Move More

Moving more may feel like a drastic change if you switch from sitting 9 hours per day to sitting just 4 or 5. Drastic changes will most likely overwhelm you, which is why we implement small consistent changes over time. These small changes will accumulate to equal the drastic change that is required to optimize your pelvic floor health. You should deploy the following steps for this strategy.

Movement Strategy 1: *Step goal*—Changing your movement patterns is easy if you have a goal associated. You may well have included step targets in the goals for your eight-phase plan and if so, this is likely a moot point. If you have not set a step goal, I encourage you first to get a pedometer and track your steps over three or four days. This gives you a baseline. Increase your daily step count by 1 k steps per week until you reach 10 k steps per day.

Movement Strategy 2: *Stand goal*—This is a small change that can make a big difference. You should set an alarm on your phone to remind you to stand up during each hour from 8 am to 8 pm. You don't have to stand for long; five minutes during a sedentary hour should be sufficient.

When I added this strategy into my toolbox, I used an adjustable desk for work. This allowed me to easily alternate between sitting and standing. Maybe you don't have a height-adjustable desk. You can prop up your monitor on reams of paper as a workaround. If standing at your desk is not an option, there are other ways to inject some movement. Take a walk, or maybe fetch a glass of water. Just get up and move rather than sitting for long periods. If the office has stairs, walk up four or five flights of stairs, and walk back down again.

If leaving your desk every hour is not an option, why not add a lunchtime walk? If you spend your days stuck in meetings, stand up and walk around the room. It might feel strange when you do this at first, but you will get used to it, and so will your colleagues. They may even join you (that's what my colleagues did).

Movement Strategy 3: *Stability ball sitting*—When sitting, you can swap your office chair for an exercise ball. This simple change ensures that you are not completely sedentary when sitting as it is not possible to remain completely still while sitting on a ball. If you sit on a ball, make sure that your pelvis is neutral (information on finding a neutral pelvis can be found in the *posture strategy 1*).

Movement Strategy 4: *Alternate sitting positions*—For this, you should use the floor sitting exercise, which is *posture strategy 2*. This is best practiced at home as sitting on the floor or squatting in the office is not always met with enthusiasm (this is the voice of experience!).

With these changes implemented, you can decrease your sedentary time dramatically. By using a ball instead of a chair, the time spent sitting in your office is more dynamic rather than static. The purpose of these changes is to create new movement habits so you can become the master of your movement patterns. That concludes the movement strategies. We will now explore diet and nutrition strategies.

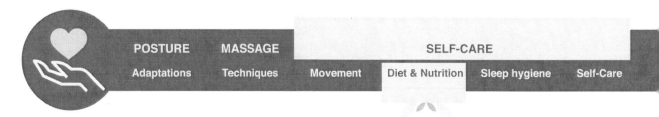

Diet plays a really important role in rehabilitation. If your body lacks the basic building blocks to rebuild muscle and other tissues, it cannot make the appropriate repairs. This is just one consideration with diet.

When it comes to PFD, we also need to consider the impact food can have on our urine and poop. Certain foods (and drinks) can irritate the bladder or make the poop hard to pass. Although this is an important consideration with PFD, it is surpassed by the increased risk associated with a high BMI.

When we reviewed the risks for developing PFD at the beginning of Chapter Eight, we learned that the risk for developing PFD is increased by 1% for every BMI point increase over 25. Another study[105] exploring obesity and urinary incontinence (UI) found that each 5-unit increase in BMI is associated with about a 20% to 70% increase in the risk of developing UI. For this reason, we will begin this section by reviewing the body measurements portion of the life pattern assessment.

If you have recorded a BMI above 24 (and are not a bodybuilder carrying excess muscle mass), I would encourage prioritizing reducing your BMI as this can help to reduce your symptoms (particularly if you are suffering from POP or stress incontinence). Reducing your BMI should also contribute to better overall health, which is a win-win. The strategies in this section can help to manage your weight and contribute to a reduction in BMI.

Diet & Nutrition Strategy 1

Increase NEAT

This first strategy can help to reduce your BMI, and that is to increase your NEAT. You may be thinking NEAT is magic weight-loss food that will strip BMI points from your body, but I am sorry to disappoint you, there is no magic food. NEAT stands for non-exercise activity thermogenesis, which is the scientific term for stimulating your metabolism through everyday activities.

These activities are not specific exercises but rather normal everyday activities such as sweeping the floor, gathering laundry from around the house, brushing your teeth, ironing in front of the television. I'm not suggesting you become a house cleaner, I am suggesting that you increase your movement through trivial activities that you may be procrastinating over. Even fidgeting falls under the NEAT label.

You may be thinking that this strategy fits better in the movement section, however, NEAT spread out over your day will contribute more to weight loss than diet or exercise activities. Figure 10.11 shows the typical daily energy expenditure for an average active adult[106].

As you can see from Figure 10.11, non-exercise activities (highlighted in green) are responsible for more energy expenditure than exercise (highlighted in blue).

A large component of NEAT comes from pottering around. It can be helpful to use a pedometer to help track NEAT activities. I use my apple watch for this purpose. I've had days where I have not left the house, and yet I have walked 30 k steps. This was due to me cleaning the house. Walking around all the rooms to gather laundry, cleaning the rooms, making beds, hoovering floors, dusting, etc. I would never

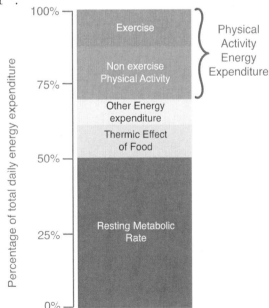

Figure 10.11: Typical daily energy expenditure in a normally active person.

have imagined that I could cover so much ground in this way. If I were to go outside to walk 30 k steps, it would feel more challenging.

Some other easy ways to clock up NEAT activity would be to park the car further from the door. To walk to the shop instead of taking the car. To take the stairs instead of the elevator. To sit on a ball in the office instead of a chair (it takes effort to sit on the ball). To alternate between sitting and standing at your desk. Use your imagination.

The best NEAT activities are the ones that don't require much of a change to your normal day, for example, you brush your teeth every day, but instead of standing still while you do this, you could walk around the bathroom. An increase in NEAT will have a very positive effect.

Of course, you may have already decided to implement the eight-phase training plan and some of the strategies that came before this one, but I really want you to understand the importance of movement if you are trying to lose weight. Not exercise, but general movement contributes more to a reduction of BMI points.

Diet & Nutrition Strategy 2
Tweak Your Diet

The second strategy is to tweak your diet. Tweaks do not always involve reducing calorie intake. If you have a BMI below 18 it is important to add calories. I would recommend working with a nutritionist if you have a high or low BMI. A nutritionist can give you a specific diet plan that is customized to your specific needs.

The objective here isn't to give you a strict diet, it is instead to offer some guidelines that can help you to ensure you are providing the basic building blocks needed for your muscles, bones, connective tissue, organs, and hormones.

Before making dietary changes, it can be useful to record a food diary over three or four "normal" days. You can use a tool such as My Fitness Pal to track your food intake or just use a notepad and pen. The benefit of using My Fitness Pal is that it will give you details on your macronutrient breakdown (otherwise known as macros).

We learned about macros in Chapter Five. Macros are the three main categories of nutrients that provide your body with fuel (energy) in the form of food. They are protein, carbohydrates, and fats. A good balance of macros will help to ensure you have the required building blocks for pelvic floor repair (through protein synthesis).

We learned in Figure 4.1 that our protein synthesis slows with age, meaning we could give the same fuel (a chicken drumstick) to a twenty and sixty-five year old but the twenty-year-old's body will produce more building blocks for repair from that same fuel source. I learned about fueling my body for muscle growth from my bodybuilding coach, John Meadows (a.k.a. Mountain Dog).

One of the key learnings was that you cannot (typically) build muscle while in a calorie deficit, so we will need to calculate the calories needed to gain muscle (a must if you are to build strength in your pelvic floor and other muscles). We will also need to calculate the macro breakdown. The following exercise will help you to do this.

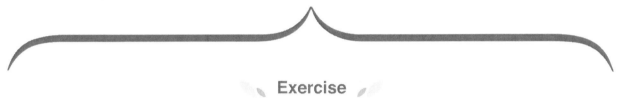

Exercise
to calculate your daily calorie intake and macro breakdown

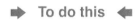

➡ To do this ⬅

1. **Calculate Total Calories**: Calculate your total calories by multiplying your body weight in pounds by fourteen. E.g., If you weigh 125 lbs. (~56 kg), this would equal *1750 calories per day.*

2. **Calculate Calories of Protein**: Multiply your bodyweight by one to calculate your protein intake in grams. E.g., if you weigh 125 lbs. (~56 kg), this would equal 125 g of protein per day. Each gram of protein is equal to 4 calories; therefore 125 g would be *500 calories of protein per day.*

3. **Calculate Calories of Fat**: Multiply your body weight by 0.5 to calculate your fat intake in grams. E.g., if you weigh 125 lbs. (~56 kg), this would equal 62.5 g of fat per day. Each gram of fat is equal to 9 calories therefore 62.6 g would be *562.5 calories of fat per day.*

4. **Calculate Calories of Carbohydrate**: Add the number of fat calories (562.5) to the

protein calories (500) and subtract the total (1062.5) from 1750 calories (the total calories for one day). This gives you 687 calories. There are 4 calories in each gram of carbs so divide 687 by 4 to find the total carbs, which is *172 grams of carbs per day.*

This is just a starting point. Having identified the macro breakdown, you need to decide what to eat. This is where food trackers like My Fitness Pal come in handy. You can look up the foods that you like to eat and see how they fit in with your macros.

Not all calories are created equal so make sure to choose more nutritious foods, avoiding processed foods as much as possible. The following table suggests some healthy proteins, carbs, and fats (this is a non-exhaustive list).

Macronutrient	Food
Protein	Eggs, beef, chicken, fish, lentils, chickpeas, beans
Fats	Avocados, nuts, olives, oils, yogurt, butter
Carbohydrates	Sweet potatoes, potatoes, rice, oats, pasta, bread

Micronutrients are also really important and that is where vegetables come in. I tend to not count calories for vegetables due to them being so low, and I try to eat plenty. My preference is for green vegetables, which I include for "free" in my own diet without counting their calories. These include spinach, broccoli, Brussel sprouts, and zucchini. These green vegetables are rich in micronutrients and exceptionally low in calories so eat some with every meal and save yourself the effort of measuring/counting calories.

I use plenty of herbs and spices for seasoning; these really add flavour to what could otherwise be considered bland food. I try to make my meals look like a rainbow on my plate, and believe I have found a healthy and nutritious balance with my food choices. When eating with a nutrition focus, you can eat so much more than if you are living on processed foods. Of course, this is just one way to eat. There are so many diets and many people have food restrictions. Some people chose to eliminate foods for environmental and other reasons.

Lots of my yoga friends are vegan. I have tried a vegan diet once, but I had problems with my skin and hair. Studies have shown that vegans have a higher fracture risk[107,108]. The benefit of a vegan or vegetarian diet is linked to the presence of lots of micronutrients rather than the absence of meat. You can simply swap out less nutritious food in your current diet with nutrient-dense vegetables and you will have all the benefits of a vegan diet without having to cut out your meat proteins.

The most important thing with your diet is to listen to your body. If something you are eating is having a negative impact on your health, change your diet. If you notice negative changes to the color of your urine or the consistency of your feces, figure out what is causing the change and correct course. Pay attention to the subtle messages that your body is sending and adjust your diet accordingly.

Diet has never been and will never be one size fits all as one man's cure is another man's poison. Find a diet that works for you, making sure you have sufficient protein to maintain your muscle. If you are unsure what you should eat, speak with a nutritionist.

Diet & Nutrition Strategy 3
Avoid Stressful Eating

What you eat is important, but equally important is how you eat. Eating when stressed impacts your body's ability to digest food. In Chapter Seven, we learned about the "rest and digest" and "fight or flight" modes of your autonomic nervous system. Digestion is slowed during "fight or flight" mode so it can be good to ensure that you are calm before eating.

The following practices can help to reduce stressful and emotional eating, which, in turn, can have a positive impact on your digestion:

Relaxed Eating
Your food is the fuel that is going to rebuild your muscles and connective tissues. It is imperative that you set yourself up for success by ensuring you are relaxed when eating so your body can make the best use of that fuel. A relaxed eating practice involves bringing the body into "rest and digest" mode

by utilizing the calming breath cycles that we have learned as part of the eight-phase training program. You should do this before each meal:

a. Sit upright with your hands rested on your lap.

b. Close your eyes.

c. Perform five to ten calming breath cycles, inhaling for a count of four and exhaling for a count of eight.

d. Gently blink open your eyes and eat your meal.

This practice was crucial for me as I have always had a tendency to eat under pressure. Extending the duration of your exhalation triggers your nervous system to activate "rest and digest" mode.

Mindful Eating

You may have heard of mindful eating. It is a practice that encourages you to pay attention while ensuring that you take sufficient time to chew your food before you swallow. This was also crucial for me as I tend to inhale my food, always finishing before everyone else.

With mindful eating, you take your time and treat eating as though it were a meditation. To enhance your focus, you can take your knife and fork in opposite hands. If you usually hold your fork in your right hand, now it will be in your left. This forces you to eat at a slower pace. Chopsticks are another great alternative to trigger mindfulness. The more mindful and calm you are when eating, the more likely you are to properly digest your food.

Avoid Emotional Eating

Did you know that emotional eating is associated with obesity? If you are obese, it is better to focus on emotional regulation skills[109] rather than following a calorie-restricted diet. Remember that food is fuel. If you need to have an emotional meal, choose one meal per week, and make that your "treat" or "reward" meal, but try to avoid eating as a way to console yourself if things don't go according to plan.

That concludes the diet & nutrition strategies. Hopefully, these strategies will empower you to fuel your body sufficiently to achieve your empowerment goals.

We will now focus on another type of nutrition that is crucial for rehabilitation—sleep!

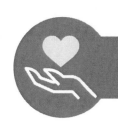
Have you ever considered the impact your sleep has on your pelvic floor? Sleep loss can lower the function of your body's immune system and is associated with an increased risk of obesity, diabetes[110], and cardiovascular disease. Quality sleep is critical to maintaining good health.

Human growth hormone, a key anabolic (muscle building) hormone, is primarily produced during the onset of sleep. Your sleep goes through a number of cycles during the course of a night. During your rapid eye movement (REM) sleep cycles, your brain is active but many of your muscles are paralyzed.

While your body is in this paralytic state, it is believed to be running in "repair" mode where your body is rebuilding and regenerating. For this repair to take place, you must have provided your body with sufficient fuel. You have learned about fueling your body for muscle growth in Diet and Nutrition Strategy 1.

It is also imperative that you have provided sufficient stimulus to your muscles and connective tissues during the day in order to promote this repair. This stimulus comes in the form of movement and exercise, which you are undertaking as part of the eight-phase training program.

If you think about sleep in relation to your pelvic floor rehabilitation, you need a diet that supports muscle repair (good proteins), you need to work the pelvic floor muscles (creating some physical stress), and you need to ensure that you have low emotional stress levels to allow your body to properly rest in order for repair to take place. Hopefully, this book is helping you with all of these actions.

The following strategies can contribute to an improved quality of sleep:

Sleep Hygiene Strategy 1:   *Sleep equipment*—The quality of your sleep is impacted by your mattress, pillows, and quilt. Choose a mattress that feels good for your body.

Pillows can usually be purchased to suit specific sleeping positions. Choose the correct pillow type for your default sleeping position.

For example, if you sleep face down on three fluffy pillows, you will eventually have back and neck pain from sleeping with exaggerated neck flexion. If sleeping face down, it is better to use a single pillow that isn't very thick.

Make sure your quilt doesn't leave you waking during the night feeling either too warm or too cold. We have a saying in Sweden; there is no such thing as bad weather, only bad clothing. I like to think it's the same for bed. If you are a naturally cold person, wear warm pajamas, fluffy socks, and have an extra blanket. If you are naturally warm, use a lighter blanket and sleep in the nude.

Sleep Hygiene Strategy 2: *Wind down before sleep*—Try to relax and take it easy for at least an hour before bed, preferably without looking at your phone or TV. Reading can help, or some form of creative task such as drawing or coloring. Pre-bed can also be a favorable time for the Mind & Meditation practice that is part of your eight-phase training plan.

Sleep Hygiene Strategy 3: *Sleep schedule*—As much as possible, you should follow a sleeping schedule. This involves going to bed around the same time each night and rising at the same time each morning. This is considered an important aspect of sleep hygiene.

Sleep Hygiene Strategy 4: *Spend time in daylight*—Did you know that spending time in daylight in the middle of your day can positively impact your circadian rhythms (sleep cycles)?[111] You should try to get at least 30 minutes of daylight during the middle of your day. Bright light close to bedtime can interrupt sleep cycles, so it is best to wind down in softer lighting before bed. This may sound obvious, but it is also important to block out light from windows for the same reason. Sleep in a pitch-black room if possible.

Sleep Hygiene Strategy 5: *Block out noise*—Noise can be very disruptive to sleep. If you are disturbed by noises during the night, purchase a good set of earplugs to block out those sounds. Bose has earplugs that block out external sounds while playing some gentle sounds that can help you to sleep.

Sleep Hygiene Strategy 6:   *Weighted blanket*—Using a weighted blanket (also known as an anxiety blanket) can give a sense of security, which can help with sleep. These blankets are believed to mimic the sensation of being held. They are also said to reduce restlessness.

If you are trying to change your sleeping position, particularly if changing from sleeping on your stomach to sleeping on your back, a weighted blanket is a great help as it places gentle pressure on the front of your body similar to what you would feel lying face down. This should make it easier to fall and stay asleep. If the weighted blanket feels uncomfortable on your feet, use a lighter blanket to cover your feet.

Sleep Hygiene Strategy 7:   *Mouth taping*—Have you heard of mouth taping? It is a practice that forces you to breathe through your nose while sleeping. As well as helping to reduce snoring, it also increases the production of nitric oxide—a chemical that helps to transport oxygen throughout the body, which is produced when you breathe in through your nose. Nitric oxide is also said to boost the immune system due to its antifungal, antiviral, and antiparasitic properties.

If you are a mouth breather, this is a really great way to encourage yourself to use nasal breathing. I am normally a mouth breather and have been mouth taping for over three years.

The first time I tried mouth taping, I was afraid I might suffocate, and I took the tape off in a panic about an hour into my sleep. Determined as I am, I tried again the following night and achieved a great night's sleep. I track my sleep using the Sleep Cycles smartphone app. It records my snore sounds as well as tracking my sleep. Since starting my mouth taping practice, my snoring has stopped.

Standard medical tape is sufficient for mouth taping. You can reduce the stickiness of the tape by applying it to your arm a few times before taping your mouth.

IMPORTANT WARNING: Although I highly recommend mouth tape when sleeping, it is extremely important that you create a little tab on one side for easy removal. I had an incident where I needed to sneeze shortly after lying down to sleep, I sat up and tried to remove the mouth tape, but I couldn't lift the edge of the tape in time. I sneezed into my closed mouth. *This created extreme intra-abdominal pressure that resulted in extreme pain on both the right and left sides of my lower abs as well as pain in my pelvic floor.* Sneezing with your mouth closed is dangerous.

You should always "sneeze out" rather than trying to hold your sneeze in. In very rare cases, it is possible to tear your throat tissue if you hold in a sneeze. I believe it is also possible to damage the tissues around your pelvic organs. If you have a hernia or POP, holding in a sneeze could make it worse. So, my advice... use mouth tape with caution and be ready to get that tape off in an instant if you need to sneeze.

My last remaining advice to help you with sleeping is to exercise more (which you should be doing if you are working on the eight-phase training). Burning more calories and getting your heart rate up during the day, can help you to rest better at night. Hopefully, the changes you are making to empower your flower are helping you to have the best sleep possible.

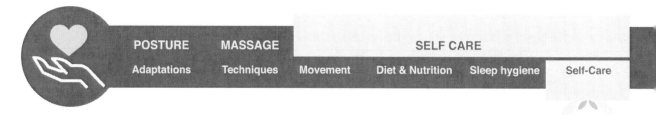

We will finish off this section with some additional strategies to help you reduce stress and create balance. During the assessments, you completed a mind assessment using the brain assessment on Dr. Amen's mybrainfitlife.com website. This assessment categorized your brain into one of sixteen different brain types using scores for brain health, sleep, memory, executive function, inner peace, mood, and flexible thinking.

The mind and meditation modules of the eight-phase plan are designed to create positive changes in your brain, which should help to improve your scores on this assessment by enhancing your thought patterns. Adopting additional strategies from this chapter should help to improve your QoL ensuring better sleep, better orgasms, and improved general wellbeing.

This final section of this chapter provides some self-care strategies that can help to further improve the overall results of your efforts and your brain health.

Self-care Strategy 1

See a Therapist

It is critical to get professional help if you need it. When you look at your mind assessment, it will give you an indication of your level of mental balance. If your mind is out of balance, you must seek professional help. You might be advised to adopt brain training exercises and that may be sufficient, or you may need to speak with a therapist every week for the next five years. You should do whatever it takes.

As I explained in Part One, stress has a negative impact on your health and your ability to heal. If you are trying to rehabilitate, stress can stand like a barrier between you and success. I am not suggesting that you should force yourself into a state where you experience eternal happiness, that is not a balanced state. It is important to allow yourself to feel all states of emotion as is part of the human experience.

What I am suggesting is that you find a balance where you allow yourself to experience the ups and downs in your life while accepting any external support you may need. In my case, that involved speaking with a therapist over several years.

My therapist was Beth Rogerson, an American psychologist based in Stockholm. She helped me to work through many of my life traumas, particularly those surrounding my childhood. The therapy helped me dramatically and improved my QoL. She has written multiple books if you are interested in reading about her approach. You can find her at bethrogerson.com.

Self-care Strategy 2

Pamper Yourself

Pampering yourself, in my opinion, is another form of therapy. Have you ever gone for a facial? Or been to the hairdressers? Did you have someone apply your makeup? These practices are quite superficial but can make you feel good. I'm not saying that you need to go to the hairdressers every week or go for regular facials (although that is lovely if you can afford it), but these practices can contribute to an improved mood.

There are a number of physical pampering practices that you can perform regularly at home to make yourself feel fresh and invigorated.

Self-massage

In the massage strategies section, you learned how to massage your vulva and vagina. In this section, we will learn about self-massage. You will need oil (I prefer coconut oil) and some privacy.

Self-massage instructions:

a. Take a pea-sized amount of oil in your hand and begin to massage your right leg starting from the foot and massage upwards. The level of pressure is a personal preference. If you find tight/sore spots apply a little extra pressure to relieve the soreness.

b. Massage your left leg, working from the foot to the hip.

c. Massage your right arm, working your way from wrist to shoulder before switching to the left arm.

d. Massage your lower back using both hands at the same time. If you have sufficient ROM to reach your upper back, massage there too, otherwise you can use a massage tool to reach your back.

e. Massage your groin and lower abdominals, ensuring that your pressure is not uncomfortable. Massage gently up toward the ribcage.

f. Use your fingers to massage in between your ribs. If you find a tight spot, go over it a few times starting at the side of your rib and working toward your center. I would suggest doing one side of the rib cage at a time.

g. Massage your breasts and decolletage (neck).

h. Massage your face using just fingertips. Pat your face gently with your fingers once you are finished.

i. Lastly, massage your hands, making sure to rub in between all the little bones on the back of your hand.

Self-massage, as well as making you feel good, also contributes to your NEAT movement goal. Of course, you can have your partner massage you instead. If you are single, you can buy a self-massage tool that allows you to reach your back, or you can place a ball behind your back rolling against a wall or on the floor.

Body exfoliation

Body exfoliation is a wonderful practice that stimulates the skin (your body's largest organ) while removing dead cells. You can use a sugar scrub for exfoliation while you are in the shower. Work the sugar scrub into your skin in place of your usual soap. Follow the same instructions as those for self-massage, starting at your feet, work your way up toward your heart. Make sure to be gentle. You can purchase pre-made exfoliation products or make your own sugar scrub using a combination of sugar and coconut oil. It can be nice to use a facecloth to remove the remaining sugar scrub before rinsing your skin. Pat the skin dry once you are fully rinsed.

Exfoliation makes the skin feel like silk. When my skin feels silky, I feel sexier, and this increases my desire to be touched. If you have been struggling with lack of desire and loss of libido, any kind of pampering that creates sexy thought trains is worth exploring.

Body brushing

Body brushing is a practice that is believed to stimulate the lymph nodes under the skin. You use a dry brush with soft bristles and follow the same trajectory as you did with self-massage, brushing gently (instead of massaging). I try to body-brush every week. It is an act of self-love and can be combined with self-affirmations to trigger positive thought trains, a most nurturing practice.

Nails, hair, makeup, etc.

After all the depth throughout the eight-phase program and this life strategies chapter, we are now coming back to the most superficial. Nails, hair, and makeup are the war-paints of our female population. You may have negative thoughts about wearing these war paints, or you may believe that it is not possible to step out of your house without them.

Either way, any empowerment plan would be incomplete without the suggestion of a good pampering session. Having your nails done, getting your hair styled, and putting on some makeup can make you feel amazing. If it's not for you, it's not for you, but if a pampering session makes you feel good, do it. Particularly if the pampered you is riding the positive thought train feeling sexy and ready to take on the world.

That brings us to the end of the section on life strategies. Hopefully, by now, your toolkit is overflowing with strategies that can help to improve your QoL as you strive to empower your flower.

Chapter Eleven will follow, with lots of information on the various conditions that fall under the umbrella term of PFD, as well as the surgical and non-surgical treatments for PFD conditions.

Chapter Eleven:
Pelvic Floor Dysfunction Treatments

Unlike chapters eight, nine, and ten, the remaining chapters are intended to be used for reference only. This chapter summarizes PFD conditions and their associated non-surgical and surgical treatments, some of which will overlap with the symptom-management strategies from Chapter Ten.

PFD should always be diagnosed by a medical professional and treatments should be based on sound professional advice. The information in this section of the book should by no means be considered a substitute for the advice of qualified medical professionals. You will find details of relevant medical professionals in Chapter Thirteen.

When we begin to explore the treatments for PFD, it is important to note that treatments can have associated side effects and carry risks. Most medicines can have side effects and every surgery carries risks including anesthetic risks, wound complications, bleeding/hematoma, and deep vein thrombosis to name a few. Risks are generally greater for open abdominal surgery than for laparoscopic (keyhole) surgeries. Common medical and surgical risks will not be listed in the pages that follow, but you should remember that they do exist.

The risks relating to mesh surgeries are ultimately what led me to bring my fingers to the keyboard to write this book so, I would like to begin by sharing what I have learned with regards to the history of mesh as a material for the surgical repair of stress incontinence and POP, a history that is marred in controversy.

The History of Mesh Used in Surgery to Treat POP and SUI

Mesh has been used as a reinforcement material in hernia surgeries since 1958 and was first used as a sling to treat stress incontinence in 1962 in the USA. That mesh device, named the Mersilene mesh, showed high tissue rejection rates[112] and complications. This Mersilene mesh didn't require clinical trials to prove its efficacy as it was on the market prior to the introduction of the risk-based classification and regulatory processes introduced by the FDA in 1976, which granted approval to existing devices automatically.

Post-1976, the requirements for market approval of *new* medical devices in the USA were more stringent, requiring premarket approval. The new regulations were designed to ensure that scientific evidence in the form of clinical trial data would be available to prove the safety and efficacy of medical devices. There was, however, an alternative path to approval, known as the 510(k), which grants approval if a medical device is *similar* to one already proven and on the market. This mechanism provides market clearance based on the safety and efficacy of a previously approved device.

The first stress incontinence mesh brought to market in the USA following the 1976 changes, was the ProteGen Sling. This was a mesh sling with pressure-injected bovine collagen. ProteGen used the 510(k) pathway, claiming to be similar to the Mersilene mesh to gain approval. The ProteGen Sling was subsequently removed from the market in 1999 due to a very high rate of erosion[113], unsurprising given that its approval was based on a device that had not itself been through a stringent approval process.

Unfortunately, even though the ProteGen Sling was removed from the market, it was subsequently used as evidence for the approval of a further sixty-one devices[114]. The Mersilene mesh was grandfather to the majority of pelvic mesh devices in the US market, with the ProteGen mesh being the father and most subsequent meshes relying on the safety and efficacy of these two faulty mesh devices for their approval.

Maybe you are based in Europe, or in Sweden like me, and you are thinking "surely the European approval processes must have been more stringent requiring studies." They were, but unfortunately, the controversy continues.

In 1997, a renowned Swedish obstetrician and gynecologist, published a small study[115] into a new procedure using mesh slings to treat stress incontinence. Seventy-five women had participated in the study, which reported an impressive 84% success rate. This made the treatment at least as successful as the Burch procedure, which was, at that time, the gold standard for treating stress incontinence.

With scientific research, small studies should be followed by larger-scale studies. Ideally, studies would be randomized (where patients are randomly selected) and controlled (where there is a control group that receives an alternative treatment or a "placebo"). Surgical studies should also be multicenter, which would mean that multiple surgeons in multiple hospitals would participate. This would help account for varying skills and the experience of surgeons as well as medical device performance.

In 1998, the Swedish gynecologist and his team published a second study[116]; this time it was a multicenter study, involving six different hospitals in Finland and Sweden, with 131 patients. The results from this study were even better than the first, showing a 91% cure rate and concluding that "[tension-free vaginal tape] TVT is a safe and effective ambulatory procedure for surgical treatment of genuine stress urinary incontinence." This study was pivotal to making TVT the "gold standard" in the surgical treatment of stress incontinence.

Had I read that multicenter study before going under the knife, I likely would have proceeded without hesitation. I mean, it sounds too good to be true, right? Unfortunately, it was indeed too good to be true.

During a US product liability case in 2014, evidence was presented proving that the same Swedish gynecologist responsible for those studies had signed an agreement in March 1997 with a medical device company, which would see him paid $1m USD on the provision that the second trial echoed the results of the first[117]. He subsequently patented the TVT, selling the patents to the medical device company for over $24m USD, and becoming a very wealthy man.

Of course, it is possible that the financial incentive did not introduce bias. The study was published at a time when it was not essential to declare conflicts of interest. Many medical device studies are funded by the companies who stand to profit from their sale, and you would hope that this funding would not impact the results. Somehow, I find it difficult to believe that financial gain can be offered without introducing bias. With native tissue surgeries, the risk of this bias is reduced as there is no substantial financial gain.

Many subsequent studies over the last twenty-five years, reference those Swedish studies to substantiate the efficacy of mesh devices. These studies re-affirm to the medical community what the gold standard should be. One such paper[118] from 2016 is titled "The New Gold Standard is Almost the Same as the Old One."

That publication concluded that, "On account of its safety and efficacy, the suburethral sling management has the highest status in incontinence surgery". This paper also stated that "[b]ecause of the changes in patient rights, in every case alternative methods such as the classic colposuspension and sling plasties should be mentioned and attention paid to a comprehensive clarification and documentation."

What does that conclusion mean? The medical community is being advised to continue to perform the mesh surgeries as the primary treatment for stress incontinence, but to make sure to "cover your ass" by mentioning alternative options and providing some clarification on the risks. It is worth noting that this paper declared conflicts of interest relating to fees and funding from multiple mesh manufacturers.

The Impact of Mesh Injuries and the Banning of Mesh Devices

It has taken years for mesh-injured women to band together around the world, shouting loudly enough to finally have their voices heard. Many mesh-injured women have been irreparably damaged. Many are wheelchair-bound due to nerve damage. Many have lost their bladder and/or bowel, and are left to live with a stoma. Some have needed obliterative surgery (requiring removal of the vagina) due to the level of damage to vaginal walls, but this is not even the worst of it.

A 42-year-old Canadian mother of two, Christina Lynn Brajcic, had a mesh sling implanted to treat mild stress incontinence in 2013. She experienced pain following surgery, which her surgeon suggested was the mesh "settling in." The pain worsened as time passed until she was eventually confined to a wheelchair, suffering recurring infections from the mesh, requiring antibiotics and painkillers. Subsequently, she developed antibiotic resistance.

She became an anti-mesh campaigner on Facebook. In October 2017, she developed sepsis and posted a video from her intensive care bed in which she said "This is insane. To almost be on your deathbed at only 42 because of mesh, it's not right." Her heart had stopped because of the sepsis infection, she considered herself lucky to be alive and was happy to have got help in time. She finished by saying, "All I want to do is get home to my kids." One month later she died.

The Canadian government had issued a position statement on the use of transvaginal mesh in June of that year[119] supporting Mesh's continued use. A subsequent safety review in 2019[120] added restrictions to its use, which could be viewed as a partial ban, leaving the use of mesh at the discretion of the surgeon.

New Zealand and Australia issued mesh bans in 2017 and, subsequently in 2018, the Australian government issued[121] a national apology to women, acknowledging decades of "agony and pain."

In 2018, following immense pressure from the UK Sling the Mesh patient support group led by Kath Sansom, the UK government instigated an inquiry into mesh. The inquiry was led by Baroness Julia Cumberlege. A mesh ban was issued in July of 2018 in order to prevent further injury while the inquiry was ongoing.

In April of 2019, new guidelines were issued by NICE (the UK's National Institute for Health and Care Excellence). However, these guidelines allowed the continued use of mesh at the surgeon's discretion and with the requirement to inform patients of the risks.

In the USA, the FDA had been aware of serious complications associated with mesh, issuing a number of communications in 2008 (regarding mesh used for POP and SUI), and in 2011 (regarding mesh used in POP). Subsequently in 2012, the FDA requested post-market surveillance studies from manufacturers of mesh. This data, a request for studies proving efficacy, was requested to help the agency better understand the safety and efficacy of mesh devices, and was needed due to the devices using the 501(k) route to market.

Between 2014 and 2017, the FDA worked on reclassifying mesh used for POP as a class three medical device, which would require that manufacturers must provide evidence of device efficacy and safety to ensure continued use. As a result of the FDA's actions, all manufacturers ceased the marketing of POP mesh for rectocele repair.

Then, an FDA advisory committee concluded that evidence into the safety and efficacy for POP mesh used for cystocele repair should be superior to native tissue repair at thirty-six months, and the safety outcomes for surgical mesh for transvaginal repair of prolapse should be comparable to native tissue repair. Manufacturers failed to provide the data proving this to be the case, so in April 2019, the FDA ordered manufacturers of cystocele mesh to immediately stop selling and distributing their products.

It does not fill me with confidence when I see that companies are willing to remove profitable devices from the market rather than providing evidence that they are safe and effective. It is beyond shocking that surgeons still believe in these devices, even when manufacturers have failed to provide the required proof.

Many surgeons continue to support the use of mesh even with bans, restrictions, high rates of injury, and the controversy surrounding its use. Those mesh-injured women, like me, who stand up to share our stories are accused of scaremongering. Surgeons still see mesh as a valuable tool in the treatment of both SUI and POP and they suggest that the reason for mesh failures could be any of the following.

1. **The skill of the implanting surgeon**: It is suggested that mesh failures are due to a lack of experience on behalf of the implanting surgeon; *however, the mesh community is filled with women whose implants were placed by world-renowned surgeons, like mine, who are performing hundreds of surgeries each month.*

2. **Patient selection**: It has been suggested that the failures could be due to patient selection, where there is a potential "ideal candidate" for mesh. It has been suggested to avoid patients with higher BMI, smokers, patients with diabetes or other pre-existing conditions, and patients who are regular steroid users. *However, that would have made me a perfect candidate, and clearly, I was not.*

After twenty-five years where mesh implantation has dominated as the "gold standard" surgical treatment for SUI and POP, many surgeons will need to retrain to learn alternative surgical techniques. If I were to provide an analogy for how this must feel for a surgeon, it would be the following.

Imagine using the Windows operating system for the first twenty-five years of your career. You are an expert in using Windows. Then you turn up to work today to find your Windows computer has been replaced with a Mac (more expensive but it will give you fewer issues when you learn how to use it). This is the equivalent of switching from mesh to traditional surgeries for a mesh surgeon.

As you read through the medical and surgical options available to treat the conditions that fall under the PFD umbrella, do so with an open mind. You have been empowered with knowledge and can speak with your medical professional without the naivety that I possessed before going under the knife myself. Together with your healthcare provider, you can agree on which treatments could be right for you. Don't be afraid to seek a second opinion if needed.

The diagnosis and treatment of PFD are typically focused on the symptoms you present with. This chapter will provide information on the conditions that fall under the PFD umbrella, and will summarize the both the non-surgical and surgical treatments for those conditions.

PFD Symptoms
and Associated Treatments

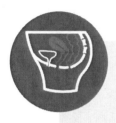

1. Urinary Conditions

a. Overactive bladder/urgency
b. Stress incontinence
c. Mixed incontinence
d. Urinary retention

2. Fecal Conditions

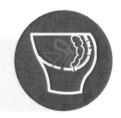

a. Fecal incontinence
b. Chronic constipation

3. POP

Pelvic organ prolapse

4. Pelvic Pain Conditions

a. Chronic pelvic pain
b. Vaginismus

Urinary Conditions

The upcoming section will step through this list starting with urinary conditions. When explaining surgical treatments, information provided includes treatment summary, procedure, efficacy data, and complications. We will begin by reviewing the overactive bladder and its associated treatments.

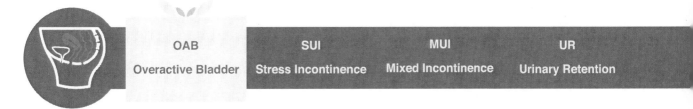

OAB	SUI	MUI	UR
Overactive Bladder	Stress Incontinence	Mixed Incontinence	Urinary Retention

Overactive bladder (OAB) also known as urgency is a condition that causes frequent urination, sometimes with urinary leakage. The average adult female urinates approximately eight to ten times per day. If you are urinating more frequently than this, your bladder may be considered to be overactive.

The condition can manifest as an urgency to urinate hence it is sometimes called urge incontinence. Those who suffer from OAB need to know where the bathroom is at all times and even then, there is a risk they may not make it. Figure 11.1 shows the overactive bladder and its associated nerves.

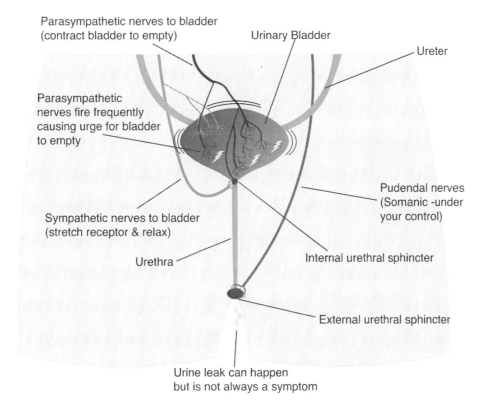

Figure 11.1: Overactive bladder (OAB) visualization.

It is believed that the parasympathetic nerves highlighted in blue in Figure 11.1, stimulate the bladder (detrusor muscle) to contract prematurely and without warning, causing a sudden urgent need to urinate. It can be difficult to control this urge.

A 2015 study[122] concluded that patients with OAB reported psychological stress levels that were significantly higher than healthy participants. Reducing your stress levels is a big focus of the Mind/ Meditation modules of the eight-phase training. If you undertake the eight-phase training, this should have a positive effect on your OAB symptoms.

Another 2015 study[123] found that OAB was common among smokers. Female smokers significantly complained of OAB, bedwetting, and peeing during sex in comparison to non-smokers. If you are suffering from OAB, reducing the amount you smoke or quitting completely could have a positive effect.

Non-Surgical Treatments
Overactive Bladder/Urgency

OAB is neurological in nature, so treatment options tend to be targeted toward the nervous system. There are six non-surgical treatments and they are detailed below.

Bladder Retraining

Bladder retraining is often offered as the primary treatment for OAB/urgency. We have already explored bladder retraining in OAB strategy 2 (Chapter Ten). It is important to complete a bladder diary to learn your urination patterns to understand if they are contributing to the condition. Bladder retraining is often combined with pelvic floor muscle training as good control over your external urethral sphincter can help you tap into your guarding reflex, which can help to relax the detrusor muscle improving OAB symptoms (which is explored in OAB strategy 1 in Chapter Ten).

Transcutaneous Posterior Tibial Nerve Stimulation (TPTNS)

TPTNS is a non-invasive treatment for OAB/urgency. It involves electrical stimulation of the tibial nerve using skin surface electrodes as shown in Figure 11.2.

The positive electrode, shown in Figure 11.2 with a red marker, is placed beneath the ankle. The negative electrode, shown in Figure 11.2 with a black marker, is placed higher up on the inside of the leg.

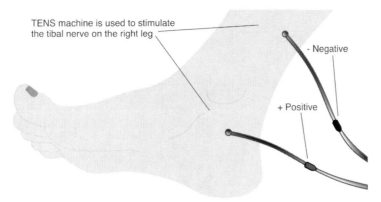

Figure 11.2: Transcutaneous posterior tibial nerve stimulation (TPTNS).

TPTNS is the least invasive of the nerve stimulation options. The skin electrodes are connected to an external device that sends electrical pulses to trigger the contraction of the muscles of the foot and lower leg.

TPTNS can be performed at home using a TENS or ESTIM device. Treatment typically takes twenty minutes, with the duration between treatments varying from 3 to 7 days between each session. **You should only undertake this treatment under the guidance of a medical health professional or, as they say in the movies "do not try this at home."**

The mechanism of action for this treatment is not fully understood, but there have been multiple small studies[124] in the past decade that suggest that TPTNS is effective in the management of severe OAB[125]. Larger-scale studies are underway.

Posterior Tibial Nerve Stimulation (PTNS)

PTNS is the more invasive version of tibial nerve stimulations for the treatment of OAB shown in Figure 11.3.

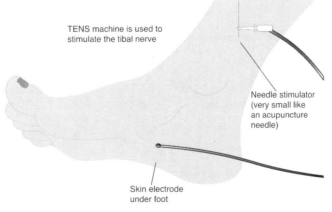

Figure 11.3: Posterior tibial nerve stimulation (PTNS).

Instead of using two skin electrodes, the negative skin electrode is replaced with a needle that is inserted into the inner leg above the ankle, as shown in Figure 11.3.

To administer the treatment, the patient is seated in a chair with legs elevated. The needle, connected to the negative feed, is inserted the width of three fingers above the ankle bone (malleolus). The positive skin electrode is placed under the foot on the heel bone (calcaneus). It is normal for the big toe to flex during treatment. Some studies suggest you should feel the contraction of your pelvic floor during treatment, although this is not always felt. Like TPTNS, studies to validate this treatment are underway.

Medication

Medication is a common treatment offered for OAB/urgency. It should be offered only when the more conservative treatments have failed. Medications to treat OAB have been used for decades but come with multiple side effects. For example, dry eyes and mouth, a side effect that can increase thirst, causing an increase in fluid intake. If fluid intake exceeds the recommended maximum of 2.7 liters per day for females (11.5 cups) the symptoms of OAB can become aggravated.

Constipation is another common side effect, which we have already learned can negatively impact the health of your pelvic floor.

Drugs for OAB/urgency are known as antimuscarinic medications. They work by inhibiting the nerves that trigger the involuntary bladder contractions that cause urgency, which we viewed in blue in Figure 11.1. You should only take medications that have been prescribed to you by a relevant medical professional. The following drugs are antimuscarinic medications:

- Tolterodine
- Oxybutynin Trospium
- Solifenacin
- Darifenacin
- Fesoterodine

Botox Injection

Botox is a more invasive treatment for OAB/urgency. You may be familiar with Botox in its cosmetic use where it relaxes the muscles of the forehead to mask wrinkles. Botox can also be used to relax the bladder muscle (detrusor) thus reducing the contractions that cause frequent urination. This treatment, like that of the forehead, is only a short-term fix, typically lasting for several months before a repeat procedure is required.

Unfortunately, the two main side effects are urine retention (which can be life-threatening) and urinary tract infections, which happen in 17% and 49% of patients respectively[126]. If conservative options have failed, your medical professional may suggest Botox. Figure 11.4 shows how Botox is administered.

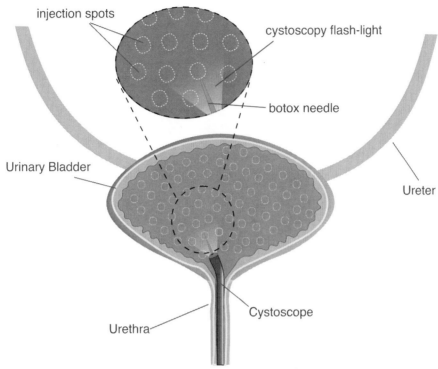

Figure 11.4: Botox bladder injection for OAB.

A cystoscope (a device with a camera) is inserted into the urethra as shown in Figure 11.4. The bladder is filled with sterile water. The detrusor muscle is then injected with many very small injections, highlighted in the zoomed image in Figure 11.4. It typically takes five to ten minutes for this treatment to be completed.

That concludes the non-surgical treatments for OAB/urgency. We will now review the surgical options.

Surgical Treatments
Overactive Bladder/Urgency

The main surgical treatment for OAB is sacral nerve stimulation, which is detailed in this section. You may also be offered stress incontinence treatments as a treatment for OAB as there is one school of thought believing that hypermobility of the neck of the bladder can trigger urgency. Most of the surgical treatments offered for stress incontinence add support around the bladder neck, hence their use. You can read about those treatments in the stress incontinence section.

Surgery Name: Sacral Nerve Stimulation (SNS)

Treatment Summary: SNS is the main surgical treatment currently offered for OAB and is the most invasive treatment available, which uses an implanted device to stimulate nerves that manage pelvic floor function.

Procedure: The procedure involves implanting a pacemaker type device under the skin of the buttocks with an electrode that is fed into the S3 sacral nerve root as shown in Figure 11.5.

The red arrow in Figure 11.5 shows the electrode connector of the device as it is

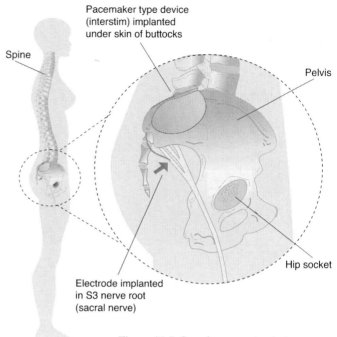

Figure 11.5: Sacral nerve stimulation.

inserted into the third branch of the sacral nerve (S3). This electrode produces a mild stimulation that helps to keep the bladder relaxed. The exact mechanism that makes this an effective treatment is not understood by the scientific community[127]. It is hypothesized that the treatment is effective due to its stimulation of the S3 nerve root, which contains sensory fibers that reach the pelvic floor and parasympathetic fibers connected to the detrusor (bladder muscle).

The device is 2 inches wide and a quarter-inch thick. Battery life is expected to last five years; however, the device manufacturer emphasizes that the more you use it, the quicker it will run out. Surgery is required to change the battery.

It is normal to undertake a two-week trial with a temporary device superficial to the skin before having the actual device implanted. During this trial period, probes are inserted into the sacral nerve, while the device is strapped to the waist instead of being implanted.

Efficacy: SNS is not effective for all forms of OAB and tends to be more effective when urge incontinence is present versus OAB without incontinence[128]. Short- and long- term efficacy is reported to be good with some studies showing a success rate higher than less invasive methods[129]. One study[130] found that patients below fifty-five tend to have higher cure rates (65%) in comparison to older patients (37%). However, the rate of complication following surgery is in the 30-40% range within the first 5 years.

Complications: Complications can include lead movement, lead fracture, high impedance in the lead, and electrical shorting. Complications typically require reoperation (either for repair or removal) so the decision to use this type of device should not be taken lightly. Unlike pelvic mesh devices, this device is not a permanent implant and can be removed.

That concludes the treatments for OAB. We will summarize stress incontinence and its treatments in the next section.

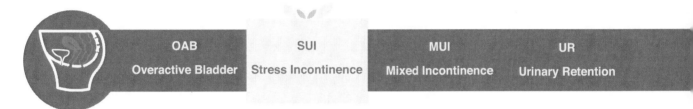

OAB	SUI	MUI	UR
Overactive Bladder	Stress Incontinence	Mixed Incontinence	Urinary Retention

Stress incontinence is the unintended leakage of urine that happens during physical movement or activity as a result of increased intra-abdominal pressure that is not matched by urethral closure pressure. Think sneeze-pee, run-pee, jump-pee, bounce-pee, or laugh-pee. This is visualized in Figure 11.6.

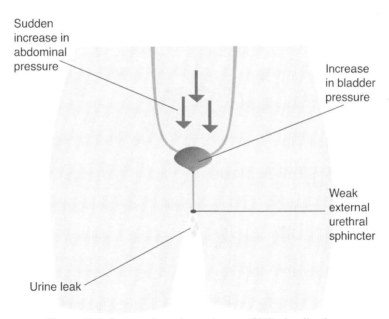

Figure 11.6: Stress urinary incontinence (SUI) visualization.

The red arrows in Figure 11.6 depict a sudden increase in intra-abdominal pressure. The yellow drips indicate urine leakage. It is almost impossible to find accurate figures on the number of people suffering from stress incontinence, but it is noted in many studies that women are twice as likely to suffer this form of incontinence than men with half of all women over the age of sixty-five suffering from the condition.

Multiple factors can contribute to SUI such as hypo-/hyper- tonic pelvic floor muscles, pelvic floor trauma (from childbirth or surgery), weak gluteus muscles, tight hamstrings, weak core muscles, imbalanced posture, dysfunctional breathing patterns, and excessive straining through bowel movements or heavy lifting.

Your risk of developing SUI is increased if you smoke more than twenty cigarettes per day, which makes a good case for quitting smoking. We have already learned that weight also has a bearing, with every unit increase in BMI over 25, increasing your risk of developing incontinence by 1%. Obese people have double the risk of developing incontinence[131] and when you add to that, obese people are three times more likely to suffer severe incontinence[132], weight management becomes a priority for SUI patients (see the diet and nutrition strategies in Chapter Ten).

Non-Surgical Treatments
Stress urinary incontinence

There are five non-surgical options for stress incontinence, which will be detailed in this section.

Pelvic Floor Muscle Training

Pelvic floor muscle training (PFMT) is the primary treatment for stress incontinence and is typically performed in a physiotherapy setting. PFMT is also the primary focus of this book.

PFMT involves exercises designed to increase strength and muscle bulk within the pelvic floor. PFMT focuses on both endurance, speed, and functional exercises. The pelvic floor module of the eight-phase program is a PFMT program.

One systematic review[133] highlighted that women with weaker pelvic floor muscles had a greater improvement in continence symptoms from PFMT than women who had stronger pelvic floor muscles to start. This should give you hope if your pelvic floor muscles are very weak, to begin with; your potential for improvement is great. That same study indicates that "cure" and "cure/improvement" rates from PFMT were 73% and 97% respectively.

Urethral Blocking

This treatment uses sticky pads to cover the urethra. This treatment does not address the symptom or prevent the condition from worsening. It simply blocks the exit of the urethra, which prevents the urine from leaking out. It does not prevent the urine from leaving the bladder and filling the urethra.

Medication

Medicine is a less frequently offered treatment for stress incontinence. A medicine called Duloxetine is sometimes prescribed to increase the activity of the nerve that stimulates your urethral sphincter to improve its function. However, a 2017 study[134] found that "[a]lthough duloxetine is effective for stress urinary incontinence in women, the rates of associated harm were high when individual patient data were analyzed, and the harms outweighed the benefits." Your medical professional should advise if this medicine is right for you.

Bulking Agents

Bulking agents have been used to plump up lips as a cosmetic procedure for many years. Those same bulking agents can also be used as a treatment for stress incontinence. Figure 11.7 shows this treatment.

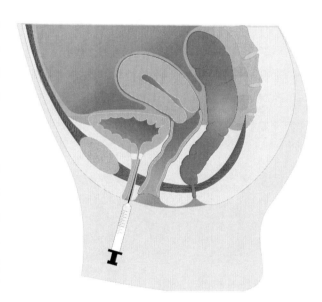

The needle is inserted through the urethra to the space around the neck of the bladder, as shown in Figure 11.7. These injections provide some additional bulk, which gives internal support). The treatment can be effective at reducing SUI symptoms with the British Association of Urological Surgeons suggesting a 50 to 70%

Figure 11.7: Bulking agent injection as treatment for SUI

success rate[135]; however, relief from SUI symptoms is temporary and the treatment would have to be regularly repeated.

There are side effects with urethral bulking, including a burning sensation, bleeding, failure to improve symptoms (20%–50% of patients), UR, urgency or OAB symptoms, and, in some cases, allergic reactions. You should weigh up these risks when you seek advice from your medical professional before considering this treatment.

LASER Treatments

LASER (Light Amplification by Stimulated Emission of Radiation) treatments are offered to treat SUI. These treatments are performed by placing a LASER device into the vaginal passage. The laser emits light that is absorbed by the skin. The light energy is converted to heat, producing tissue damage similar to a burn on vaginal tissues in order to promote regrowth of new tissues.

Originally, LASER vaginal treatment was used in plastic surgery with terms like "rejuvenation" and "vaginal tightening" promoting these treatments. This caused some medical professionals[136] to raise concerns as to whether these procedures were ethical.

A 2015 study[137] showed some promising results, with 77% of SUI patients showing an improvement in symptoms at one-year follow-ups. Side effects have not been fully documented and it is not yet clear of long-term efficacy.

The most recent review in April 2020[138] concluded "based on the available scientific evidence and on the lack of long-term follow-up, the use of LASER should, so far, not be recommended for the treatment of vaginal atrophy, vulvodynia, lichen sclerosis, stress urinary incontinence, vaginal prolapse, or vaginal laxity." More studies are needed before I would consider this option.

That concludes the non-surgical treatments for stress incontinence. We will now review the surgical options.

Surgical Treatments
Stress urinary incontinence

We will review four surgical treatments that are generally offered for stress incontinence. These are the following:
1. Retropubic suspension (urethropexy)
    a. Burch colposuspension
    b. Marshall-Marchetti-Krantz (MMK)
2. Anterior colporrhaphy/Kelly plication
3. Biological slings
4. Mesh slings
    a. TVT-sling
    b. TVT-O/Trans obturator tape (TOT) sling
    c. SIS/Mini-sling

The choice to have surgery is not one to be taken lightly. All surgeries carry risks that need to be weighed up against the benefits. Surgery will introduce scar tissue that can negatively impact the balance of tension within the pelvis. There is also a chance that the symptoms will appear again, as surgery often addresses symptoms rather than root cause (in the case of SUI, the root cause is an inability to manage intra-abdominal pressure by producing sufficient urethral closure pressure).

If you are suffering from incontinence, you should not consider surgery without first trying conservative treatments *with consistency* for at least eighteen months (in my opinion). This will also ensure you are as strong as possible should you require surgery, as this strength is likely to improve your recovery prospects.

Retropubic Suspension

There are two varieties of retropubic suspension (urethropexy) surgeries offered to treat stress incontinence, which are detailed below:

Surgery name: Burch Colposuspension

Treatment summary: Burch colposuspension is a retropubic suspension surgery that uses sutures to improve urethral positioning by lifting the neck of the bladder. The procedure was first performed in the late 1950s.

Procedure: Burch colposuspension was originally performed as open abdominal surgery but is now performed using a laparoscopic approach (keyhole surgery). The surgery is performed by making a small incision in your lower abdomen, just above your pubic bone, and placing the sutures as shown in Figure 11.8.

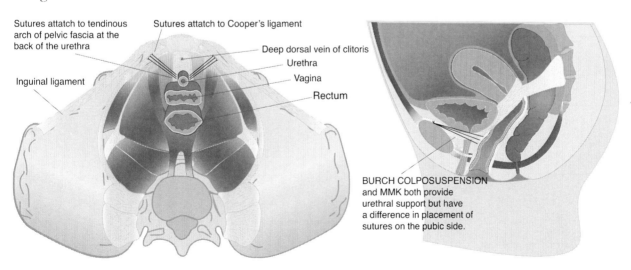

Figure 11.8: Burch colposuspension surgical procedure for stress incontinence.

Figure 11.8 shows the pelvis viewed from above, highlighting sutures attached to Cooper's ligament, providing support underneath the urethra.

Efficacy: There have been many long-term studies into these procedures and the success of the Burch procedure[139] is reported to be 90% after a five-to-ten-year follow-up and 69% after a ten-to-twenty-year follow-up. Retropubic suspension was considered to be the gold standard for SUI when the cause was urethral hypermobility.

Complications: Complications following the Burch procedure can include voiding difficulties or UR, development of OAB/urgency, and pelvic pain.

Surgery name: Marshall-Marchetti-Krantz (MMK)

Treatment Summary: The MMK is a retropubic suspension surgery that uses sutures to improve urethral positioning by lifting the neck of the bladder. The procedure was first performed in the mid-1940s.

Procedure: The main difference between the Burch procedure and the MMK is the placement of the sutures on the pubic side. Figure 11.9 shows the MMK procedure.

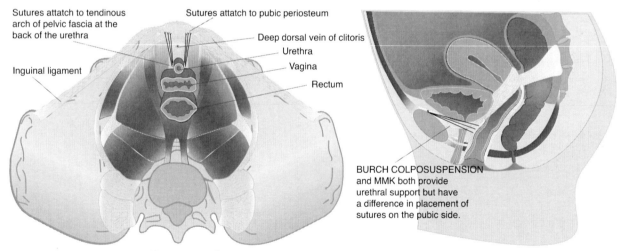

Figure 11.9: The MMK surgical procedure for stress incontinence.

Figure 11.9 shows the pelvis viewed from above, highlighting sutures attached to the pubic periosteum, providing support underneath the urethra.

Efficacy: The MMK procedure has been shown to be less efficacious in some studies in comparison to the Burch procedure, however, one long-term study[140] into the longevity of the MMK procedure found that failure tends to occur within the first two years and stated that patients who are still continent after two years will maintain continence in the long-term.

Complications: Complications following MMK are similar to the Burch procedure, including voiding difficulties or UR, development of OAB/urgency, and pelvic pain. However, an additional complication from MMK is a condition known as osteitis pubis[141]. This is an inflammation of the pubic bones, and, for this reason, the Burch procedure is preferred.

Anterior Colporrhaphy (AC)

This surgical treatment falls under one of two names, anterior colporrhaphy (AC) or Kelly plication. This procedure, detailed below, is also used in the treatment of cystocele (prolapse of the front vaginal wall), which we will discuss later in this chapter.

Surgery name: AC/Kelly plication

Treatment Summary: The use of AC or Kelly plication to treat stress incontinence (and POP) is one of the oldest gynecological procedures first performed in 1913. The surgery reinforces the tissues on the posterior side of the urethra (anterior vaginal wall), which is the space between the vagina and the urethra.

Procedure: A surgical incision is made inside the vaginal opening, exposing the space behind the urethra. There are multiple layers of tissue including the epithelium (vaginal tissue) and the endopelvic fascia (the connective tissue between the vagina and the urethra). The tissues are folded in on themselves (like a pleat) and stitched together to add support. You can visualize taking a wide thin piece of tissue pleating/stitching it so that it forms a narrower thicker piece of tissue.

Efficacy: This treatment has had varying rates of efficacy in studies but generally reports lower rates of success in the longer-term versus the Burch procedure. One study[142] showed AC with a 56% success rate at sixty months versus the Burch procedure, which showed 89%.

Complications: Complications following AC include voiding difficulties or UR, development of OAB/urgency, and pelvic pain

Biological Slings

This surgical treatment involves the use of biological materials for use as slings to support the urethra. The treatment is detailed below.

Surgery name: Biological Pubovaginal Sling (PVS)

Treatment Summary: Biological slings were the first slings used to treat SUI back in 1907 when Giordano used the gracilis (a muscle from the inner thigh) to support the bladder neck. Over subsequent years, other muscles were used until eventually, it was realized that muscles were not an ideal graft material due to difficulty with maintaining good blood and nerve supply.

The focus turned to using fascia, harvested either from the rectus abdominis (lower abs) or the fascia lata (large band of fascia down the outside of the leg). The first major study to confirm that fascial slings were safe and effective was in 1978 by McGuire et al.[143]

As well as using your own fascia (autologous slings), biological slings can be created using fascia from human cadavers (allograft slings) or from animals such as pigs (xenograft slings). The common name given to these slings is pubovaginal sling or PVS for short.

Procedure: The PVS procedure will either use a biological allo- or xeno- graft, or connective tissue harvested from your body at the beginning of the surgery. If your own connective tissue is used, it will be taken from just below your abs or alternatively from the fascia lata, which runs down the outside of your thigh.

The biological graft is soaked in an antibiotic solution before implantation. The implantation portion of the surgery involves two incisions, one in your lower abdomen just above the pubic bone, and one inside the vagina on the front (anterior) wall. Some surgeons perform this surgery using a laparoscopic keyhole approach, resulting in a faster-expected recovery period. Figure 11.10 shows the placement of the PVS.

You can see from Figure 11.10 that the sling reaches around behind the neck of the bladder to provide urethral support.

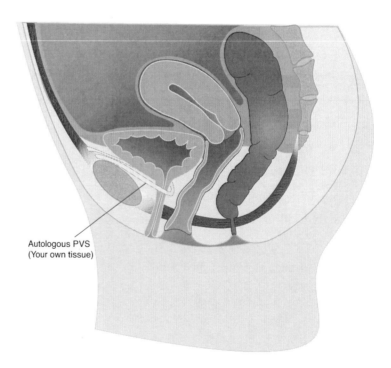

Autologous PVS
(Your own tissue)

Figure 11.10: Biological pubovaginal sling (PVS) placement.

If having abdominal surgery, you can expect to be in hospital overnight. Abdominal surgery typically lasts about an hour and has an expected recovery time of six weeks[144].

Efficacy: According to the British Association of Urological Surgeons (BAUS), success rates for PVS are the same as for mid-urethral slings (mesh) procedures but without mesh complications. A 2018 study[145] puts success rates for the autologous fascial sling at 87.8% with the remaining 12.2% of women seeing an improvement in symptoms.

Allograft slings (from a cadaver) and xenograft slings (from an animal) were introduced around the same time as synthetic mesh; however, they didn't receive the same level of uptake. A study in 2014[146] found that the costs of repair with synthetic mesh were roughly a quarter of that of biologic mesh, which likely contributed to its lower uptake, particularly in the USA where healthcare is for profit.

When it comes to efficacy for allograft slings, multiple early studies have shown high failure rates[147,148]. Xenograft slings have similarly shown high failure rates. In many cases, the small intestinal submucosa of pigs is used as a sling. Studies[149,150] have shown cure rates from 79 to 93% however, one study[151] suggests the small intestinal submucosa tissues (which are chemically treated) may still contain pig DNA.

Complications: There are some common complications with biological slings including voiding difficulties or UR, development of OAB/urgency, pelvic pain, and dyspareunia. There are additional complications specific to the type of graft:

For autologous slings, there is increased risk due to the operation time, potential infection, or pain at the site where the graft has been removed (e.g.: side of leg if harvesting fascia lata).

For allograft slings, there is a risk of transmission of illness from the cadaver tissue such as CJD (Creutzfeldt-Jakob prion disease), hepatitis, or HIV (human immunodeficiency virus). This type of tissue is also believed to have less tensile strength.

For Xenograft slings, there is a risk of encapsulation/contracture (where your body produces excess scar tissue around the graft). There is also a risk of developing a foreign body reaction that can prevent healing.

Mesh Slings

There are three Mesh surgeries offered to treat stress incontinence. The main difference between these surgeries is the placement of the mesh. These sling surgeries do not require major abdominal surgery, so operation time is reduced, and as a result, general surgery risks are reduced and recovery times are perceived to be shorter. These surgeries are detailed below:

Surgery Name: TVT-Sling

Treatment summary: The transvaginal tape or TVT sling is a mid-urethral sling also known as a retropubic sling due to its method of placement. This is the type of sling that was implanted into me. These slings use the same polypropylene material that is used to make blue IKEA bags.

Procedure: Implantation of the TVT can be bottom-up or top-down. For top-down, it is implanted by first making two incisions just above the pubic bone on the left and right side, and one inside the vagina in front of the urethra. The sling is attached to two large needles (known as trocars). Figure 11.11 shows the TVT-sling's placement when implanted.

One of the trochars is blindly inserted into one of the incisions above the public bone and guided past the bladder, blood vessels, and nerves, eventually reaching the vaginal incision. It is then guided to the inscision above the public bone on the opposite side. The blind insertion increases the risk of bladder perforation.

Bottom-up implantation involves the same incisions, but the needles are blindly fed through the incision in the vagina finally exiting at the site of the incisions above the public bone.

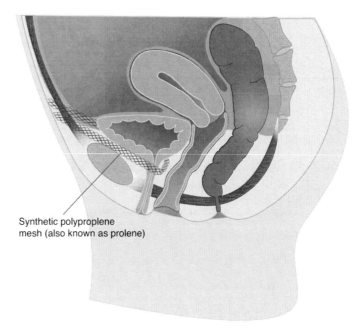

Synthetic polyproplene mesh (also known as prolene)

Figure 11.11: Mesh sling—TVT mesh placement.

Bottom-up implantation is the preferred route with one study[152] suggesting a lower number of bladder perforations with this approach versus top-down. In some cases, a small camera may be used to help guide the needles.

The mesh lies flat against the urethra and is checked to ensure there is no tension (hence sometimes calling it "tension-free vaginal tape"). The incisions are then closed.

Efficacy: A multi-study review[153] of eighty-one trials with 12,113 women comparing both TVT and TOT slings found long-term subjective cure rates ranging from 51% to 88% in the TVT group.

Complications: Complications are common with mesh slings. A 2017 study[154] including 92,246 women found that 9.8% of women will suffer complications thirty days to five years after the initial surgery. Mesh slings share common complications with other incontinence surgeries. These include voiding difficulties or UR, development of OAB/urgency, pelvic pain, and dyspareunia.

Mesh slings also share complications with xenografts, including encapsulation/contracture, and risk of foreign body reaction.

The most common complication with mesh materials is erosion (also called exposure, extrusion, or protrusion) where the mesh cuts through tissues. This can lead to damage to the vaginal wall, urethra, and/or bladder.

Erosion is more common with retropubic placement than with other placements. Erosion can lead to a fistula (a hole between the urethra and vagina allowing urine to leak into the vagina). If the mesh breaks through the vaginal wall, it can be felt by male partners as "something sharp" in the vagina, in some cases resulting in injury to the penis during intercourse[155].

Complications during surgery including bladder perforation and bleeding are more common with TVT than the other mid-urethral mesh slings.

Surgery Name: TVT-O / TOT

Treatment Summary: The TVT-O (Transvaginal Tape obturator) and TOT are mid-urethral slings made from a synthetic mesh (like the TVT). The sling provides support beneath the urethra but unlike the TVT, placement of TVT-O/TOT is from the inside of one thigh to the inside of the other.

Procedure: These devices are implanted in the space between the left and right obturator foramen (these are the holes in the hip bones that we visualized in Figure 2.7). Figure 11.12 shows the placement of TVT-O/TOT.

Figure 11.12 shows the pelvic floor muscles from beneath the skin with the blue mesh sling visible. TVT-O is implanted inside-out whereas TOT is implanted outside-in.

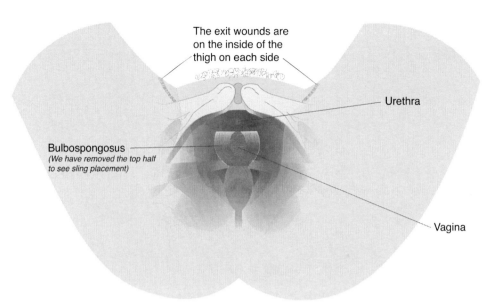

The exit wounds are on the inside of the thigh on each side

Urethra

Bulbospongosus
(We have removed the top half to see sling placement)

Vagina

Figure 11.12: Mesh Sling—TVT-O/TOT mesh placement.

For TVT-O, an incision is made inside the vagina in front of the urethra. The sling is attached to two large needles (known as trocars). With the inside-out approach, the first needle is inserted into the vagina and guided past muscles, blood vessels, and nerves until the fascia at the obturator membrane is perforated.

The curved needle is then rotated toward a small mark the surgeon has made on the inside of the patient's leg close to the groin. The needle is pushed through the obturator externus muscle, two of the adductor muscles (magnus & brevis), and the gracilis muscle, before coming through the skin. This procedure is repeated on the other side.

For TOT with the outside-in approach, two incisions are made on the inside of the legs close to the groin and one in the front wall of the vagina. The needle is fed in through the groin on one side, going through the same muscles and past the nerves, blood vessels, and connective tissue.

Once the needle makes it to the hole in the vaginal wall, the needle is then guided up through the tissues to come out at the groin on the opposite side.

With both approaches, the tape lies flat against the urethra and is checked to ensure there is no tension. The incisions are closed following implantation.

Efficacy: Most studies[156] found no significant difference[157] in efficacy between these two approaches with cure rates of 76% to 92%.

Complications: As well as the complications listed for TVT, patients TVT-O/TOT often suffer neuromuscular pain that can radiate down the leg. This can create walking difficulties. Groin pain and vaginal injuries are also more common with this treatment[158]. I believe these issues are due to the mesh being implanted through the adductor muscles.

Surgery Name: Mid-urethral sling (SIS)

Treatment Summary: The single incision sling (SIS), also known as the mini-sling, is a version of the TVT-O/TOT sling. Unlike the TVT-O/TOT, however, the mini-sling attaches to the obturator membrane (connective tissue) rather than going through the muscles to come out at the inside of the legs.

Procedure: This type of sling requires only a single incision in the vagina, beneath the urethra, which makes this a faster surgery with less surgery risk and a faster recovery time. The mini-sling placement is shown in Figure 11.13.

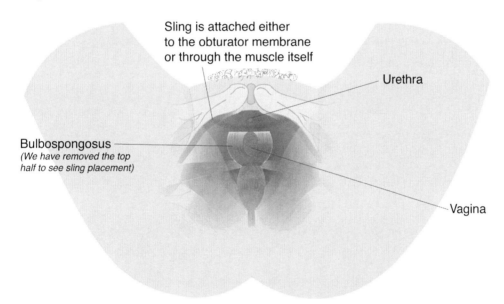

Figure 11.13: Mesh Sling—SIS (Mini-sling) placement.

Figure 11.13 shows the mini-sling in blue. Like the TOT, the SIS mini-sling application needle is inserted through an incision in the vagina just behind the urethra. The needle is guided past muscles, blood vessels, and nerves.

Depending on the specific sling (there are multiple brands), it will either be guided to the obturator muscle or into the obturator membrane (connective tissue). The mesh is placed flat against the urethra with no tension. There are no additional incisions required with this surgery.

Mini-slings and SIS devices need some form of adhesion to ensure they attach and stay in place. Some have an adhesive surface, while others have anchors or barbs that have some abrasion allowing them to grip or hook onto the muscle or connective tissue to which they should attach (a little like a fishhook).

Efficacy: The first of these devices to be brought to market was the TVT-Secur (also known as the TVT-S), which had multiple studies showing positive results[159,160]. However, the device was withdrawn from the market with some studies concluding it was inferior to TVT-O[161] and had a high recurrence rate of stress incontinence[162].

Another European randomized study[163], comparing single-incision slings with TVT-O slings also found the SIS to be inferior to TVT-O in both objective and subjective cure rates but superior in respect to postoperative pain.

Since the removal of the TVT-S from the US market, other SIS devices have been brought to market through the 501(k) mechanism with the TVT-Secur as the "similar" device to prove efficacy due to it being the most studied single incision sling. If you opt for this type of surgery, you must be aware that you are effectively a guinea pig due to the lack of studies.

Complications: The SIS has the same common risks as other mesh devices and an increased risk of failure leading to a return of stress incontinence.

Summary of Surgery to Treat Stress Incontinence

Having reviewed the surgical options, I feel it is important to summarize the information. *Surgery as a treatment for SUI should be the very last resort.* In many countries, surgery using mesh is offered as a first-line treatment, even though medical guidelines advise otherwise. This is due to the perception by a lot of surgeons that the "gold standard" mesh surgeries are quick, easy, effective, and safe.

With one in every ten women implanted[164] suffering mesh-related complications, you should consider your options carefully. Patient support groups across the world are filled with thousands of mesh-injured women who were not offered alternatives, nor alerted to the dangers. Current bans and restrictions require that you are alerted to the dangers and offered non-mesh alternatives.

Please also be aware that women are commonly told "this is a different mesh" or "this is not one of those problem devices." This is like saying "It's not Coke. It's different. It's Pepsi." *All mesh devices* are mesh and carry a very high risk. In my opinion, their use should be avoided (and banned). Ask for a second opinion if you feel you are being pressured or ignored when you discuss your concerns.

The true rate of mesh injuries is not known as no country has tracked implantation, even though mesh has been used for 25 years. I am mesh-injured and have not been counted in any mesh-injury database. The true extent of harm from mesh may never be understood.

Non-mesh surgeries offer similar levels of efficacy but without the extra risks associated with mesh materials. All surgeries have the potential to fail, which would mean a return of incontinence. I have spoken to many women who have had repeat surgeries where second and third mesh slings were added on top of the original sling to try to address the failure, often without success. Be mindful of this should you find yourself in that position.

If you have a mesh sling and are considering a removal, I have written an article sharing eighteen considerations for mesh removal, which can be found on theflowerempowered.com. Partial removals and dissections (where the mesh is cut in half) are inadvisable and often lead to multiple further surgeries.

If you do have your mesh removed, there is a 50%[165] chance your pain will continue following its removal. Removal of mesh is like removing chewing gum from hair. It is not possible to take it away without removing a lot of your own tissues with it and the result can leave you severely incontinent. Removal is not a decision to be taken lightly and needs to be performed by a skilled surgeon due to the risk of further injury or even death. There are few surgeons skilled at mesh removal, so waiting lists tend to be long and many women have to travel long distances for removal.

Many surgeons don't want to accept that the graft material is at fault. I personally have debated with a mesh implantation surgeon who felt justified in continuing to perform the surgeries as she felt that helping those other nine women was worth the risk of injuring one in ten. With all of this information to hand, you will have to decide for yourself if you would be willing to take the risk.

That concludes the surgical treatments for SUI. We will now review mixed incontinence.

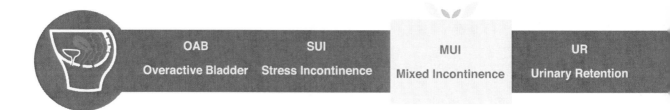

OAB
Overactive Bladder

SUI
Stress Incontinence

MUI
Mixed Incontinence

UR
Urinary Retention

Mixed incontinence combines the symptoms of OAB and SUI, where you can suffer both urgency, frequent urination, and leakage. The treatments offered are the same as those that have already been reviewed for OAB and SUI, so refer to those sections for details.

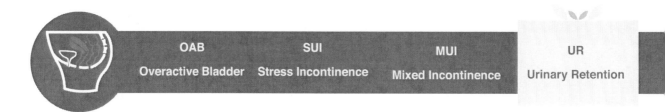

OAB
Overactive Bladder

SUI
Stress Incontinence

MUI
Mixed Incontinence

UR
Urinary Retention

UR is the inability to partially or completely empty the bladder. Acute UR can be life-threatening, so it is critical to seek medical advice should you display symptoms of retention. Men are ten times more likely to suffer retention versus women[166], and as such, studies into UR in women are limited.

UR can be caused by obstruction, for example from kidney stones, tumors blocking the urethra, or obstruction caused by POP (cystocele) creating a kink in the urethra. UR can be a symptom of other conditions such as multiple sclerosis, diabetes, or Parkinson's disease.

Antimuscarinic drugs, such as muscle relaxants (including those used to treat OAB), non-steroidal anti-inflammatory drugs (NSADs), and antidepressants, can also cause UR.

Chronic UR is a condition that tends to develop over a long period of time. With this condition, it can feel like you constantly need to urinate (similar to OAB) but are unable to start the stream or have a slow/weak stream once it gets started. This can be due to an inability to fully relax the external urethral sphincter. It can also be due to stiffness or scarring of the bladder or a lack of coordination with the reflexes of urination.

Regardless of the cause, it is important to seek medical care for this condition as it can be life-threatening and can also cause urinary tract and kidney infections.

Non-Surgical Treatments
Urinary retention

There are multiple treatment options available for UR, depending on the case.

Pelvic Floor Muscle Down-Training

When retention is due to hypertonicity (rare), reverse Kegels can be used to train the pelvic floor to relax. You will find reverse Kegels in the Phase 1 pelvic floor module of the eight-phase training. Biofeedback devices can also be used to complement down-training. These therapies are typically offered in a physiotherapy setting.

Medications

Most medications used in the treatment of UR are only for use in men, with the exception of Terazosin[167] and Doxazosin (which can cause incontinence[168]). Studies into these drugs have focused mostly on the treatment of males.

Catheterization

A catheter is a device that is inserted through the urethra into the bladder to allow emptying. A little bit like a straw, a catheter will create a channel for the urine to flow out. Catheters can also be used for urethral dilation to widen the urethra if the tissues are restricted. There are two main types of catheters as listed below.

1. **Indwelling catheter (also known as a Foley catheter)**: Indwelling catheters are fitted and remain in place for up to 3 months. An inflatable balloon on the bladder side of the tube stops it from sliding back out of the urethra. The catheter tube can be drained into a bag (strapped to the leg) or can be emptied by a release valve into the toilet.

2. **Intermittent catheter**: An intermittent catheter is a short-term catheter that you insert for the purpose of bladder emptying and then it is immediately removed. It can be used by a professional or for self-catheterization. You will be trained in self-catheterization if needed.

Bladder Retraining

Bladder retraining and lifestyle modifications may also be proposed as a treatment of UR. This has been detailed in the OAB non-surgical treatments.

Surgery for UR may be performed if there is an obstruction from kidney stones, a tumor, or a POP (cystocele). You can read more on the surgical treatment for Cystocele in the POP surgical treatments section later in this chapter.

That concludes the treatments for urinary symptoms.

Fecal Conditions

We will now explore fecal symptoms, many of which have similar treatments to urinary symptoms.

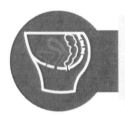

FI
Fecal Incontinence

CC
Chronic Constipation

FI is the unintentional leakage of poop. As well as being a symptom of PFD, it can also be a symptom of neurological diseases like multiple sclerosis or spina-bifida. FI can also present as a symptom of inflammatory bowel disease such as ulcerative colitis or Crohn's disease. Tearing from childbirth can damage the anal sphincter resulting in muscle dysfunction, which can also contribute to FI.

Severe diarrhea can result in fecal leakage but is not an indication of FI. Rather, it is a symptom of the gastrointestinal issue causing the leakage. Chronic diarrhea and rectal urgency however are both risk factors[169] for developing FI, and these conditions are impacted by bowel habits and nutritional/lifestyle choices.

With FI, you cannot hold your poop under normal circumstances. It can be an indication of a weak anal sphincter, although it can also happen in cases of extreme intra-abdominal pressure increases (such as lifting very heavy weights or pushing out a baby).

Those with stress incontinence are at an increased risk of developing FI. You should seek medical advice if you are suffering from FI.

Non-Surgical Treatments

Fecal incontinence

There are six non-surgical FI treatments detailed in this section. They are as follows:

Pelvic Floor Muscle Training

PFMT for FI is usually managed in a physiotherapy setting and generally combines additional therapies such as biofeedback, neuro-muscular electrical stimulation (NMES), and neuro-galvanic electrical stimulation (NGES). Studies into pelvic floor rehabilitation show 50% to 80% success in the treatment of FI[170]. Biofeedback has been reported to relieve symptoms in 72% of patients[171]. *Note*: Information on biofeedback and electrical stimulation devices will be provided in Chapter Twelve.

Bowel Retraining

Bowel retraining, like bladder retraining, may be offered as a treatment for FI if disordered bowel habits have contributed to the condition. Bowel retraining involves setting timed intervals to use the bathroom and staying on the toilet for a set time (usually fifteen to twenty minutes) following either coffee or a meal. You should not strain excessively to poop. If defecation does not happen normally, go about your business.

It may be suggested to use an enema following three days without defecation during bowel retraining. If so, your doctor will prescribe a pre-made enema. Bowel retraining should only be undertaken under the guidance of your healthcare provider.

Medication

Drugs are not typically offered to treat fecal incontinence, but they can be used to treat diarrhea or constipation, both of which can have an impact on FI.

Anal Plug

Anal plugs are similar to tampons but for the anus; shown in Figure 11.14, the anal plug sits beyond the pelvic floor muscles with the removal string hanging from the body. This can be viewed as a management tool rather than a treatment (FI pads are also available for this purpose). You can read more on plugs and pads in Chapter Twelve.

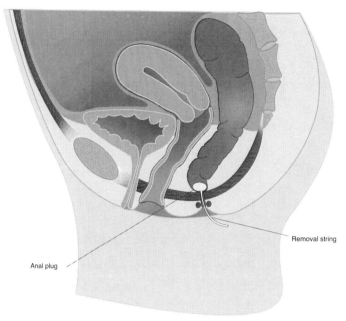

Figure 11.14: Anal plug for the management of FI.

Bulking Agents

Bulking agents can be used to provide bulk around the anal sphincter. Figure 11.15 shows the placement of bulking agents to treat FI.

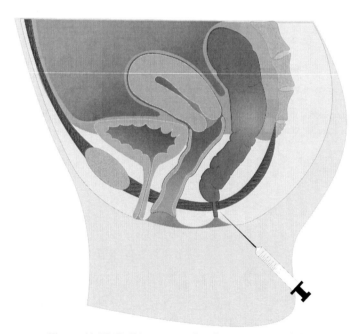

Figure 11.15: Bulking agents for the treatment of FI.

Figure 11.15 shows how a needle is used to inject bulking agents into the area surrounding the anal sphincter to increase passive outlet resistance. The treatment has not proven to be completely effective, with most studies[172] reporting only a 15% to 50% improvement.

TPTNS/PTNS

TPTNS and PTNS are nerve stimulation modalities that we reviewed as OAB non-surgical treatments. These modalities are also offered in the treatment of FI. One study[173] found 63% of patients reported some degree of improvement following an at-home course of TPTNS treatment over three months. Another study[174] suggested that PTNS was an effective treatment for FI, however, these studies were both small. Further studies into these treatments are needed and you should only use this treatment if prescribed by your healthcare provider.

Surgical Treatments
Fecal incontinence

There are three non-surgical options for FI and they are detailed in this section.

Sacral Nerve Stimulation

Sacral nerve stimulation is an OAB treatment also used to treat FI. The procedure, efficacy, and complications are detailed earlier in this chapter. Sacral nerve stimulation has been used to treat FI since 1995 and is considered to have "revolutionized" the treatment of FI[175]. One multicenter prospective study[176] reported a 90% success rate with test implantation and 85% success at twenty-four months.

Anal Sphincter Repair Surgeries

Anal sphincter repair surgeries are sometimes performed and, on rare occasions, a treatment known as a dynamic graciloplasty is performed. This is where part of the gracilis muscle is mobilized and used to form a new sphincter (while ensuring the nerve bundle for the muscle remains intact). Learning to voluntarily contract this muscle is difficult so this procedure typically includes implantation of a small electrical stimulation device, similar to the SNS device, to stimulate contractions to control the muscle. Severe complications are frequent with graciloplasty. One study[177] showed 92% having severe treatment-related complications so, get a second opinion if this treatment is offered.

Fecal Diversion

Fecal diversion surgery is an extreme option that can be considered the very last resort. It is a surgical intervention in which a colostomy, an opening in the large intestine, is created. Fecal matter is diverted through the colostomy to an external bag (stoma). It is a permanent treatment that cannot be reversed.

That completes the surgical options for FI. We will now review the treatments for CC.

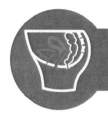

FI
Fecal Incontinence

CC
Chronic Constipation

CC is a functional gastrointestinal disorder that results in persistently hard-to-pass stools (Types 1 or 2 on the Bristol stool scale, which we viewed in Figure 5.7). CC can lead to excessive straining, which is detrimental to pelvic floor function. This condition is typically diagnosed if you have fewer than three defecations a week for six months or more.

There are many potential causes including nutritional deficiencies, dehydration, allergies, medications (for example antidepressants, narcotics, and iron tablets), vitamin deficiencies, irritable bowel syndrome (IBS), and diseases (multiple sclerosis, Parkinson's, etc.). It is important to seek medical advice if you are suffering from constipation. Constipation can be a symptom of an NR-PFD where hypertonic pelvic floor muscles can obstruct defecation. It can also be a symptom of a POP (rectocele). Whereas management of constipation as a symptom of PFD is covered in Chapter Ten, treatments for the condition are beyond the scope of this book.

That completes the treatments for fecal symptoms. We will now explore the treatment of POP.

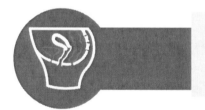

POP
Pelvic Organ Prolapse

POP is a hernia within the pelvis. The name given to the specific hernia is based on the organ that is prolapsing. For example, a rectocele is a hernia where the rectum is prolapsing into the vagina. "Cele" means hernia. A hernia is the area that provides the path of least resistance when there is an increase in pressure; or, to put it another way, the area that produces the least tension in resisting pressure.

Our bodies are pressure chambers formed mostly from soft tissues. We learned about these pressure chambers when we explored Figure 3.1, which showed the body's cavities. Herniation can happen not just in these cavities, but also elsewhere in the body. I would expect that most people have some degree of herniation in their body, whether that be as small as a varicose vein or as large as a full diastasis recti (abdominal separation). It is estimated that 50% of parous women (mothers) will have some degree of POP[178].

The Balloon Analogy to Explain POP

Many POPs are asymptomatic (they produce no symptoms). This is to be expected, particularly with stage 1 and 2 prolapses as the tissues are likely to be in an anatomically correct position unless they are being exposed to excess intra-abdominal pressure.

We can use the analogy of a balloon to demonstrate this. An empty balloon is under no pressure and therefore has no "bulge." If you blow air into the balloon, you put the balloon's tissues under pressure, which creates a "bulge."

Now think about the balloon. If it was made from really tough material but had a weak spot, the tough tissue would resist expansion from the increase in pressure more than the weak spot, causing the weak spot to expand excessively and creating a small bulge with lighter balloon tissues.

The balloon functions more efficiently if it has consistent tension throughout, as does the body. This is one of the reasons why myofascial release has a positive impact on POP. Releasing taut tissues increases the elastic potential of those tissues allowing for more even expansion when exposed to pressure increases. Better for everything to stretch a little than for one point to stretch a lot.

The eight-phase program uses a combination of practices that adhere to this principle. We use yin yoga to release both taut connective tissues and muscle hypertonicity, encouraging a rebalancing of tension. This can reduce the impact of herniation by improving elasticity in tissues surrounding the weak point, so they resist a little less, which can reduce the amount of excess pressure placed on the point of herniation.

The eight-phase program also teaches you to increase your strength in order to manage intra-abdominal pressures. Good pelvic floor muscle control is the equivalent of placing your hand over the weak point in the balloon to prevent it from excessively expanding. Pelvic floor training creates the strength that provides support beneath the pelvic organs to help resist against pressure increases. If you can understand these principles, you are empowered to live your best life without POP defining you.

We reviewed the POP-Q measuring system in Figure 8.7. Measurements using this grading system are performed by trained medical professionals. They typically communicate your stage of POP after this evaluation. POP herniations are measured in four stages, with each stage being incrementally worse than the previous stage, where stage four has a herniation that protrudes outside the vagina.

When you look at the visualizations of these POP images, I would like you to realize that they are the equivalent of the herniation when under pressure (so the POP balloon has been blown-up). This isn't necessarily the all-day everyday position. If you can understand this, particularly if you have a grade 1 or 2 POP, you are empowered to learn to avoid "blowing up the POP balloon" unnecessarily. There are four main categories of POP that are listed below.

Rectocele

A rectocele is a herniation where the path of least resistance is on the back wall of the vaginal passage between the rectum and the vagina. Figure 11.6 shows the first three stages of rectal prolapse.

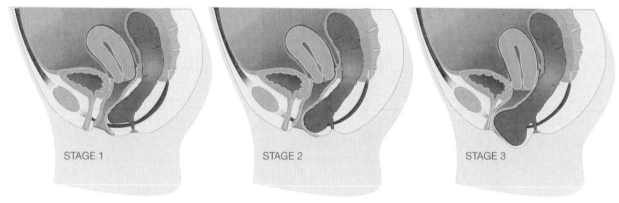

STAGE 1   STAGE 2   STAGE 3

Figure 11.16: Pelvic organ prolapse—The first three stages of a rectocele.

Figure 11.16 shows the progress of herniation as the condition worsens, allowing more pressure to fill the POP balloon when there is excess intra-abdominal pressure. Remember, these images are showing the "filled balloon" rather than the all-day, everyday position.

In the case of a rectocele, pressure comes not only in the form of intra-abdominal pressure but also from the build-up of feces within the rectum. The rectocele can create a pocket that prevents complete emptying, leaving you needing to splint to fully defecate (we detailed splinting in POP Fecal Strategy 3, Chapter Ten).

One study[179] estimated that 80% of rectoceles are asymptomatic so the prevalence of this type of condition is potentially underestimated. It is critical with this type of prolapse to ensure that you avoid constipation and learn to listen for the subtle messages from your bowel telling you that it is time to empty. The POP symptom management advice in Chapter Ten should help you to manage rectocele.

Cystocele

A cystocele is a herniation where the path of least resistance is on the front wall of the vaginal passage between the urethra and the vagina. Figure 11.17 shows the first three stages of a cystocele.

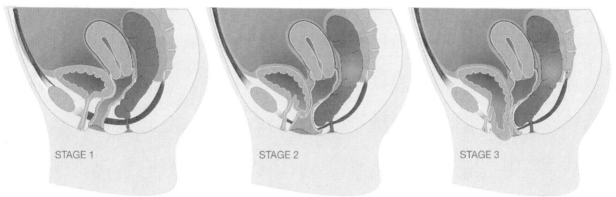

Figure 11.17: Pelvic organ prolapse—The first three stages of a cystocele.

Figure 11.17 shows how the bladder can get pulled into the vaginal passage with an increase in intra-abdominal pressure. This can cause a kink in the urethra (which can lead to UR or difficulty in starting a void) and can also prevent full emptying of the bladder. You can try UR Strategy 4 (the HCDV) in Chapter Ten to help you to empty if you have this issue.

Once again, you should remember that these images show the hernia when under pressure (either from tension in tissues pulling or intra-abdominal pressures pushing). Training to rebalance tension in your tissues and learning to manage intra-abdominal pressures will make a big difference to your symptoms and help you to avoid "blowing up the POP balloon."

Uterine Prolapse

A uterine prolapse is a herniation where the path of least resistance exists around the ligaments that support the cervix at the neck of the womb. We viewed these ligaments in Figure 3.12.

Figure 11.18, on the next page, shows the first three stages of a uterine prolapse where the uterus can descend into the vaginal cavity when under excess intra-abdominal pressure.

It is important to remember that the position of the cervix (the opening of the uterus) changes during a normal monthly cycle as we saw in Figure 8.14. This fluctuation should not be confused with uterine prolapse; however, you should remember that the fluctuation could make your prolapse feel more symptomatic at different stages during your cycle.

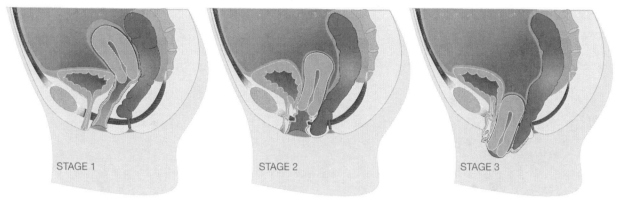

STAGE 1   STAGE 2   STAGE 3

Figure 11.18: Pelvic organ prolapse—The first three stages of uterine prolapse.

Figure 11.18 shows how the tissues of the vagina can kink as the uterus descends.

Enterocele

An Enterocele is a herniation that can happen around the vaginal fornix, which is the tissue at the top of the vagina surrounding the neck of the cervix. It causes the tissues of the small bowel (intestines) to protrude into the vaginal cavity or the space between the vagina and the rectum (where the apex, the upper back part of the vagina, collapses). Remember that the prolapse occurs when there is excess pressure. Figure 11.19 shows a stage four enterocele.

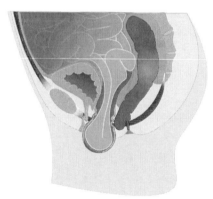

Figure 11.19: Pelvic organ prolapse—The fourth stage of an enterocele.

You can see in Figure 11.19 there is no womb present, this is to highlight that this type of prolapse is more common following hysterectomy and it often requires further surgical repair.

Hysterectomy is one of the most frequently performed gynecological surgeries globally with up to 90% of hysterectomies being performed to treat benign conditions[180]. Following hysterectomy, the path of least resistance exists due to destabilization surrounding the ligaments of the uterus due to uterine removal. Some techniques that add support when removing the womb are believed to help prevent enterocele following hysterectomy.

One such method, recommended by a systematic review in Nov 2020[181], is known as a "McCall culdoplasty" (or a variation of that method), which sutures different parts of the vagina to their respective uterosacral ligaments. Hysterectomies that save the cervix are also considered to be less prone to this type of prolapse. If you are considering a hysterectomy, you should discuss the associated risk of developing an enterocele with your surgeon.

It is not uncommon for more than one type of POP to be diagnosed at the same time and I want to assure you, if you receive a diagnosis of multiple POPs, you can still empower yourself to manage those POPs and live a healthy life.

One important point, when it comes to the avoidance of *"blowing up the POP balloon"*, is that there is a positive correlation between intra-abdominal pressure and BMI[182]. If you have any herniation (whether it be POP, DR, abdominal hernia, rectal prolapse, or inguinal hernia), you should carefully manage your weight to eliminate unnecessary excess pressure from an unhealthy BMI.

Having explained the various types of POP, we will now explore the non-surgical treatments offered for POP. Overlap exists between these treatments and the symptom-management strategies listed in Chapter Ten. I would encourage you to work with a pelvic floor PT if you have POP as this will greatly enhance your prospect of managing and possibly overcoming the condition.

 ## Non-Surgical Treatments
Pelvic organ prolapse (POP)

There are three non-surgical options for POP detailed in this section. They are as follows:

PFMT
PFMT is typically the primary treatment for POP, which is usually offered in a physiotherapy setting and is the primary focus of this book. PFMT is shown to both improve subjective POP symptoms and objective POP severity[183].

Hypopressive exercises
Hypopressives are offered as a treatment for POP and they are included as part of the eight-phase training in this book. However, as I mentioned in Part One, evidence for its efficacy as a treatment for SUI or POP has not been forthcoming.

A randomized control trial published in April 2020[184], included ninety-four women in three groups. One PFMT group, one PFMT + hypopressives group and one hypopressives-only group. The study did not find statistical differences in outcomes between the three groups. However, the hypopressives-only group was also trained to practice *the knack*, which is a pelvic floor exercise (this is covered in SUI Strategy 2) so, it could not be concluded that their gains were the result of the hypopressive exercises. I have heard many hypopressive teachers say that the exercises strengthen the pelvic floor. However, I do not believe that to be the case, and nor do I believe that to be the benefit of these exercises.

In Chapter Three, we learned how the pattern of connective tissue fibers depends on your movement patterns, and how this movement leaves slug-like collagen trails, which eventually form new connective tissue fibers through which tension is distributed. In my opinion, the movement of connective tissues within the intra-abdominal space when performing hypopressives has the potential to stimulate the formation of new fibers. Consistency over an extended period would be absolutely required for this to lead to an improvement in POP and I would hope that eventually there would be evidence to substantiate this hypothesis.

Myofascial release

Myofascial release of the pelvic floor was discussed when reviewing the ligaments of the uterus in Chapter Three. This technique releases excess tension from tissues that surround the point of herniation. This restores elasticity to those tissues, and reduces stiffness, which enables a better distribution of pressure. A UK study[185], with participants having a blend of different types of prolapse, of which, 70% of participants had more than one prolapse, reported meaningful reductions in prolapse symptoms following treatment. Further research is underway.

Pessaries

Pessaries provide intravaginal structural support covered in POP Heaviness Strategy 1, in Chapter Ten. Pessaries are either supportive or space-filling. A multicenter randomized controlled trial of women with stage two or greater POP found that there was a significant improvement in symptoms reported by the group using pessaries as a treatment for POP[186].

Pessaries can be very beneficial when there is a lot of tissue laxity within the vaginal passage, as may be the case if you have a connective tissue disorder such as Ehlers-Danlos syndrome. Your healtcare provider can confirm if a pessary is right for you. Figure 11.20 shows a visualization of pessaries in place within the vagina. There are three different pessaries shown in Figure 11.20; a ring pessary, Gellhorn pessary, and ring pessary with a knob.

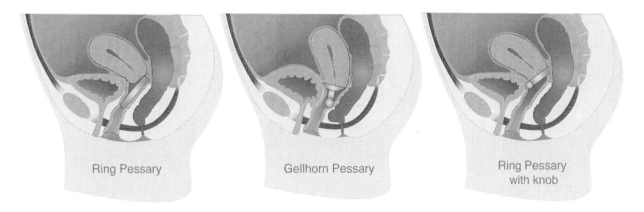

Figure 11.20: Pessaries for pelvic organ prolapse—supportive or space-filling.

Ring pessaries are support pessaries, which are commonly used for the early stages of prolapse. They can also be used to prevent stress incontinence. The silicone ring is folded in half for insertion and unfolds to provide support. Sometimes a string is attached to aid removal. There are many more shapes and structures of supportive pessaries available, including gehrung and mar-land. Support pessaries can remain in place during intercourse.

Gellhorn pessaries are space-filling and commonly used for more advanced prolapses where the patient is no longer sexually active. There are many more shapes and structures of space-filling pessaries such as donuts and cubes. It is not possible to have intercourse with a space-filling pessary in place.

Pessaries are designed to be persistently worn. They can be removed and cleaned weekly, or even daily if the patient is comfortable with removal and refitting. If the patient is unable to remove the pessary, they will likely have the cleaning performed by their healthcare provider every two to three months. It is common for pessaries to be either plastic or silicone, with silicone pessaries going through a high-temperature process to ensure sterilization.

There are some potential complications with pessaries, the mildest of which being vaginal discharge or odors. More severe complications such as fistula (ulcer/sore) or erosion can occur. The use of local estrogen creams may be advised to reduce the risk of fistula or tissue damage.

One study presented two cases where pessaries had been neglected, leaving them in place for an extended period causing fibrosis. That study concluded that "resulting fibrosis can cure the prolapse"[187]. Fibrosis is the thickening or scarring of tissues. I would not suggest that you "forget" your pessary in the hopes that it will cure you, but do consider the support of a pessary if you need it and continue to work on rebalancing the tension in your body while utilizing that support.

Surgical Treatments

Pelvic organ prolapse (POP)

An Oxford study[188] showed that women who have POP repair surgery have a 10.8% risk of requiring further surgery within the following eleven years, although it is noted that it will most likely be for a different prolapse. This is unsurprising, given what we have learned with the balloon analogy.

Surgery adds scar tissue, which is taut (less elastic) in comparison to the surrounding tissues. You should understand by now that adding stiff inflexible tissues in the pelvis is counterproductive to proper function and will expose other tissues to weakness. Surgery does not train you to manage the intra-abdominal pressure that was responsible for "blowing up the POP balloon" in the first place. Intra-abdominal pressure will find the new path of least resistance and, *hey, presto*…a new POP balloon will be filled.

The surgical treatments offered for POP tend to fall into mesh and non-mesh varieties. POP surgeries that use mesh are now banned (in the USA, New Zealand, and Australia) due to a lack of evidence on their safety and efficacy. Even with the ban, many surgeons still prefer to use mesh as they believe it has superior results versus native tissues or biological grafts.

One 2019 study[189] assessed reoperation rates between biologic and synthetic grafts for POP repair over a 6-year period. They found reoperation rates to be the same, although the reason for reoperation with biological grafts was the recurrence of POP. With mesh grafts, reoperation was due to mesh complications. Another study[190] found both native tissue and POP repairs to be successful but with reoperation for native tissue being 5% compared to 9% for mesh repairs.

If you are suffering from POP, you should visit a pelvic floor PT, preferably one who is trained in myofascial release. Consider non-surgical options, such as having a pessary fitted and try everything in your power to avoid surgery. In my opinion, surgery should only be considered in late-stage prolapses, and only after conservative treatments have been tried with consistency for an extended period, without success.

There are many names given to the surgeries for POP and a blend of techniques are often used in each surgery. Surgeries can be open abdominal varieties, laparoscopic (keyhole), or vaginal. Sometimes surgeries are performed directly by a surgeon and sometimes they are robotically performed (where the surgeon is nearby using a robot-controlled device to perform the tasks).

Surgeries often involve the use of tissue grafts (as reviewed in the stress incontinence section of this chapter), with biological issues more likely to undergo tissue remodeling and less likely to cause erosion[191].

Covering all the possible options would be beyond the scope of this book, but we will explore two main surgery types in both their native tissue and mesh versions. These surgeries are designed to add support either to the vaginal walls (to repair cystocele or rectocele) or to the apex of the vaginal passage (to repair uterine prolapse or enterocele).

As it is possible to have more than one prolapse simultaneously, repair surgeries can sometimes include multiple repairs within the same operation.

Vaginal Wall Repairs

Vaginal wall repairs are typically performed on the front (anterior) walls of the vagina to treat cystocele, or on the back (posterior) walls of the vagina to treat rectocele. They can be performed using native tissues or using biological grafts (allograft or xenograft) or synthetic mesh. Vaginal wall surgeries are detailed below as follows:

Surgery Name: Biological Cystocele Repairs

Treatment Summary: Anterior vaginal wall repair can be performed with native tissue or a biological graft. This surgery is referred to as an anterior colporrhaphy (AC—like the Kelly plication technique used for stress incontinence) and is shown in Figure 11.21.

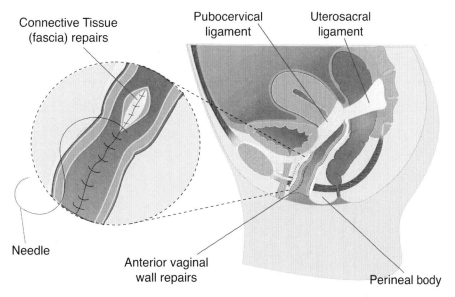

Figure 11.21: Surgical repair of cystocele (anterior wall repair) using native tissue.

In the zoomed-in image in Figure 11.21, you can see how the connective tissue and vaginal mucosa are sutured for additional support along the anterior wall.

Procedure: This procedure is typically performed vaginally. The prolapsed vaginal wall is dissected off the underlying connective tissue. Plicating sutures are used to augment support in connective tissue and subsequently, the vaginal tissues are sutured. There are many techniques that may be used to suture the layers of tissue to provide support (like the pleating in Kelly plication). Sutures can be either permanent or absorbable.

Efficacy: Results in studies vary and no consensus on the efficacy seems to exist. One study[192] assessed long-term efficacy and satisfaction rate following native tissue repair. That study assessed both objective success (physical grading 0 or 1 for Cystocele) and subjective success (the patient's satisfaction with the procedure). They found that objective success was 13.2% whereas subjective success was 68.7%. A whopping 98.5% of patients reported being satisfied with the procedure.

Complications: Anterior repair procedures without the use of grafts (native tissue only) report few side effects aside from those associated with general surgery. Occasionally, there can be some voiding difficulties or UR, pelvic pain, and dyspareunia. There have also been reported cases of de novo incontinence following this procedure (stress incontinence that did not exist prior to the repairs) with one study[193] finding 22% (sixteen out of twenty-three women) developed stress incontinence following repairs.

Additional complications with biological graft materials are the same as those with biological graft materials used to treat SUI, which have been detailed earlier in this chapter.

Surgery Name: Biological Rectocele Repairs

Treatment Summary: Posterior vaginal wall repair can be performed with native tissue or a biological graft. This surgery is referred to as a posterior colporrhaphy (PC), with the native tissue version shown in Figure 11.22.

In the zoomed-in image in Figure 11.22, you can see how the connective tissue and vaginal mucosa are sutured for additional support along the posterior wall. This was the type of prolapse repair that I had during the surgery when the mesh sling was implanted. A perineal repair was performed during the same surgery.

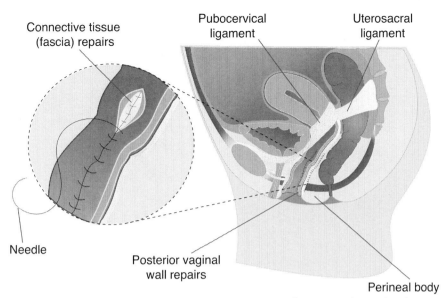

Figure 11.22: Surgical repair of rectocele (posterior wall repair), using native tissue.

Efficacy: As with cystocele repairs, results into studies into PC vary and consensus on the efficacy is sketchy. One long-term study[194] into sexual function and QoL for patients with native-tissue rectocele repairs concluded that "[v]aginal native tissue repair is a safe and effective procedure for symptomatic rectocele, with a low rate of complications, and improves pelvic organ prolapse-related symptoms, QoL, and sexual function."

From my own perspective, I was subjectively satisfied with my repairs, even though an objective assessment during my mesh removal revealed I still had the rectocele. My rectocele is symptomatic only when I allow myself to become constipated. It was not symptomatic at all prior to the first surgery, nor was I aware of its existence at that stage.

Complications: PC repair procedures without the use of grafts, (native tissue only) have few side effects other than those associated with general surgery. Occasionally, there is pelvic pain and dyspareunia (painful sex). Additional complications with biological graft materials are the same as those with biological mesh materials used to treat incontinence, as have been detailed in this chapter.

Surgery Name: Cystocele Repairs with Synthetic Mesh

Treatment Summary: AC can be performed using synthetic mesh. This is shown in Figure 11.23 on the following page.

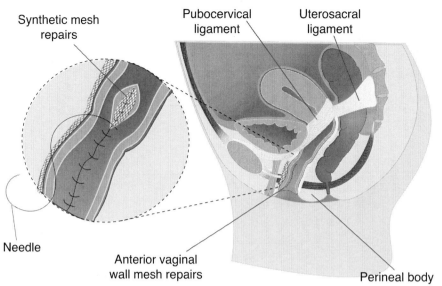

Figure 11.23: Surgical repair of cystocele (anterior wall repair) using synthetic mesh.

In the zoomed-in image in Figure 11.23, you can see how the mesh is placed along the anterior wall and sutured there.

Efficacy: AC with mesh has been reported to have a 75.7% cure rate in a study[195] involving thirty-seven patients with grade four cystoceles. A systematic review, including eleven randomized controlled trials and four prospective studies, showed a mean complication rate of 17% with anterior mesh repairs. Another randomized control trial[196] comparing native tissue with mesh for cystocele repair showed a higher objective cure after three years for the mesh group (91.4%) versus the native tissue group (41,2%), however, no difference was observed in the subjective outcomes between these groups. 14,7% of the mesh group had mesh exposure.

Complications: Anterior repair with mesh carries the risks of general surgery, along with the risk associated with AC using native tissue (voiding difficulties, UR, and pelvic pain). De novo incontinence is also a risk for anterior mesh repair, with some studies showing the risk to be significantly higher when using mesh.

This type of repair also includes additional risks associated with mesh including erosion, with one study[197] showing a mesh erosion rate of 19% for this procedure. A meta-analysis[198] that studied 110 articles, including 11,785 patients, found the mean incidence of erosion to be 10.3%. Patients with mesh are also at a higher risk of infection.

Surgery Name: Rectocele Repairs with Synthetic Mesh

Treatment Summary: PC can be performed using synthetic mesh, which is shown in Figure 11.24.

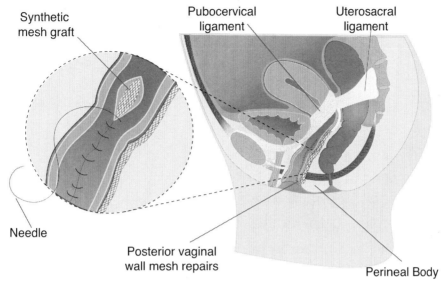

Figure 11.24: Surgical repair of rectocele (posterior wall repair) using synthetic mesh.

In the zoomed-in image in Figure 11.24, you can see how the mesh is placed along the posterior wall and sutured there.

Efficacy: Posterior colporrhaphy with mesh has not been shown to be superior to native tissue repair. The 2018 Cochrane review[199], including ten randomized controlled trials, found that using mesh as a graft material offered no benefits for rectocele repair.

Complications: Posterior repair with mesh carries the risks of general surgery, along with the risk associated with posterior colporrhaphy using native tissue (pelvic pain and dyspareunia), as well as constipation and difficulty defecating.

This type of repair also includes additional risks associated with mesh including erosion, encapsulation, and contracture, with one study[200] showing a mean complication rate of 20%. It has also been reported that there is a higher reoperation rate (11%) than with native tissue repairs (3.7%)[201].

That concludes the vaginal wall repairs. We will now review apical repairs that are used to provide support at the apex of the vaginal passage (the back top side of the vaginal passage) as a treatment for uterine prolapse or enterocele.

Apical Repairs

Apical repairs are typically performed to provide structural support to the top of the vaginal vault (apex). This can be performed with the uterus still in place or following a hysterectomy. Apical surgeries are detailed below.

Surgery Name: Uterosacral ligament suspension

Treatment Summary: A uterosacral ligament suspension is typically performed when the womb is still in place, although it can also be performed in the absence of the uterus.

Procedure: The procedure was traditionally performed with open abdominal surgery but is now more commonly performed using either laparoscopic or transvaginal surgery. The apex of the vagina is sutured to the uterosacral ligament on both sides to help support the vagina during increases in intra-abdominal pressure. Figure 11.25 shows the placement of the sutures from two views.

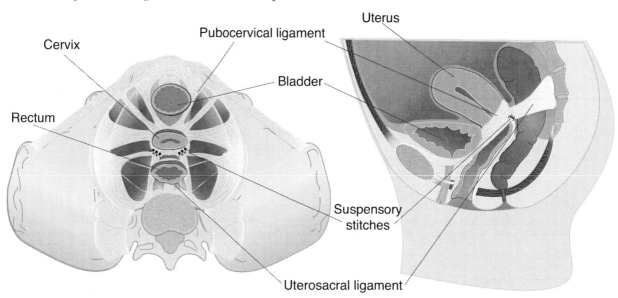

Figure 11.25: Surgical repair of vaginal apex using uterosacral ligament suspension.

The image on the left in Figure 11.25 shows a view of the pelvis from above with the apex of the vagina attached to the uterosacral ligament on both the left and right sides with three sutures. The image on the right shows a side view with sutures visible at the apex of the vagina on the uterosacral ligament.

Efficacy: Long-term efficacy for uterosacral ligament suspension in one study[202] was reported to be 87.5% with a patient satisfaction rate of 91.1%. Some studies show high reoperation rates following this treatment, with one Danish study showing 19% having a symptomatic apical prolapse and 9% having symptomatic subsequent prolapse in another compartment (e.g., cystocele or rectocele).

Complications: This surgery carries the risks of general surgery, along with a small risk of pelvic pain or dyspareunia. Additionally, one study[203] found that there was a risk of urethral kinking (2.6%).

Surgery Name: Sacrospinous fixation

Treatment summary: A sacrospinous fixation is an apical repair procedure to treat vaginal vault prolapse (where the uterus is no longer present). Figure 11.26 shows two views of this procedure.

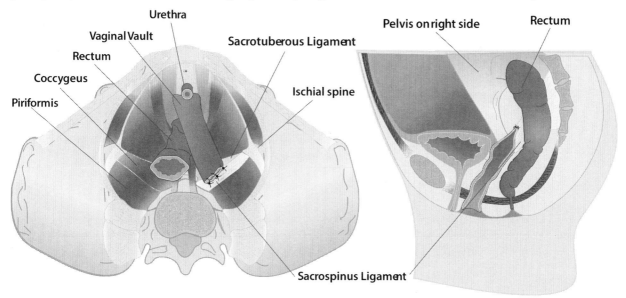

Figure 11.26: Surgical repair of vaginal apex using sacrospinous fixation.

The image on the left in Figure 11.26 shows a view of the pelvis from above with the vagina attached to the sacrotuberous ligament on the right side. This treatment can also be done using bilateral fixation.

Procedure: The procedure was first performed in 1950 and was further refined in 1968. It was traditionally performed using abdominal surgery but is more commonly performed using laparoscopic or transvaginal surgery. This technique can suspend the vagina from the sacrotuberous ligament on one side (as shown in Figure 11.26), bilateral sacrotuberous suspension, or iliococcygeus suspension, where the vaginal vault is sutured to the connective tissue surrounding the iliococcygeus muscle.

Efficacy: A 2013 systematic review reported an overall cure rate of 84.6% for this technique with some studies showing high recurrence rates. A 2018 study that evaluated the efficacy and impact on QoL and sexuality, was focused on twenty patients who had failed monolateral sacrospinous fixation and were subsequently reoperated with bilateral sacrospinous fixation. At twelve-month follow-ups, 90% of patients were cured and showed a significant improvement in sexual function with the greatest improvement being for "physical factor."

Complications: This surgery carries the risks of general surgery. One study[204] highlighted a high risk of bleeding and prolonged surgery with the laparoscopic approach. This surgery also carries a risk of pelvic pain, dyspareunia, or urinary tract infection. It has also been reported that buttock pain on the side of the sacrospinous sutures can impact 5–10% of women but this typically subsides within six weeks.

Surgery Name: Sacrocolpopexy (with mesh)

Treatment Summary: A sacrocolpopexy is an apical repair using mesh without uterus present. A sacrohysteropexy is the same procedure but with the uterus in place. Figure 11.27 shows two views of the sacrocolpopexy.

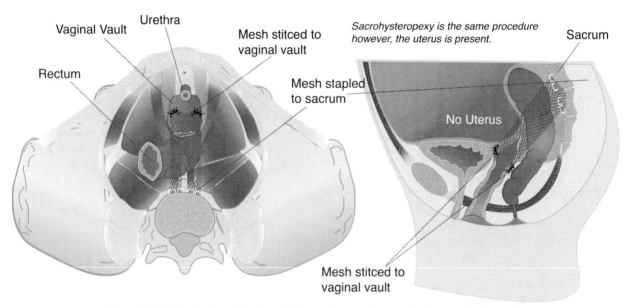

Figure 11.27: Surgical repair of vaginal apex (sacrocolpopexy) using synthetic mesh.

The image on the left in Figure 11.27 shows a view of the pelvis from above with the mesh sutured to the top of the vagina. The image on the right shows the side profile.

Procedure: The procedure involves stitching mesh into the top of the vaginal fault if there is no uterus present, or into the top portion of the vagina when the uterus is present. The mesh is stitched both on the front and back side of the vagina in both cases. The opposite end of the mesh is then stapled (with titanium staples) into the sacrum.

Complications: This surgery carries the risks of general surgery and the risks associated with native tissue apical repairs (pelvic pain, dyspareunia, etc.). This surgery also includes the common mesh complications (including erosion, pain, etc.). Additionally, this procedure carries a rare and severe risk of developing lumbosacral spondylodiscitis[205]. Spondylodiscitis is a condition that includes a spectrum of spinal infections such as discitis, osteomyelitis, epidural abscess, meningitis, subdural empyema, and spinal cord abscess. Symptoms of this condition include low blood pressure, fever, radiating pain, and loss of mobility. That concludes the apical repairs for POP.

Summary of Surgery to Treat POP

Having reviewed the surgical options for POP repair, I feel it is important to summarize the information. Surgery as a treatment for POP should be the very last resort. In many countries, surgery using mesh is offered as a first-line treatment, even though the use of mesh for POP has been banned in multiple countries and medical guidelines advise that a conservative approach should be offered first.

I have spoken at length in this chapter about the risks associated with mesh and I mentioned that removal of mesh is like removing chewing gum from hair in that it cannot be done without also removing your own tissues. Unlike the mesh slings used for incontinence, which are smaller and placed in spaces between organs, the meshes for prolapse are generally larger and often sutured to vaginal walls for support.

Removal of prolapse mesh can result in obliterative surgery, where the vagina is removed. Given that there is no definitive way to identify which patients will suffer adverse events requiring removal, I do not believe that it is worth taking the risk. Neither the short nor long-term implication of mesh removal (for POP or SUI) has been studied. As a consequence, the risk of developing subsequent prolapse, incontinence, or other PFDs following mesh removal is unknown.

The impact of aging and menopause following mesh removal is also unknown. I have yet to reach my own menopause and can only hope that my continued dedication to the management of my prolapse and maintenance of my pelvic floor strength will see me come out the other side still continent and unimpaired.

If you are contemplating surgery that uses mesh, you *must* consider the implications should it require removal. However bad you may feel it is now, I can almost guarantee that post mesh removal you will be in a worse situation. With so many unknowns, I doubt any potential gains from using mesh as a graft material will ever be worth the unnecessary and unavoidable risks.

Pelvic Pain Conditions

We will now review pelvic pain conditions and their associated treatments.

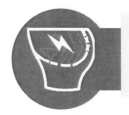
Chronic pelvic pain syndrome (CPPS) is a debilitating condition that negatively impacts QoL. It is defined as persistent, pelvic pain in the absence of pathology, lasting for a period greater than six months. CPPS is believed to affect 2% of the female population.

Pain can be neurologic, gynecologic, urologic, gastrointestinal, or musculoskeletal. This book is focused on PFD, so we will focus on musculoskeletal conditions relating to non-relaxing pelvic floor dysfunction (NR-PFD), which is a condition that gets even less attention than PFD. With NR-PFD, some of the pelvic floor muscles remain in a hypertonic state for extended periods. Sometimes the condition can be given other names, such as hypertonic PFD, or LAS.

CPPS can impact urination, sexual function, and defecation. The pain can manifest in many different ways and can radiate to other areas. Pain can be constant or intermittent (for example, cramping in pelvic floor muscles following orgasm). The pelvic floor can have a mix of hypo- and hyper- tonic muscles. According to a 2012 study[206], referral patterns for pelvic pain from pelvic floor muscles can produce the symptoms shown in Table 11.1.

The referral pattern for each muscle within the pelvic floor, and the associated symptoms are listed in table 11.1. Pain is complex and can differ from person to person. You should not self-diagnose the source of your pain and should consult with a pelvic floor PT if you are suffering from pelvic pain.

The understanding of pain has shifted with the latest scientific research defining new understandings that will fundamentally change how the treatment of pain is approached. A 2020 article[207] highlighted three key understandings. These are as follows:

1. Pain is not a signal originating from bodily tissues. Rather, it is a compelling perceptual experience generated on the basis of an apparent need to protect tissues from harm.
2. Pain is not an accurate measure of tissue damage.
3. The plasticity of the nervous system means that the nervous system itself is a viable target of treatment.

PELVIC FLOOR Muscle	Referral Pattern	Potential Symptom
Bulbospongiosus	Perineal pain or urogenital pain	Painful sex, pain with orgasm, or clitoral pain
Ischiocavernosus	Perineal pain or urogenital pain	Painful sex, pain with orgasm, or clitoral pain
Superficial transverse perineal	None documented	Painful sex
Anal sphincter	Pain in posterior pelvic floor, rectum/anus, or pubic pain	Increased urgency and/or frequency. Painful sex or painful urination after sex
Pubococcygeus / Puborectalis	Low-belly pain, bladder pain, or pain in perineum	Increased urgency and/or frequency. Painful sex or painful urination after sex
Iliococcygeus	Pain toward the sacrum or deep in the vagina, rectum, or perineum	Pain before, during, or after pooping. Painful sex, particularly with thrusting
Coccygeus	Pain toward the sacrum or buttock pain	Pain on sitting. Pain during pooping. Intestinal fullness and anal pressure/pain
Obturator internus	Pain in anus, coccyx, vulva or vagina. Pain on back of thighs	Generalized pelvic pain, often with burning or aching
Piriformis	Pain in sacrum, pain on one side of buttock	Buttock or leg pain. Sometimes sciatic pain

Table 11.1: Pelvic floor muscles—Referral patterns and pain symptoms.

What I would add to this is, as I have said repeatedly throughout this book, what you think (in this case "about your pain"), will impact what manifests in your body. So long as you believe the cause of your pain to be sinister, its impact will be dramatic. If you have done the rounds to multiple healthcare providers, having an ultrasound, MRI, urodynamics, and a host of other assessments that all turn up no tissue pathology or underlying disease, you should do "the work" on the sinister thoughts on your pain and begin the process of getting safety messages through to your nervous system.

We will begin our pain treatment review with the non-surgical treatments for CPPS.

 # Non-Surgical Treatments
Chronic pelvic pain syndrome (CPPS)

Pain is complex, and treatments can be quite varied. We will review six non-surgical treatments in this section.

Pelvic Floor Muscle Down-Training
CPPS due to NR-PFD can benefit from reverse Kegels (detailed in Phase 1 of the pelvic floor module of the eight-phase training), which trains the pelvic floor to relax. Biofeedback devices can be used to complement this training. Electromuscular (EMS) and electrogalvanic stimulation (EGS) therapies are also offered when the underlying condition is LAS.

A 1987[208] study found that 60% of patients had a good or excellent response to High-voltage EGS as a treatment for LAS. Other studies showed pain relief in up to 90% of patients[209]. The mechanism of pain relief is believed to be the intensity of the contractions tiring out the muscle allowing a release of hypertonicity. These therapies are generally combined with manual therapy and myofascial release and are offered in a physiotherapy setting.

Medications
Medications are commonly prescribed for patients suffering from pelvic pain. As well as standard over-the-counter pain medications, tricyclic antidepressants, anticonvulsants, opiates, muscle relaxants, antibiotics, alpha-blockers, and pentosan polysulfate may also be offered. It should be noted that all medications come with side effects, some of which can be severe. Potential side effects should be understood before commencing any course of treatment.

Cognitive Behavioral Therapy

CBT as a treatment for CPPS is usually combined with physiotherapy and other manual therapy treatments. You may feel offended or insulted when CBT is suggested as a treatment. Maybe I have also offended you by suggesting you do "the work" on your pain thoughts. Please do not feel offended.

In Part One of this book, you learned about the business of your body's movement, and how the nervous system utilizes inhibitory reflexes to protect tissues. You learned that old functional patterns are not returned to by default, requiring some conscious intent to return to functional patterns. The same is true with pain. The nervous system sends pain signals to protect you and will not necessarily stop sending those signals when the original condition that triggered the protective response has resolved.

Fear (and stress) adds tension to the system, which can prolong pain unnecessarily. CBT helps you to calm the nervous system, getting messages of safety through, which can help to circumvent the protective pain patterns that are the default. Whereas this may not stop your pain completely, it should help to reduce the degree and frequency of your pain and thus help to increase the quality of your life.

Botox

Botox has already been mentioned as a treatment for OAB. It is also sometimes offered as a treatment for CPPS where hypertonic muscles can be injected in an attempt to relax them thus reducing pain. A double-blinded randomized, placebo-controlled trial[210] found a significant reduction in dyspareunia for both the Botox and placebo groups as well as reporting lower pelvic floor muscle pressures in both groups. Your healthcare provider should be able to confirm if this may be a valid treatment for you.

Sitz baths

Use of heat or cold has often been used to treat pain conditions. Sitz baths, where you submerge your pelvis in a shallow bath or basin of water, have been discussed as part of *Sexual Pain Strategy 1* in Chapter Ten. In that case, it was a salty sitz bath. One study[211] found that sitz baths with a temperature of 40 degrees Celsius were found to reduce anal canal pressures in those with anorectal pain. In that study, it was just water without salt.

Alternative Therapies

Alternative therapies such as acupuncture, are also offered in the treatment of CPPS. One systematic review[212] found that acupuncture combined with conventional therapies significantly reduced CPPS, however, that same study concluded that there was insufficient evidence to conclude that acupuncture could be recommended as a complementary and alternative treatment suggesting further study would be needed.

Surgical Treatments
Chronic pelvic pain syndrome (CPPS)

Whereas certain pelvic pain conditions, such as endometriosis, human papillomavirus (HPV), pelvic inflammatory disease (PID), cervical stenosis, polyps, interstitial cystitis (IC), bowel adhesions, and ovarian cysts (to name a few) may require some form of surgical treatment. They are not musculoskeletal pelvic floor related conditions and thus are beyond the scope of this book.

Only two relevant surgical treatments were found in the literature. They are as follows:

Sacral Nerve Stimulation (SNS)

We have already explored SNS as a surgical treatment option for OAB and FI. SNS can, in extreme cases, also serve as a treatment for CPPS. One small study[213] using SNS on patients with chronic intractable pelvic pain found that severity of pain was decreased with its use. On a scale of 1 to 10, with 10 being the highest, the average reported pain was 9.7 at baseline and 4.4 following treatment. Details on the SNS procedure, efficacy, and complications are detailed earlier in this chapter.

Posterior Division of the Puborectalis Muscle

Division of the PC muscle has been used in some extreme cases, particularly where CC is prevalent, however, this type of surgery comes with a high risk of developing FI. One study[214] into the procedure included nine female patients. Only two patients reported improvement following surgery and five patients developed FI. If you are offered this treatment for your CPPS, seek a second opinion.

That concludes the treatments for CPPS.

We will now explore one further pelvic pain condition known as vaginismus. Vaginismus was one of three sexual pain conditions that were covered in the symptom-management strategies in Chapter Ten with the other two being dyspareunia (painful sex) and vulvodynia. The treatments for CPPS are also generally offered for vaginismus, dyspareunia and vulvodynia. The pages that follow detail some extra treatment options offered for vaginismus.

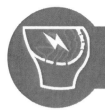
Vaginismus is a condition in which involuntary muscle spasms interfere with vaginal penetration, whether that be through sexual intercourse or simply attempting to insert a tampon or a period cup. This condition can make sexual intercourse difficult or impossible having a dramatic impact on QoL. Vaginismus can be considered to be a type of dyspareunia (painful intercourse); however, it can also prevent the use of tampons or can prevent gynecological exams.

We have already discussed the complexities associated with pain, and the impact negative thoughts can have on exacerbating or prolonging pain. A 2020 study[215] into vaginismus found that treatment is less effective in patients who believed, "It's my fault." I believe this highlights how thoughts can impact what manifests in the body. If you suffer from this condition, you should do "the work" on these thoughts. It is also important to address any past abuses (sexual or otherwise) that may be contributing to this protective response from the nervous system.

Vaginismus is either primary, where penetration has never been achieved, or secondary, where penetration was once possible but is no longer possible. This can be due to pelvic radiation therapy.

There aren't so many treatments for vaginismus, aside from those we have already detailed for pelvic floor hypertonicity and CPPS. This section will summarize the treatment options.

Non-Surgical Treatments

Vaginismus

The non-surgical treatments offered for CPPS are also offered in the treatment of vaginismus. In addition to those treatments, vaginal dilation is also offered as a treatment. We have explored vaginal dilation through the *sexual pain strategy 2* in Chapter Ten. Vaginal dilation is a primary treatment offered in the treatment of vaginismus. I view this treatment as a method to communicate safety to the nervous system to release its protective tone.

One study[216] into vaginal dilation found that although dilation is effective in minimizing hypertonicity, adherence is poor with many ceasing to continue with dilation after just 90 days. *Consistency is key* when you are trying to change protective patterns, and it is likely that you will need to be consistent for a long period if you suffer from vaginismus or any other PFD for that matter.

Surgical Treatments
Vaginismus

Surgical treatments are not recommended for vaginismus. In cases where the hymen is still intact and cannot be broken by normal penetration, a hymenectomy may be performed. That is a treatment where the hymen is dissected to enable penetration.

Vaginismus, by its nature, is driven by the "fight or flight" response. The results of a 2001 study[217] highlighted that "[p]hysicians often opt for hymenectomy with episiotomy and labiaectomy when treating vaginismus in the hope of easing penetration and allowing for the consummation of marriages and relationships. Unfortunately, although such surgical management exposes the introitus, it fails to address the mechanism of vaginismus, leaving the patient with an unresolved problem yet with the added trauma of the surgery coupled with visible physical alterations."

That study concluded that "If a rigid, imperforated hymen is suspected, conclusive evidence as to its presence must be obtained before turning to surgical intervention, which, in itself, has to be minimal and targeted. Otherwise, surgery is to be reserved for correcting structural deformities, not vaginismus, because the psychophysical nature of vaginismus will not respond to such intervention."

Consequently, if you are offered surgical treatment for your vaginismus, you should seek clarification as to the reasoning for this surgery and get a second opinion prior to going under the knife.

That concludes the treatments for vaginismus, which was the last condition to be explored. You should now have an understanding of what treatment options are available as well as some indication as to the safety and efficacy of available treatments. This information should empower you further, helping to ensure you can make informed decisions under the guidance of your healthcare provider to achieve the best possible outcomes.

The next chapter will cover devices and tools that may be used in the management and treatment of pelvic floor conditions.

Chapter Twelve:
Devices and Tools

There are many devices and tools on the market to help deal with the symptoms of PFD. The information provided in this section is just a short summary based on my own personal opinion of the devices, many of which I have purchased for myself and have tried over the years.

This is by no means a definitive list of what is available, but I hope you find the information useful in your endeavors to manage and overcome your condition. You will find more information on products and devices on theflowerempowered.com and you can also watch product review videos on the YouTube channel.

Panty Liners, Pads, and Disposable Incontinence Pants

Panty liners, pads, and disposable incontinence pants are sold to help manage stress incontinence and FI. It is important to realize that the pads that are used to manage your period are not sufficient for SUI or FI. Differences in material, degree of soakage, and location of that soakage material vary depending on the intended use of the products.

Many companies make products not only for women but also for men. Not only do these companies provide products that give much-needed protection against embarrassment, but they also work hard to advertise and raise awareness of these issues. Awareness is key to breaking the taboo.

Incontinence pads and pants (whether for urinary or fecal incontinence) will not improve or eliminate your incontinence symptoms. They are simply an aid to manage your symptoms. Many of these products also prevent noticeable odors that can be a big source of embarrassment. Let's face it, there isn't much benefit to being dry if you smell like a toilet. Another consideration is that these products are single-use and as such, will contribute to landfill and are not environmentally friendly.

When you regain continence, it is likely that you will still want to use some sort of product JIC. When I regained my continence, I still had the fear—what if I leak again? I like to call this post-incontinence

PTSD. It took a long time for me to trust my bladder enough to go without that shield of protection. When I did eventually ditch the panty liners, I had to work to calm my nerves during the wet days of my cycle, when the volume of vaginal fluids naturally increased. If you are trying to wean yourself off pads and panty liners, give yourself time; just like you gave yourself time to rehabilitate.

Reusable Incontinence Pants
Reusable incontinence pants are made from materials that are designed to soak up mild leakage while preventing odors. They claim to absorb leakages of 25 to 50 ml, which is well below typical incontinence pads where the small pads absorb 115 ml of liquid with disposable incontinence pants absorbing between 1100 ml and 4099ml of liquid. They are marketed as a sustainable alternative to disposable incontinence pads. I have not personally tried them and cannot vouch for their efficacy.

Disposable Pessaries
When looking at symptom-management strategies and treatments for SUI and POP, we discussed disposable pessaries, both in Chapter Ten and Chapter Eleven. These products have come to the market within the last decade and are gaining ground as tools to manage symptoms while patients work to overcome their PFD.

Product availability is very much dependent on your location. You can usually buy a starter pack with different sizes allowing you to find the right size for you. Sites like Amazon should present you with options if you search for disposable pessaries.

Urethral Blockers
Urethral blockers are small sticky pads that cover the exit of the urethra. They do not stop urine from entering the urethra, so I would not use them frequently. I would imagine that, if used excessively, they may cause the urethra to expand due to filling. I would suggest that they could be useful for very occasional use. For example, if you had a wedding to attend and wanted to dance without fear of leaking or without having to wear a bulky pad, urethral blockers could support you in doing that.

Fecal Plugs
Fecal plugs are like anal tampons designed to help prevent fecal leakage. They are available in a few different shapes and are typically prescribed by a doctor. Like incontinence pads and pants, disposable pessaries, and urethral blockers, anal plugs are designed to help with symptom managment. They should be viewed as support tools to use while you undertake other treatments. They are for single use only and as such are not sustainable or environmentally friendly.

Perineometer and Biofeedback Devices

Periniometers and biofeedback devices are designed to measure muscular tension. These are also known as electromyography (EMG) devices. When we learned about the business of the body's movement in Chapter Three, we learned that the nervous system is the body's electrical system that turns muscle contractions on. It is these *on* signals that are recorded by the EMG.

You can imagine that the muscle bundles (that we viewed in Figure 2.2) have their own *on* switches. The EMG reading, which measures millivolts, will be higher if more muscle bundles are switched on. Hypertonic muscles will have most of their *on* switches triggered and thus will show higher readings that indicate a higher level of tone. These devices allow you to see the strength of your contraction, the depth of your relaxation, and your resting tone.

Physiotherapists use biofeedback devices in the treatment of conditions both with hypo- and hypertonicity. The first biofeedback device for pelvic floor use was pioneered in 1948 by Dr. Kegel. He designed a biofeedback device that also provided some resistance, as he promoted the use of progressive resistance exercises to build muscular strength.

Biofeedback devices use a vaginal probe, which is inserted into the vagina. Some also require a skin electrode. These devices can cost anywhere from 100 to 500 $. Some biofeedback devices use a vaginal probe that inflates (like a balloon) after being inserted into the vagina. These devices do not record resting tone, instead reading the pressure on the baloon. They tend to score strength on a scale of 1 to 10 rather than millivolts.

Other biofeedback devices connect to your smartphone via Bluetooth. They are gamified, meaning that you play a game using the strength of your pelvic floor muscles to move a pointer on the screen. These biofeedback devices record your resting tone and will prompt you to relax in between contractions. They typically have programs for both sustained endurance contractions and "quick flick" speed contractions in order to train both slow and fast-twitch fibers.

The nice thing about gamified apps is that they record your performance (usually to the cloud) so you can easily monitor your progress over time. The readings they record are not always in millivolts and as they set a "starting" level based on your strength, it is not possible to compare your scores with your neighbor as their "starting" level will be different (like the RPE-scale).

A few words of caution on home-use of biofeedback devices. They will show higher readings if you contract other muscle groups, such as glutes and core. It is also possible to show higher readings when bearing down, which can give you a false sense of security. Another caution when gamifying exercises; it is easy to get "lost in the game," focusing on the screen, and incorrectly performing exercises in order to achieve a better score. For this reason, I suggest gaining some control and strength before turning to these devices (completing Phase 4 of the training before using), or use them under the guidance of your physiotherapist who can ensure that you are performing the exercises correctly.

Wands and Dilators

Pelvic Wands and Dilators are used to help release hypertonic pelvic floor muscles. They are generally either plastic or silicone. The purpose of a pelvic wand is to enable you to reach pelvic floor muscles from within the vagina. The wand is typically shaped with curves such that you can adjust the angle easier than if you were to use fingers. With dilators, they are typically straight. They are used to mimic vaginal penetration. They come in varying sizes and are typically used in the treatment of vaginismus, which we reviewed in the symptom management strategies for vaginismus in Chapter Ten.

Vaginal Weights, Cones, and Eggs

Vaginal weights, cones, and eggs are devices that add weighted resistance to help strengthen the pelvic floor. There are many varieties of these devices on the market. Some come with an "indicator" tail to show that you are contracting properly. This is simply a length of plastic that reaches outside the body like a little flag pole. When you contract, it should move toward your backside. If the indicator moves toward your clitoris, you are not contracting correctly. These indicator devices can come with or without weight.

With vaginal weights, there are different shapes, sizes, and weights available. Weights are typically sold in sets ranging from 5g to 125g. I really like the Intimate Rose weights as they are a nice texture (silicone) and a shape that fits well in my vagina. You should always wash weights before and after use. Do not wear a weight for more than twenty minutes. If your weight is a jade egg, you will need to boil it thoroughly, making sure it cools before use, rather than washing it with soap and water. These eggs are permeable and so they can hold bacteria.

If you research weights online, you will find some sites recommending all day continual use. Michelle Kenway, a leading Australian pelvic floor physiotherapist, advises against this, advising instead that the weights be inserted, Kegels performed, and weights removed. Wearing weights for longer than twenty minutes could cause the pelvic floor muscles to spasm (like a vaginismus response) resulting in a visit to the emergency room to have them removed.

It is possible to add weights to the standing version of your pelvic floor exercises from Phase 6 of the eight-phase program. You should only add weight on the guidance of your healthcare provider.

Remember you are trying to achieve a balance between strength, tension, flexibility, alignment, and relaxation throughout the whole body and not just the pelvic floor. Meet yourself in the middle as that is where true health and wellbeing exists.

Electrical Stimulation Devices (E-Stim)

Electrical Stimulation devices (E-Stim) can also be called Electronic Muscle Stimulators (EMS) and Neuromuscular Electrical Stimulation (NMES), but all are essentially the same thing so, we will refer to them as EMS devices in this section. These devices work by creating a local electrical charge that switches *on* muscle contraction.

EMS devices can be used with skin electrodes, internal probes (both intravaginal and anal) or they can be connected to shorts that you wear. Maybe you have seen advertisements for EMS devices that proclaim to create six-pack abs? Well, these devices are basically the same but for your pelvic floor, and you should no more be fooled into thinking a device will give you six-pack abs than thinking it will give you a strong pelvic floor.

My relationship with the EMS devices is a long one. I first purchased an EMS device in 2005 when my increased triathlon training first highlighted my issue with mild SUI. I thought EMS would be a "quick fix" and loved that it required no effort. I was already doing so much with my life; I was looking after my three children, keeping the house in great order, progressing in my career as a software engineer (involving a lot of travel), AND training for triathlons. I didn't have time for my pelvic floor.

I wanted a quick fix for this worrying issue. The impact on my QoL was minimal so, I wasn't overly concerned. Therefore, I didn't prioritize putting in the time and effort to resolve my issue. I did feel some changes after using the device for a few weeks; there was definitely more awareness of sensation in that part of my body, and I believed that my muscles were "tighter." I assumed then that my issues were resolved

One thing that commonly happened when I used my EMS device was that muscle contractions on the left side of my pelvic floor would reach out through my left buttock and travel down my leg causing it to externally rotate while my toes curled upwards. I expect that my piriformis was contracting, while the strength of the stimulation was sending the *on* signals all the way through my leg down to my toes.

In Chapter Two (Figure 2.1.2), we learned that the piriformis is a deep hip flexor, which also participates in posture and pelvic floor stability. The very fact that this muscle was in spasm while using the device, highlights a potential issue. There is every chance that I was making my PFD worse and adding hypertonicity rather than just increasing strength.

I cannot emphasize strongly enough the importance of speaking with a doctor or physiotherapist before deciding to self-prescribe an EMS device. EMS has its place in the treatment of PFD, but, in my opinion, that place is not in the hands of an uninformed woman. Your pelvic floor PT can show you how to properly use such a device and can guide you to the right settings on the device to treat your specific issues.

EMS devices may seem like a quick fix and it is tempting to use them, but EMS contractions **ARE NOT THE SAME** as functional contractions. These devices are typically used by physiotherapists to help trigger motor unit recruitment when the patient is struggling to find the mind-to-muscle connection. Following the use of these devices, the patient will be encouraged to perform exercises without stimulation to ensure they actually regain control.

Functional EMS, where the device creates a contraction as the client tries to simultaneously contract the pelvic floor, is another practice that is sometimes utilized by pelvic floor PTs. Again, though, it is the PT who should decide if this treatment could be helpful for you.

In some countries, these types of devices are available on prescription and in most countries, you can purchase them online as a consumer. They vary quite dramatically in price ranging from ~50 $ to ~300 $. You should always follow the manufacturer's instructions, which typically indicate that you should increase the milliamps to a level that is tolerable. If you turn the milliamps (mA) up high, the stimulation can cause co-contractions that reach all the way down to your toes like mine did (your focus shouldn't be toe strength!).

My advice is to seek the advice of your healthcare provider before trying EMS as a treatment; they will know if this treatment is right for you.

That concludes the section on devices and tools. We will now proceed to the final, short chapter, which details the various healthcare providers that can assist you on your journey of rehabilitation.

Chapter Thirteen:
Medical Professionals and Therapists

In this chapter, we will explore the different types of therapists who can help you if you are suffering from PFD. A specialist directory has been created on specialists.theflowerempowered.com to ensure you can find local help and support. Below are some descriptions of the types of therapists you will find in the database. Bear in mind that, often, specialists will have trained in multiple disciplines and different countries may place responsibility for treating PFD with specialists other than those listed below.

General Practitioners (GP)

A general practitioner is your general doctor who can confirm if your symptoms are likely to be caused by PFD and can refer you to other specialists who can carry out tests and treat your conditions.

Gynecologists

Gynecologists are medical doctors who specialize in women's reproductive issues. They treat women of all ages and are often trained to perform gynecological surgeries. They commonly perform surgeries to treat female stress incontinence and POP.

Obstetricians

Obstetricians are medical doctors for women during pregnancy and just after birth. They are often trained to perform gynecological surgeries and commonly perform surgeries to treat female stress incontinence and POP.

OBGYN

An OBGYN is a medical doctor trained in both gynecology and obstetrics. They have the same functions as both obstetricians and gynecologists.

Urologist

A Urologist is a medical doctor trained in diseases of the urinary tract. Urologists primarily focus on male urological disorders. They perform both surgical and medical treatments for diseases of the male urinary tract. It is less common for them to perform surgery for stress incontinence in females

Urogynecologist

A urogynecologist is a medical doctor trained in both gynecology and urology. These doctors typically perform surgeries to treat incontinence and POP.

Midwifes and Doulas

These are specialists who support women through pregnancy and during birth.

Physiotherapist/Physical Therapist (PT)

A physiotherapist (UK) /physical therapist (USA) is a therapist trained in the musculoskeletal system. They provide manual therapies and prescribe exercises to treat physical disabilities and conditions, affecting movement and biomechanical functions. PTs can also hold a doctorate, in which case they may be referred to as a doctor of physical therapy.

Pelvic Floor PT

A pelvic floor PT is a physiotherapist/physical therapist who is trained to specialize in the management and treatment of pelvic floor disorders. They should be the primary health care provider responsible for the assessment and treatment of PFD.

Chiropractor

A chiropractor is a therapist trained to perform spinal manipulations (sometimes referred to as "back-cracking") to treat neuromuscular and postural conditions. Sometimes PTs will also have training in these treatments.

Rolfer

A rolfer is a manual therapist who performs structural integration, which is a form of myofascial release, which is used to correct postural imbalances. Many rolfers are also trained as PTs.

Structural Integrator (Anatomy Trains)

A structural integrator is a manual therapist who performs structural integration. This is a form of myofascial release used to correct postural imbalances. Structural integrators are also commonly trained in other disciplines (e.g., physiotherapy).

Osteopath

An Osteopath is an alternative medicine practicioner who offers musculoskeletal treatments, similar to a physiotherapist and a chiroractor.

Visceral Mobilisation Practicioner

Typically, therapists offering visceral mobilisations are physiotherapists, osteopaths or other manual therapists who have taken further training to specialise in visceral mobilisation, a type of connective tissue release that focuses on tissues within the abdominopelvic cavities.

Yoga Teachers and Other Fitness Professionals

Specially trained yoga teachers, personal trainers and Pilates instructors, can also work, along with your primary healthcare provider, to help you as you undertake your journey toward rehabilitation.

Other Specialists

Other specialists including nutritionists, sexologists, and psychologists can help when dealing with PFD. You can find some of these various professionals in the specialist directory at theflowerempowered. com.

Empower Your Flower

Having read through the book and the eight-phase training, you may feel that this is not the right program for you. Maybe my words don't resonate with you. If so, I encourage you to go out and find someone who speaks a language that you understand.

There are so many great pelvic health programs out there that can help you to overcome your pelvic floor dysfunction. You will find books, pelvic floor programs and other resources by Dr. Brianne Grogan, Michelle Kenway, Dr. Sarah Duval, Jeanice Mitchell, Amanda Olsen, Jen Torborg, Louise Field, Jessie Mundell, Laura Arndt, Haley Shevener, Annemarie Everett, Tracey Sher, Dr. Sara Reardon, Katy Bowman, and Kim Vopni to name just a few.

The most important thing is that you seek help rather than suffering in silence, and remember to talk about pelvic floor dysfunction. If we talk about these taboo subjects, we can create chage that will benefit future generations.

Together we can and will make a difference.

References

1. Crosby, E. C., Abernethy, M., Berger, M. B., DeLancey, J. O., Fenner, D. E., & Morgan, D. M. (2014). Symptom resolution after operative management of complications from transvaginal mesh. Obstetrics and gynecology, 123(1), 134–139. https://doi.org/10.1097/AOG.0000000000000042

2. Benham, W. (1887). The Dictionary of Religion. PP. 1013 Retrieved from: https://archive.org/details/dictionaryofreli00benhuoft/page/n1024/mode/2up

3. Mackenzie, J. (2017). " Vagina surgery 'sought by girls as young as nine'". BBC News. Retrieved from: http://www.bbc.com/news/health-40410459

4. McCartney, J. (2013). "The Great Wall of Vagina". Retrieved from: http://www.greatwallofvagina.co.uk/great-wall-vagina-panel-1-0

5. Ensler, E. (n.d.) "The Vagina Monologues". Retrieved from: https://www.eveensler.org/pf/plays-the-vagina-monologues/

6. Llewellyn-Jones, D. (1999). "Everywoman, A gynelogical guide for life"(9). Page 3.

7. Dobbeleir, J. M., Landuyt, K. V., & Monstrey, S. J. (2011). Aesthetic surgery of the female genitalia. Seminars in plastic surgery, 25(2), 130–141. https://doi.org/10.1055/s-0031-1281482

8. Azadzoi, K. M., & Siroky, M. B. (2010). Neurologic factors in female sexual function and dysfunction. Korean journal of urology, 51(7), 443–449. https://doi.org/10.4111/kju.2010.51.7.443

9. Pastor, Z., & Chmel, R. (2018). Differential diagnostics of female "sexual" fluids: a narrative review. International urogynecology journal, 29(5), 621–629. https://doi.org/10.1007/s00192-017-3527-9

10. KEGEL A. H. (1952). Stress incontinence and genital relaxation; a nonsurgical method of increasing the tone of sphincters and their supporting structures. Ciba clinical symposia, 4(2), 35–51.

11. Bø, K., Talseth, T., Holme, I. Single blind, randomised controlled trial of pelvic floor exercises, electrical stimulation, vaginal cones, and no treatment in management of genuine stress incontinence in women BMJ 1999; 318 :487 https://doi.org/10.1136/bmj.318.7182.487

12. Lothian J. A. (2004). Do not disturb: the importance of privacy in labor. The Journal of perinatal education, 13(3), 4–6. https://doi.org/10.1624/105812404X1707

13. Schmid, V. (2005). "About physiology in pregnancy and childbirth" Page 54.

14. Park, H., & Han, D. (2015). The effect of the correlation between the contraction of the pelvic floor muscles and diaphragmatic motion during breathing. Journal of physical therapy science, 27(7), 2113–2115. https://doi.org/10.1589/jpts.27.2113

15. Ashton-Miller, J. A., Howard, D., & DeLancey, J. O. (2001). The functional anatomy of the female pelvic floor and stress continence control system. Scandinavian journal of urology and nephrology. Supplementum, (207), 1–125. https://doi.org/10.1080/003655901750174773

16. Bernardes, B. T., Resende, A. P., Stüpp, L., Oliveira, E., Castro, R. A., Bella, Z. I., Girão, M. J., & Sartori, M. G. (2012). Efficacy of pelvic floor muscle training and hypopressive exercises for treating pelvic organ prolapse in women: randomized controlled trial. Sao Paulo medical journal = Revista paulista de medicina, 130(1), 5–9. https://doi.org/10.1590/s1516-31802012000100002

17. Resende, A. P., Stüpp, L., Bernardes, B. T., Oliveira, E., Castro, R. A., Girão, M. J., & Sartori, M. G. (2012). Can hypopressive exercises provide additional benefits to pelvic floor muscle training in women with pelvic organ prolapse?. Neurourology and urodynamics, 31(1), 121–125. https://doi.org/10.1002/nau.21149

18. Day, B. L., Marsden, C. D., Obeso, J. A., & Rothwell, J. C. (1984). Reciprocal inhibition between the muscles of the human forearm. The Journal of physiology, 349, 519–534. https://doi.org/10.1113/jphysiol.1984.sp015171

19. Hu, H., Meijer, O. G., van Dieën, J. H., Hodges, P. W., Bruijn, S. M., Strijers, R. L., Nanayakkara, P. W., van Royen, B. J., Wu, W. H., & Xia, C. (2011). Is the psoas a hip flexor in the active straight leg raise?. European spine journal : official publication of the

European Spine Society, the European Spinal Deformity Society, and the European Section of the Cervical Spine Research Society, 20(5), 759–765. https://doi.org/10.1007/s00586-010-1508-5

20. Benias, P.C., Wells, R.G., Sackey-Aboagye, B. et al. (2018). Structure and Distribution of an Unrecognized Interstitium in Human Tissues. Sci Rep 8, 4947. https://doi.org/10.1038/s41598-018-23062-6

21. Crowle, A., & Harley, C. (2020). Development of a biotensegrity focused therapy for the treatment of pelvic organ prolapse: A retrospective case series. Journal of bodywork and movement therapies, 24(1), 115–125. https://doi.org/10.1016/j.jbmt.2019.10.008

22. Diez-Itza, I., Aizpitarte, I., & Becerro, A. (2007). Risk factors for the recurrence of pelvic organ prolapse after vaginal surgery: a review at 5 years after surgery. International urogynecology journal and pelvic floor dysfunction, 18(11), 1317–1324. https://doi.org/10.1007/s00192-007-0321-0

23. Dillon, Edgar. (2012). Nutritionally essential amino acids and metabolic signaling in aging. Amino acids. 45. 10.1007/s00726-012-1438-0.

24. Hansraj K. K. (2014). Assessment of stresses in the cervical spine caused by posture and position of the head. Surgical technology international, 25, 277–279.

25. Jacobson E. (2011). Structural integration: origins and development. Journal of alternative and complementary medicine (New York, N.Y.), 17(9), 775–780. https://doi.org/10.1089/acm.2011.0001

26. Nguyen, J. K., Lind, L. R., Choe, J. Y., McKindsey, F., Sinow, R., & Bhatia, N. N. (2000). Lumbosacral spine and pelvic inlet changes associated with pelvic organ prolapse. Obstetrics and gynecology, 95(3), 332–336. https://doi.org/10.1016/s0029-7844(99)00561-x

27. Mattox, T. F., Lucente, V., McIntyre, P., Miklos, J. R., & Tomezsko, J. (2000). Abnormal spinal curvature and its relationship to pelvic organ prolapse. American journal of obstetrics and gynecology, 183(6), 1381–1384. https://doi.org/10.1067/mob.2000.111489

28. Fowler, C. J., Griffiths, D., & de Groat, W. C. (2008). The neural control of micturition. Nature reviews. Neuroscience, 9(6), 453–466. https://doi.org/10.1038/nrn2401

29. Shafik A. (1999). A study of the continence mechanism of the external urethral sphincter with identification of the voluntary urinary inhibition reflex. The Journal of urology, 162(6), 1967–1971. https://doi.org/10.1016/s0022-5347(05)68080-9

30. Farrell, D. J., & Bower, L. (2003). Fatal water intoxication. Journal of clinical pathology, 56(10), 803–804. https://doi.org/10.1136/jcp.56.10.803-a

31. Hisano, M., Bruschini, H., Nicodemo, A. C., & Srougi, M. (2012). Cranberries and lower urinary tract infection prevention. Clinics (Sao Paulo, Brazil), 67(6), 661–668. https://doi.org/10.6061/clinics/2012(06)18

32. Schwalfenberg G. K. (2012). The alkaline diet: is there evidence that an alkaline pH diet benefits health?. Journal of environmental and public health, 2012, 727630. https://doi.org/10.1155/2012/727630

33. Markland, A. D., Dunivan, G. C., Vaughan, C. P., & Rogers, R. G. (2016). Anal Intercourse and Fecal Incontinence: Evidence from the 2009-2010 National Health and Nutrition Examination Survey. The American journal of gastroenterology, 111(2), 269–274. https://doi.org/10.1038/ajg.2015.419

34. Pecora, P., Suraci, C., Antonelli, M., De Maria, S., & Marrocco, W. (1981). Constipation and obesity: a statistical analysis. Bollettino della Societa italiana di biologia sperimentale, 57(23), 2384–2388.

35. Ursell, L. K., Metcalf, J. L., Parfrey, L. W., & Knight, R. (2012). Defining the human microbiome. Nutrition reviews, 70 Suppl 1(Suppl 1), S38–S44. https://doi.org/10.1111/j.1753-4887.2012.00493.x

36. Morten O.A. Sommer, George M. Church & Gautam Dantas (2010) The human microbiome harbors a diverse reservoir of antibiotic resistance genes, Virulence, 1:4, 299-303, https://doi.org/10.4161/viru.1.4.12010

37. Zhang, Y. J., Li, S., Gan, R. Y., Zhou, T., Xu, D. P., & Li, H. B. (2015). Impacts of gut bacteria on human health and diseases. International journal of molecular sciences, 16(4), 7493–7519. https://doi.org/10.3390/ijms16047493

38. Rao, K., & Young, V. B. (2015). Fecal microbiota transplantation for the management of Clostridium difficile infection. Infectious disease clinics of North America, 29(1), 109–122. https://doi.org/10.1016/j.idc.2014.11.009

39. Alang, N., & Kelly, C. R. (2015). Weight gain after fecal microbiota transplantation. Open forum infectious diseases, 2(1), ofv004. https://doi.org/10.1093/ofid/ofv004

40. Marotz, C. A., & Zarrinpar, A. (2016). Treating Obesity and Metabolic Syndrome with Fecal Microbiota Transplantation. The Yale journal of biology and medicine, 89(3), 383–388.

41. Mitchell, N. S., Catenacci, V. A., Wyatt, H. R., & Hill, J. O. (2011). Obesity: overview of an epidemic. The Psychiatric clinics of North America, 34(4), 717–732. https://doi.org/10.1016/j.psc.2011.08.005

42. L. Elaine Waetjen, Shanmei Liao, Wesley O. Johnson, Carolyn M. Sampselle, Barbara Sternfield, Siobán D. Harlow, Ellen B. Gold, for the Study of Women's Health Across the Nation, Factors Associated with Prevalent and Incident Urinary Incontinence in a Cohort of Midlife Women: A Longitudinal Analysis of Data: Study of Women's Health Across the Nation, American Journal of Epidemiology, Volume 165, Issue 3, 1 February 2007, Pages 309–318, https://doi.org/10.1093/aje/kwk018

43. Flegal KM, Kruszon-Moran D, Carroll MD, Fryar CD, Ogden CL. (2016). Trends in Obesity Among Adults in the United States, 2005 to 2014. JAMA. 315(21):2284–2291. https://doi.org/10.1001/jama.2016.6458

44. Galland L. (2014). The gut microbiome and the brain. Journal of medicinal food, 17(12), 1261–1272. https://doi.org/10.1089/jmf.2014.7000

45. Ochoa-Repáraz, J., & Kasper, L. H. (2016). The Second Brain: Is the Gut Microbiota a Link Between Obesity and Central Nervous

System Disorders?. Current obesity reports, 5(1), 51–64. https://doi.org/10.1007/s13679-016-0191-1

46. Martinez, C. S., Ferreira, F. V., Castro, A. A., & Gomide, L. B. (2014). Women with greater pelvic floor muscle strength have better sexual function. Acta obstetricia et gynecologica Scandinavica, 93(5), 497–502. https://doi.org/10.1111/aogs.12379

47. Darling C, Haavio-Mannila E, Kontula O. (2001). Predictors of orgasmic frequency: A case of Finland. Scandinavian Journal of Sexology. 4(2):89–106.

48. Kontula O. The Population Research Institute D49/2009. Helsinki: The Family Federation of Finland; 2009. Between Sexual Desire and Reality: The evolution of Sex in Finland.

49. Shirazi, T., Renfro, K. J., Lloyd, E., & Wallen, K. (2018). Women's Experience of Orgasm During Intercourse: Question Semantics Affect Women's Reports and Men's Estimates of Orgasm Occurrence. Archives of sexual behavior, 47(3), 605–613. https://doi.org/10.1007/s10508-017-1102-6

50. Nicholas, A., Brody, S., de Sutter, P., & de Carufel, F. (2008). A woman's history of vaginal orgasm is discernible from her walk. The journal of sexual medicine, 5(9), 2119–2124. https://doi.org/10.1111/j.1743-6109.2008.00942.x

51. Corliss, J. (2019). " How it's made: Cholesterol production in your body". Retrieved from: https://www.health.harvard.edu/heart-health/how-its-made-cholesterol-production-in-your-body

52. Carmichael, M.S., Warburton, V.L., Dixen, J. et al. (1994). Relationships among cardiovascular, muscular, and oxytocin responses during human sexual activity. Arch Sex Behav 23, 59–79. https://doi.org/10.1007/BF01541618

53. Fan, X., & Markram, H. (2019). A Brief History of Simulation Neuroscience. Frontiers in neuroinformatics, 13, 32. https://doi.org/10.3389/fninf.2019.00032

54. Komisaruk, B. R., Wise, N., Frangos, E., Liu, W. C., Allen, K., & Brody, S. (2011). Women's clitoris, vagina, and cervix mapped on the sensory cortex: fMRI evidence. The journal of sexual medicine, 8(10), 2822–2830. https://doi.org/10.1111/j.1743-6109.2011.02388.x

55. Sukel, K. (2011). " I had an orgasm in an MRI scanner". Retrieved from: https://www.theguardian.com/science/blog/2011/nov/16/orgasm-mri-scanner

56. Sukel, K. (2011). " Sex on the brain: Orgasms unlock altered consiousness". Retrieved from: https://www.newscientist.com/article/mg21028124-600-sex-on-the-brain-orgasms-unlock-altered-consciousness/

57. Georgiadis J. R. (2012). Doing it … wild? On the role of the cerebral cortex in human sexual activity. Socioaffective neuroscience & psychology, 2, 17337. https://doi.org/10.3402/snp.v2i0.17337

58. Daily Mail Reporter (2011). " Secrets of the female orgasm revealed: Scientists discover new hope for women who can't climax". Retrieved from: https://www.dailymail.co.uk/news/article-1386186/Its-brain-Scientists-discover-orgasm-leads-altered-state-conciousness.html

59. Sandler, L. (2012). " Naomi Wolf sparks another debate (on sex, of course)". Retrieved from: https://www.nytimes.com/2012/09/20/fashion/naomi-wolf-on-her-new-book-vagina.html

60. Adams, C. (2014). " Scientists discover that just IMAGINING exercises can make you stronger, tone your muscles and delay or stop muscle atrophy". Retrieved from: https://www.dailymail.co.uk/news/article-2887151/Scientists-discover-just-IMAGINING-exercising-make-stronger-tone-muscles-delay-stop-muscle-atrophy.html

61. Clark, B. C., Mahato, N. K., Nakasawa, M. Law, T. D., Thomas, J. S. (2014). The power of the mind: the cortex as a critical determinant of muscle strength/weakness. Journal of Neurophysiology 112:12, 3219-3226. https://doi.org/10.1038/ajg.2015.419

62. Conway, D. (2014). " 6 Mindful ways to calm your mind and heal your heart". Retrieved from: https://tinybuddha.com/blog/6-mindful-ways-calm-mind-heal-heart/

63. Amen, D. (n.d.). " ANT Therapy, How to develop your own internal anteater to eradicate Automatic Negative Thoughts". Retrieved from: https://ahha.org/selfhelp-articles/ant-therapy/

64. Katie, B. (n.d.) "The Work is a Practice". Retrieved from: https://thework.com/instruction-the-work-byron-katie/

65. Marciniak, R., Sheardova, K., Cermáková, P., Hudeček, D., Sumec, R., & Hort, J. (2014). Effect of meditation on cognitive functions in context of aging and neurodegenerative diseases. Frontiers in behavioral neuroscience, 8, 17. https://doi.org/10.3389/fnbeh.2014.00017

66. Cox, B., Forshaw, J. (2011). The quantum universe: everything that can happen does happen. 11:211.

67. Gardner, B., Lally, P., & Wardle, J. (2012). Making health habitual: the psychology of 'habit-formation' and general practice. The British journal of general practice : the journal of the Royal College of General Practitioners, 62(605), 664–666. https://doi.org/10.3399/bjgp12X659466

68. Lally, P., van Jaarsveld, C.H.M., Potts, H.W.W. and Wardle, J. (2010), How are habits formed: Modelling habit formation in the real world. Eur. J. Soc. Psychol., 40: 998-1009. https://doi.org/10.1002/ejsp.674

69. Subak, L. L., Richter, H. E., & Hunskaar, S. (2009). Obesity and urinary incontinence: epidemiology and clinical research update. The Journal of urology, 182(6 Suppl), S2–S7. https://doi.org/10.1016/j.juro.2009.08.071

70. Wetle, T., Scherr, P., Branch, L. G., Resnick, N. M., Harris, T., Evans, D., & Taylor, J. O. (1995). Difficulty with holding urine among older persons in a geographically defined community: prevalence and correlates. Journal of the American Geriatrics Society, 43(4), 349–355. https://doi.org/10.1111/j.1532-5415.1995.tb05806.x

71. Wysocki, S., Kingsberg, S., & Krychman, M. (2014). Management of Vaginal Atrophy: Implications from the REVIVE Survey.

Clinical medicine insights. Reproductive health, 8, 23–30. https://doi.org/10.4137/CMRH.S14498

72. Waetjen, E. L. Liao, S., Johnson, W. O., Sampselle, C. M., Sternfield, B., Harlow, S. D., Gold, E. B. (2007). Factors Associated with Prevalent and Incident Urinary Incontinence in a Cohort of Midlife Women: A Longitudinal Analysis of Data: Study of Women's Health Across the Nation. American Journal of Epidemiology, 165(3), 309–318. https://doi.org/10.1093/aje/kwk018

73. Poświata, A., Socha, T., & Opara, J. (2014). Prevalence of stress urinary incontinence in elite female endurance athletes. Journal of human kinetics, 44, 91–96. https://doi.org/10.2478/hukin-2014-0114

74. Hannestad, Y. S., Rortveit, G., Daltveit, A. K., & Hunskaar, S. (2003). Are smoking and other lifestyle factors associated with female urinary incontinence? The Norwegian EPINCONT Study. BJOG : an international journal of obstetrics and gynaecology, 110(3), 247–254.

75. Olsen, A. L., Smith, V. J., Bergstrom, J. O., Colling, J. C., Clark, A. L. (1997). Epidemiology of surgically managed pelvic organ prolapse and urinary incontinence. Obstetrics & Gynecology 89(4), 501-506. https://doi.org/10.1016/S0029-7844(97)00058-6

76. United States Food and Drug Administration. (2019). "Urogynecologic Surgical Mesh Implants".Retrieved from: https://www.fda.gov/medical-devices/implants-and-prosthetics/urogynecologic-surgical-mesh-implants

77. Rankin, L. (2011). " 15 Crazy things about lady parts". Retrieved from: https://www.psychologytoday.com/ie/blog/owning-pink/201104/15-crazy-things-about-lady-parts

78. Naess, I., & Bø, K. (2018). Can maximal voluntary pelvic floor muscle contraction reduce vaginal resting pressure and resting EMG activity?. International urogynecology journal, 29(11), 1623–1627. https://doi.org/10.1007/s00192-018-3599-1

79. Da Roza, T., Brandão, S., Mascarenhas, T., Jorge, R. N., & Duarte, J. A. (2015). Volume of training and the ranking level are associated with the leakage of urine in young female trampolinists. Clinical journal of sport medicine : official journal of the Canadian Academy of Sport Medicine, 25(3), 270–275. https://doi.org/10.1097/JSM.0000000000000129

80. Ansari R. M. (2016). Kapalabhati pranayama: An answer to modern day polycystic ovarian syndrome and coexisting metabolic syndrome?. International journal of yoga, 9(2), 163–167. https://doi.org/10.4103/0973-6131.183705

81. Fitzgerald, M. P., Stablein, U., & Brubaker, L. (2002). Urinary habits among asymptomatic women. American journal of obstetrics and gynecology, 187(5), 1384–1388. https://doi.org/10.1067/mob.2002.126865

82. Lukacz, E. S., Sampselle, C., Gray, M., Macdiarmid, S., Rosenberg, M., Ellsworth, P., & Palmer, M. H. (2011). A healthy bladder: a consensus statement. International journal of clinical practice, 65(10), 1026–1036. https://doi.org/10.1111/j.1742-1241.2011.02763.x

83. Meinders, A. J., & Meinders, A. E. (2010). Hoeveel water moeten we eigenlijk drinken? [How much water do we really need to drink?]. Nederlands tijdschrift voor geneeskunde, 154, A1757.

84. Jácome, C., Oliveira, D., Marques, A., & Sá-Couto, P. (2011). Prevalence and impact of urinary incontinence among female athletes. International journal of gynaecology and obstetrics: the official organ of the International Federation of Gynaecology and Obstetrics, 114(1), 60–63. https://doi.org/10.1016/j.ijgo.2011.02.004

85. Geynisman-Tan, J., Kenton, K., Leader-Cramer, A., Dave, B., Bochenska, K., Mueller, M., Collins, S. A., & Lewicky-Gaupp, C. (2018). Anal Penetrative Intercourse as a Risk Factor for Fecal Incontinence. Female pelvic medicine & reconstructive surgery, 24(3), 252–255. https://doi.org/10.1097/SPV.0000000000000408

86. Adibmoghaddam, E., Sourinejad, H., Dehkordi, Z., Beigi, M., Hadian, M. (2019). The Use of Flaxseed in Gynecology: A Review Article. Journal of Midwifery & Reproductive Health. 7. https://doi.org/10.22038/JMRH.2019.31820.1345

87. Morrison, O. (2019). "Europe's food safety watchdog plays down flaxseed cyanide danger". Retrieved from: https://www.foodnavigator.com/Article/2019/08/21/Europe-s-food-safety-watchdog-plays-down-flaxseed-cyanide-danger

88. Ohkusa, T., Koido, S., Nishikawa, Y., & Sato, N. (2019). Gut Microbiota and Chronic Constipation: A Review and Update. Frontiers in medicine, 6, 19. https://doi.org/10.3389/fmed.2019.00019

89. Song, B. K., Cho, K. O., Jo, Y., Oh, J. W., & Kim, Y. S. (2012). Colon transit time according to physical activity level in adults. Journal of neurogastroenterology and motility, 18(1), 64–69. https://doi.org/10.5056/jnm.2012.18.1.64

90. Crowle, A., & Harley, C. (2020). Development of a biotensegrity focused therapy for the treatment of pelvic organ prolapse: A retrospective case series. Journal of bodywork and movement therapies, 24(1), 115–125. https://doi.org/10.1016/j.jbmt.2019.10.008

91. Arya, L. A., Novi, J. M., Shaunik, A., Morgan, M. A., & Bradley, C. S. (2005). Pelvic organ prolapse, constipation, and dietary fiber intake in women: a case-control study. American journal of obstetrics and gynecology, 192(5), 1687–1691. https://doi.org/10.1016/j.ajog.2004.11.032

92. InformedHealth.org [Internet]. Cologne, Germany: Institute for Quality and Efficiency in Health Care (IQWiG); 2006-. Pelvic organ prolapse: Overview. 2018 Aug 23. Available from: https://www.ncbi.nlm.nih.gov/books/NBK525783/

93. Son, H., Song, H. J., Seo, H. J., Lee, H., Choi, S. M., & Lee, S. (2020). The safety and effectiveness of self-administered coffee enema: A systematic review of case reports. Medicine, 99(36), e21998. https://doi.org/10.1097/MD.0000000000021998

94. Latthe, P., Latthe, M., Say, L. et al. WHO systematic review of prevalence of chronic pelvic pain: a neglected reproductive health morbidity. BMC Public Health 6, 177 (2006). https://doi.org/10.1186/1471-2458-6-177

95. Butler, D. S., Moseley, L. G., (2020). Explain Pain Second Edition Retrieved from: https://www.noigroup.com/product/explain-pain-second-edn-epub/

96. Johnson M. (2007). Transcutaneous Electrical Nerve Stimulation: Mechanisms, Clinical Application and Evidence. Reviews in pain,

1(1), 7–11. https://doi.org/10.1177/204946370700100103

97. Sharma, N., Rekha, K., & Srinivasan, J. K. (2017). Efficacy of transcutaneous electrical nerve stimulation in the treatment of chronic pelvic pain. Journal of mid-life health, 8(1), 36–39. https://doi.org/10.4103/jmh.JMH_60_16

98. Lahaie, M. A., Boyer, S. C., Amsel, R., Khalifé, S., & Binik, Y. M. (2010). Vaginismus: a review of the literature on the classification/diagnosis, etiology and treatment. Women's health (London, England), 6(5), 705–719. https://doi.org/10.2217/whe.10.46

99. Binik Y. M. (2010). The DSM diagnostic criteria for vaginismus. Archives of sexual behavior, 39(2), 278–291. https://doi.org/10.1007/s10508-009-9560-0

100. Cichowski, S. B., Dunivan, G. C., Komesu, Y. M., & Rogers, R. G. (2013). Sexual abuse history and pelvic floor disorders in women. Southern medical journal, 106(12), 675–678. https://doi.org/10.1097/SMJ.0000000000000029

101. Cottrell B. H. (2010). An updated review of of evidence to discourage douching. MCN. The American journal of maternal child nursing, 35(2), 102–109. https://doi.org/10.1097/NMC.0b013e3181cae9da

102. Zhoolideh, P., Ghaderi, F., Salahzadeh, Z. (2017). Are there any relations between posture and pelvic floor disorders? A literature review. Crescent Journal of Medical and Biological Sciences. 4(4), 153-159.

103. Baddeley, B., Sornalingam, S., & Cooper, M. (2016). Sitting is the new smoking: where do we stand?. The British journal of general practice : the journal of the Royal College of General Practitioners, 66(646), 258. https://doi.org/10.3399/bjgp16X685009

104. Hamilton, M. T., Healy, G. N., Dunstan, D. W., Zderic, T. W., & Owen, N. (2008). Too Little Exercise and Too Much Sitting: Inactivity Physiology and the Need for New Recommendations on Sedentary Behavior. Current cardiovascular risk reports, 2(4), 292–298. https://doi.org/10.1007/s12170-008-0054-8

105. Owen, N., Sparling, P. B., Healy, G. N., Dunstan, D. W., & Matthews, C. E. (2010). Sedentary behavior: emerging evidence for a new health risk. Mayo Clinic proceedings, 85(12), 1138–1141. https://doi.org/10.4065/mcp.2010.0444

106. Subak, L. L., Richter, H. E., & Hunskaar, S. (2009). Obesity and urinary incontinence: epidemiology and clinical research update. The Journal of urology, 182(6 Suppl), S2–S7. https://doi.org/10.1016/j.juro.2009.08.071

107. Melanson E. L. (2017). The effect of exercise on non-exercise physical activity and sedentary behavior in adults. Obesity reviews : an official journal of the International Association for the Study of Obesity, 18 Suppl 1(Suppl 1), 40–49. https://doi.org/10.1111/obr.12507

108. Appleby, P., Roddam, A., Allen, N., & Key, T. (2007). Comparative fracture risk in vegetarians and nonvegetarians in EPIC-Oxford. European journal of clinical nutrition, 61(12), 1400–1406. https://doi.org/10.1038/sj.ejcn.1602659

109. Iguacel, I., Miguel-Berges, M. L., Gómez-Bruton, A., Moreno, L. A., & Julián, C. (2019). Veganism, vegetarianism, bone mineral density, and fracture risk: a systematic review and meta-analysis. Nutrition reviews, 77(1), 1–18. https://doi.org/10.1093/nutrit/nuy045

110. van Strien T. (2018). Causes of Emotional Eating and Matched Treatment of Obesity. Current diabetes reports, 18(6), 35. https://doi.org/10.1007/s11892-018-1000-x

111. Knutson, K. L., & Van Cauter, E. (2008). Associations between sleep loss and increased risk of obesity and diabetes. Annals of the New York Academy of Sciences, 1129, 287–304. https://doi.org/10.1196/annals.1417.033

112. Blume, C., Garbazza, C., Spitschan, M. (2019). Effects of light on human circadian rhythms, sleep and mood. Somnologie. 23, 147-156. https://doi.org/10.1007/s11818-019-00215-x

113. Wohlrab, K. J., Erekson, E. A., & Myers, D. L. (2009). Postoperative erosions of the Mersilene suburethral sling mesh for antiincontinence surgery. International urogynecology journal and pelvic floor dysfunction, 20(4), 417–420. https://doi.org/10.1007/s00192-008-0787-4

114. Kobashi, K. C., Dmochowski, R., Mee, S. L., Mostwin, J., Nitti, V. W., Zimmern, P. E., & Leach, G. E. (1999). Erosion of woven polyester pubovaginal sling. The Journal of urology, 162(6), 2070–2072. https://doi.org/10.1016/s0022-5347(05)68103-7

115. Heneghan, C. J., Goldacre, B., Onakpoya, I., Aronson, J. K., Jefferson, T., Pluddemann, A., & Mahtani, K. R. (2017). Trials of transvaginal mesh devices for pelvic organ prolapse: a systematic database review of the US FDA approval process. BMJ open, 7(12), e017125. https://doi.org/10.1136/bmjopen-2017-017125

116. Ulmsten, U., Henriksson, L., Johnson, P. et al. (1996). An ambulatory surgical procedure under local anesthesia for treatment of female urinary incontinence. Int Urogynecol J 7, 81–86. https://doi.org/10.1007/BF01902378

117. Ulmsten, U., Falconer, C., Johnson, P., Jomaa, M., Lannér, L., Nilsson, C. G., & Olsson, I. (1998). A multicenter study of tension-free vaginal tape (TVT) for surgical treatment of stress urinary incontinence. International urogynecology journal and pelvic floor dysfunction, 9(4), 210–213. https://doi.org/10.1007/BF01901606

118. Gornall J. (2018). The trial that launched millions of mesh implant procedures: did money compromise the outcome? BMJ. 363:k4155. https://doi:10.1136/bmj.k4155

119. Viereck, V., Bader, W., Lobodasch, K., Pauli, F., Bentler, R., & Kölbl, H. (2016). Guideline-Based Strategies in the Surgical Treatment of Female Urinary Incontinence: The New Gold Standard is Almost the Same as the Old One. Geburtshilfe und Frauenheilkunde, 76(8), 865–868. https://doi.org/10.1055/s-0042-107079

120. Welk, B., Carlson, K. V., Baverstock, R. J., Steele, S. S., Bailly, G. G., & Hickling, D. R. (2017). Canadian Urological Association position statement on the use of transvaginal mesh. Canadian Urological Association journal = Journal de l'Association des urologues du Canada, 11(6Suppl2), S105–S107. https://doi.org/10.5489/cuaj.4579

121. Government of Canada, Drugs, health & consumer products, review decisions. (2019). "Summary Safety Review - Surgical mesh products made from non-absorbable synthetic (polypropylene) material that are used for the transvaginal repair of pelvic organ prolapse (POP) - Health Canada". Retrieved from: https://hpr-rps.hres.ca/reg-content/summary-safety-review-detail.php?lang=en&linkID=SSR00229

122. BBC News. (2018). " Vaginal mesh implants: Australia apologises for 'decades of pain'". https://www.bbc.com/news/world-australia-45806324

123. Lai, H., Gardner, V., Vetter, J., & Andriole, G. L. (2015). Correlation between psychological stress levels and the severity of overactive bladder symptoms. BMC urology, 15, 14. https://doi.org/10.1186/s12894-015-0009-6

124. Madhu, C., Enki, D., Drake, M. J., & Hashim, H. (2015). The Functional Effects of Cigarette Smoking in Women on the Lower Urinary Tract. Urologia internationalis, 95(4), 478–482. https://doi.org/10.1159/000438928

125. Amarenco, G., Ismael, S. S., Even-Schneider, A., Raibaut, P., Demaille-Wlodyka, S., Parratte, B., & Kerdraon, J. (2003). Urodynamic effect of acute transcutaneous posterior tibial nerve stimulation in overactive bladder. The Journal of urology, 169(6), 2210–2215. https://doi.org/10.1097/01.ju.0000067446.17576.bd

126. de Sèze, M., Raibaut, P., Gallien, P., Even-Schneider, A., Denys, P., Bonniaud, V., Gamé, X., & Amarenco, G. (2011). Transcutaneous posterior tibial nerve stimulation for treatment of the overactive bladder syndrome in multiple sclerosis: results of a multicenter prospective study. Neurourology and urodynamics, 30(3), 306–311. https://doi.org/10.1002/nau.20958

127. Orasanu, B., & Mahajan, S. T. (2013). The use of botulinum toxin for the treatment of overactive bladder syndrome. Indian journal of urology : IJU : journal of the Urological Society of India, 29(1), 2–11. https://doi.org/10.4103/0970-1591.109975

128. Das, A. K., White, M. D., & Longhurst, P. A. (2000). Sacral nerve stimulation for the management of voiding dysfunction. Reviews in urology, 2(1), 43–60.

129. Abello, A., & Das, A. K. (2018). Electrical neuromodulation in the management of lower urinary tract dysfunction: evidence, experience and future prospects. Therapeutic advances in urology, 10(5), 165–173. https://doi.org/10.1177/1756287218756082

130. Siegel, S., Noblett, K., Mangel, J., Griebling, T.L., Sutherland, S.E., Bird, E.T., Comiter, C., Culkin, D., Bennett, J., Zylstra, S., Berg, K.C., Kan, F. and Irwin, C.P. (2015), Results of a prospective, randomized, multicenter study evaluating sacral neuromodulation with InterStim therapy compared to standard medical therapy at 6-months in subjects with mild symptoms of overactive bladder. Neurourol. Urodynam., 34: 224-230. https://doi.org/10.1002/nau.22544

131. Stothers, L., & Friedman, B. (2011). Risk factors for the development of stress urinary incontinence in women. Current urology reports, 12(5), 363–369. https://doi.org/10.1007/s11934-011-0215-z

132. Hannestad, Y.S., Rortveit, G., Daltveit, A.K. and Hunskaar, S. (2003), Are smoking and other lifestyle factors associated with female urinary incontinence? The Norwegian EPINCONT Study. BJOG: An International Journal of Obstetrics & Gynaecology, 110: 247-254. https://doi.org/10.1046/j.1471-0528.2003.02327.x

133. Neumann, P. B., Grimmer, K. A., & Deenadayalan, Y. (2006). Pelvic floor muscle training and adjunctive therapies for the treatment of stress urinary incontinence in women: a systematic review. BMC women's health, 6, 11. https://doi.org/10.1186/1472-6874-6-11

134. Maund, E., Guski, L. S., & Gøtzsche, P. C. (2017). Considering benefits and harms of duloxetine for treatment of stress urinary incontinence: a meta-analysis of clinical study reports. CMAJ : Canadian Medical Association journal = journal de l'Association medicale canadienne, 189(5), E194–E203. https://doi.org/10.1503/cmaj.151104

135. The British Association of Urological Surgeons (BAUS). (2020). "Urethral bulking injections for stress urinary incontinence (SUI)". Patient information leaflet No: 16/148. Page 1. Retrieved from: https://www.baus.org.uk/_userfiles/pages/files/Patients/Leaflets/Urethral%20bulking.pdf

136. Barbara, G., Facchin, F., Buggio, L., Alberico, D., Frattaruolo, M. P., & Kustermann, A. (2017). Vaginal rejuvenation: current perspectives. International journal of women's health, 9, 513–519. https://doi.org/10.2147/IJWH.S99700

137. Ogrinc, U. B., Senčar, S., & Lenasi, H. (2015). Novel minimally invasive laser treatment of urinary incontinence in women. Lasers in surgery and medicine, 47(9), 689–697. https://doi.org/10.1002/lsm.22416

138. Preti, M., Vieira-Baptista, P., Digesu, G. A., Bretschneider, C. E., Damaser, M., Demirkesen, O., Heller, D. S., Mangir, N., Marchitelli, C., Mourad, S., Moyal-Barracco, M., Peremateu, S., Tailor, V., Tarcan, T., De, E., & Stockdale, C. K. (2019). The Clinical Role of LASER for Vulvar and Vaginal Treatments in Gynecology and Female Urology: An ICS/ISSVD Best Practice Consensus Document. Journal of lower genital tract disease, 23(2), 151–160. https://doi.org/10.1097/LGT.0000000000000462

139. Cevasco, Juan & Colorado, Esther & Barco, Laura. (2007). Burch procedure: Experience of 45 years of history. Ginecología y obstetricia de México. 75. 155-63.

140. Hegarty, P. K., Power, P. C., O'Brien, M. F., & Bredin, H. C. (2001). Longevity of the Marshall-Marchetti-Krantz procedure. Annales chirurgiae et gynaecologiae, 90(4), 286–289.

141. Mainprize, T. C., & Drutz, H. P. (1988). The Marshall-Marchetti-Krantz procedure: a critical review. Obstetrical & gynecological survey, 43(12), 724–729. https://doi.org/10.1097/00006254-198812000-00003

142. LIAPIS, A. E., ASIMIADIS, V., LOGHIS, C. D., PYRGIOTIS, E., ZOURLAS, P.A. (1996). A Randomized Prospective Study of Three Operative Methods for Genuine Stress Incontinence. Journal of Gynecologic Surgery 12(1): 7-14. https://doi.org/10.1089/gyn.1996.12.7

143. McGuire, E. J., Lytton, B. (1978). Pubovaginal Sling Procedure for Stress Incontinence. Journal of Urology 1(119), 82-84. https://doi.org/10.1016/S0022-5347(17)57390-5

144. The British Association of Urological Surgeons (BAUS). (2020). "Urethral bulking injections for stress urinary incontinence (SUI)". Patient information leaflet No: 17/145. Page 6. Retrieved from: https://www.baus.org.uk/_userfiles/pages/files/Patients/Leaflets/Autologous%20female%20sling.pdf

145. Osman, N. I., Hillary, C. J., Mangera, A., Aldamanhoori, R., Inman, R. D., Chapple, C. R. (2018). The Midurethral Fascial "Sling on a String": An Alternative to Midurethral Synthetic Tapes in the Era of Mesh Complications. Surgery in Motion 74(2), 191-196. https://doi.org/10.1016/j.eururo.2018.04.031

146. FitzGerald, J. F., & Kumar, A. S. (2014). Biologic versus Synthetic Mesh Reinforcement: What are the Pros and Cons?. Clinics in colon and rectal surgery, 27(4), 140–148. https://doi.org/10.1055/s-0034-1394155

147. Huang, Y. H., Lin, A. T., Chen, K. K., Pan, C. C., & Chang, L. S. (2001). High failure rate using allograft fascia lata in pubovaginal sling surgery for female stress urinary incontinence. Urology, 58(6), 943–946. https://doi.org/10.1016/s0090-4295(01)01430-3

148. Fitzgerald, M. P., Mollenhauer, J., & Brubaker, L. (1999). Failure of allograft suburethral slings. BJU international, 84(7), 785–788. https://doi.org/10.1046/j.1464-410x.1999.00246.x

149. Jones, J.S., Rackley, R.R., Berglund, R., Abdelmalak, J.B., Deorco, G. and Vasavada, S.P. (2005), Porcine small intestinal submucosa as a percutaneous mid-urethral sling: 2-year results. BJU International, 96: 103-106. https://doi.org/10.1111/j.1464-410X.2005.05576.x

150. Rutner, A. B., Levine, S. R., Schmaelzle, J. F. (2003). Processed porcine small intestine submucosa as a graft material for pubovaginal slings: durability and results. Adult Urology 62(5), 805-809. https://doi.org/10.1016/S0090-4295(03)00664-2

151. Zheng, M.H., Chen, J., Kirilak, Y., Willers, C., Xu, J. and Wood, D. (2005), Porcine small intestine submucosa (SIS) is not an acellular collagenous matrix and contains porcine DNA: Possible implications in human implantation. J. Biomed. Mater. Res., 73B: 61-67. https://doi.org/10.1002/jbm.b.30170

152. Chang, J., & Lee, D. (2017). Midurethral slings in the mesh litigation era. Translational andrology and urology, 6(Suppl 2), S68–S75. https://doi.org/10.21037/tau.2017.04.06

153. Ford, A. A., Rogerson, L., Cody, J. D., Aluko, P., & Ogah, J. A. (2017). Mid-urethral sling operations for stress urinary incontinence in women. The Cochrane database of systematic reviews, 7(7), CD006375. https://doi.org/10.1002/14651858.CD006375.pub4

154. Keltie, K., Elneil, S., Monga, A. et al. Complications following vaginal mesh procedures for stress urinary incontinence: an 8 year study of 92,246 women. Sci Rep 7, 12015 (2017). https://doi.org/10.1038/s41598-017-11821-w

155. Steinbuch, Y. (2017). " My new vagina almost ruined my partner's penis". New York Post. Retrieved from: https://nypost.com/2017/03/20/my-improved-vagina-nearly-cut-off-my-partners-penis/

156. Lee, K. S., Choo, M. S., Lee, Y. S., Han, J. Y., Kim, J. Y., Jung, B. J., & Han, D. H. (2008). Prospective comparison of the 'inside-out' and 'outside-in' transobturator-tape procedures for the treatment of female stress urinary incontinence. International urogynecology journal and pelvic floor dysfunction, 19(4), 577–582. https://doi.org/10.1007/s00192-007-0487-5

157. Leone Roberti Maggiore, U., Finazzi Agrò, E., Soligo, M., Li Marzi, V., Digesu, A., & Serati, M. (2017). Long-term outcomes of TOT and TVT procedures for the treatment of female stress urinary incontinence: a systematic review and meta-analysis. International urogynecology journal, 28(8), 1119–1130. https://doi.org/10.1007/s00192-017-3275-x

158. Latthe, P.M., Singh, P., Foon, R. and Toozs-Hobson, P. (2010), Two routes of transobturator tape procedures in stress urinary incontinence: a meta-analysis with direct and indirect comparison of randomized trials. BJU International, 106: 68-76. https://doi.org/10.1111/j.1464-410X.2009.09051.x

159. Bernasconi, F., Napolitano, V., Natale, F., Leone, V., Lijoi, D., & Cervigni, M. (2012). TVT SECUR System: Final results of a prospective, observational, multicentric study. International urogynecology journal, 23(1), 93–98. https://doi.org/10.1007/s00192-011-1520-2

160. Sandhu, J. S., Karan, S. C., Maiti, G. D., & Dudeja, P. (2017). To evaluate the safety and efficacy of the TVT-Secur procedure in the treatment of stress urinary incontinence in women. Medical journal, Armed Forces India, 73(1), 36–41. https://doi.org/10.1016/j.mjafi.2016.07.010

161. Song, B., He, Y., Shen, R., Shao, H., He, X., Wang, X., Sheng, T., Zhu, X., & Jiang, D. (2020). TVT-O vs TVT-S for female stress urinary incontinence: A systematic review and meta-analysis. International journal of clinical practice, 74(9), e13506. https://doi.org/10.1111/ijcp.13506

162. Cornu, J. N., Sèbe, P. Peyrat, L., Ciofu, C., Cussenot, O., Haab, F. (2010). Midterm Prospective Evaluation of TVT-Secur Reveals High Failure Rate. Female Urology - Incontinence. 58(1): 157-161. https://doi.org/10.1016/j.eururo.2010.04.021

163. Schellart, R. P., Rengerink, K. O., Van der Aa, F., Lucot, J. P., Kimpe, B., de Ridder, D. J. M. K., Dijkgraaf, M. G. W., Roovers, J. P. W. R. (2014). A Randomized Comparison of a Single-incision Midurethral Sling and a Transobturator Midurethral Sling in Women with Stress Urinary Incontinence: Results of 12-mo Follow-up. European Urology. 66(6): 1179-1185. https://doi.org/10.1016/j.eururo.2014.07.027

164. Keltie, K., Elneil, S., Monga, A. et al. Complications following vaginal mesh procedures for stress urinary incontinence: an 8 year study of 92,246 women. Sci Rep 7, 12015 (2017). https://doi.org/10.1038/s41598-017-11821-w

165. Crosby, E. C., Abernethy, M., Berger, M. B., DeLancey, J. O., Fenner, D. E., & Morgan, D. M. (2014). Symptom resolution after operative management of complications from transvaginal mesh. Obstetrics and gynecology, 123(1), 134–139. https://doi.

org/10.1097/AOG.0000000000000042

166. Ugare, U. G., Bassey, I. A., Udosen, E. J., Essiet, A., & Bassey, O. O. (2014). Management of lower urinary retention in a limited resource setting. Ethiopian journal of health sciences, 24(4), 329–336. https://doi.org/10.4314/ejhs.v24i4.8

167. Kessler, T. M., Studer, U. E., & Burkhard, F. C. (2006). The effect of terazosin on functional bladder outlet obstruction in women: a pilot study. The Journal of urology, 176(4 Pt 1), 1487–1492. https://doi.org/10.1016/j.juro.2006.06.009

168. Menefee, S. A., Chesson, R., & Wall, L. L. (1998). Stress urinary incontinence due to prescription medications: alpha-blockers and angiotensin converting enzyme inhibitors. Obstetrics and gynecology, 91(5 Pt 2), 853–854. https://doi.org/10.1016/s0029-7844(97)00497-3

169. Bharucha, A. E., Zinsmeister, A. R., Locke, G. R., Seide, B. M., McKeon, K., Schleck, C. D., & Melton, L. J., 3rd (2006). Risk factors for fecal incontinence: a population-based study in women. The American journal of gastroenterology, 101(6), 1305–1312. https://doi.org/10.1111/j.1572-0241.2006.00553.x

170. Scott K. M. (2014). Pelvic floor rehabilitation in the treatment of fecal incontinence. Clinics in colon and rectal surgery, 27(3), 99–105. https://doi.org/10.1055/s-0034-1384662

171. Norton, C., & Kamm, M. A. (2001). Anal sphincter biofeedback and pelvic floor exercises for faecal incontinence in adults--a systematic review. Alimentary pharmacology & therapeutics, 15(8), 1147–1154. https://doi.org/10.1046/j.1365-2036.2001.01039.x

172. Luo, C., Samaranayake, C. B., Plank, L. D., & Bissett, I. P. (2010). Systematic review on the efficacy and safety of injectable bulking agents for passive faecal incontinence. Colorectal disease : the official journal of the Association of Coloproctology of Great Britain and Ireland, 12(4), 296–303. https://doi.org/10.1111/j.1463-1318.2009.01828.x

173. Eléouet, Marianne & Siproudhis, Laurent & Guillou, Nelly & Couedic, Jocelyne & Bouguen, Guillaume & Bretagne, Jean. (2010). Chronic posterior tibial nerve transcutaneous electrical nerve stimulation (TENS) to treat fecal incontinence (FI). International journal of colorectal disease. 25. 1127-32. 10.1007/s00384-010-0960-3.

174. Peña Ros, E., Parra Baños, P. A., Benavides Buleje, J. A., Muñoz Camarena, J. M., Escamilla Segade, C., Candel Arenas, M. F., Gonzalez Valverde, F. M., & Albarracín Marín-Blázquez, A. (2016). Short-term outcome of percutaneous posterior tibial nerve stimulation (PTNS) for the treatment of faecal incontinence. Techniques in coloproctology, 20(1), 19–24. https://doi.org/10.1007/s10151-015-1380-8

175. Saldana Ruiz, N., & Kaiser, A. M. (2017). Fecal incontinence - Challenges and solutions. World journal of gastroenterology, 23(1), 11–24. https://doi.org/10.3748/wjg.v23.i1.11

176. Wexner, S. D., Coller, J. A., Devroede, G., Hull, T., McCallum, R., Chan, M., Ayscue, J. M., Shobeiri, A. S., Margolin, D., England, M., Kaufman, H., Snape, W. J., Mutlu, E., Chua, H., Pettit, P., Nagle, D., Madoff, R. D., Lerew, D. R., & Mellgren, A. (2010). Sacral nerve stimulation for fecal incontinence: results of a 120-patient prospective multicenter study. Annals of surgery, 251(3), 441–449. https://doi.org/10.1097/SLA.0b013e3181cf8ed0

177. Matzel, K. E., Madoff, R. D., LaFontaine, L. J., Baeten, C. G., Buie, W. D., Christiansen, J., Wexner, S., & Dynamic Graciloplasty Therapy Study Group (2001). Complications of dynamic graciloplasty: incidence, management, and impact on outcome. Diseases of the colon and rectum, 44(10), 1427–1435. https://doi.org/10.1007/BF02234593

178. Patel, P. D., Amrute, K. V., & Badlani, G. H. (2007). Pelvic organ prolapse and stress urinary incontinence: A review of etiological factors. Indian journal of urology : IJU : journal of the Urological Society of India, 23(2), 135–141. https://doi.org/10.4103/0970-1591.32064

179. Kim, S., Pollock, G. R., Twiss, C. O., & Funk, J. T. (2019). Surgery for Posterior Compartment Vaginal Prolapse: Graft Augmented Repair. The Urologic clinics of North America, 46(1), 87–95. https://doi.org/10.1016/j.ucl.2018.08.015

180. Aarts, J. W., Nieboer, T. E., Johnson, N., Tavender, E., Garry, R., Mol, B. W., & Kluivers, K. B. (2015). Surgical approach to hysterectomy for benign gynaecological disease. The Cochrane database of systematic reviews, 2015(8), CD003677. https://doi.org/10.1002/14651858.CD003677.pub5

181. Carlin, G.L., Bodner-Adler, B., Husslein, H. et al. The effectiveness of surgical procedures to prevent post-hysterectomy pelvic organ prolapse: a systematic review of the literature. Int Urogynecol J 32, 775–783 (2021). https://doi.org/10.1007/s00192-020-04572-2

182. Smit, M., Werner, M., Lansink-Hartgring, A. O., Dieperink, W., Zijlstra, J. G., & van Meurs, M. (2016). How central obesity influences intra-abdominal pressure: a prospective, observational study in cardiothoracic surgical patients. Annals of intensive care, 6(1), 99. https://doi.org/10.1186/s13613-016-0195-8

183. Li, C., Gong, Y., & Wang, B. (2016). The efficacy of pelvic floor muscle training for pelvic organ prolapse: a systematic review and meta-analysis. International urogynecology journal, 27(7), 981–992. https://doi.org/10.1007/s00192-015-2846-y

184. Navarro-Brazález, B., Prieto-Gómez, V., Prieto-Merino, D., Sánchez-Sánchez, B., McLean, L., & Torres-Lacomba, M. (2020). Effectiveness of Hypopressive Exercises in Women with Pelvic Floor Dysfunction: A Randomised Controlled Trial. Journal of clinical medicine, 9(4), 1149. https://doi.org/10.3390/jcm9041149

185. Crowle, A. Harley, C. (2019). Development of a biotensegrity focused therapy for the treatment of pelvic organ prolapse: A retrospective case series. Journal of Bodywork and Movement Therapies. 24(1): 115-125. https://doi.org/10.1016/j.jbmt.2019.10.008

186. Barber, M. D., Walters, M. D., Cundiff, G. W., & PESSRI Trial Group (2006). Responsiveness of the Pelvic Floor Distress Inventory (PFDI) and Pelvic Floor Impact Questionnaire (PFIQ) in women undergoing vaginal surgery and pessary treatment for pelvic

organ prolapse. American journal of obstetrics and gynecology, 194(5), 1492–1498. https://doi.org/10.1016/j.ajog.2006.01.076

187. Fernando, R. J., Sultan, A. H., Thakar, R., & Jeyanthan, K. (2007). Management of the neglected vaginal ring pessary. International urogynecology journal and pelvic floor dysfunction, 18(1), 117–119. https://doi.org/10.1007/s00192-006-0089-7

188. Price N, Slack A, Jwarah E, Jackson S. The incidence of reoperation for surgically treated pelvic organ prolapse: an 11-year experience. Menopause International. 2008;14(4):145-148. https://doi:10.1258/mi.2008.008029

189. Sohlberg, E.M., Dallas, K.B., Weeks, B.T. et al. Reoperation rates for pelvic organ prolapse repairs with biologic and synthetic grafts in a large population-based cohort. Int Urogynecol J 31, 291–301 (2020). https://doi.org/10.1007/s00192-019-04035-3

190. Lee, U., Wolff, E. M., & Kobashi, K. C. (2012). Native tissue repairs in anterior vaginal prolapse surgery: examining definitions of surgical success in the mesh era. Current opinion in urology, 22(4), 265–270. https://doi.org/10.1097/MOU.0b013e32835459bb

191. Dällenbach P. (2015). To mesh or not to mesh: a review of pelvic organ reconstructive surgery. International journal of women's health, 7, 331–343. https://doi.org/10.2147/IJWH.S71236

192. Šumak, R., Serdinšek, T. & But, I. Long-term follow-up of native tissue anterior vaginal wall repair: does the POP-Q stage really reflect patients' satisfaction rate?. Int Urogynecol J 31, 2081–2088 (2020). https://doi.org/10.1007/s00192-020-04353-x

193. Borstad, E., & Rud, T. (1989). The risk of developing urinary stress-incontinence after vaginal repair in continent women. A clinical and urodynamic follow-up study. Acta obstetricia et gynecologica Scandinavica, 68(6), 545–549.

194. Schiavi, Michele & D'oria, Ottavia & Faiano, Pierangelo & Prata, Giovanni & Pinto, Anna & Sciuga, Valentina & Colagiovanni, Vanessa & Giannini, Andrea & Zullo, Marzio & Monti, Marco & Muzii, Ludovico & Benedetti Panici, Pierluigi. (2017). Vaginal Native Tissue Repair for Posterior Compartment Prolapse: Long-Term Analysis of Sexual Function and Quality of Life in 151 Patients. Female Pelvic Medicine & Reconstructive Surgery. 24. 1. https://doi.org/10.1097/SPV.0000000000000463

195. Ng, C. C., & Chong, C. Y. (2006). The effectiveness of transvaginal anterior colporrhaphy reinforced with polypropylene mesh in the treatment of severe cystoceles. Annals of the Academy of Medicine, Singapore, 35(12), 875–881.

196. Rudnicki, M, Laurikainen, E, Pogosean, R, Kinne, I, Jakobsson, U, Teleman, P. A 3–year follow–up after anterior colporrhaphy compared with collagen-coated transvaginal mesh for anterior vaginal wall prolapse: a randomised controlled trial. BJOG 2016; 123: 136– 142.

197. Nieminen, K., Hiltunen, R., Takala, T., Heiskanen, E., Merikari, M., Niemi, K., & Heinonen, P. K. (2010). Outcomes after anterior vaginal wall repair with mesh: a randomized, controlled trial with a 3 year follow-up. American journal of obstetrics and gynecology, 203(3), 235.e1–235.e2358. https://doi.org/10.1016/j.ajog.2010.03.030

198. Abed, H., Rahn, D. D., Lowenstein, L., Balk, E. M., Clemons, J. L., Rogers, R. G., & Systematic Review Group of the Society of Gynecologic Surgeons (2011). Incidence and management of graft erosion, wound granulation, and dyspareunia following vaginal prolapse repair with graft materials: a systematic review. International urogynecology journal, 22(7), 789–798. https://doi.org/10.1007/s00192-011-1384-5

199. Mowat, A., Maher, D., Baessler, K., Christmann-Schmid, C., Haya, N., & Maher, C. (2018). Surgery for women with posterior compartment prolapse. The Cochrane database of systematic reviews, 3(3), CD012975. https://doi.org/10.1002/14651858.CD012975

200. Barski, D., Otto, T., & Gerullis, H. (2014). Systematic review and classification of complications after anterior, posterior, apical, and total vaginal mesh implantation for prolapse repair. Surgical technology international, 24, 217–224.

201. Ladd M, Tuma F. Rectocele. [Updated 2020 Dec 27]. In: StatPearls [Internet]. Treasure Island (FL): StatPearls Publishing; 2021 Jan-. Available from: https://www.ncbi.nlm.nih.gov/books/NBK546689/

202. Wang, W., Zhang, Y., Shen, W., Niu, K., Lu, Y. (2020). Long-term efficacy of transvaginal high uterosacral ligament suspension for middle-compartment defect-based pelvic organ prolapse. Annals of Translational Medicine. 8(24). https://doi.org/10.21037/atm-20-7296

203. Milani, R., Frigerio, M., Cola, A., Beretta, C., Spelzini, F., & Manodoro, S. (2018). Outcomes of Transvaginal High Uterosacral Ligaments Suspension: Over 500-Patient Single-Center Study. Female pelvic medicine & reconstructive surgery, 24(3), 203–206. https://doi.org/10.1097/01.spv.0000533751.41539.5b

204. Kong, W., Cheng, X., & Xiong, G. (2018). A Posterior Approach to Laparoscopic Sacrospinous Ligament Suspension. JSLS : Journal of the Society of Laparoendoscopic Surgeons, 22(2), e2017.00105. https://doi.org/10.4293/JSLS.2017.00105

205. Qu, Da-Cheng MS; Chen, Hong-Bin MS; Yang, Mao-Mei BD; Zhou, Hong-Gui MS. Management of lumbar spondylodiscitis developing after laparoscopic sacrohysteropexy with a mesh, Medicine: December 2019 - Volume 98 - Issue 49 - p e18252. https://doi.org/10.1097/MD.0000000000018252

206. Pastore, E. A., & Katzman, W. B. (2012). Recognizing myofascial pelvic pain in the female patient with chronic pelvic pain. Journal of obstetric, gynecologic, and neonatal nursing : JOGNN, 41(5), 680–691. https://doi.org/10.1111/j.1552-6909.2012.01404.x

207. Parker, R., & Madden, V. J. (2020). State of the art: What have the pain sciences brought to physiotherapy?. The South African journal of physiotherapy, 76(1), 1390. https://doi.org/10.4102/sajp.v76i1.1390

208. Billingham, R.P., Isler, J.T., Friend, W.G. et al. Treatment of levator syndrome using high-voltage electrogalvanic stimulation. Dis Colon Rectum 30, 584–587 (1987). https://doi.org/10.1007/BF02554802

209. Ng C. L. (2007). Levator ani syndrome - a case study and literature review. Australian family physician, 36(6), 449–452.

210. Abbott, J. A., Jarvis, S. K., Lyons, S. D., Thomson, A., & Vancaille, T. G. (2006). Botulinum toxin type A for chronic pain and pelvic

floor spasm in women: a randomized controlled trial. Obstetrics and gynecology, 108(4), 915–923. https://doi.org/10.1097/01.AOG.0000237100.29870.cc

211. Dodi, G., Bogoni, F., Infantino, A., Pianon, P., Mortellaro, L. M., & Lise, M. (1986). Hot or cold in anal pain? A study of the changes in internal anal sphincter pressure profiles. Diseases of the colon and rectum, 29(4), 248–251. https://doi.org/10.1007/BF02553028

212. Sung, S. H., Sung, A. D., Sung, H. K., An, T. E., Kim, K. H., & Park, J. K. (2018). Acupuncture Treatment for Chronic Pelvic Pain in Women: A Systematic Review and Meta-Analysis of Randomized Controlled Trials. Evidence-based complementary and alternative medicine : eCAM, 2018, 9415897. https://doi.org/10.1155/2018/9415897

213. Paszkiewicz, E & Siegel, S & Kirkpatrick, C & Hinkel, B & Keeisha, J & Kirkemo, Aaron. (2001). Sacral nerve stimulation in patients with chronic, intractable pelvic pain. Urology. 57. 124. 10.1016/S0090-4295(01)01080-9.

214. Barnes, P. R., Hawley, P. R., Preston, D. M., & Lennard-Jones, J. E. (1985). Experience of posterior division of the puborectalis muscle in the management of chronic constipation. The British journal of surgery, 72(6), 475–477. https://doi.org/10.1002/bjs.1800720623

215. Anğın, A. D., Gün, İ., Sakin, Ö., Çıkman, M. S., Eserdağ, S., & Anğın, P. (2020). Effects of predisposing factors on the success and treatment period in vaginismus. JBRA assisted reproduction, 24(2), 180–188. https://doi.org/10.5935/1518-0557.20200018

216. Law, E., Kelvin, J. F., Thom, B., Riedel, E., Tom, A., Carter, J., Alektiar, K. M., & Goodman, K. A. (2015). Prospective study of vaginal dilator use adherence and efficacy following radiotherapy. Radiotherapy and oncology : journal of the European Society for Therapeutic Radiology and Oncology, 116(1), 149–155. https://doi.org/10.1016/j.radonc.2015.06.018

217. Katz, D., Tabisel, R. L. (2001). Is surgery the answer to vaginismus?. Obstetrics & Gynecology. 97(4,1):S27. https://doi.org/10.1016/S0029-7844(01)01203-0

Table of Abbreviations

PFD:	Pelvic Floor Dysfunction		*PNF:*	Proprioceptive Neuromuscular Facilitation
NR-PFD:	Non Relaxing Pelvic Floor Dysfunction			
POP:	Pelvic Organ Prolapse		*ATP:*	Adenosine Triphosphate
SUI:	Stress Urinary Incontinence		*ROM:*	Range of Motion
FI:	Fecal Incontinence		*BPS:*	Bladder Pain Syndrome
IUD:	IntraUterine Device		*BMI:*	Body Mass Index
PDF:	Portable Document Format (editable document format we use for assessments)		*NEAT:*	Non Exercise Activity Thermogenesis
			REM:	Rapid Eye Movement
QoL:	Quality of Life		*NICE:*	National Institute for Health and Care Excellence
OAB:	Overactive Bladder			
F-SMART:	Functional, Specific, Measurable, Achievable, Realistic and Timed		*FDA:*	Food and Drug administration
			TPTNS:	Transcutaneous Posterior Tibial Nerve Stimulation
RPE :	Rate of Perceived Effort			
ASIS:	Anterior Superior Iliac Spines		*PTNS:*	Posterior Tibial Nerve Stimulation
EDS:	Ehlers-Danlos Syndrome		*PFMT:*	Pelvic Floor Muscle Training
PCOS:	Polycystic Ovary Syndrome		*SNS:*	Sympathetic Nervous System
IC:	Interstitial Cystitis		*PNS:*	Parasympathetic Nervous System
HCDV:	Hokey Cokey Double Void		*LASER:*	Light Amplification by Stimulated Emission of Radiation
CPP:	Chronic Pelvic Pain			
CPPS:	Chronic Pelvic Pain Syndrome		*PVS:*	Pubovaginal Sling
DIMs:	Danger in Me		*BAUS:*	British Association of Urological Surgeons
SIMs:	Safety in Me			
TENS:	Transcutaneous Electrical Nerve Stimulation		*SIS*	Single Incision Sling
			CJD	Creutzfeldt-Jakob prion disease

FMT:	Fecal Matter Transplant
HIV:	Human Immunodeficiency Virus
TVT:	Trans Vaginal Tape or Tension-free Vaginal Tape
TVT-O:	Trans Vaginal Tape - Obturator
TOT:	Trans Obturator Tape
UR:	Urinary Retention
NSAID:	Non Steroidal Anti-Inflammatory Drugs
FI:	Fecal Incontinence
NMES:	Neuromuscular Electrical Stimulation
NGES:	Neurogalvanic Electrical Stimulation
EMS:	Electro Muscular Stimulation
EGS:	Electrogalvanic Stimulation
LAS:	Levator-Ani Syndrome
PTSD:	Post Traumatic Stress Disorder
EMG:	Electromyography
EStim:	Electrical Stimulation
EMS:	Electrical Muscle Stimulation
OBGYN:	Obstetrician and Gynecologist
PT:	Physiotherapist/Physical Therapist

About the Author

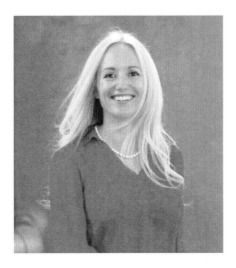

" *Together we can and will make a difference.*
#breakthepfdtaboo "

With her passion for pelvic health, Denise has helped and inspired many people to overcome their pelvic floor dysfunction.

She is a qualified yoga teacher who has studied various styles of yoga including: Ashtanga, Vinyasa Flow, Restorative, Yin Yoga, SUP Yoga, Prenatal Yoga, Pranayama and Meditation.

She is also a certified personal trainer. She has studied courses in anatomy, psychology, neurology, urology, hypopressives, and the management and treatment of pelvic floor dysfunction. She has also completed multiple *Anatomy Trains* courses and has participated in human dissection as part of her studies.

She is the founder of theflowerempowered.com with a mission to break the taboo surrounding pelvic floor dysfunction.

Made in United States
North Haven, CT
15 February 2023

32610402R00348